W9-AUJ-546

PHYSICIAN
ASSISTED
SUICIDE

Reflective Bioethics

Series Editor:

Hilde Lindemann Nelson, and James Lindemann Nelson

Do We Still Need Doctors?
John D. Lantos, M.D.

The Patient in the Family: An Ethics of Medicine and Families
Hilde Lindemann Nelson, and James Lindemann Nelson

Stories and Their Limits: Narrative Approaches to Bioethics
Hilde Lindemann Nelson

PHYSICIAN

ASSISTED

SUICIDE

Expanding the Debate

Edited by

Margaret P. Battin, Rosamond Rhodes, and Anita Silvers

ROUTLEDGE

New York and London

Published in 1998 by
Routledge
29 West 35th Street
New York, NY 10001

Published in Great Britain in 1998 by
Routledge
11 New Fetter Lane
London EC4P 4EE

Copyright © 1998 by Routledge

Printed in the United States of America on acid-free paper.
Design and typography: Jack Donner

All rights reserved. No part of this book may be reprinted or reproduced or utilized in any form or by any electronic, mechanical, or other means, now known or hereafter invented, including photocopying and recording, or in any information storage or retrieval system without permission in writing from the publishers.

Cynthia B. Cohen, "Christian Perspectives on Assisted Suicide and Euthanasia: The Anglican Tradition," originally appeared in *Journal of Law, Medicine, & Ethics* 24, 1996: 369–79. Patricia King, "African-Americans and Physician-Assisted Suicide," originally appeared in *Minnesota Law Review,* Spring 1998.

10 9 8 7 6 5 4 3 2 1

Library of Congress Cataloging-in-Publication Data

Physician assisted suicide: expanding the debate / edited by Margaret P. Battin,
    Rosamond Rhodes, Anita Silvers.
    p.   cm.
Includes bibliographical references and index.
ISBN 0–415–92002–7 (hbk). — ISBN 0–415–92003–5 (pbk.)
1. Assisted suicide—Miscellaneous.   I. Battin, M. Pabst.
    II. Rhodes, Rosamond.   III. Silvers, Anita.
R726.P496   1998
174'.24—dc21   97–52070
                                                                         CIP

To Joe, for getting us through it.

Contents

Introduction   1

Part One: Conceptual Issues   9

1. **Meanings of Death**   11
   PATRICIA S. MANN

2. **Physician-Assisted Suicide, Euthanasia,**   28
   and Intending Death
   FRANCES M. KAMM

3. **Physician-Assisted Suicide**   63
   Safe, Legal, Rare?
   MARGARET P. BATTIN

Part Two: Considering Those at Risk   73

4. **Assisted Suicide**   75
   Are the Elderly a Special Case?
   LESLIE PICKERING FRANCIS

5. **Lessons for Physician-Assisted Suicide**   91
   From the African-American Experience
   PATRICIA A. KING AND LESLIE E. WOLF

6. **Why Suicide Is Like Contraception**   113
   A Women-Centered View
   DENA S. DAVIS

7. **Disability and Life-Ending Decisions**   123
   JEROME E. BICKENBACH

8. **Protecting the Innocents**   133
   From Physician-Assisted Suicide
   Disability Discrimination and the Duty
   to Protect Otherwise Vulnerable Groups
   ANITA SILVERS

9. **Assisted Suicide, Terminal Illness, Severe Disability,**   149
   and the Double Standard
   FELICIA ACKERMAN

Part Three: Considering the Practice of Medicine   163

10. **Physicians, Assisted Suicide, and the Right**   165
    to Live or Die
    ROSAMOND RHODES

11. **Physician, Stay Thy Hand!**   177
    BERNARD BAUMRIN

12. **An Alternative to Physician-Assisted Suicide**   182
    A Conceptual and Moral Analysis
    BERNARD GERT, CHARLES M. CULVER,
        AND K. DANNER CLOUSER

13. **Not in the House**   203
    Arguments for a Policy of Excluding Physician-Assisted Suicide
    from the Practice of Hospital Medicine
    MICHAEL TEITELMAN

Part Four: Considering the Impact of Legalization   223

14. **Physician-Assisted Suicide**   225
    To Decriminalize or to Legalize, That Is the Question
    LANCE K. STELL

15. **From Intention to Consent**   252
    Learning from Experience with Euthanasia
    HELGA KUHSE

16. **The Weakness of the Case for Legalizing**   267
    Physician-Assisted Suicide
    DON MARQUIS

17. **Physician-Assisted Suicide**   279
    A Tragic View
    JOHN D. ARRAS

18. **The Supreme Court and Terminal Sedation**   301
    An Ethically Inferior Alternative to Physician-Assisted Suicide
    DAVID ORENTLICHER

19. **Would Physician-Assisted Suicide**   312
    Save the Healthcare System Money?
    (Or, Is Jack Kevorkian Doing All of Us a Favor?)
    MERRILL MATTHEWS, JR.

Part Five: Considering Religious Perspectives   323

20.   A Catholic Perspective on Physician-Assisted Suicide   324
      JOHN J. PARIS AND MICHAEL P. MORELAND

21.   Christian Perspectives on Assisted Suicide and Euthanasia   334
      The Anglican Tradition
      CYNTHIA B. COHEN

22.   A Protestant Perspective on Ending Life   347
      Faithfulness in the Face of Death
      ALLEN VERHEY

23.   Jewish Deliberations on Suicide   362
      Exceptions, Toleration, and Assistance
      NOAM J. ZOHAR

Part Six: Appendices   373

A.   *Washington et al. v. Glucksberg et al.*   377
     Text of the Supreme Court Decision
        Delivered by Chief Justice Rehnquist.
     Concurring Opinions by Justices O'Connor, Stevens,
        Souter, Ginsburg, Breyer

B.   *Vacco et al. v. Quill et al.*   423
     Text of the Supreme Court Decision
        Delivered by Chief Justice Rehnquist.
     Concurring Opinions by Justices O'Connor, Stevens,
        Souter, Ginsburg, Breyer

C.   The Philosophers' Brief   431
     Ronald Dworkin, Thomas Nagel, Robert Nozick,
     John Rawls, Thomas Scanlon, and Judith Jarvis Thomson

D.   The Oregon Death With Dignity Act   443
     Ballot Measure No. 16

Contributors   449

Index   455

Introduction

MARGARET P. BATTIN, ROSAMOND RHODES,
AND ANITA SILVERS

O NE WEEK BEFORE THE END OF ITS SPRING TERM, on June 26, 1997, the
United States Supreme Court issued decisions in two cases that claimed
constitutional protection for physician-assisted suicide, *Washington* v.
Glucksberg and *Vacco* v. *Quill*, by a single 9–0 vote covering both cases. "The bell
tolls for a constitutional right to physician-assisted suicide," announced one
observer, but many others insisted that the Court's decision marks the beginning of what is likely to clearly be a long period of social ferment and that even
the constitutional issues are by no means fully resolved.[1] By issuing a decision
that had the legal effect of recognizing states' decisions in the matter of physician-assisted suicide, the Court seemed to invite a deepening of the dispute and
to ensure that it would be fought out over and over again in the light of the differing values, historical circumstances, religious commitments, and political
and economic environments of the people in each of the fifty states. Although
its ruling was technically limited to the question of whether state laws prohibiting assistance in suicide were unconstitutional, the Court itself appeared to recognize that this would be a consequence of its decision, concluding its majority
opinion with these words:

> Throughout the Nation, Americans are engaged in an earnest and profound
> debate about the morality, legality, and practicality of physician-assisted suicide.
> Our holding permits this debate to continue, as it should in a democratic society.[2]

Furthermore, less than half a year after the Supreme Court's ruling, voters in
Oregon refused to repeal their Death With Dignity Act, known as Measure 16.
Originally passed in 1994, this Act makes it legal for a physician to provide a terminally ill patient who requests it, for the purpose of ending his or her own life,
a prescription for lethal drugs. Despite a variety of political and legal challenges,
physician-assisted suicide has thus become legal in Oregon. Many observers
regard this as the first of the "state-by-state experiments" envisioned by the
Supreme Court and expect that other states will follow Oregon's lead within the
near future. (The Supreme Court decisions and Measure 16 are included in the
appendices to this volume.)

In this volume, as encouraged by the Supreme Court and made far more
urgent by Oregon's vote to uphold Measure 16, the debate continues. Virtually

all of the pieces in this collection take explicit account of the Court's decision, and many consider conceptual, ethical, clinical, public-policy, and religious issues in light of the prospect of legalization. It may be a decade, we think, before the full implications of the Court's decision and Oregon's action are clear. As several justices recognized, it may even be the case that a future, more focused constitutional case will be heard by the Court and, as at least one justice intimated, decided in a different way.

Whatever the future, it is important to understand that the debate over physician-assisted suicide is not just a legal debate, but a moral, medical, social, political, and religious debate as well. It is particularly important to understand how the ground has shifted as the debate has evolved. The papers in this volume address issues that are familiar but, in subtle yet crucial ways, are also quite new.

Two or three decades ago, the twin issues of physician-assisted suicide and euthanasia began to emerge as philosophic issues. Among many other early contributions to the discussion, James Rachels's powerful essay on the (non)distinction between killing and letting die appeared in the prestigious *New England Journal of Medicine*, igniting a vigorous intellectual debate. The questions of physician-assisted suicide and euthanasia arose as public and practical issues too: Derek Humphrey wrote an account of helping his first wife, dying of cancer, end her life; he then founded the Hemlock Society and eventually published the best-selling book *Final Exit*, with its explicit list of drugs that could be used for "self-deliverance." Groups emerged to oppose the legalization of these practices: the International Anti-Euthanasia Task Force, activist groups within the Catholic Church and Hospice, and the disabled-advocacy group, Not Dead Yet. Throughout this time, Jack Kevorkian, M.D., achieved increasing notoriety by providing assistance in suicide to a number of people, some terminally ill and some not demonstrably so. He survived repeated trials in which Michigan juries refused to convict him. Timothy Quill, M.D., also entered the public debate after he published an account in the *New England Journal of Medicine* of the careful, thoughtful assistance in dying he gave his leukemia patient, Diane. Quill was seen as the "good doctor" counterpart to Kevorkian's maverick. During these years, one by one, states had been developing legislation providing for advanced directives—proxy forms, living wills, and durable powers of attorney for healthcare—and discussion increased over the role a person might play in ending his or her own life. Initiatives to legalize physician-assisted suicide appeared on the ballot in Washington in 1991, California in 1992, and Oregon in 1994. Washington's and California's measures, which would also have legalized physician-performed euthanasia, failed by narrow margins; Oregon's Measure 16, which covered only physician assistance in suicide by means of prescribing a lethal drug, passed by an equally narrow margin. Measure 16 was kept from going into effect by a series of legal challenges until after the Supreme Court's 1997 decision, when the repeal measure failed by a 60 to 40 percent margin and physician-assisted suicide became permissible under Oregon law.

Other more subtle changes have accompanied this increasingly vigorous public discussion and the more direct involvement of the courts. This complex pattern of shift, displacement, concurrence, and evolution is crucial to understanding the papers in this collection and why they illuminate so vividly the American political landscape in the wake of the Supreme Court's decision. These changes are happening in areas corresponding to the sections of this volume: philosophical and conceptual issues, social issues, clinical issues, public-policy and economic issues, and religious issues.

The Philosophical Landscape

Shift, displacement, concurrence, and gradual evolution have all contributed to the increasingly nuanced character of philosophical argumentation over physician-assisted suicide. Some combatants in the debate have attempted to shift the argument to other topics or displace it onto related but more controversial topics, as some have tried to move the argument about physician-assisted suicide to an argument about euthanasia. Some have tried to identify elements of mutual agreement—for instance, agreement that pain should be controlled. Many have tried to move the discussion along in a pattern of intellectual evolution, exploring disagreement, seeking compromise where possible, recognizing the subtly shifting character of values and facts. In the early stages of public discussion of physician-assisted suicide, positions were staked out rather starkly: proponents on one side, opponents on the other, arguing their cases in absolutist terms. Proponents had insisted that values of autonomy and the right to avoid suffering were central; opponents had insisted that killing, unlike letting die, was intrinsically wrong, that the integrity of the profession would be compromised, and that the obscure boundary that might accomodate a few sympathetic cases of physician-assisted suicide would be easily crossed into widespread mistreatment.

But these starkly stated positions are becoming more nuanced and subtle as the discussion continues. Parties on opposite sides now claim the same values. Autonomy, for example, is championed by proponents of physician-assisted suicide as securing patients' free, voluntary choice; but opponents claim that they too respect the same principle, autonomy, insisting that depression, fear, and social pressure impair and preclude autonomous choice. Even if genuinely autonomous choice should be respected where it occurs, opponents insist that in this sombre context it is simply not possible. Similarly both sides claim to protect the integrity of the medical profession: Opponents argue that prohibiting physician-assisted suicide will prevent physicians from succumbing to its temptations, while proponents argue that legalization will allow physicians to be honest and aboveboard about what they must already do to provide adequate, humane care to the dying. Both sides claim to extend mercy and to prevent suffering; proponents by granting patients an easy, hastened death, opponents by protecting patients against the fears that would plague their last weeks and days if they thought their physician might kill them. Both sides claim that only the social vision they see, legalization or legal prohibition, can provide a realistic bulwark against the slippery slope and the possibility of abuse. And both sides also recognize that there are no longer just two sides in this debate, pro and con, but a range of sensitivities and views all relevant in exploring the issues.

The Clinical Landscape

At the same time that the philosophical debate has been evolving into more subtle and nuanced discussions, the clinical landscape has been changing in three significant ways. First, there is greater realism and honesty about the dilemmas that arise in differentiating between already accepted medical practices and those still under discussion. During the last two decades, there has been increasing recognition that it is ethically and legally appropriate for patients, their families, and physicians to make decisions about the end of life, including decisions about withholding and withdrawing care, even with the foreseeable result that death will occur. The conditions for doing so have been outlined by the courts in a series of cases, from *Quinlan* through *Cruzan*. But the actual techniques involved in withholding and particularly withdrawing treatment have come under greater and greater scrutiny. Is disconnecting a respirator, thereby allowing a patient to die of an underlying lung disease, merely permitting the patient to refuse treatment, or is it killing the patient by cutting off an effective air supply? What does the physician "really" do in withdrawing the ventilator, especially when lavish amounts of morphine are supplied for pain control? Is it killing, or just allowing to die, to withdraw treatment and artificial nutrition and hydration with the certain result that the patient's death will occur? And is the provision of adequate pain relief with the foreseeable result that the patient will die (explicitly acknowledged by the Supreme Court as permissible) actually euthanasia? However this question is resolved, the debate is forced to become more honest and forthright as the technology of modern medicine and the specific mechanisms of withdrawing care and negotiating death come into the open.

The second factor in the evolving sophistication of the debate is the recognition that the way people now die is seriously problematic. The immense 1995 SUPPORT study shocked the country by revealing that 50 percent of the thousands of patients in the five major tertiary-care hospitals it studied were reported to have suffered moderate to severe pain at least 50 percent of the time during the last two or three days before they died.[3] This revelation has forced another clinical issue into the open: the dichotomy between the claim that most pain can be adequately controlled—a claim that is largely true—and the claim that most pain is adequately controlled, a claim that is clearly and tragically false.

Third is the greater realism about what is happening in end-of-life care. Previously, the issue seemed to be whether to permit physician-assisted suicide or euthanasia at all. But a number of recent surveys have revealed that the issue can no longer be conceptualized as whether to permit it, but what to do about the assisted suicide, physician-assisted suicide, and nurse-assisted suicide that occurs. In the eyes of many, the issue of physician-assisted suicide has come to seem rather like the issue of abortion prior to the *Roe* v. *Wade* decision; the practice is already occurring underground, and the question is whether to legalize and control the conditions under which it is practiced, to attempt to suppress it, or to continue to wink at the current situation of "private arrangements" between patients and physicians who are willing to break the law. Some theorists believe that we should prohibit physician-assisted suicide completely, others that the current practice should be decriminalized; still others favor full legalization under a set of reasonable safeguards. It is even possible to imagine a future in which the practice becomes the normal, ordinary way of ending life, preferred on rational grounds to a situation in which withdrawing or withholding treatment is the standard way of ending life, as is now the case. Almost all partisans in these debates, however, recognize that physician-assisted suicide will continue to be part of the landscape, and the real question is what moral, medical, and legal status it should have.

The Social, Political, and Public Policy Landscape

Evolution on the political landscape has also produced pictures of greater diversity in attitude. Physicians and other health professionals, who once seemed monolithically opposed, have been revealed by surveys to be strikingly divided on the issue. Surveys of the public show that as much as three-quarters of the population say that they favor allowing physicians to assist terminally ill patients to end their lives. Furthermore, it has become increasingly evident, as similar debates simmer in Canada, Australia, Great Britain, the Netherlands, and other countries, that this is not an issue solely for the United States, but for any developed country with an advanced healthcare system, a long lifespan, and an epidemiologic pattern of most people dying of diseases with long, deteriorative terminal courses.

Meanwhile, patient-related interest groups have entered the debate to focus the public's attention on the potential consequences to patients of legalizing physician-assisted suicide. Particularly effective have been groups focusing on categories of patients regarded as vulnerable, especially those said to be at particular risk because of specific features of their physical or social characteristics or circumstances. These groups include people with disabilities, people who are members of racial minorities, the elderly, women, patients who are not competent or never have been competent. The danger of abuse is at issue: Would legalizing physician-assisted suicide put members of these groups at greater risk of "receiving assistance" when they did not want it?

Concern with the impact on vulnerable groups is rooted in part in concern over recent changes in the economics of medicine. With the failure of the healthcare reform initiative that would have assured health coverage to virtually all Americans, a more cutthroat climate of competitive cost cutting and institutional competition has developed among United States healthcare providers and institutions. Countering the previous patterns of patient overtreatment, patients have now begun to worry that they will be undertreated: denied diagnostic investigation, denied life-saving surgery or therapy, denied comfort care and symptom control, and, most pointedly, be manipulated or forced into requesting assistance in suicide. Many organizations concerned with the impact on vulnerable groups of persons filed amicus briefs before the Supreme Court. The Court itself remarked on these concerns, approvingly quoting the New York State Task Force on Life and the Law's report, *When Death Is Sought*:

> The risk of harm is greatest for the many individuals who are ill and vulnerable. . . . [and] for the many individuals in our society whose autonomy and well-being are already compromised by poverty, lack of access to good medical care, advanced age, or membership in a stigmatized social group.[4]

With this attention to issues concerning vulnerable groups has come the heightened realization that not all people identified with a minority group see the issue of physician-assisted suicide in the same way. The politics of interest groups is too crude and too likely to ignore individual differences of perception and value to decide such a deeply personal issue for all members.

The discussion of the costs of care has also led to the violation of a particularly strong taboo, a taboo on the discussion of the economic consequences of permitting physician-assisted suicide. Fears that patients would be manipulated or coerced into requesting assistance in suicide have an economic root: They assume that physicians, hospitals, or healthcare insurers will calculate that a dead patient costs less than a living one, especially one with a lengthy terminal illness or an expensive disability, and will structure incentives accordingly. Opponents fear that these incentives will be too much to resist and that patients will be pressured for purely economic reasons; proponents argue that any potential savings would be so small as a proportion of total healthcare budgets that they could not play this role.

The social and political landscape also reveals new evidence about the way in which the practice of terminal care can evolve in response to open debate and the prospect of legal change. Despite the highly polarized political climate in Oregon leading up to and following the original passage of Measure 16, there has been a sincere commitment to improving the care of the dying. The Oregon Health Sciences University has developed dramatically enhanced programs in terminal care and has devoted extensive efforts to the education of physicians throughout the state about advanced directives and pain and symptom control, and many measures of the adequacy of terminal care have improved dramatically. Yet there are controversies in Oregon and elsewhere, including controversies about the setting in which physician-assisted suicide, even if legal, might take place, in the hospital, or in the patient's home? Some think an institutional environment is inherently dangerous; a few distrust the secrecy of the domestic situation.

Evidence has also been accumulating about how the provision of assistance in suicide to terminally ill patients could function in at least a partly open way. It is known that assistance in dying is being provided to many patients by their physicians, but this occurs largely out of public view and is not described or reported as suicide. Very little is known about the character of these deaths. However, Compassion in Dying, a group originally founded in Seattle, gives open support to terminally ill patients seeking an easy death. Working carefully within the law, Compassion in Dying provides counseling, advice on drugs, support, and companionship for patients electing an assisted death. Compassion has zealously protected the identities and confidentiality of the patients who have used its services, but it has made available information about the characteristics of their choices, the drugs they have used, and the nature and duration of their deaths.[5] It is to be expected that more extensive empirical information about both underground and legal assisted suicides will be available in the future.

The Religious Landscape

In many ways, religious groups can be the most conservative of institutions, committed as they typically are to a long tradition and central body of doctrine. Yet there has been fairly significant change even in those religious groups that might seem most conservative. For example, although the Catholic Church has been and remains resolutely opposed to suicide and euthanasia, Pope Pius XII's articulation of the teaching that heroic measures are not required to prolong the life of a dying patient, and that analgesics may be used to control pain even though it is foreseen, though not intended, that death may result, has meant in practice that Catholic patients or patients in Catholic hospitals have been able to receive terminal care very close to what others might call "aid-in-dying": Treatment may be withdrawn and morphine used to suppress pain or other symptoms involved in dying. Other religious groups have debated extensively whether assisted suicide is religiously permitted or not. Particularly interesting are the variations in the degree to which different groups appeal to scripturally or doctrinally based considerations or, instead, to considerations of the impact and effects of these practices.

Products of the continuing shift, displacement, concurrence, and evolution in the discussion of physician-assisted suicide, the papers in this collection reflect the long distance this discussion has already moved since its beginnings. On the one hand, as the issue has come before the voters and before the highest court, the public debate has intensified enormously, and the political volatility of the issue has greatly increased. On the other hand, there has been a great deal of progress in the debate: The conceptual issues are framed with greater clarity; there is greater perceptiveness about the realities of current medical practice; there is greater sensitivity to fears of abuse; there is more experience in the design and implementation of programs of terminal care and support both for choices of comfort care and of hastened death; and there is more direct attention to these issues among religious groups. Thus the debate is both larger and louder, but at the same time deeper, more profound, and more sensitive to patients, their physicians, and the realities of modern medicine. The essays in this book are dedicated to encouraging this continuing evolution in the public conversation.

Practical Notes

A few remarks on the design of this collection are in order. First, intended as they are to reflect the discussion in the wake of the Supreme Court's decision, many of the essays in this volume describe the decision or relevant parts of it. It might have seemed more efficient to provide a comprehensive, overall review of the Court's opinion at the beginning of the volume. Even cursory inspection of these essays, however, will reveal something important: They interpret the Court's decision in quite different ways. We think these differences are crucial to understanding the character of the overall argument about physician-assisted suicide in the wake of the Court's decision, and thus have preferred to let each author present that picture of the decision he or she sees as appropriate.

Also reflecting the increasingly nuanced and complex character of the recent discussion, many of the pieces in this volume discuss the interrelation of multiple issues, and so could have been placed in sections other than those in which they appear. As a modest convenience to the reader, the chapters are divided into categories concerned with philosophical, social, clinical, public policy, and religious considerations, but many of these essays would be at home in more than one section. We think this is a good sign; it shows that these authors recognize how complex and multifaceted the issues are.

Finally, although we have sought to provide a collection of writings fairly evenly balanced between "pro" and "con" views, the reader will also discover that such easy allegiances are not always readily apparent. True, some essays announce a position for or against legalization or social acceptance or rejection with straightforward vigor. But others reflect at length on ambiguous features of the situation or on the ambivalent feelings of their authors, and some adopt compromise positions which attempt to reduce the conflicts between pro and con views. The papers are also quite different in tone. Some are analytic or reflective in character, while other have a distinctly rhetorical flavor, advocating specific policies or solutions. We think these differences reflect the more varied character of the contemporary discussion, a discussion which is discovering that the issue is not so simple and that it is more than a theoretical debate, but a broad political, public, practice-affecting one. Indeed, it is precisely because the issue is no longer so simple that we expect the public debate, openly encouraged by the Supreme Court's own decision and confronted with the reality of legalization in Oregon, to continue for an extended period of time.

Notes

1. Annas, George J., "The Bell Tolls for a Constitutional Right to Physician-Assisted Suicide," *The New England Journal of Medicine* 337 (15) (Oct. 9, 1997).
2. *Washington v. Glucksberg* 117 Sup. Ct. 2258 (1997); bench opinion 32.
3. The SUPPORT Principal Investigators, "A Controlled Trial to Improve Care for Seriously Ill Hospitalized Patients," *Journal of the American Medical Association* 274 (20) (1995): 1591–98.
4. The New York State Task Force on Life and the Law, *When Death Is Sought: Assisted Suicide and Euthanasia in the Medical Context*, May 1994.
5. Thomas A. Preston and Ralph Mero, "Observations Concerning Terminally Ill Patients Who Choose Suicide," in Margaret P. Battin and Arthur G. Lipman, eds., *Drug Use in Assisted Suicide and Euthanasia* (New York and London: Pharmaceutical Products Press/The Haworth Press, 1996), pp. 183–92.

Part One

Conceptual Issues

PHYSICIAN-ASSISTED SUICIDE is a poignant and troubling issue for individuals and their families in the face of serious illness, pain, and suffering. Their personal stories move us emotionally and incline us towards taking a particular position on each individual case. However, when we are asked to develop policy for the place where we live, or to adopt laws that will be the rule for every case, we need a fuller and more nuanced understanding of the issues. A reasonable person will want to explore a broad range of relevant background considerations before attempting to arrive at a position on the legalization of physician-assisted suicide. Some of these are germane to practice, others reflect on our culture, still others are theoretical.

Up until the 1997 Supreme Court decisions in the cases of *Washington* v. *Glucksburg* and *Vacco* v. *Quill*, one of the central themes of the debate was whether people have a constitutionally protected right to die. In the 1997 cases the Court reiterated its previously established view that people have the right to refuse invasive medical treatment, even though doing so may cause their deaths from underlying disease. The Court did not similarly acknowledge that people have a right to control the time and means of their deaths if they are in any other circumstance. Consequently, the debate about physician-assisted suicide has shifted focus to emphasize other concepts that are relevant to whether it is the state or individual citizens who should have ultimate control over how each of us dies. The papers in this section further this broad conceptual analysis.

First, it is useful to consider how our conceptualization of and attitudes toward death affect our understanding of physician-assisted suicide. Patricia Mann's essay, "Meanings of Death," explores how our philosophical and cultural explanations of death account for our passive attitudes toward our own deaths. She proposes that we consider adopting attitudes that will permit us to be more active in relation to our own deaths. She hypothesizes that legalizing physician-assisted suicide would involve us all in a dynamic evolution of cultural rituals and social relations to the deaths of people who are close to us, while death itself would remain something of a mystery.

Arguments about the legalization of physician-assisted suicide rely upon several technical philosophical concepts and theoretical distinctions. For this reason, it is also important to become fluent in the language of the debate and to understand the arguments at its core. Frances Kamm's essay, "Physician-Assisted Suicide, Euthanasia, and Intending Death," analyzes a number of the concepts at the heart of the debate—intending, foreseeing, double effect, killing, letting die, intending lesser evil, action, omission—and presents arguments for taking a particular position on these crucial distinctions. Because these key conceptual issues play such a central role in the theoretical debate, many of them are also discussed later in the volume by other authors. Kamm's analyses should be assessed in juxtaposition to the expositions and applications found in the chapters of succeeding sections.

Finally, the issue of physician-assisted suicide should be viewed in a larger cultural and temporal context. In formulating their own positions on physician-assisted suicide, people are likely to want to take into account not only the immediate future but the distantly foreseeable consequences of legalization. In her chapter, "Physician-Assisted Suicide: Safe, Legal, and Rare?," Peggy Battin addresses the question of whether assisted suicide is likely to be a rarely chosen option or to be a common occurrence—the usual and preferred way of dying, and what cultural changes might lead to such evolution in practice.

These three chapters set out some of the most basic conceptual issues, the leitmotif of the debate in light of the Supreme Court decisions. They also frame the questions that we need to answer: Should we change? Can we adapt to change? Do we understand the conceptual and practical implications of change? As the debate expands, more conceptual issues will be introduced and the richness of the discussion will grow.

Chapters in later sections of this volume introduce additional concepts. Felicia Ackerman raises issues of double standards that suggest prejudice; Dena Davis compares suicide to sterilization; Jerome Bickenbach and Anita Silvers explore how concepts imported from antidiscrimination law and policy play out in the context of physician-assisted suicide; Rosamond Rhodes explains the relationship of rights and duties; and Lance Stell and Bernard Gert, Charles Culver and Danner Clouser question whether language itself plays a role in this debate. All of the essays in this volume add to the analysis of concepts that have moved to the foreground of the debate about whether to permit physicians and other medical personnel to be involved in their patients' suicides without threat of prosecution. All of these efforts add to the complexity of what has to be understood and taken into account within the ongoing debate.

1

Meanings of Death

PATRICIA S. MANN

In this chapter, I do not take a position for or against assisted suicide. Instead, I examine the ways in which our cultural expectations with respect to death are likely to be transformed by the legalization of assisted suicide. I suggest the inadequacy of the philosophical framework currently taken as the basis for discussing the advantages as well as the dangers of legalizing assisted suicide, denying that individual autonomy is any sort of possibility for dying patients insofar as our individual agency in this situation is necessarily intertwined with that of various relevant others. By means of a theory of agency relations, I attempt to show the dynamic ways in which we may all adjust to the option of assisted suicide as a preferred end-of-life option. My theoretical goal is to explain the qualitative complexity of individual choices, as well as the dynamic social process by which both cultural values and individual choices are likely to evolve if we legalize assisted suicide.

*   *   *

What is the tie between two instants that have between them the whole interval, the whole abyss, that separates the present and death, this margin at once both insignificant and infinite, where there is always room enough for hope?"

—Emmanuel Levinas, *Time and the Other*

Is death possible? *Can* I die? Can I say "I can" with respect to death? Can I?"

—Simon Critchley, *Very Little . . . Almost Nothing*

Comprehending Death: The Limits of Philosophy

We philosophers are always trying to get a grip on death, and always failing. Anthropologists and social historians are likely to do better than philosophers in their efforts to characterize death, insofar as they can investigate the many faces of death in different cultural contexts: Death in battle may be heroic; death in youth may be tragic; death in old age benign. In different times and different cultures death means very different things, as is clear when we read of suttee, the Hindu widow's immolation of herself on her husband's funeral pyre, or of seppuku, the suicidal disembowelling done by Japanese for infractions of honor.[1]

Yet all these so-called meanings of death are more precisely identified as different social practices and associations surrounding death. Death itself is an event that exceeds our human capacity to wrest meaning from occurrences in the world. Strangely in our world and of it, death is also elusively yet absolutely not of our world. As when we speak of God, we speak of death in self-consciously metaphoric ways. We speak of a loved one's dying in terms of their "leaving us," "passing," or "passing away." But when we say they have left us, we mean only that they are no longer capable of interacting with us in daily physical interactions. We didn't really see them leave, and we have no real idea of where they have gone, even if we believe in heaven and the immortality of the soul. And they do not fully leave us, remaining present in our memories, or in books or letters they have written or in sweaters they have knitted or in projects they have begun for us to finish.

Similarly, when we say someone has passed away, we experience their physical absence, but we don't experience their actual passing to another place, whether to nothingness or some spiritual realm. The event of death is one that we only understand from the side of the living. A person who dies passes out of our culture, but its not clear how they go, or where. We have no physical, temporal, or conceptual grasp upon where they are going, and so there is also no obvious border between our world and death. As Jacques Derrida remarks, "The crossing of a border always announces itself according to the movement of a certain step—and of the step that crosses a line. . . . Consequently, where the figure of the step is refused to intuition, where the identity or indivisibility of a line is compromised . . . the crossing of the line—becomes a *problem*."[2] For this reason, Derrida designates the boundary that is death as an "aporia," a site of interminable confusion. So long as we live, we see only life and living, and so we speak necessarily with metaphors and elliptical partiality of our experience of another person's death and passage from life.

While it is impossible to speak about death as a destination in any literal sense, it might seem obvious that we can speak of it as a cessation of our human agency or efficacy in the world. From the perspective of materialism, we as human agents simply cease to exist. But what does that mean? It turns out that we also require metaphors to express an end of our worldly agency. To the Greek philosopher Epicurus, for example, death is a matter of ceasing to experience pleasure and pain; whereas Socrates in the *Apology* suggests that death may be a dreamless sleep.[3] I am not sure these notions of a cessation of our human agency are any more imaginable, however, than is a deathly destination beyond life. I do not know what it would be to experience an end of pleasure and pain. And while I often fail to remember dreaming, it is only when I awake from sleep that I experience my dreamless sleep. I cannot imagine the dreamless sleep of death because I cannot imagine failing to wake up from sleep. Quite generally, I cannot understand the end of my experience, except as another experience. So these references to the end of my experience of agency leave me with a sense of interminable confusion, or in Derrida's terms, aporia.

The philosopher Emmanuel Levinas argues that Epicurus misunderstands the whole paradox of death, insofar as he "effaces our unique relationship with death," which involves precisely our inability as living agents to experience the nothingness of this future state. Levinas suggests that death announces itself in suffering, in "an experience of the passivity of the subject which until then had been active." But even this is not quite right, he points out, insofar as a subject who experiences passivity still experiences the alternative possibility of initiative and activity. So finally, he posits, "the unknown of death signifies that the [subject] . . . is in relationship with mystery."[4] In fact, Levinas's philosophical project involves emphasizing the radical alterity or mystery of other persons. So, the almost tangible mystery of death provides a metaphoric pathway to the otherness or mystery of other persons.

For Martin Heidegger, on the other hand, death provides a unique possibility for self-conscious reflection upon one's individual life. According to Heidegger, a human subject (Dasein) exists fundamentally as a "potentiality-for-Being" in the world. "It is essential to the basic constitution of Dasein that there is constantly something still to be settled . . . something still outstanding in one's potentiality-for-Being." In death, of course, our human potentiality comes to an abrupt and absolute end. In anticipating death, or Being-towards-death, Heidegger believes we discover in a primordial way our potentiality-for-Being, insofar as we attempt to imagine an end of our potentiality. In anticipating death, we must imagine an impossible wholeness of Dasein insofar as nothing is left outstanding; we imagine a heady freedom from human entanglements insofar as nothing remains to be settled. Death, Heidegger emphasizes, is the only worldly phenomenon which is nonrelational, and so very much our own, our "ownmost possibility."[5] So, in properly confronting the fact that we will die, we have access to a more authentic knowledge of ourselves as individuals.

Both Levinas and Heidegger offer accounts of our living agency in relation to dying. Dying itself remains beyond. Death for these philosophers illuminates aspects of living, but they have no more access to death itself than do nonphilosophers. And so it seems that they can tell us little about our relationship to death when we are actually dying. Philosophers are limited by their commitment to the articulable; insofar as death is finally an inarticulable aspect of experience, they have no obvious recommendations about how we should reckon with dying.

Religions and other self-consciously spiritual narratives offer a more literal relationship with death, insofar as they see death as a continuation of life. Or rather, not seeing at all, they counsel faith that death is a continuation of life. In positing an immortal soul, religions within the Judeo-Christian tradition, for example, offer various narratives of how our human agency can, in some mysterious sense, continue after death. These narratives counsel both a responsibility to live well prior to death, and then when death beckons, a responsibility to die well, in God's hands. Insofar as these narratives require faith in God and an afterlife, they posit a culture on either side of the border of death, to utilize one of Derrida's metaphors.[6] Religions offer comfort in the face of death insofar as they accept our human inability to imagine our own end, and offer a narrative of how life continues after death. Religions prepare us to face death by denying its most fearful and unimaginable implications, an absolute end to our human agency.

Philosophers and theologians, alike, in our Western cultural tradition have assumed that people will have a passive relationship with their own deaths, dying of natural causes or perhaps at the hands of another in battle. While not unthinkable, suicide has remained an exceptional, highly dramatic personal statement.[7] With recent proposals that we legalize assisted suicide, we must envision the normalization of a very much more active relationship with our own deaths. Given the inarticulability of the experience of death, we may wonder what it will mean for individuals to actively choose it.

Given Heidegger and Levinas's belief that death illuminates aspects of our life prior to death, we may ask how proposals for legalizing assisted suicide illuminate the lives we are leading today prior to death. While I am not opposed to legalizing assisted suicide, I believe that we have not yet begun to grapple with important social implications of such a policy decision. Advocates of assisted suicide currently emphasize the value of an autonomous choice at the end of one's life, while opponents are concerned with categories of individuals—the poor, the disabled, minorities—who may be coerced rather than autonomous in their "choice" of assisted suicide. By contrast, I will suggest that the very notion of an autonomous choice at the end of one's life is problematic and misleading. We need a more complicated framework for evaluating the agency of dying individuals today, as well as for tracking changes in agency if assisted suicide becomes an option.

The Case for Assisted Suicide:
Ronald Dworkin and the Philosophers' Brief

The much debated issue of assisted suicide corresponds with a rather paradoxical social situation in our late twentieth century. On the one hand, a combination of social and technological forces have combined to give individuals an unprecedented sense of control over their physical narratives. When we are hungry we may nonchalantly satisfy our hunger with fruits from Peru or condiments from India. When it becomes very hot, we move from one air conditioned environment to another. When we experience allergies, we take medications that eliminate our symptoms. We utilize contraception of various sorts so that sexual interactions cease to be organically related to reproduction. When a hip, knee, or shoulder joint fails, we replace it. We even replace such basic organs as kidneys and hearts. It seems consistent with this extraordinary level of control over our physical options that we would also exercise greater control over the time and place of our death. It is in this spirit that six contemporary moral philosophers have referred to an individual's death as "the final act of life's drama," in a recent amici curiae brief submitted to the Supreme Court in support of a constitutional right to assisted suicide.[8]

On the other hand, many people are discovering that it can be difficult to retain any sense at all of personal control over the end of one's life within a high-powered medical context. Medical technology has developed amazing resources for dealing with the failure of various bodily functions and organs; and the institutional commitment to life-saving treatment of the medically ill tends to move into high gear as patients become sicker and nearer death. The medical technology for curing bodily ills is on a continuum with the technology for extending life through deferring systemic bodily failures. A high-minded medical commitment to preserving individual lives can sometimes today lead to a tortuous standoff between powerful medical technologies capable of deferring immediate death and a bodily self whose physical resources have dwindled to the point where the continuation of life seems futile. Yet the dying individual may experience herself as caught up in a force field of medical technology, and she may be frustrated in efforts to extricate herself. Indeed, she may experience intolerable pain and seek help in dying more quickly, to no avail. As legal philosopher Ronald Dworkin declares, these are situations we all dread today, and he believes that individuals require the right to assisted suicide in order to properly exercise self-determination in the face of a medical establishment which often seems implacably and impersonally committed to the extension of life.[9]

As one of the foremost public intellectuals addressing this issue today, Ronald Dworkin brings the philosophical resources of our liberal democratic tradition to bear on this problem in a clear, incisive manner in his book *Life's Dominion*. Assisted suicide involves an effort to restore to individuals a conscious relationship to their own process of dying and death. Assisted suicide is defended as an extension of the individual autonomy or self-determination we seek to enact throughout our lives. As Dworkin explains it, we act in the course of our lives in response to various convictions about what makes life worth living, and these convictions about how to live tend to color our views about when and how we should die.[10] An aggressive medical establishment may treat our bodily ills while disregarding these personal views about how and when we should die. Our sense of personal autonomy may be compromised in such instances, and assisted suicide is proposed as a means of restoring a sense of control to individuals nearing the end of their life. It is thus envisioned as a logical extension of our individual freedom to pursue our lives as we please, so long as we do not harm others. Poignantly, if also a little oddly, assisted suicide is viewed as a way of making our individual death a meaningful concluding act in our own individual life.

In the Philosophers' Brief, Dworkin joins with five other contemporary moral philosophers to argue that assisted suicide should be added to the list of controversial personal decisions protected by the Fourteenth Amendment's due process clause. Over the last thirty years, the Supreme Court has concluded that a number of socially contested personal decisions (from contraception and abortion to the right to request removal of a feeding tube) are constitutionally protected as aspects of the "ordered liberty" mentioned in the due process clause.

The Supreme Court very recently responded to this and other arguments by ruling that there are not currently sufficient grounds to conclude that such a constitutional right to assisted suicide exists.[11] But while they did not deny the right of states to make assisted suicide illegal, they also did not prohibit states from legalizing it. Oregon voters approved an assisted suicide policy by referendum in 1994, but it never went into effect due to constitutional challenges upheld by a federal court. Oregon voted again on an assisted suicide referendum in November 1997, rejecting a repeal measure. We may be sure that "the earnest and profound debate on the morality, legality, and practicality of physician-assisted suicide" encouraged by Justice Rehnquist and others in the recent Supreme Court decisions will take place over the next few years in many state legislatures and popular referenda.[12] It is appropriate to consider the philosophical adequacy of arguments for and against the legalization of assisted suicide at this point.

Many theorists have pointed out dangers in legalizing assisted suicide, as effectively giving a social sanction to a form of killing people. Instead of enhancing individual autonomy, such a policy might result in various pressures for particular sorts of people to "choose" to die. While these results are not intended by the proponents of assisted suicide, philosopher Richard Doerflinger maintains that they are inherent in the policy. The idea is that once assisted suicide becomes a legal option, individuals who are very sick or very old will become vulnerable to various sorts of pressures by those caring for them. Those with limited economic resources may feel great pressure from either healthcare organizations or from relatives to simply call it quits, insofar as efforts to preserve their life and care for them are likely to be very expensive. Even those with substantial economic resources may feel pressure from families to free them from the psychologically draining aspects of tending a dying person. In addition, the families of wealthy patients may be impatient to claim their portions of the patient's estate. For a variety of reasons then, there are grounds to fear that laws intended to increase the autonomy of individuals at the end of their lives may, in fact, make them vulnerable to new forms of social coercion.[13]

Proponents of assisted suicide respond to these concerns by arguing that legal safeguards are capable of protecting dying individuals from these pressures. Indeed, Ronald Dworkin makes a persuasive case that laws allowing assisted suicide can be written so as to include various features encouraging other sorts of patient options that are often in short supply today. Improved forms of pain control and hospice care can be mandated as legal alternatives to assisted suicide, and may thereby become more available than they currently are.[14]

Yet it is not clear why laws encouraging various sorts of ameliorative care at the end of life should be linked with laws allowing assisted suicide. It will be beneficial if the debate over assisted suicide promotes greater patient welfare by encouraging greater attention to various sorts of ameliorative care at the end of life. But one would hope that improved forms of pain control as well as hospice facilities will become available regardless of policy decisions about assisted suicide. Moreover, one suspects that the mere existence of palliative care and pain medication does not really address what Richard Doerflinger has referred to as the "loose cannon" social consequences of legalizing assisted suicide, although it is difficult to articulate these consequences within a paradigm of patient autonomy.

Rethinking the Philosophical Framework of Agency at the End of Life

I assigned Ronald Dworkin's *Life's Dominion* in an upper-level philosophy seminar recently, and it inspired some very interesting discussions. Indeed, as we analyzed Dworkin's very reasonable examination of how and why individuals might want to bring their life to a close through assisted suicide, Heather, one of my students, burst into tears, saying, "It just doesn't work like that." Her grandmother had died recently, and Heather was certain, in a way that she could not articulate, that there was something very much missing from Dworkin's apparently judicious discussion of individual choices at the end of one's life.

As we addressed Heather's experience, as well as the experiences of other students in the class, what was missing from Dworkin's analysis became more evident. Dworkin's defense of assisted suicide refers exclusively to issues of the individual patient's agency at the end of his or her life. In the context of the autonomy framework, the agency of others, whether family or doctors, is seen only as a potential problem insofar as it threatens to impinge upon the sick individual's agency.

However, as we discussed situations of death and dying in the context of our own families and friends, we noticed a rather more complicated and dynamic quality of interpersonal agency in these situations. In fact, little about a dying person's situation supports a sense of their autonomy, in any but the most formal sense. A dying person's sense of agency is fundamentally bound up with their relationships to other family members or friends. Perhaps a dying woman wants to remain alive long enough to see a grandchild graduate. Or perhaps she has come to a point where she cannot accept being a burden on family and friends any longer. In addition, the wishes of family and friends inevitably affect the dying person's sense of their own agency. A spouse's desire that the dying person continue to live may be an overriding concern. By contrast, the recent death of a spouse may mean that the patient feels little further reason to live. All these relationships, and many more, impact immediately and inevitably on a sick person's agency in the face of death.

The discussion of assisted suicide has centered on notions of individual autonomy and self-determination, as the values ideally characterizing an individual's decision to seek an end of his or her life. And criticisms of assisted suicide have focussed on social and political reasons why various groups of people—the poor, the disabled, minorities—are not likely to be allowed to exercise an autonomous choice. I want to suggest that the whole notion of an autonomous choice at the end of one's life is problematic and misleading. I believe that we need a richer framework for understanding the agency of dying individuals.

Indeed, as I have argued at greater length in my book *Micro-Politics*, we require a theoretical framework that addresses the social as well as the more self-referential dimensions of action, if we are to adequately understand individual agency in most circumstances.[15] Because of our idealization of individual autonomy as a basic perspective of liberal individualism, we rarely notice the complex social motivations of individual actions. But end-of-life situations provide a particularly powerful demonstration of the inadequacy of self-referential notions of individual agency and the need for a more socially nuanced conception of individual actions and choices.

Our modern philosophical and political tradition of individualism is founded on a rationalist Cartesian theory of knowing selfhood and a radically physicalist Hobbesian theory of individual action. While it would have made no sense within the classical tradition of Plato and Aristotle to conceive of individuals or their actions apart from a larger social framework, the powerful modern philosophical worldview that began to be articulated in the writings of Rene Descartes and Thomas Hobbes gave a thorough-going metaphysical priority to individual selves. Thus, for a Cartesian self, knowledge of the world is premised upon a foundational consciousness of oneself. And for a Hobbesian self, even the most complicated social projects can all finally be traced back to physically based categories of individual "appetite" and "aversion." While he notes that the Greek use of concepts of desire and aversion to express more complex social aims was merely "metaphorical," Hobbes insists that his terminology be understood quite literally: "But whatsoever is the object of any man's Appetite or Desire; that is it, which he for his part calleth Good. . . ." For Hobbes, even the most general social norms should be understood as founded upon individual desires and aversions.[16] Sigmund Freud eventually complicates this Hobbesian theory of agency, embedding Hobbes's physicalist narrative within a psychoanalytic narrative of sexual desire that, perhaps surprisingly, serves only to strengthen the self-referential quality of individual agency within our liberal tradition.[17]

What I will hereafter refer to as the Hobbesian/Freudian tradition of "desiring agency" provides one of the foundation-stones for liberal political theory. A politics of liberal individualism highlights the value of autonomy, or lack of interference from others, insofar as our desiring agency, our individual appetites and desires, are likely to place us in conflict with others.[18] While a number of contemporary philosophers have criticized Cartesian notions of unitary selfhood and rationality, the Hobbesian/Freudian tradition of desiring individual agency, as well as the liberal framework of autonomy, have as yet escaped serious critique.[19]

I first began to have doubts about the adequacy of the one-dimensional Hobbesian theory of desiring agency when I sought to analyze gender relations and the agency of women within familial settings over the last several centuries. Women's actions as wives and mothers frequently failed to accord with Hobbesian or Freudian paradigms of desiring individual agency. Freud famously declared women "a dark continent" insofar as it was not clear what they desired. While some feminists equated the oppression of women under patriarchy with a suppression of their agency, women in traditional roles frequently manifest a sense of personal efficacy. In order to take such women seriously I had to broaden my vision of agency in several respects. A major portion of these women's actions originated in a sense of responsibility or obligation to others, and so I posited that feelings of responsibility could be as basic to a sense of individual agency as self-referential desires. Indeed, this dimension of agency illuminated actions of men in relation to their families, as well. In addition, I found a third dimension of agency necessary to fully comprehend individual actions; individuals act out of expectations of recognition and reward, often quite apart from their immediate desires. Moreover, actions not properly recognized and rewarded never attain full status as acts of agency, as women found when they began moving outside their traditionally designated roles. And this is surely the case today with respect to unacknowledged acts of assisting and assisted suicide.

I concluded that in order to fully comprehend individual agency, we must recognize the three potential dimensions of any individual action. Individual agency may be comprised of self-referential desires, of other-directed feelings of responsibility, as well as by expectations of recognition and reward that are directed toward others while also referring to oneself. One is empowered when one has agency involving all three dimensions. But, quite typically, these dimensions are distributed among different individuals within a situation, often in accord with prevailing power relations. We care about the desires of the dominant person, and we offer them recognition and rewards. The subordinate person's agency, by contrast, involves primarily the dimension of responsibility. Servants, slaves, minimum wage workers, women in traditional roles may have important duties and responsibilities, but they receive relatively little recognition and reward for them, and people rarely inquire after their desires.

An important consequence of this distribution of the dimensions of agency is that we can only understand the agency of particular individuals insofar as we understand their relationships with other individuals. The binary opposition of self and other encouraged by the Hobbesian schema of competing desires no longer makes sense; each of the dimensions of agency are about self-other relations in constitutive but different ways. Whether we act out of desires, or out of a sense of responsibility, or with an expectation of recognition and reward, we are acting in relation to relevant others. Autonomy, understood as freedom from interference of others, ceases to be a meaningful value, insofar as it ignores the fabric of relationships, good and bad, within which our actions necessarily occur. (We could, of course, still use a notion of autonomy to refer to situations in which we were free from overt forms of physical or mental coercion. But we would have to be very careful not to let this slip back into a vision of being free from the influence of others.)

Agency Relations As We Live and Die

My three-dimensional social theory of agency relations allows us to discuss the situation of sick or dying individuals in terms of the various relationships that affect their senses of living and dying. And it enables us to consider how these relationships will be affected by legalizing assisted suicide.

We may begin by reassessing the end-of-life situation that, as Ronald Dworkin points out, many people most dread. Suppose we become very ill, perhaps unto death, and we are in the care of a highly respected doctor at a major medical institution. The agency of this doctor is quite clear. Everything in her medical training and practice promote in her a strong desire, compounded by a sense of medical duty via the Hippocratic oath, to find a method of returning us to health. Moreover, her recognition and rewards in the world of medicine are based upon her reputation for overcoming the forces of disease and physical decline. The hospital stands behind her in this. The agency of our doctor is well-defined in terms of her commitment to the care and maintenance of life.

As a patient, we are often less certain of our goals, and almost always less certain of how to go about achieving them. As we experience bodily decline, it is common to be ambivalent and confused about our own desires. And even if we have a firm commitment either to fighting for life to the very end, or alternatively, a commitment to die with dignity while we still have all of our faculties about us, we are likely to require a great deal of help in accomplishing either goal. We also may have a strong sense of responsibility, quite apart from our desires, to either continue living, or to die as rapidly as possible. But here, too, we may be conflicted, and we will require aid in accomplishing our goals. Expectations of recognition and reward may add to our sense of anxiety and ambivalence. We may be horrified at the thought of losing our mental and physical capacities and being remembered in that way. We may thus desire to die as quickly as possible, but at the same time we may not want to be remembered as having made the cowardly choice of killing ourselves. There is no end to our possible conflicts about living and dying at this stage of our lives.

Our physical situation makes us extremely dependent upon others, in a society in which dependency is not recognized as a basic and constant human reality. Only children are acknowledged as legitimately dependent, and so we may feel like children when we are ill. Our society also emphasizes the value of having clearly articulated goals, on a daily as well as longer-range basis. But with death approaching, we must establish a very different sort of relationship with our future. As Levinas observed, our relationship to death is a relationship with mystery. And as Derrida said, death is fundamentally confusing and paradoxical. Our sense of being out of control at the end of our life has as much to do with our extreme dependency and with our sense of uncertainty in relation to the approach of our death as it does with an aggressive medical establishment denying our wishes.

The potential appeal of assisted suicide to dying individuals in our society is almost too clear. As a dying person, we are, as Levinas pointed out, experiencing a final form of passivity. Our agency is waning, objectively and painfully. We confront mystery, uncertainty, aporia. Yet our culture teaches us that mature adults are supposed to struggle against all forms of uncertainty and dependency. Accordingly, in choosing suicide, we marshall our waning powers aggressively in order to put an end to uncertainty and dependency in the only way possible. We may congratulate ourselves upon seizing back, not just from an overwhelming medical establishment, but from God him- or herself, the power of death. We refuse the fundamental and continuing fact of human potentiality and hope in order to control the moment and the site of our final breaths of life. As Heidegger would point out, however, we seek to create a final act which we can never experience as a final act, insofar as our human subjectivity ends when its potentiality ends.

Let's examine the other agency relations surrounding such a death. In the first place, if we are asking assistance in this suicide, there is at least one medical doctor involved. If assisted suicide becomes legal, some doctors will no doubt assert their continuing commitment to the Hippocratic oath and refuse to participate in it. But many doctors will adjust their practices, and gradually their values, as well. Initially, some will simply desire to help patients in this final act, and some will feel it part of their medical responsibility to do so, regardless of their personal desires. Insofar as assisted suicide is a cost-efficient means of death, doctors are also likely to be rewarded by healthcare companies for participating in it. As institutional expectations and rewards increasingly favor assisted suicide, expectations and rewards within the medical profession itself will gradually shift to reflect this. Medical students will learn about assisted suicide as an important patient option from the beginning of their training. We may expect that a growing proportion of doctors will find themselves sympathetic to this practice, and will find themselves comfortable with recommending it to their patients.

Families will also be affected by the legalization of assisted suicide. Familial agency in the context of a dying loved one is likely to be as confused and conflicted as that of the patient. Family members may want a loved one to remain alive as long as possible, while also harboring secret desires to be done with this painful process. Many people today are ashamed of such secret desires, regarding the very thought of hastening a loved one's death as wrongful and blameworthy. But if assisted suicide becomes legal, such desires will cease to be wrongful in such an obvious way. If patients themselves may decide to put an end to this painful process of dying, then it is not blameworthy for relatives of such a patient to inquire whether he or she may be thinking along these lines, and to offer sympathetic support for the idea.

As dying individuals begin to articulate their desires to be done with the painful process of suffering and decline, relatives will participate in the dialogue, adding their own perspectives on the option of assisted suicide. They may quite reasonably desire to get on with their lives, and in this new context of considering assisted suicide, they may experience these desires more strongly. Where they once felt great responsibility to put up with the pains and inconveniences of an extended process of dying, they may no longer feel it necessary to hide their impatience with the process. And they may even find themselves emphasizing their competing responsibilities to healthy children and spouses. Where they would once have felt ashamed to feel these things, and may even now be surprised to hear themselves saying them, they may come to feel free to have them recognized. Once assisted suicide ceases to be illegal, its many advantages to busy relatives will become readily apparent. More than merely an acceptable form of ending, relatives and friends may come to see it as a preferred or praiseworthy form of death. They will become comfortable with considering the merits of assisted suicide in relation to their loved ones because it will be designated a socially good end.

Managed-care organizations will also be involved. If dying sooner is more cost efficient, their profit-based concerns will make them prefer patients to choose assisted suicide, and their sense of responsibility to shareholders will reinforce this preference. Economic interests may still seem crass in relation to dying patients, and yet we are already accustomed to recognizing them in the context of treatment, as well as in all other contexts of daily life. When we legalize assisted suicide, it too becomes a part of daily life. Everyone is allowed to have and to express their own interests in relation to acts of assisted suicide, once it is viewed as an accepted patient alternative, as an established, approved ending.

The appeal of assisted suicide to relatives and friends and to healthcare organizations is easy to comprehend. In legalizing assisted suicide, we will be legalizing a method of death which will be very much more convenient as well as more cost-effective than current methods of dying. In our society, where almost everyone is pressed for time, and many are pressed for money, individual notions of agency and the fabric of social agency relations may evolve very quickly to reflect its conveniences and cost efficiency.[20] The agency of medical doctors is likely to remain more conflicted, insofar as healing remains their primary role. Many doctors may find it difficult to change hats and aid people in dying. But as doctors come to be employed primarily by managed-care organizations, they will inevitably come to reflect the efficiency concerns of their employers.

Now let us consider the dynamic fabric of agency relations surrounding a dying person in a society where assisted suicide has become an accepted practice. Patients may still have the legal right to exercise options for aggressive treatment, or for transferral to a hospice, as well as for assisted suicide. But those who are dying will be aware—sometimes keenly, sometimes dimly—of the wishes of their family and friends, their doctors and managed care organizations, as well as the general cultural expectations for one in their circumstances. Some relatives may speak frankly and not necessarily unkindly about their burdensome work or family obligations and their inability to devote much more time to caring for the ill person. They may gently propose assisted suicide as the best solution for everyone at this point (as children today sometimes gently propose to elderly parents that it would be appropriate to enter a nursing home). Other relatives may say they desire the patient to live as long as possible, while at the same time making clear that they deem it the responsibility of the patient to choose assisted suicide to relieve them of this ordeal of dying. It will be legitimate for families to have and express these feelings.

Some doctors may enthusiastically recommend assisted suicide in a variety of circumstances, while others may evince desires to keep fighting for the patient's life. All, however, will be operating within a framework of managed care organizations' holding medical doctors responsible for making reasonable decisions about when to encourage the patient to give up. Healthcare providers will surely create guidelines and rules about when it ceases to be rational to treat illnesses, and when hospice care or assisted suicide become the appropriate choices. Of course, wealthy patients will retain the right to pay for further aggressive care, and rules designating the limits of rational treatment will be most stringent in the health plans of the most impoverished.

Assisted suicide will offer all patients a way to escape overwhelming and unpleasant feelings of dependency and uncertainty as they experience serious bodily and, perhaps, mental decline. And the undeniable convenience of avoiding a lingering, painful, indeterminate period of dying will have great advantages for the friends and relatives of almost everyone. In a society where an ever larger portion of our population is becoming elderly, the cost efficiency of cutting short a potentially extended process of dying is readily apparent and desirable. A lingering death may come to seem an extravagance, a frivolous indulgence. If you doubt that our views on death could change so rapidly, remember, or try to remember, how strong the expectations were for even highly educated women to become fulltime homemakers during the '50s and '60s. And consider how rapidly we have come to consider it somewhat indulgent and eccentric for such a woman to decide today to give up work and remain at home fulltime caring for her children and house. We can be relatively certain that our views of dying will change quite radically if and when assisted suicide is legalized.[21]

Further Thoughts on the Social Relations of Assisted Suicide

My aim in this paper is to make a radical intervention in the current debate over assisted suicide, to insist on a dynamic analysis of the social relations surrounding death in our society. To put my argument in terms suggested by the anthropologist Cheryl Mwaria, our cultural expectations with respect to death, our beliefs about "what is considered proper, moral, or even sane," will be transformed if assisted suicide is legalized.[22] There will be new arguments for and against legalizing assisted suicide in the context of such envisioned cultural changes. My goal here is to demonstrate the need for such arguments, not to make them. I will conclude by outlining the dynamics of the prospective cultural changes.

Such cultural changes may occur quite rapidly insofar as a social practice of assisted suicide seems very compatible with four of our most basic existing societal values.

1. The fast pace of our lives, what sociologist Arlie Hochschild has evocatively termed "the time bind" so many of us find ourselves in on a daily basis, makes us less patient with indefinite or extended processes of dying. Life-extending medical technology is ironically juxtaposed to fast-paced lives that leave little time for dying. The convenience of assisted suicide will be perhaps its most compelling feature.[23]

2. Americans have long exhibited a low tolerance for ambiguity and mystery. As

a society, we turn to the quantitative measurements and analytic descriptions of social science rather than the metaphoric evocations or figures of poetry or literature. As philosopher Simon Critchley explains, suicide is "an attempt to abolish both the mystery of the future and the mystery of death." Critchley quotes Maurice Blanchot as opining that "this tactic is in vain," insofar as one's death remains ungraspable and strange so long as one remains sentient ("the suicide feels the tightening of the rope that binds him more closely than ever to the existence he would like to leave").[24] But this is a case where metaphysical subtleties are at odds with pragmatic meanings. In controlling the time and place of their deaths, many people will experience a diminution if not an end of the ambiguity and mystery of those deaths.

3. Dependency relations are discouraged in our society. Dying is painful insofar as it involves a degree of dependency we are unused to in our lives up to this point. Moreover, with the recent movement of large numbers of women into the workplace, the social ethic for the twenty-first century seems to impose a heightened ideal of autonomy; there is a cultural expectation that every adult man and woman will be responsible for the economic maintenance of themselves. As Hochschild has shown, women and men alike engaged in ever longer workplace hours, have little time to devote to children or other dependents. We increasingly pay others to care for our children, as well as the elderly and unwell, making dependency an impersonal, costly relationship.

4. Our concerns with costs and with cost efficiency hardly need be elaborated. Individuals as well as institutions in our market-driven society cease to appear rational when they wander even a little from concerns with economic efficiency.

These four current social values taken together allow us to predict that proposals for assisted suicide will appear compelling to a great many people in our society.

I have suggested the inadequacy of the philosophical framework currently taken as the basis for discussing the advantages as well as the dangers of legalizing assisted suicide. I do not believe that individual autonomy is any sort of possibility for dying patients, regardless of the social policies that surround death in a society, insofar as our individual agency in this situation is necessarily intertwined with that of various relevant others. I do acknowledge that an ideal of autonomy and a fear of its opposite, dependency, play a large role in the current debate about assisted suicide. But rather than misrepresenting the capabilities of a policy of assisted suicide to guarantee autonomy, I believe we need to confront the qualities of dependency and relatedness that are inevitable in this situation. By means of my three-dimensional theory of agency relations, I have attempted to show the dynamic ways in which we will all be likely to adjust to the option of assisted suicide as a preferred end-of-life option. My theory of social agency relations does not deny individual choice; rather it explains the qualitative complexity of individual choice, as well as its dynamic social process of evolving.[25]

To speak once again in anthropological terms, my theory of agency relations seeks to show the shaping power of cultural dynamics in this situation. According to the picture I am presenting, if assisted suicide is legalized, strong social expectations are likely to develop for individuals to choose assisted suicide as soon as their physical capacities decline to a point where they become extremely dependent upon others in an expensive, inconvenient way. I am not making a "slippery slope" argument about likely abuses of this policy. And I am not suggesting that dying patients will be manipulated by relatives, doctors, and health-care organizations in choosing assisted suicide. Rather, I am attempting to show how current social values will encourage a dramatic alteration in our attitudes and practices surrounding death, such that a large proportion of individuals will choose assisted suicide once it has been legalized. While not at all denying the relevance of individual choice, I am theorizing about the social factors that will bring about a change in the quality of individual choices in a society like ours that legalizes assisted suicide. It will be appropriate to say that individuals are choosing assisted suicide, with society's blessing, in order to avoid an extended period of dependency and uncertainty during the process of dying. As Margaret Battin points out, there seem to have been a number of societies throughout history within which individuals similarly felt a social responsibility to die when they became sufficiently old and infirm.[26] Our twenty-first-century American society will be yet another.

In legalizing assisted suicide, we will be ushering in a whole new set of relationships between dying individuals and their friends, relatives, and healthcare providers. Various end-of-life rituals may develop around this new process of dying. Surely the ultimate mystery surrounding death will remain; the abyss between life and death will not be altered by our new practices of assisted suicide. But insofar as we accept assisted suicide, we will believe that there is a moment when the element of hope and potentiality that philosophers identify with human life is properly extinguished by those who might continue to live with hope and potentiality somewhat longer.

My analysis does not indicate whether assisted suicide is an appropriate social option at this time within our culture. As the elderly make up a growing proportion of our populace, the costs and inconveniences of the dying process are already growing astronomically. Assisted suicide is a very efficient way of dying. Perhaps the Supreme Court will reverse its recent holding in *Washington* v. *Glucksberg* and find it a constitutionally sanctioned liberty interest within the next few years. If so, assisted suicide may become a ubiquitous form of death within the next quarter of a century. That may be a good thing, or it may not. Insofar as it is clear that our agency relations with relatives, friends, medical caregivers, and institutional providers will be transformed, it will be important to evaluate the quality of the new relationships, something I cannot do here. What I hope to have done, however, is shift the grounds of evaluation away from an illusory goal of autonomy, and towards the new social relations that will develop if we legalize assisted suicide.

Notes

1. See Margaret Pabst Battin, *The Least Worst Death* (New York: Oxford University Press, 1994), p. 190.
2. Jacques Derrida, *Aporias*, trans. Thomas Dutoit (Stanford: Stanford University Press, 1993), p. 11–12, 16.
3. See Epicurus, "Letter to Menoeceus," and Plato's *Apology*, trans. G.M.A. Grube, in *Plato: Five Dialogues* (Indianapolis: Hackett Publishing Co., 1981), line 40d.
4. Emmanuel Levinas, *Time and the Other*, trans. Richard Cohen (Pittsburgh: Duquesne University Press, 1987), pp. 69–70.
5. Martin Heidegger, *Being and Time*, trans. John Macquarrie and Edward Robinson (New York: Harper and Row, 1962), pp. 279, 308–309, 354.
6. See Jacques Derrida, *Aporias*, pp. 6, 8, 62, 74.
7. As Margaret Battin notes, the Greek and Roman Stoics were exceptional within our western philosophical tradition, in recommending an active, or what Battin terms an "autonomist" approach to one's own death. While the goal of exercising control over one's own death did not always require suicide, in the cases of such well-known Stoics as Cato, Lucretia, and Seneca suicide was their way of responsibly acting to bring their lives to an end. See Battin's *The Least Worst Death*, pp. 95, 189, 232.
8. See "Assisted Suicide: The Philosophers' Brief," authored by Ronald Dworkin, Thomas Nagel, Robert Nozick, John Rawls, Thomas Scanlon, and Judith Jarvis Thomson, in *New York Review of Books*, March 27, 1997, p. 44. See also appendix B of this volume.
9. Ronald Dworkin, *Life's Dominion* (New York: Random House, 1994), pp. 179–80.
10. Dworkin, *Life's Dominion*, p. 211.
11. See *Washington* v. *Glucksberg*, 117 Sup. Ct. 2293 (1997); No. 96–110 and *Vacco* v. *Quill*, 117 Sup. Ct. 2293 (1997); No. 95–1858.
12. New York and several other states legalized abortion several years before *Roe* v. *Wade* made abortion a constitutional right in 1973. Many proponents of assisted suicide envision a similar pattern of building popular support for a controversial new social policy.
13. Richard Doerflinger, "Assisted Suicide: Pro-Choice or Anti-Life?" in Joseph Howell and William Frederick Sale, eds., *Life Choices: A Hastings Center Introduction to Bioethics* (Georgetown: Georgetown University Press, 1995), pp. 240–48.
14. Ronald Dworkin cites the Coalition of Hospice Professionals as saying, "Removing legal bans on suicide assistance will enhance the opportunity for advance hospice care for all patients because regulation of physician-assisted suicide would mandate that all palliative measures be exhausted as a condition precedent to assisted suicide." See Ronald Dworkin's introduction to "Assisted Suicide: The Philosophers' Brief," p. 42.
15. Patricia S. Mann, *Micro-Politics: Agency in a Postfeminist Era* (Minneapolis: University of Minnesota Press, 1994).
16. Thomas Hobbes, *Leviathan*, C. B. MacPherson, ed. (New York: Penguin, 1981), pp. 118–20. See also my discussion of this in *Micro-Politics*, chapter four, particularly pp. 131–36.
17. See my analysis of Freud's contribution to this tradition in *Micro-Politics*, pp. 73–78.
18. The Kantian ideal of moral autonomy, whereby the freedom of each individual is premised upon his acting in accordance with the categorical imperative to "give laws' to himself, is also part of this picture. I am not dealing with this issue of abstract moral autonomy in this paper.
19. Margaret Battin remarks upon recent critiques of autonomy in cultural studies and literary theory, and acknowledges that they have "real bite," despite their failure to make much headway in bioethics so far. See her *The Least Worst Death*, p. 25. In fact, the Hobbesian/Freudian account of our desiring agency is so naturalized, so taken for granted within our tradition at this point that it is the rare philosopher, such as Battin, who retains the capacity to even speculate upon other possibilities. It is also important to state that a denial of autonomy does not require a denial of individual agency. I believe that it is the *quality* of individual agency that is the issue at this point. See my analysis of how Freud complicates while extending the Hobbesian tradition of desiring agency in *Micro-Politics*, chapter two.

20. See Arlie Hochschild's *The Time Bind* (New York: Henry Holt and Co., 1997) for a penetrating sociological analysis of what Hochschild judges a general shift in social priorities in American society today. Women and men alike are spending increasing time in the workplace. Women are finding various ways to decrease absolutely or to "outsource" all the traditional domestic duties they once performed, including childcare, as well as care of the sick and elderly. See also Arthur and Joan Kleinman, "Cultural Appropriations of Suffering in Our Times," *Daedalus*, vol. 125, no.1 (Winter, 1996), pp. 14–15. As anthropologists, the Kleinmans find shifts in the American cultural rhetoric of illness which correspond with Hochschild's findings as to the devaluation of traditional domestic duties of women. Our cultural rhetoric, the Kleinmans remark, "is changing from the language of caring to the language of efficiency and cost; it is not surprising to hear patients themselves use this rhetoric to describe their problems. Thereby, the illness experience, for some, may be transformed from a consequential moral experience into a merely technical inexpediency."

21. See Robert Kastenbaum, "Suicide as the Preferred Way of Death," in Edwin S. Shneidman, ed., *Suicidology: Contemporary Developments* (New York: Grune and Stratton, 1976), pp. 425–41, for a much earlier analysis predicting that our society would readily embrace suicide as a desirable way of dying.

22. Cheryl Mwaria, "Physician-Assisted Suicide: An Anthropological Perspective," *Fordham Urban Law Journal* (forthcoming). Mwaria focusses particularly on our attitudes towards the disabled, warning that existing prejudices against dependence and disability may become heightened within a culture which encourages assisted suicide.

23. Hochschild, *The Time Bind*.

24. Simon Critchley, *Very Little ... Almost Nothing*: Death, Philosophy, Literature (New York: Routledge, 1997), p. 70.

25. Margaret Battin addresses many of the issues I take up here by maintaining that choices of assisted suicide may be both rational and "manipulated," i.e., to some degree a product of outside influences. While acknowledging the morally repugnant character of manipulation, she finally concludes that so long as patients experience their choice as free, rational, and voluntary, we should accept their right to make such a choice. See *The Least Worst Death*, pp. 201–202.

    Battin comes to the right conclusion despite operating from within a framework idealizing autonomous individual rationality. My argument is that the framework has now outlived its several centuries of usefulness. In order to deal with a number of contemporary problems, I believe we require new theories of selfhood and agency.

26. Battin, pp. 58–59.

2

Physician–Assisted Suicide, Euthanasia, and Intending Death

FRANCES M. KAMM

This article presents a three-step argument for the moral permissibility of physician-assisted suicide (PAS) and euthanasia (E). The article begins by providing criteria for distinguishing passive and active PAS from passive and active E, and for determining whether and when each is a killing or a letting die. After a brief discussion of how death could sometimes be in a person's best interests and a lesser evil than other bad things that might happen to her, I present the Three-Step Argument. (In addition, I suggest another argument for the permissibility of PAS and E and one for the duty of a physician to perform PAS or E.) Among the criticisms of the Three-Step Argument that I consider are that it condones killing and that it involves treating a person as a mere means. In trying to deal with the latter objection, I examine in detail the idea of treating a person as a mere means, and offer a test for the particular circumstances in which PAS or E is permissible. In conclusion, I compare the Three-Step Argument with arguments given by Ronald Dworkin and several other distinguished philosophers and I reflect on who has responsibility for the deaths in PAS and E.

*   *   *

What Are PAS and E?

Terminology and Conceptual Distinctions

EUTHANASIA (E) involves a *death that is intended* (not merely foreseen) in order to benefit the person who dies. It differs from physician-assisted suicide (PAS) undertaken in the interest of the person who dies partly in that it involves a final act or omission by someone other than the patient (e.g., the doctor) in order to end the patient's life. I speak of act or omission because there can be passive as well as active euthanasia, and at least some passive euthanasia occurs by omission. In a clear case of the latter, the doctor does not provide lifesaving treatment, intending the patient's death for the patient's good. In active euthanasia, the doctor introduces the cause of the patient's death, e.g., a lethal injection. It also is possible for someone to commit suicide passively or actively. A clear case of the former is when someone refuses his lifesaving medicine because he intends to die; a case of the latter is when someone shoots himself intending to die. Active PAS can involve, for example, the provision of means of death, like pills, that a patient may use. However, it might also involve giving the patient a stimulant to keep him awake so that he can shoot himself. That is, the active assistance need *not* involve giving a lethal substance.

Is there is a passive form of *assisting* suicide? When a doctor terminates treatment that sedates a patient who wants to be sufficiently awake to shoot himself, we have a case of passively assisting (active) suicide. The doctor may simply not give the next dose of sedating medicine that he would otherwise have given. Suppose he terminates sedation by interfering with a machine that delivers sedation, because the patient intends to shoot himself. Is it appropriate to call this *passive* assisted suicide even though it involves a doctor's *act*? I believe that ending treatment by an act is commonly referred to as passive because it involves removing a barrier to some end state (like being awake) rather than inducing it (as by giving a stimulant). For the same reason ending lifesaving treatment (even by an act) can be considered passive E; it is the removal of a barrier to death, rather than a way to induce it (unless, for example, stopping the machine causes sudden fatal trauma).

Notice that the active/passive distinction drawn in this way is different from the killing/letting die distinction *and* that both these distinctions are different from the distinction between permissible and impermissible conduct. If a doctor gives a patient a lethal injection, actively inducing death, he kills the patient, whether he intends the death or not. But *passive E could also be a killing* when someone terminates lifesaving treatment *without the patient's permission,* by disconnecting a machine that is neither his nor something he is running. This passive killing might or might not be permissible. Let me expand on the difference between the three distinctions.

When a doctor withholds treatment, she lets a patient die. She can let die, intending that the patient die, as when she refuses to give an antibiotic, so that he will die, because she thinks this is better for him. Or she can let die, foreseeing that the patient will die without intending it, as when she decides to save five other people and lets one die because she is busy. Sometimes, letting die is morally permissible (as in the latter case) and sometimes it is impermissible (as it may be in the former case). If a patient is already receiving life-saving treatment and a doctor must actively terminate it by, for example, pulling out tubes, an act rather than an omission is required to terminate aid, yet, I have said, I consider this passive E. Furthermore, if the doctor is terminating aid that she (or the organization of which she is a part) is providing or that is provided by means that belong to them, then I think she *lets* die rather than kills.

Consider the following analogy: I am saving someone from drowning and I decide to stop. Even if I must actively push a button on my side to make myself stop, I still let the person die rather than kill him.[1]

If a machine providing life-saving treatment belongs to the person who stops it, then even if he leaves it and returns to stop it, he is letting die in stopping *his* aid. Does this mean that one will have killed whenever one stops a machine belonging to someone else (which one is not running)? No, for if one has the permission either of the machine's owner or the person receiving aid to stop it, and one is then seen as their agent carrying out their will, one will be letting die. This is because if the owner of the machine or the receiver of aid would stop the aid, he would be letting (either another or himself) die. Notice that even if the *receiver of aid does not own the life support machine from which he disconnects himself,* he lets himself die rather than kills himself. This is because the recipient stands in an ownership-like relation to his own body and he is withdrawing its use from the process of life support.

Still, even when a doctor pulls the plug on aid he is giving, the fact that he acts makes him a partial *cause* of death, the disease being the other partial cause. So, there is the following difference between not beginning treatment and terminating the aid that either one provides or one's device provides: Only in the latter case does *letting die cause a death,* at least in part. Still, only a killing introduces an *original cause* which induces death, rather than merely removing the barrier to a cause of death that is or will be present.[2]

Returning to PAS, there can be cases of passive or active PAS, in which the patient goes on to *passively* refuse food and water in order to starve himself to death. One contrast between passive PAS and passive E involves it being true that in the E case there is no need for the patient to act or deliberately desist from some further action such as eating, in order for what the doctor does to suffice for allowing death to come about.

In *voluntary* E, both the patient and doctor intend the death. In PAS, the doctor only *may* intend the death, while the patient does intend it. (This is supposed to insure its voluntariness.) Only "may," since some doctors provide lethal pills or disconnect sedation only in order to give patients a choice whether to live or die. For example, Dr. Timothy Quill claims that he only intended to give his patient an option to kill herself.[3] I believe that a doctor will not be, strictly speaking, assisting in suicide if he gives drugs prior to the patient forming an intention to use them. If the patient does not subsequently attempt suicide, the doctor certainly does not assist in it, though he did make possible the choice between doing it and not doing it.[4] If the patient takes the drug, having formed the intention to do so after the doctor gave her the drug, he has helped her do what kills her, but this is not quite the same as assisting in suicide. If he gave drugs to give a choice (i.e., before he knew an intention was formed), then if he is present at the time she takes the drug, this is also not assistance in suicide, even if he does not stop the suicide. However, if a doctor gives the lethal drug knowing the patient has formed the settled intention to use it and she uses it, he assisted in suicide, perhaps only intending to help a person, not intending death. If he gives a medicine that keeps the patient alert in order that she can commit suicide, he also assists in suicide. (This may also mean that there are really two persons who engage in a killing, even if only the patient gives himself the lethal medicine.)[5]

To summarize a bit, active euthanasia is killing. Passive euthanasia by omission is letting die. Passive euthanasia by action can be a killing or it can be a letting die (that helps cause death), depending on such factors as who owns the life-support machine and who is running it. Once a patient forms an intention to commit suicide, he can do so actively which involves killing himself or passively (either by an omission or act which terminates life support) and this involves letting himself die. If a doctor actively assists an active suicide (either by, for example, giving lethal drugs or giving drugs to facilitate a patient's suicidal act), he assists in killing; if he actively assists a passive suicide, he assists a letting die. If a doctor passively assists an active suicide (either by, for example, omitting sedation or terminating it), he assists a killing; if he passively assists a passive suicide, he assists a letting die.

Death As a Benefit

Some have argued that the idea of E makes no sense because it is logically impossible to seek to benefit someone by seeking his death, given that death eliminates the person. We cannot produce a benefit if we eliminate the potential beneficiary, it is argued. One of the ways conceptual analysis can be useful in the ethical examination of E is by making clear how someone can be benefited by death even if it involves his nonexistence, just as someone can be harmed by death even though it involves his nonexistence. To be benefited or harmed, one need not continue on in a state of good experience or bad experience. If one's life would have included important basic goods if it had continued, then at least *one* of the ways in which one is harmed by death is that it interferes with those important basic goods; as a result of death, one has had a less good life, a life that is seriously worse overall than one would have had, and whatever leads us to have such a worse life harms us. The shorter life is not worse because it contains an additional intrinsic evil (e.g., pain). It is comparatively worse than it might have been.[6]

But are we harmed whenever our life is worse than it might have been?[7] If my life would have been better if I had been able to fly, is it a harm to me not to be able to fly? It might be argued that it is only when the goods I lack are crucial to my well-being that their absence is a harm. But if something interferes with even a noncrucial good that I could have had, e.g., if a chemical in the air makes it impossible for me to fly, does not the *chemical* harm me, even if the good it deprives me of is not such that its absence is a harm to me? I am inclined to think so. In any case, it certainly makes me worse off than I would have been. Furthermore, if the chemical deprived me of a basic component of a good life, such as all human relations, it would clearly harm me. The goods of which death deprives us *are* such basic ones, whose absence is a harm to us; and so death harms us.

If one's life would have gone on containing only misery and pain with no compensating goods, then, it might be argued, one will be benefited in having had a shorter life containing fewer of such bad things rather than a longer one containing more of such uncompensated-for bad things. The shorter life is not better because it contains more intrinsic goods. It is better because it has fewer intrinsic evils and so is comparatively better. In this sense, it might be argued, it is possible for death to benefit a person.

But we said that *one* of the ways death harms us is by depriving us of basic goods of life. If there is *another way* in which death harms us, then even if death eliminates uncompensated misery, it may still overall harm us. Suppose the *end of the person* independent of its causing the end of more goods of life is a separate harm to the person that death causes. Then it is possible that this harm could outweigh the elimination of life's miseries.[8] But it is also possible that the elimination of the miseries is such an important good that it overrides the harm of the end of the person. Suppose this is so. This does not show that it is ever morally permissible to benefit a person by helping to end his life even when he requests it. That is our next question.

Arguments for PAS and E

An Argument for the Permissibility of PAS or E

Doctors may, at least with the consent of a terminally ill patient, give morphine for the relief of severe pain otherwise not manageable, even if they foresee *with 100 percent certainty* that death would thereby soon occur, and sooner than it would without morphine.[9] Notice that this could be true even if the morphine put the patient in a deep unconscious state when he was alive, from which he never awoke before he died, so that he did not experience conscious, pain-free time alive. Why may doctors do this? One reason given is that, in this particular type of case, the *greater good is relief of pain*, and the *lesser evil is the loss of life* given that life would end soon anyway and is not of very good quality. This means the patient is overall benefited by a shorter pain-free life rather than a longer, painful life.[10] The absence of pain is a comparative good; that is, it is better than pain, though it is not an intrinsic good (like pleasure), but this does not stop it from outweighing an evil. (Similarly, relief of pain could outweigh brief nausea as a side effect of a painkiller.) In this *morphine for pain relief* case (MPR), furthermore, the lesser evil of death is only a foreseen side effect. It is not intended, hence this is not a case of euthanasia. (The fact that death will occur with certainty does not mean it is intended. If I have a drink to soothe my nerves and foresee that it will certainly cause a hangover tomorrow, that does not mean that I intend the hangover.) Still, in the MPR case, the doctor gives a drug which is inducing death, so I see no reason not to call this a case of killing, though the doctor does not intend the death. (It is quite possible to kill without intending death, as when one runs over someone while driving a car.)

However, it might be argued that there is another reason why giving the morphine in MPR is permissible. This reason does not require one to accept the view that death sometimes involves a lesser evil while pain relief is a greater good. (Hence, while this view is sufficient to explain the permissibility of MPR, it is not necessary.) This other reason is that doctors may give MPR foreseeing death because death will occur soon anyway if the patient is terminal.[11] Therefore, even if death were always a greater evil than pain, when it will occur imminently no matter what we do, it is permissible to produce an overall better state of affairs by giving MPR to at least eliminate the pain, which is avoidable.

The two premises—death involves a lesser evil and imminence of death—have different implications in cases in which the patient is not terminal. Only if death involves a lesser evil would we permit a doctor to give a painkiller that will hasten death even if the patient would not otherwise die soon anyway, but would live on in great pain for a long time. To know for sure whether we are relying on death as involving a lesser evil to justify the use of MPR, it would be best to consider nonterminal cases.

In what follows, I will assume that death can involve a lesser evil. But I shall also say something about how we might proceed if it were always a greater evil.

Now suppose the morphine has lost its pain-relieving effects on the patient. It can still be used to kill the patient as a means to ending his pain, and the patient requests its use to kill him in order to end his pain. Call this the *morphine for death* case (MD). It is said by some that we may not give the morphine in this case. This is so, even though relief of pain is still the greater good and death the lesser evil, and though the consequences of killing him are *essentially* the same as in MPR. It is said to be impermissible to *intend the lesser evil* as a means to a greater good. Those who say this may support what is called the Doctrine of Double Effect (DDE), according to which there is a large moral difference between acting with the foresight that one's conduct will have some evil consequence and acting with the intent to produce that same evil as a means to a greater good. (Though not all supporters of some version of DDE would rule out killing in MD).

I said the consequences in MPR and MD were *essentially* the same. It is worth pointing out a way in which the cases differ somewhat. When morphine is a painkiller, it produces at least a short span of life without pain. The death that is the side effect might be the effect of (a) the morphine itself, that is, a side effect of our means to the greater good, or (b) it might be the result of the greater good itself produced by morphine. The former is what actually occurs. The latter would occur (though it does not in fact occur) if pain relief, rather than morphine, altered the body's chemistry in such a way as to lower the heart rate and lead to death. In both these scenarios, the death is clearly a causal effect of either the morphine or the pain relief, and the pain relief is caused by the morphine. In MD, where death is the means to pain relief, the pain relief does not involve a span of life without pain. Furthermore, the good of absence of pain does not follow as a *causal effect* of the death, even though the death is intended as a means to pain relief.[12] For the nonexistence of pain is best described as a part of the whole which consists of nonexistence of the person, that is, as a part of death. The elimination of life has as one of its parts, not as its causal after-effect, the absence of any experience and hence the absence of bad experience (e.g., pain).

Given this, in what sense do we intend the lesser evil in MD? If an evil of death is the absence of a few more of the good experiences of life, and this is also a part of nonexistence, we need not necessarily be intending *it* if we aim at death in order to achieve its other part, namely the absence of the bad experiences. If we nevertheless are intending a lesser evil in MD—as is commonly thought—and not just foreseeing it, this must be because future nonexistence of the person (or end-of-life) is itself an evil, in addition to the loss of further goods that would have been made possible by life. Hence, we intend an evil in intending death only if there is an evil to death aside from the loss of goods of life. (It is surprising, I

believe, that this view about what is bad about death is implied by the view that
to intend death is not merely to foresee an evil.) By contrast, if we thought that
the only thing that makes death bad is the absence of more goods of life, then we
would not be able to say that in intending death, and foreseeing the absence of
these goods, we would be intending an evil. And the DDE then could not be used
as an objection to killing in MD.

One alternative is to say that if we intend the whole (nonexistence), then we
do intend all its parts, including the lesser evil of a few less good experiences. I
do not think this is correct. Another alternative, already discussed, is to say that
intending death is not per se to intend an evil. I suspect this is not right either.
But, to repeat, if it were, the DDE could not be used to argue against the administration of morphine in MD.[13]

Let us assume that we do intend an evil in MD.[14] Without denying that sometimes the distinction between intending and foreseeing death makes a moral difference, here is an argument to show that it provides no reason against
performing E or PAS when death is the lesser evil. The first step is to show that
on many other occasions already, doctors (with the patient's consent) *intend the
lesser evil* to a person in order *to produce his own greater good*. For example, it is
permissible for a doctor to intentionally amputate a healthy leg (the lesser evil)
in order to get at and remove a cancerous tumor, thereby saving the patient's life
(the greater good).[15] It would be permissible for her to intentionally cause blindness in a patient if seeing would somehow destroy the patient's brain. It would
be permissible for her to intentionally cause an hour of nausea if this is necessary to stop unbearable pain. Furthermore, it is permissible for her to intentionally cause someone pain, thereby acting contrary to a doctor's duty to relieve
physical suffering, if this is a means to saving the person's life. For example, she
might permissibly cause pain if this alone keeps a patient awake during lifesaving surgery that requires his responsiveness for success. The duty to save life
sometimes just outweighs the other duty. Blindness, nausea, and pain are presumably intrinsic evils, so intending them is clearly intending lesser evil.

The Principle of Totality, a part of natural law theory (which also contains the
DDE), permits us to destroy a part to save the whole and so seems to account for
some of the above cases. But it also seems to conflict with, or override, the DDE.
For insofar as the DDE is at issue, there should be a moral distinction not only
between intending death and merely foreseeing it, but also between intending to
destroy sight and merely foreseeing its destruction. Insofar as we are not anymore
dealing with a doctrine that denies the permissibility of intending all lesser evils,
we are not really concerned with the DDE. (Rather, we shall find ourself focusing
on the specialness of intending death, for it is only then that we do not intend
the destruction of a part to preserve the whole.) This is an important point for,
in interpersonal, as opposed to intrapersonal cases, that is, in cases where we
intend an evil to a person for the good of others rather than for his own good, it
may be correct to still focus on the DDE. For example, we may omit to aid one
person, *foreseeing* that he will go blind, in order to help five avoid blindness, but

it would be wrong to omit helping him *intending* that he go blind because his being blind will (somehow) prevent five others from going blind. Yet, as I have noted, we think it is permissible to intend such a lesser evil to a person for his own greater good.[16]

Now, we come to the next step in the argument for E and PAS: Why cannot doctors likewise intend death when *it* is the lesser evil in order to produce the greater good of no pain, thereby benefiting the patient by giving her a shorter, less painful life rather than her enduring a longer, more painful one? Recall that in MPR, it was assumed that death would be the lesser evil and pain relief the greater good. That was one reason we could give the morphine. Indeed, one important reason we use the MPR case in this argument is to establish in a less controversial case the possible *relative values* of pain relief and death. Why cannot doctors sometimes act against a duty to preserve life in order to relieve pain, just as they can sometimes act against a duty to relieve pain in order to save a life in cases where pain is the lesser evil and life the greater good? It is true that when we intend the destruction of the leg or cause blindness, we save the whole person, and in aiming at death, we destroy the whole person. But, as argued above, this may still overall benefit the patient.

To summarize, we have constructed a three-step argument for PAS and E: Assuming patient consent, 1) we may permissibly cause death as a side effect if it relieves pain, because *sometimes death is a lesser evil and pain relief a greater good*; 2) we may permissibly *intend other lesser evils* to the patient, for the sake of her greater good; 3) therefore, *when death is a lesser evil*, it is sometimes *permissible for us to intend death* in order to stop pain. Call this the Three-Step Argument.[17]

Recall that we considered the possibility that death might always be a greater evil, and yet it would be permissible to act in MPR because of the unavoidable imminence of death. Using this premise we could construct an Alternative Three-Step Argument. The second premise is that doctors could permissibly intend greater evils other than death that will occur imminently anyway in order to produce a lesser good. For example, suppose it is worse to be blind than to be deaf. If a patient will shortly be blind anyway, it would be permissible to intentionally cause his blindness if only this would prevent him from also going deaf. The conclusion is that it is permissible for doctors to intentionally kill a terminally ill patient in order to stop pain, even if death is the greater evil and relief of pain the lesser good.

In this article I will focus on the Three-Step Argument since I assume that death is sometimes a lesser evil relative to certain possible ways of living, and not to be avoided at all costs to the patient.

An Argument for a Duty to Perform PAS and E

Before considering possible objections to this argument, I want to add another set of considerations that support E and PAS.

According to the Three-Step Argument, a doctor is *permitted* to give the morphine though she knows it will kill the patient. But we may be able to say more:

If her killing the patient does not serve as a reason to prevent her giving morphine as a painkiller, it may also not be a justification for her refusing to give morphine as a painkiller. That is, she may have a duty to give it. This is because a doctor, I assume, has a duty to relieve physical suffering, and so the doctor has a *duty* to relieve such suffering by giving the morphine if the patient requests this; she cannot refuse to give the morphine on the ground that she will be a killer if she does. The case in which morphine is a painkiller shows that patients have some right to be physically invaded, for example, with pain medication when they request it for pain relief.

If doctors have a duty to relieve pain, and even being a killer does not override this when the patient requests morphine, then maybe they also have a duty, not merely a permission, to kill their patients, or to aid in their being killed, intending their deaths in order to relieve suffering. Now, we have a new argument: Assuming patient consent, 1) there is a *duty* to treat pain even if it foreseeably makes one a killer, when death is the lesser evil and no pain is the greater good. 2) There is a *duty* to intend other lesser evils (e.g., blindness) for a patient's own greater good. 3) There is a *duty* to kill the patient or assist in his death, intending his death, when death is the lesser evil and pain relief the greater good. Call this the Duty Argument.[18]

While I find the Duty Argument worth considering, I shall, in this paper, focus on the Three-Step Argument for permissible E and PAS.

Criticism and Objections

The Killing Objection to the Three-Step Argument

Objections may be raised to the Three-Step Argument. First, it may be said that the doctor who intends the death of his patient in PAS or E is *killing*. Even if intending a lesser evil for a greater good is permissible when this does not involve killing, when it does involve killing, it is impermissible. One way of understanding this objection is that the killing is what makes things wrong. But how can one object to the Three-Step Argument solely on grounds that it involves killing when giving the lethal injection in MPR also involves killing, and we approve of giving the morphine there?

A patient's right to life includes a right not to be killed, but, some have argued, the right to life is a discretionary right—that is, it gives one a protected option whether to live or die, an option with which others may not interfere; it does not give one a duty to live. If a patient decides to take morphine for pain though he knows it will kill him, he is waiving his right to live, as someone may waive her right to speak on a given occasion. By waiving his right, he releases others from their duty not to do what will kill him, *insofar as their duty not to do what will kill him stems from his right to live.*[19] More particularly, he may exercise a power that his discretionary right to life gives him so that another person now has the right (i.e., a permission with which others may not interfere) to kill him. Does this power stem from a right the patient has to kill himself, so that if he had no right to kill himself, he could not give to another a right to kill him? Not necessarily, for someone might be prohibited from killing himself on his own, but still have the moral power to designate someone else to kill him or to perform the act with him. So the right, with which others may not interfere, to give someone the right (with which others may not interfere) to perform euthanasia or to assist in one's suicide need not be based on a general right to suicide, although it might be.

Furthermore, a person's right to life may be discretionary only in certain conditions, for example, when life gets bad enough, and the right to empower others to kill him may be limited to those conditions. Others may also be limited in what they can do because their duty not to do what will kill someone stems not only from his right not to be killed, but from their *duty not to harm him*, even if he wishes them to do what harms him. This may be a duty from which he has no power to release them, even if he waives his right not to be killed. But I have stipulated that the doctor is to kill only when death is the lesser evil and so no harm overall is done to the patient.

If a patient may permissibly waive his right to life insofar as it protects him from others doing things to him that lead to his death (e.g., giving morphine as a painkiller), it is not the inability to waive this right (nor the duty others have not to harm) that stands in the way of deliberately killing him.[20]

Notice that I have emphasized this waiver is morally necessary even when the doctor wishes to give morphine that will kill as a side effect. This means doctors should get permission for giving the morphine as a painkiller if it will kill as a side effect, as well as for giving it to deliberately kill. I do not believe they always do so.

The Intending-Death Objection to the Three-Step Argument

What other reason could there be for the impermissibility of intentionally killing a patient to end his pain? Rather than pointing to the killing alone, we might point to the distinctiveness of intending death rather than intending other lesser evils, or perhaps the combination of intending death and killing.

In one revisionist proposal for distinguishing morally between intending and foreseeing harm to people other than ourselves, *without those other's consent*, Warren Quinn distinguishes between 1) not treating people as ends, and 2) treating them as mere means.[21] We do the former, he says, when we pursue our projects without constraining our behavior in the light of the foreseen harm to others. We do the latter when we treat people as being available for our purposes, as something we can take charge of and use to meet our goals, even when this involves harm to them. He thinks the latter is worse than the former when the harm is equal. (He here divides the Kantian injunction to treat persons as ends in themselves and not merely as means into two components.) On Quinn's analysis, *intending the involvement* of a person in a way which we foresee will lead to uncompensated harm to him is taken to be as wrong as *intending uncompensated harm* to him (and hence, treating such *harm* to him as available for our purposes). The traditional DDE would distinguish these two, ruling out only the latter, since it is aiming at such harm (an evil) with which it is particularly concerned. (The traditional doctrine, but not necessarily Quinn, also seems to rule out intending the harm when it leads to overall good for the person himself as well, even when he consents to it, as in the MD case. As noted above, it does not distinguish between *intra*personal harm for benefit—intending lesser harm to the same person who will greatly benefit from it—and *inter*personal harm for benefit—intending harm to someone for another's benefit.) I agree with Quinn that intending involvement of another with foreseen harm is worse than merely causing such foreseen harm, but I also think that intending *the harm* itself is a distinctive concern. Before I deal with this issue, however, I wish to first focus on the idea of using a person in the intrapersonal context in objecting to the Three-Step Argument.

If it is permissible for a person to take, or direct another to take, his life as a means to stopping his pain, this implies that it is permissible for people to take control of and destroy their own persons for their own purposes; the whole of their being is not off limits to be used to stop their pain. If morality has a special interest in insisting that people not see themselves as under their control to be used for their purposes in this way, this would be consistent with its not having as much interest in their making attempts to preserve their lives when death is merely foreseen. Furthermore, it is possible that taking control of one's life can only be done actively; if one intends a death and so *omits* to stop a deadly natural event that one has not set in motion (or one *removes a barrier* to it that belongs to one or that one was maintaining), the element of control is less. This is one reason why the *combination* of killing and intending death is often more significant than the combination of omitting or terminating treatment and intending death. (We shall consider two other reasons to morally distinguish killing and terminating treatment below.)[22]

Obviously, people can take control of their whole lives and devote their beings to the pursuit of certain goals within the living of their lives. But, it is claimed, when this is appropriate, they do not aim to destroy their persons, but rather set them in one direction or another. So, in PAS or E, we treat the *destruction of a person* as available for use in achieving a good. (Now we have moved from merely taking control of the person to taking control of the person in order to cause an evil, the destruction of the person. We intend not only involvement of the person, but her destruction.) The Three-Step Argument says that we may intend death if it is a lesser evil and if we may intend other lesser evils. Part of the objection to this argument suggested here is that acting with the intention to bring about the lesser evil of death is different because it requires us to have a further intention, namely to treat our whole selves (or another person, if we are doctors) as destructible in order to achieve good. We do not have this further intention when we intend such other lesser evils as blindness.

More specifically, in voluntary E and PAS, we use a rational being—a being who judges, aims at goals, and evaluates how to act. One of the things that seems odd about killing only someone who is capable of rationally deciding to be killed—this is the point of complicated controls on E and PAS—is that one is *making sure* that one is destroying a being of great worth—a reasoning, thinking being. This will not be so if the person is unconscious or vegetative or otherwise no longer functioning as a rational being.[23]

The idea that there are limits on what we may do to ourselves as persons is Kantian. Kant thought that rational humanity in ourselves and in others is (and should be treated as) *an end in itself, and not a mere means* to happiness or other goals.[24] (It is important to emphasize that treating someone as a means is not the same as treating him as a *mere* means.) Even if bads outweigh what in our life is *good for us*, the fact that one is a rational agent in life—judging, aiming, evaluating—has worth in itself. To have this status as a person is more like an honor which brings with it responsibilities (Kant called it "dignity") than a benefit that answers to some interest or desire of ours. Thus, I (and, in that sense, my life) may have worth, even if my life does not provide benefits to me that outweigh bads to me. The worth *of me* as a person is not measured solely by its worth *to me* in satisfying my interests and desires, or its worth to others in satisfying theirs.[25]

This means that whether our life is a benefit to us (or death instead would benefit us) is a different question from whether we have worth (or death would end something of worth). Still, being a creature that has this worth *may be part of what makes* my life *worth living*, even if the bads *to me* outweigh the goods to me in my life. Or, put another way, even if the bads outweigh goods *other than the good of being a person*, my life may be worth living because I am a person. (This is why euthanasia might be right for cats but not for persons.) If my life is *worth living* (in part because I am a being of a certain sort), then death will not be a lesser evil, even though it *would* remove things that are in important ways bad *for* me and not eliminate things that are in important ways good *for* me. However, if it were possible for my life *not* to be worth living, despite the fact that I am a being of a particularly significant sort, then death could be a lesser evil, and it could benefit me.[26] Notice that this would still be consistent with its eliminating a creature of worth, only one whose life is not worth living. The apparent oddity of making sure one only kills a being of worth who has reasonably chosen to die might thus be explained away. This analysis would also show that when one says someone's life is not worth living, one is not necessarily saying that they are not worthwhile as persons or are disposable entities.

According to Kant, however, it is wrong for others to treat me as a mere means for their ends, and equally wrong for me to treat myself as a mere means for my own ends such as eliminating pain. As others should respect my worth as a person by not using me merely as a means for their purposes, I should have proper regard for my own worth as a person, and not simply treat myself as a means to achieving goods and avoiding harms. (Perhaps he believes this even if one's life is not worth living, or maybe he believes it can never be true of a rational being that her life is not worth living.) But, it is said, that is precisely what I do when I aim at my own death as a way to eliminate pain. So I ought not to pursue that aim, and therefore ought not to consent to a morphine injection aiming at death, or give one to a patient who has consented.

Killing and Intending Death

Before assessing this Kantian argument, I want to justify focusing on intentional killing rather than other ways of intentionally contributing to a death. I have already noted one possible reason—the combination of intention and killing involves greater control than intending death and only omitting to stop a cause of death one does not start. But there is a second, and, I believe, a more important reason for focusing on intentional killing. Consider a patient who intends his death to eliminate pain and therefore wants life support of any sort removed. Suppose for the sake of argument that we disapprove of this intention. We may also disapprove of a doctor's agreeing to remove treatment because she also intends this patient's death. But while we may disapprove of these intentions and conduct, acting on that disapproval would require us to *force* life support on the patient, and this he has a right that we not do.[27] Our supposed opposition to his intentions and the doctor's is trumped, I believe, by our opposition to forced invasion of the patient.[28] So, we permit the patient and doctor to act—to remove treatment—intending death. In this analysis, I am distinguishing between (1) the (supposed) impermissibility of the agents intending, (2) the permissibility and even obligatoriness of the doctor acting to stop treatment, and (3) the permissibility and even obligatoriness of our allowing doctor and patient to intend death and act on their intentions.

Consider, in contrast, a patient who intends his own death and, therefore, requests a lethal injection or pills. Here, too, suppose we oppose the intention. In this case, acting on our opposition would require us to refrain from administering a lethal injection or the pills. But it seems clear that the right *not* to be invaded with treatment against one's will is stronger than the right to be given a lethal injection or pills. Does the patient have a *right* to a lethal injection at all? We said he had a right to have a painkiller (the doctor had a duty to give it) if this would stop pain, even though it was also a lethal injection. But this does not mean that he has any right to a lethal injection per se. So, the fact that the doctor must terminate treatment and we must allow termination of treatment, even when the patient and his doctor intend his death, does not show that it is permissible to kill the patient or assist him in killing himself, or required of us to allow these acts, when the patient and doctor intend his death. Correspondingly, an objection to intentional killing need not imply an objection to terminating treatment for someone who intends his own death.

This shows that while the Kantian argument against PAS and E with which we are concerned focuses on the distinction between intending and foreseeing death, it also hooks onto the distinction between killing and letting die. For the wrong intention is not allowed to carry weight when the opposite to *letting die* is forcing treatment on the patient, but the wrong intention *is* allowed to carry weight when the opposite to *killing* is just leaving the patient alone. The objection raised here is not to killing per se but to the intention, yet this objection can play itself out only when killing is at issue.[29] (Below I shall suggest a third reason some might be especially opposed to killing combined with intending death.)

We have considered how a supposed objection to a patient or doctor intending death could work itself out differentially in cases of killing or letting die. It might be thought that another way to interpret these cases is that we (the State?) are more concerned with the doctor not intending the patient's death than with the patient not intending his own death. For when the doctor terminates treatment on a patient who intends his death, she *need not* intend anything except not imposing on a patient against his will. But, of course, it is possible that a doctor who terminates treatment does so because *she also intends the death*. This will not make her stopping treatment impermissible, since regardless of her actual aim, it is still true that if she doesn't terminate treatment she will be imposing on a patient against his will. It seems that even if we were opposed to a doctor intending death, our opposition could show itself in our behavior only in a context where there is no other acceptable reason that could justify the doctor's action.[30]

In contrast to cases so far discussed, suppose that a patient who intends his own death is also suffering great pain that only morphine can stop. Death is the lesser evil, pain relief the greater good. But he asks for the morphine, not because it will stop the pain, but because he knows it will kill him. If the morphine would not kill him, he would not ask for it. (Call this the Death Drip Case.)[31] Does he have a right that the doctor give him the morphine? If he does, then here we have a case where the doctor is not at liberty to refuse a lethal injection simply because of the *patient's intention*, anymore than he could refuse to terminate treatment because of the patient's intention. But again, this is a case where invasion with a lethal injection could be given a clearly acceptable justification (pain relief) by the patient, even if intending death is his actual rationale.

In other cases somewhat analogous to this one, doctors *would* have a duty to provide a treatment. Suppose, for example, that being made blind will save a person's life. The patient is not at all interested in having his life saved, but he nevertheless wants the surgery because he intends his own blindness (Blindness Case). The doctor must still produce the greater good of saving life, even though this involves his *intending* the lesser evil of blindness (not merely foreseeing it). Why then should not the doctor in the Death Drip Case produce the greater good of pain relief at the cost of what, from his point of view, is just the foreseen lesser evil of death, even though his patient intends the death?

But now suppose the doctor in the Death Drip Case also intends the patient's death. If the patient still has a right to the morphine as painkiller, we would not be permitted to interfere with the doctor's giving morphine, despite the doctor's (supposedly) improper intention. Once again, we see that, so long as there is another factor in the situation that could provide a clearly acceptable justification, the patient and/or doctor are free to act on any intention.[32]

In sum, we might permissibly express an opposition to intending death only when killing is at issue, and then only if there is not another factor that could provide an acceptable justification for doing what induces death.

Using a Person As a Mere Means

In order to evaluate the Kantian argument against aiming at one's death or aiming at another's death as a means to greater good for the person who would die, I believe it is important to distinguish *three* different ways in which one may treat a person as a mere means:

1. Calculating the worth of living on in a way which gives insufficient (even no) weight to the worth of being a person *in itself*, rather than as a means to other goods.
2. Treating the death of a person as a mere means to a goal, e.g., ending pain.
3. Using a person merely in order to bring about his own end.

The first idea is that a person has worth in himself and is not merely a means to an overall balance of other goods over evils in his life. On this interpretation, we treat persons as a mere means if we give no weight in our decisions to the intrinsic value of our existence as persons; if we do this, then death may seem a lesser rather than a greater evil. But even when there are few goods in life, the capacity to be a rational agent may make the loss of life—and therefore the loss of that capacity—a greater evil than pain. This analysis implies that the fact that one treats one's rational humanity (what makes one a person) as a way to achieve a good for *onself* (no pain) is not enough to constitute not treating one's person as a *mere* means. One may still fail to respect oneself, to take oneself seriously as a person. That we are satisfying our interests rather than those of others is not enough to rebut the charge of treating our rational humanity as a mere means.

Though I do not doubt that this idea has force, it can equally well be given as a reason for not terminating a course of treatment, or not taking a painkiller, *even when one merely foresees one's death*. That is, we might decide to ask for morphine as a painkiller despite its foreseen deadly effects because we underestimate the importance of being a person and think that if our life is painful that is sufficient reason not to resist its passing. That is, we assign incorrect weight and so our calculation is flawed. Because this way of treating persons as a mere means does not distinguish *the morality of intending and merely foreseeing death*, it cannot be used to explain why intentional killing in particular is impermissible.[33]

It might be said that this observation should prompt us to rethink the permissibility of ever killing in the case of morphine for pain relief, where death is foreseen but not intended. For it might be said that the concern to treat people not as mere means can be met only by giving *overriding* weight to the importance of rational humanity, and that this requires that we refrain from acting in ways that we foresee as leading to death, and not simply from intentional killing. This response seems unjustified, though there are different ways to argue this point. Suppose life involves such unbearable pain that one's whole life is focused on that pain. Some may claim that when this happens, one's status as a rational being is compromised,[34] and so when we kill we no longer destroy rational humanity; even that we kill in order to end an insult to rational humanity. The point here is to argue that rational humanity is overriding, not merely a value that can be outweighed; whenever it seems to be outweighed, it has already been undermined, and killing is permissible. But, we may ask, if the person who asks for morphine as pain relief is still able to rationally weigh considerations and is in control of his faculties, why is his rationality undermined by pain?

If we think that the *diminished opportunity* to exercise one's rationality (because one is always focusing on one's pain) counts as the relevant sort of compromise of rationality, shall we condone suicide for someone who sleeps most of the time? This is an odd view, and certainly not one that can be justified on the ground that rational humanity itself no longer exists. Most importantly, in situations where there is a great pain and where rationality is present but has great limits on its exercise, is it these limits or the great pain that would be the real reason for tolerating the end of life? My sense is that the pain would be the most important reason for doing what would end life, not the limits on exercising rationality.

A final thought experiment may help in this regard: Suppose someone's life alternates between days when he is fully rational and able to exercise his rationality and days of intense pain when he is still rational but limited in his ability to do anything but focus on the pain.[35] In this case, one cannot argue that death by painkiller is tolerated because of limits on rational activity, since every other day one can engage in rational activities. The pain may still reasonably drive one to take medication that foreseeably causes death.

I conclude that when pain justifies taking the medication, it is not always a matter of the deterioration or humiliation of rational nature or the absence of dignity, just the burden of living. Hence, one must argue that in such circumstances one does not lack self respect if one does what will cause one's end, for in so doing we do not treat our life as *mere* means to a balance of good for us over bads for us. We might acknowledge the great (and normally overriding) importance of being a person and believe it is right in many cases to go on in life even if it has more pain than other goods besides rational agency. Though we reject the thought that rational agency is merely a means to happiness, we allow that some bad conditions may overshadow its very great value.

Notice that I say "allow" rather than "insist," since it does not seem *ir*rational to be so committed to continuing life as a person that one puts up with pain that others see as outweighing the worth of their persons. (It may be that some of those who go on are just better able to cope with pain rather than that they are more committed to living.) Suppose we allow that acting while intending or foreseeing one's death does not always indicate a failure of self respect or a failure to accord sufficient weight to being a person in itself. This does not imply that we think acting while intending or foreseeing one's death is the only rational step to take. Similarly, suppose we allow that taking morphine for pain relief when it is known to lead to death does not always indicate a failure to accord sufficient weight to being a person. This in itself does not imply that taking the morphine is required by reason. In this sense, being a person is still an unconditional good: It is *always available* to be an overriding reason for going on in the face of great evils, even if it need not always be one's overriding reason.

Still, we can learn something from the attempt to give overriding weight to rational humanity. It proposed that death can be less bad than a life in which rationality is severely undermined. This can still be true, even if death can also sometimes be less bad than a life in which rationality is not so undermined. If death is less bad than a life in which reason is so undermined, this suggests that we should prefer some ways of ending rational humanity over others—for example, death rather than mental deterioration—when this is necessary to avoid great evils such as great pain.

Suppose that to relieve intense pain there are two drugs. One has the side effect of eliminating personhood irreversibly, but not killing the patient. The other has the side effect of certainly killing the patient. It is possible that one should prefer the second drug. Likewise, if the only two ways to eliminate pain were to intentionally eliminate personhood (because neurons responsible for it also control pain) or to intentionally kill, it is possible that one should prefer the second way. Living on in a severely subrational state might be worse than having one's life end so that there is complete physical absence. It is even possible that it would be *wrong* (not only less good) to deliberately destroy rationality in a still-living human being or do what destroys rationality in a still-living human being as a side effect in order to end pain. If so, it would indicate that death has specific virtues as a way of eliminating a person that play a role in our allowing that ending pain may outweigh the value of personhood.

If the value of one's rational humanity can be overshadowed by pain, does this have implications for *inter*personal as well as *intra*personal decisions; does it imply that we may sometimes sacrifice a person for the sake of stopping other people's pain, as well as implying that we may sacrifice him to stop his own pain? I do not believe so, any more than the fact that we may blind someone to save his life means that we may blind him to save other people's lives. The Kantian claim that one may not treat oneself, any more than others, solely as a means may conceal some strong asymmetries between the interpersonal and intrapersonal cases.

Kant thought we had a duty to actively preserve rational humanity and hence we should not too lightly do what we foresee will lead to its end. Still, he allows that we may sometimes engage in conduct though we foresee it will result in our deaths, but not aim at our deaths in the same circumstances. Our discussion so far has shown that, to explain this distinction, we must move beyond the first sense of treating oneself as a mere means. But other arguments that Kant provides, or that a Kantian might provide to support this distinction, also fail to distinguish between taking the morphine foreseeing that one will die and intending the death. For example, Kant claims that it is not rational to destroy the ground of the disvalue of pain in order to eliminate pain. That is, if there were no rational humanity, it would not be important that there be no pain (he seems to think). But if it were true, that we should not destroy the ground of the disvalue of pain, this would also rule out taking medication in MPR, for one would foresee the destruction of rational humanity, and hence be eliminating the (supposed) ground of disvalue of pain.

Consider another Kantian argument for not intending one's death: One cannot justify not doing one's duty simply by showing that it is burdensome to do it.[36] For example, if one has children to care for, one cannot just abandon them because it is burdensome to care for them. Similarly, one has a duty to go on living; then, even if life becomes very burdensome, one may not be relieved of this duty. To this argument, someone might respond by asking whether we do have a duty to go on living, rather than a duty not to evade other duties by escaping life. One might also ask whether some degree of burden *can* serve as a justification for not doing one's duty. But my concern here is different: If I have a duty, not only must I not deliberately abandon it to avoid the burden of carrying it out, I also must not do what will ease my burden when I foresee that this will interfere with my doing my duty. For example, suppose I have a duty to play my violin but this causes me pain. If I must not stop playing to avoid the pain, I also must not take the only drug that will stop the pain when I know it will put me to sleep, thus disabling me from playing the violin. Once again, this Kantian argument does not distinguish between taking the morphine for pain relief or for death.

What, then, about the second and third interpretations I offered of the idea of using persons as mere means? Can they justify the distinction between engaging in conduct though we foresee it will result in our deaths, and aiming at our deaths? To see the difference between the second and the third interpretations, consider an analogy: My radio is a device for getting good sounds and filtering out bad sounds. It is a mere means to a balance of good sounds over bad ones. Suppose it stops performing well, that it only produces static, but cannot be turned off. I can wait until its batteries run down and not replace them, or I can smash it now, thus using the radio itself to stop the noise it produces. Either way, I would see its death as I saw its life, as a mere means to a better balance of good over bad sounds. While I have always seen my radio as a mere means to an end, if I smash it, I use it as a mere means to its end (termination). This is sense 3. (If I see someone else destroy it and do not interfere, I may be intending its use as a means to its own end, although *I* do not use it.) If I let the radio run down, intending its demise, but do not smash it—I see it wasting away and do not replace its batteries—then I do not see it as a mere means to its own end, but I do *see its end (termination) as a mere means* to a better balance of sounds. This is sense 2.

The sort of use of the person as a means that takes place in active suicide or euthanasia is analogous to the smashing of the radio: The person uses himself, or another uses him, as a mere means to his own death. Some people find this complete taking control of a life particularly morally inappropriate, perhaps because they think our bodies belong to God and that we have no right to achieve the goal of our own death by manipulating a "tool" that is not ours (or intending that others manipulate it). This objection is not present if—here we have sense 2—we terminate medical assistance with the intention that the system run down, aiming at its death, for then we achieve the goal of death by interfering with what is ours (the medication), not God's. This is another reason why someone may not object to terminating treatment even when intending death as a means 2 is present, but may object to killing: Terminating treatment, unlike intentional killing, does not involve 3. Some say, though, that sense 2 is also more objectionable than merely foreseeing the death. They say that if we terminate medical assistance, intending death, then though we may not treat our person merely as a means to a balance of greater good for us over bads for us (sense 1), we do treat *our death (the end of our life, destruction of our person)* as a mere means to greater good over bad.

Another way to show that the sense of using as a means in 1 differs from those in 2 and 3 is to consider *interpersonal* cases of treating people as mere means. Suppose I intend A's death in order to save B and C and D, and then kill him or let him die intending his death, but I would not kill him or let him die in order to save just B and C. It might be argued that I give him weight in his own right and do not see him merely as a tool for maximizing good, because it takes more than two people to override his life. Hence, perhaps I do not literally run afoul of 1. But in another sense, I do treat him as a mere means, because on the occasion that I use him for B, C, and D's sakes, it is *not at all in his interest to be used in this way.* Now, when someone intends his death as a means to avoid great pain, it may be in his interest to do so, but nevertheless he treats rational humanity as available for his purposes when this purpose does not serve rational humanity at all, in himself. Even if termination of the person is the lesser evil for the person, this does not alter the fact that we see rational humanity as available to be used for a purpose that doesn't serve rational humanity per se. This sense of treating someone as a means occurs in both 2 and 3.

In the interpersonal case, A also does not consent to being used. But suppose he did. Then he makes the lives of B, C, and D one of his goals in life. If his consent meant that he (or rational humanity in him) was not being used as a mere means in senses 2 and 3, then killing someone with his consent for his *own* greater good would also not involve using him (or rational humanity in him) as a mere means. Sense 2 and 3 would then be eliminated as objections to PAS and E. I shall not assume that this is so, for it would completely eliminate any Kantian objection to intending one's death.

How much weight, then, should be placed on the second and third senses of "use a person as a means?" Should they really stand in the way of PAS or E? Here are some reasons for saying no. It cannot be argued, at least with secular moral arguments, that one's body belongs to someone else and that one cannot, therefore, use it as a means to achieve death. Notice also that if your body belonged to someone else, it isn't clear why you should be permitted to use it in order to administer morphine as a painkiller when you foresee that this will destroy the body. We aren't usually permitted to treat other people's property, even property they have loaned to us for our use, in ways that certainly lead to its destruction. Hence, an objection based on sense 3 also does not distinguish between morphine in MPR and MD. This eliminates sense 3 as an objection, if MPR is permissible. That leaves us with the question whether treating one's death as available for one's purposes (sense 2) is necessarily a morally inappropriate attitude to take to oneself if one has not undervalued the importance of just being a person (not violating sense 1). I must admit that when I consider all we may permissibly intend (destruction of parts) and all we may permissibly bring about with mere foresight (death), I find it hard to see why we may not intend destruction of the entire person for his own greater good. If this is so, then at least sometimes a patient would do no wrong in intentionally causing his death. At least sometimes, a doctor who helped him by giving pills would also do no wrong merely because he killed, or assisted killing, aiming at death. Suppose this is true.

Particular Reasons for PAS and E

The strongest case can be made for doing this, I believe, if the overriding aim is to end physical pain (or other physical suffering, e.g., persistent nausea) whether the patient is otherwise terminal or not. The need to do this may be rare with modern techniques of pain control, but still the patient would have a *disjunctive right* either to adequate pain control *or* to the assistance of a willing doctor in assisted suicide or euthanasia. Might we extend the argument for PAS and E to the permissibility of killing a person as a means to achieving any end which is such that it is considered a greater good for him relative to his death, *and* which a doctor might permissibly achieve by giving a medication that had death as a side effect? Perhaps so, but we must be careful how we argue. The danger that we will extend ourself beyond what we are allowed is exemplified in Peter Singer's discussion of euthanasia. He describes the rules governing the practice in the Netherlands, as follows:

- Only a medical practitioner should carry out euthanasia.
- There should be an explicit request from the patient that leaves no room for doubt about the patient's desire to die.
- The patient's decision should be well-informed, free, and persistent.
- The patient must be in a situation of unbearable pain and suffering without hope of improvement.
- There must be no other measures available to make the patient's suffering bearable.
- The doctor must be very careful in reaching the decision and should seek a second opinion from another independent doctor.[37]

He then gives as an admirable example of a real-life instance of that practice the following case:

> In the case of Carla, too, though she had a continuous infusion of morphine, she did not want to die by a gradually increasing dose, which would most likely have put her into a state of drowsy confusion for some days before death came. She preferred to die at a time of her own choosing, with her family around her.[38]

But this very case which he gives to illustrate the practice does not clearly fall under the rules he cites. The rules say that lethal medicine is to be administered only if there is unbearable pain and suffering. Apparently the Dutch take this to include psychological suffering and the sense that one's dignity will be lost. This woman could have had her pain relieved by morphine; she received a lethal injection because she did not want to die from an increased dosage of morphine in drowsy confusion. Is dying in drowsy confusion a threat to one's dignity? Does the thought of it cause unbearable psychological suffering? This is not clear. It is striking that Singer himself does not notice—was not on the lookout for?—a possible transgression of the supposed rules. Even if the rules should be changed to allow that such a case is permissible, what worries many people is that violations of extant rules suggest that there will be insufficient attention paid to *any* rules.

All the steps of a variant of the Three-Step Argument may not be satisfied even when death is a lesser evil. Suppose a person will produce great paintings if he is given a drug that will soon cause his death, and truly producing great paintings is a greater good for his life and death a lesser evil. Still, it is not appropriate for a doctor to give drugs for such a reason, if death is a side effect of the drug; and so we could not use a Three-Step Argument to justify giving someone a lethal injection for the purpose of killing him, if he requests it because it will also prompt a flurry of last-minute brilliant painting. This case shows that it is only if the greater good is a *medically appropriate* goal that a Three-Step Argument works. Hence we should understand the argument-type in this way.

How about death to end psychological suffering, which is a reaction to one's beliefs about a state of affairs (i.e., propositional attitude suffering)?[39] The test I am suggesting is: Would we give a drug that narcotizes to treat such psychological suffering if we *foresee* that the drug would rapidly kill as a side effect with no improved quality of life first? If not, then giving pills to a patient intending that they kill him in order to end such psychological suffering would not be sanctioned by a Three-Step Argument.[40] Would we give a patient a drug that, as a side effect, will soon cause death (rather than a safer drug) if it will save him money? If not, then a Three-Step Argument does not imply that we may perform E or PAS to stop the drain on his family finances (Finances Case). (Of course, the application of the test I have suggested may yield positive responses rather than negative ones to these questions.)[41]

The general point is that to get a Three-Step Argument going, we have to have the first step: a case in which it is permissible to do what foreseeably leads to death. (I do not say that a different argument could not be constructed to justify killing where a Three-Step Argument fails.) But now it is important to show that if we fail to get the first premise *for certain special reasons*, it is still possible to use a Three-Step Argument. These two reasons are: (1) giving the drug that has death as a side effect makes things worse than they would be if the patient just died, and (2) giving the drug that has death as a side effect makes no positive difference for the patient, aside from that produced by death. Let us consider cases that illustrate these points.

In the first case, suppose the patient is totally paralyzed. If we had a drug that would cure him, but speeded up his death greatly and he requested the drug, would we give it? Suppose we would. If our reason for doing this is that the person can then live well without paralysis for a while, our behavior has no necessary implications for E or PAS. This is so because *they* do not produce a period of life during which the patient lives well in an improved condition. Suppose our reason for ending paralysis is just so that the person not be paralyzed, even if he goes into an immobile, unconscious state as a result of a second drug and then dies. What we may permissibly do or not do in *this case* may be relevant to E and PAS because the drug, like death, does not provide a period of higher quality life. But would we give the drug, foreseeing that it will kill the patient if it merely puts him in the immobile, unconscious state? Probably not.

One disanalogy between this last drug case and the death case remains, however: If we give the second drug, the patient remains in a totally dependent subrational condition before death. In the opinion of some, this could be a reason for not giving the drug that could not be raised against killing. So if we can get the first premise needed for a Three-Step Argument—showing that we may do what foreseeably causes death—by *subtracting* what makes the case of foreseen death *worse* than the case of intended death, a Three-Step Argument is still successful in justifying intentional killing.

Here is another case. Assuming we had an advance directive, would we give a demented patient a drug that unraveled the tangled neurons that caused his dementia but that we foresaw would put him in an unconscious, undemented state and then rapidly kill him as a side effect? As a preface to answering this question, consider that a doctor might well give the patient the drug if it had the side effect of causing death after a few moments of conscious, undemented life, because the patient considered a few moments of conscious, undemented life a greater good and death a lesser evil. This leads us to consider how large a benefit, *besides that producible by death itself*, might be needed in order to make giving the drug permissible when it kills as a side effect. Suppose very little besides what is provided by death is needed, e.g., a few undemented minutes with friends and family in addition to the end of dementia. This would show that the value of living in the demented state is rated very low indeed. This in turn means that death, intended or not, does not deprive one of very much (even taking into account the value of being a person or life itself).

This also suggests that if, in our original scenario where the drug unravels neurons but puts the patient in an unconscious state and soon kills, one refused to give the drug, this may be because one has *no positive reason at all for action*. That is, one does not refuse to give the drug because life is a greater good and death is a greater evil; it is rather that, in giving the drug, one would not be aiming to make any positive difference to a patient's life at all, since the unraveled unconscious state is no better than the conscious demented state. For example, even if it had no fatal side effect, one would seem to lack a positive reason for giving a drug that untangles the neurons of a calm, demented person, knowing that he will only then go into a coma. So, sometimes at least, a "no" answer to the questions raised about giving a drug that we foresee will cause death may only reflect the absence of bare requirements of rational action.

But just because a rational agent cannot act to give a drug that has death as a side effect unless the drug produces some positive change that gives one reason to act, this does not mean that seeking to *end a life* of a certain sort is not sufficient justification for action, because death is a lesser evil and remaining alive is not a greater good. For example, being calm and demented may be no better and no worse than being undemented and in a coma, so one wouldn't give a drug to produce the latter state, but the elimination of either one of these states might still be a permissible goal in itself.[42] For, as noted above, both of these states, because they involve a period of dependence in a subrational state before death, might be greater evils than death.

In sum, to get the first premise for a Three-Step Argument, we must *subtract* what makes giving a drug with foreseen death worse than death and also *compensate* for the absence of any positive reason for acting aside from seeking death.

The Philosophers' Brief

I have argued that if it is permissible to treat someone when he consents, though we *foresee* that this treatment will rapidly cause death, it is permissible to kill or assist in killing someone *intending* his death. (Consent is required in both cases.) In their recent Philosophers' Brief, Ronald Dworkin, Thomas Nagel, Robert Nozick, John Rawls, Thomas Scanlon, and Judith Jarvis Thomson take a different approach to this issue: They argue that if it is permissible to omit or *terminate treatment* with the intention that the patient die, it is permissible to assist in *killing* with the intention that the patient die, at least when the patient consents.[43] One reason they give for this is that there is no intrinsic moral difference between killing and letting die. Another reason is that they think a person has a right to make important personal choices about his own life, and whether to be killed or let die could equally be a means to facilitating these choices.

Dworkin *et al.* wrote as amicus curiae in the "assisted-suicide cases" that the Supreme Court heard in December 1996.[44] The cases came on appeal from two circuit courts, which had both ruled that governments cannot simply prohibit doctors from prescribing medication that would hasten the death of patients who request such medication. The philosophers urged the Supreme Court to uphold those decisions.

One part of their argument builds on the Court's 1990 decision in *Cruzan* v. *Missouri,* in which the Court majority assumed (if only for the sake of argument) that patients have a constitutional right to refuse life-preserving treatment.[45] According to these philosophers, the existence of a right to refuse treatment also implies a right to assistance in suicide: If, as *Cruzan* indicates, it is permissible for doctors to let a patient die even when the patient and the doctor intend the patient's death, then it is permissible for doctors to assist in killing. In a preface to the Philosophers' Brief written after the Supreme Court heard oral arguments on the case, Ronald Dworkin notes that several justices rejected this link between *Cruzan* and the assisted suicide cases. They sought to distinguish them by reference to a "common-sense distinction" between the moral significance of acts and omissions: Assisting suicide is an act and thus requires a compelling moral justification; in contrast, not providing treatment is an omission, a matter of "letting nature take its course," and can be justified more easily. Dworkin says that "the brief insists that such suggestions wholly misunderstand the 'common-sense' distinction, which is not between acts and omissions, but between acts or omissions that are designed to cause death and those that are not."[46] This means that Dworkin believes that common sense denies that there is ever a moral difference between action and omission per se, and only a moral difference between intending and foreseeing death. Presumably, the latter moral distinction will only matter sometimes, and not always, since sometimes, he thinks, intending death is justified.

I agree that the *act/omission* distinction will not bear much moral weight in this setting: When a doctor removes life-sustaining treatment by pulling a plug, he acts, though he does not necessarily kill. As I argued above, if the doctor is terminating aid he (or the organization of which he is a part) or what he is providing, then I think he *lets* die rather than kills. Remember the following analogy: I am saving someone from drowning and I decide to stop. Even if I must actively push a button on my side to make myself stop, I still let the person die rather than kill him. When a doctor gives morphine to ease pain, foreseeing it also causes death, he also acts and even kills, yet it is permissible to do this.[47] But I part company with these philosophers when they argue that, once a patient has consented, we can *always* move from the permissibility of letting the patient die intending his death to the permissibility of assisted suicide. Killing and assisted killing are not, in general, on a moral par with letting die. Let me explain by reference to cases.

In the first set, doctors act *against* their patients' wishes to live. Dworkin, *et al.* agree that a doctor may permissibly deny an organ to a patient in order to give it to another, but *not* kill a patient to get his organ for another. But, they say, this is not because of a moral difference between letting a patient die and killing him, but because the doctor merely foresees death in the first case, whereas he intends it in the second. But if this showed that killing made no moral difference, it would imply that it is permissible for a doctor, in order to transplant an organ into some patients, to use a chemical that he *foresees* will seep into the next room where another patient lies, killing that patient. For in this case, the doctor does not intend the death of the patient in the other room, but only foresees his death as a side effect of the chemical. Presumably, though, transplanting with this effect is wrong, even if it cannot be done otherwise, because it is a killing, albeit foreseeable rather than intended. So, in cases in which we merely foresee death, killing may be wrong, even if letting die is not. This shows that there is a per se moral difference between killing and letting die that can determine differential moral judgments in at least some cases.

In addition, killing can be a significant factor in cases where a patient does not want to die because letting die with the intention that death occur might be permissible, even if killing with such intention is not. It is true, as the brief says, that a doctor who lets his patient die of asphyxiation against the patient's will, intending that he die so that his organs are available for use in others, has done something wrong, as has a doctor who kills the same sort of patient, intending him to die. This is because both doctors aim against the welfare of their patients and violate their rights. The first doctor violates the positive right to treatment; the second doctor violates the negative right against being killed. But this does not always imply, as Dworkin et al. think, that "a doctor violates his patient's rights whether the doctor acts or refrains from acting *against the patient's wishes* in a way that is designed to cause death" (p. 45). For example, suppose that someone does not want to die, but it would be in his interest to die. If a treatment is experimental, or in general something to which the patient has no positive right, it may be permissible to deny it to him because death would be in his own best interest. I do not believe the patient acquires a right to have the experimental therapy merely because the doctor's reason for refusing it is that he aims at the patient's death. But it would be morally wrong to kill the patient if he did not want to die, even if it were in his interest to die.[48] Once again, we see a case where a moral difference between killing and letting die surfaces.

Next, consider the type of case in which the patient consents to death. The distinction between killing and letting die makes a moral difference when deciding on the *scope* of permissible refusal of treatment versus permissible assistance to killing. Dworkin et al. seem to suggest that the scope should be the same, saying that if a doctor can turn off a respirator, he can prescribe pills. But a mentally competent patient may legally refuse treatment, intending to die, even when it is *not in his best interest* to do so and, on many occasions, even when he could be cured. Presumably, in many of these cases, he could also insist on the doctor terminating treatment, even if his intention is to die. Furthermore, even if the doctor in these cases improperly intends that the patient die, the treatment must be terminated. *This is because the alternative to letting the patient die is forcing treatment on him.* We think the right of a mentally competent patient not to be physically invaded against his will is typically stronger than our interest in the patient's well-being (even if it could be overridden for considerations of public safety). But if he asks for assistance in killing himself when it is not in his medical interest to be killed, it might well be morally *im*permissible to assist in killing him. Certainly, if his reason for wanting to die is to sacrifice himself as a political protest, it would be ludicrous to go to a doctor for assistance, though he could have a doctor terminate treatment. Even if his best interests were at stake, but they concerned his having to die in order to ensure his glorious post mortem reputation, it would be inappropriate for a physician to assist in his killing. So, contrary to what Dworkin says, a doctor might in some cases be permitted and even required to turn off a respirator but not permitted to give pills.[49]

So, the alternative to letting die has such a morally objectionable feature—forcing treatment, which he has a right we not do—that even if we think the competent patient's and doctor's goals are wrong, we must terminate aid. In contrast, the competent alternative to assisted suicide may simply be leaving the patient alone; this often does not violate any of his rights against us, and so we can, and sometimes we should be required to, refuse to help because we disapprove of his goals. Many people—including Supreme Court justices whom Dworkin cites—might, then, reasonably distinguish refusing treatment, and a doctor letting a patient die, from assisting in a suicide. The move from *Cruzan's* right to refuse treatment to the permissibility of assisted suicide is, therefore, not generally available, especially since *Cruzan* did not base its decision on a judgment as to when death would be a lesser evil and so not against the patient's interests. In sum, I have argued that the approach of the Philosophers' Brief does not succeed. In particular, I argued that it is not always permissible to assist killing, intending death, when it is permissible to let die, intending death. Even if it is sometimes permissible to assist killing, intending death, when it is permissible to let die, intending death, this would not be because there is no intrinsic moral difference between killing and letting die, since, I tried to show, an intrinsic difference shows up in several cases.

The case-based arguments in the brief for the conclusion that killing and letting die do not matter per se contrast with the second, more theoretical argument that Dworkin *et al.* make in favor of physician-assisted suicide. Dworkin *et al.* adopt the view proposed in *Planned Parenthood* v. *Casey*—that a person has a right to self-determination in the most intimate and important matters in his life—and from that view deduce a right to determine the time and manner of death, by implication whether by letting die or killing.[50] But does their theory then endorse the conclusion that a person has a right to assisted suicide from a willing physician if he decides his medical treatment is consuming too much of his family's finances or if he wishes to give up his life for some noble causes, given that he would have a right to refuse treatment for these reasons? I suggest this theoretical argument is too broad if it yields these conclusions.

There is a third type of argument that we might construct to show that if we may let die intending death, it is also permissible to assist killing intending death. When *death is a lesser evil*, the greater good is a medically appropriate aim (e.g., no pain versus post-mortem glory), and the patient consents, assisting killing with the intention to bring about death will be permissible if letting die intending death is permissible. This is (I believe) a different argument from those presented in the brief. Notice that while we have to add the qualifier "when death is a lesser evil" to get a certain moral equivalence of killing and letting die, this qualifier is not necessary in a Three-Step Argument. This is because letting die may be permissible even when death is not a lesser evil (or imminent), but giving a medicine with merely foreseen fatal effects will not be permissible unless death is a lesser evil (or imminent). Because in a Three-Step Argument we *cannot* get the first step without death being the lesser evil (or imminent), we *can* move more easily from it to the conclusion that intentional killing is permissible. Because we *can* get the first step in the Philosophers' Brief argument (i.e., letting die while intending death is permissible) without death being the lesser evil (or imminent), we *cannot* move so easily to the conclusion that assisting killing, too, is permissible.

Still, it is true that in those circumstances (i.e., when death is a lesser evil and the greater good is a medically appropriate aim) in which a Three-Step Argument is sound, it will also be true that killing or assisting killing is as acceptable a means to death as letting die. I have not denied this. Why, then, focus on the Three-Step Argument rather than the (Assisting) Killing-Equals-Letting-Die-When-Death-Is-A-Lesser-Evil Argument? My sense is that showing that it is permissible to intend the patient's death is a crucial moral issue. When we allow that it is permissible to let die intending death, we can do so without inquiring into the morality of intending death per se, since (as argued above) the alternative to allowing termination of treatment is forcing treatment on someone, and this we may not do. But when we want to kill or assist in killing someone, forcing treatment is not the alternative, so then what we must do is show *why*, when death is a lesser evil, intending death is morally acceptable. This is what we are forced to do by the Three-Step Argument, whereas the alternative argument threatens to conceal the importance of doing this by deluding us into thinking that we *have* already argued for the permissibility of intending death when we conclude that letting die while intending death is permissible.

Moral Responsibility for PAS and E

Responsibility for Death

Suppose a doctor performs PAS or E because it is at least permissible to do so, and so she is either partially or completely *causally* responsible for death. What does this imply about who has moral responsibility for the patient's death? I want to suggest that when the doctor does what is permitted to intentionally kill her patient or assist in killing, she does not necessarily have moral responsibility for the death.

There are at least two ways in which PAS and E are typically presented. The first takes the view that doctors have a duty of medical mercy. That is, one of the projects to which they commit themselves is the relief of the physical suffering of their patients, when their patients consent. This may even imply, as is suggested in the Duty Argument, the commitment to kill the patient to relieve pain. The second way in which PAS and E are typically discussed emphasizes the patient's autonomy. In certain contexts, at least, patients may decide that it is best for them to die and then, it is said, it is at least permissible for the doctor to serve the patient's will, when it is not obviously against the patient's interest to do so. On some people's view, this implies it is at least sometimes permissible for a doctor to kill a patient as a patient's agent in carrying out her wishes. This is analogous to a lawyer who acts for his client. On the first view, the doctor commits herself to the *project of doing what is best for the patient in her judgment, so long as this is in accord with the patient's wishes.* On the second view, the doctor commits herself to the *project of being the patient's agent, so long as this is not obviously against the patient's interests.*

There is a reversal of emphasis in these two accounts. Only the second does not imply that the doctor agrees with the patient's decision to die, or that she is fulfilling her own project to do well by the patient in seeking the patient's death.

My claim is that in the second "agent model," moral responsibility for negative consequences of killing the patient (in active E) or providing lethal drugs (in PAS) lie at the patient's doorstep, even though the doctor shares causal responsibility with the patient in some PAS and has complete causal responsibility for death in active E. This is analogous to what happens when a lawyer acts for his client: If the client wants a tenant evicted and it is wrong to evict, it may still be permissible for a lawyer to act on his client's request because it is morally permissible for people to have agents even in such circumstances, as an aid to autonomy. But it is the client who bears full moral responsibility for the eviction. In the first "beneficence model," the doctor and patient at least share moral responsibility for negative consequences, as seeking the death in particular (as opposed to just doing whatever the patient wants) is a joint project of theirs, a goal they both decide best fulfills their projects. The fact that moral responsibility for negative consequences will be at the patient's doorstep in the agent model might not unreasonably lead a doctor to act when she otherwise would not. Does the doctor in her role as agent get moral responsibility for good consequences? Not if she only acts in her role as the patient's agent and the good consequences are intended by the patient.

The distinction I have drawn between two ways of conceiving the doctor's behavior is sometimes not recognized in discussions of these topics, and ignoring the difference can lead to inconsistencies. For example, at one point in Dan Brock's discussion, he says that "Both physician and family members can instead be helped to understand that it is the patient's decision and consent to stopping treatment that limits their responsibility for the patient's death and that shifts responsibility to the patient."[51] But, at another point, he says, "Seeking a physician's assistance, or what can almost seem a physician's blessing, may be a way of trying to remove that stigma and show others that ... the decision for suicide was ... justified under the circumstances. The physician's involvement provides a kind of social approval. . . ."[52] But what makes it true that the doctor's moral responsibility is limited makes it false that a doctor gives approval of patients' seeking death. For, I suggest, it is only when the doctor is merely the patient's agent and does not necessarily endorse her decision—as the lawyer does not necessarily endorse his client's decision—that moral responsibility for the killing lies so heavily with the patient, and then helping the patient die does not imply that the doctor agrees that the patient has chosen the correct course.

Brock also argues that if someone assists in suicide, he has moral responsibility for a killing, and as much moral responsibility as if he performed active euthanasia. His argument claims that if A gives B a lethal drug knowing that B will give it to C, A shares moral responsibility for killing C. Hence, if A gives B a lethal drug knowing that B will give it to himself, A must also have moral responsibility for killing B.[53] But I think the substitution of B for C changes matters, for if B is the legitimate authority over his own life and may appoint A as his agent,

A does not necessarily have moral responsibility for a killing. (This will be true of A and B if C may appoint them as *his* agents.) Brock's claim that there is not necessarily more moral responsibility for active voluntary euthanasia than for physician-assisted suicide may be true, but that might only mean that there is no moral responsibility in *either* case if it is permissible for one to be another's agent in these circumstances.

None of this is altered by the fact that the doctor intends the patient's death. A doctor may intend the patient's death in the course of being the patient's agent, and, if the patient is permitted to have an agent, then the doctor still may not share moral responsibility for the death. But a doctor may well intend a patient's death because he thinks it is best for the patient to die and he is doing what is best for the patient, and then he shares moral responsibility with the patient who requests his help.

Notes

This paper is a longer version of "A Right to Die" that appeared in *The Boston Review*, Summer 1997. I want to thank for their comments Seana Shiffrin, Tim Hall, Joshua Cohen, as well as the audience at the UCLA Department of Philosophy Colloquium.

1. Notice that my analysis of terminating aid differs from Dan Brock's analysis in "Voluntary Active Euthanasia," reprinted in *Life and Death* (New York: Cambridge University Press, 1993). Brock believes that if a greedy nephew, in order to get his aunt's inheritance, pulls out the plug on her life support machine without her consent or anyone else's, he kills. Brock notes that a doctor who pulls a plug at the request of the patient in the patient's interest may make the same exact physical movements as the nephew. Brock concludes from this that if the nephew kills, the doctor does. Their motives and intention are not the same and the permissibility of their behavior may differ, but they both kill. I disagree that they both kill. It might be thought that an explanation for this is that one must extend one's *temporal perspective* in order to determine who kills and who lets die. That is, one cannot just look at the behavior at the time of terminating treatment; one must check to see what the person did at t^1-n, e.g., did he set up the machine to help the aunt and is he now disconnecting it? But this is not correct as the following cases show. Suppose the nephew set up the machine to help his aunt, but the machine does not belong to him and he goes away, leaving it running on its own. If he returns and turns off the machine without permission of his aunt or the owner of the machine, he kills. On the other hand, suppose someone else takes a machine that belongs to the nephew (with or without his permission) and sets it up to give life support. If the nephew stops it, he will have let his aunt die, not killed her. (I owe the last two cases and the emphasis on the importance of ownership of the means to Timothy Hall.) Suppose a life support machine is not the nephew's and he didn't start it, but he remains running it. If he pushes a button to stop his doing so, he lets die. In sum, if one stops aid one is providing or that one's means provide, one lets die, permissibly or impermissibly. For a more detailed presentation of this analysis see my *Morality, Mortality*, vol. 2 (Oxford University Press, 1996) and unpublished work by Timothy Hall.
2. See *Morality, Mortality*, vol. 2 (Oxford University Press, 1996).
3. *New England Journal of Medicine* 329 (14) (Sept. 30, 1993): 1039.
4. Does he aim at the person's death, though he waits for her to make the choice? No, he only aims to give her the choice. Doctors may even give the option because they think having the option will reduce a patient's eagerness to commit suicide. So, some doctors may give the option to commit suicide, intending to prevent the desire to commit suicide.
5. This is suggested by Dan Brock in "Voluntary Active Euthanasia," p. 204.
6. A comparative analysis of the badness of death is offered by Thomas Nagel in "Death,"

reprinted in *Mortal Questions* (Cambridge: Cambridge University Press, 1979). I discuss it in *Morality, Mortality*, vol. 1 (New York: Oxford University Press, 1993).

7. This point was pressed on me by Gertrude Ezorsky.

8. In *Morality, Mortality*, vol. 1, pp. 19–22, I argued that the simple coming to an end of the person was itself an evil to the person. See note 13 below for more on this.

9. There is some question about whether high doses of morphine do actually kill the patient. Hence, our question is whether, if they did, giving morphine would be permissible

10. When death is the lesser evil, will this always mean that the death benefits the patient? Perhaps not—if it is right that someone be executed for murder, his death may be the lesser evil relative to his staying alive, but it does not benefit him.

11. I owe this point to Rivka Weinberg.

12. This point was emphasized to me by Timothy Hall.

13. I said that Thomas Nagel thinks that death is bad because it makes impossible the goods of life, but he seems to think that mere existence is such a good. In *Morality, Mortality, Vol. 1*, I have provided one account of the badness of death that might bear on whether future nonexistence itself is a bad thing. I there consider what I call the Limbo Man. This is someone who will have a fixed amount of goods in his life, but rather than have these continuously, he has them separated by long periods of unconsciousness which extend his life so that he thereby puts off his future nonexistence. I argue that someone might rationally prefer to live in this "interrupted fashion," and if he does so, it is because he is avoiding some evil. But what evil? Fewer goods of life? No, since the Limbo Man does not want to put off death because this reduces the degree to which death deprives him of further goods of life, for, by hypothesis, he does not gain *more* goods of life by putting off death. Rather, the evil he puts off is that of having his life and the goods in it be all over forever.

14. In other cases, it may not be clear whether or not the doctor intends an evil, because there is a fine line between intending and foreseeing. For example, suppose a doctor wants to give her patient the only drug that will alleviate his pain. Unfortunately, one side effect of the drug is convulsions. Because a life with convulsions is more unbearable for this patient than is a life of pain, the doctor and patient decide to use the drug *only* because in the presence of convulsions the drug also has the side effect of quickly ending the patient's life. While the patient finds pain preferable to convulsions, he finds death preferable to pain. If the drug would not also cause death when it produces convulsions, the doctor would not give the painkiller and, if she gives it, it is in part *because* death will be *the cause of* ending convulsions. Nevertheless, I believe, the doctor does not *intend* the death of her patient; she intends the end of pain and gives the drug to end it only because it causes death. She does not intend the death of the patient, *because she would not do anything additional to bring it about that the painkiller results in death*. If it doesn't, she simply will not use it. And if she uses it, it is because she intends its painkilling properties. Similarly, a doctor may give a painkiller that helps only temporarily, and that would leave the patient in more pain than he was in to begin with when it wears off, only *because* the drug also causes death before the painkiller wears off. Here the doctor also does not intend the death. That we use the drug only because it has an effect does not mean that we intend this effect.

   The structure of these Painkiller Cases is that the means (painkiller) to the greater good (no more pain) causes the lesser evil (death) and this lesser evil sustains the greater good that would otherwise end. These cases involve *intending under a condition* but not intending the condition. That is, *if* death occurs (the condition), one will *intend* no more pain, but one doesn't intend that death occur or even that no more pain occur in the presence of death. (Suppose the doctor had a choice of drugs: One causes death when it causes convulsions and one does not. If she chooses the first drug, she makes a choice driven by the intention that if pain relief occurs, death would, too. This still does not mean that she intends death. If she creates a new painkilling drug, so that it also causes death, she will be intending death. (I discuss the distinction between intending an effect and acting because the effect will occur in *Morality, Mortality*, vol. 2, in analyzing the Trolley Problem and the killing of innocents in wartime. See chapter 7 of that book.) One common test for whether we intend rather than merely foresee an effect is that we would not continue to act if the effect did not come about. This is known as the Counterfactual Test. But that test turns out not to be discriminating enough to test for intention, since the doctor in the Painkiller Cases would not give the painkiller if it did not also cause death but she does not intend the death. (Is it possible that it is correct to describe, the doctor's *aim* as giving pain relief free of convulsions? *If so, then death is the means to that end*, and yet it seems the doctor does *not* intend the means to her end. This would show that rational agents need not always intend the means to their end. [I thank Calvin Normore for discussion of this point.])

15. Is the loss of a limb itself a lesser evil, or is it merely the absence of the good effects of having a limb that is a lesser evil? If only the latter, then this would not be a case of intending a lesser evil, but I do think loss of a limb is itself a lesser evil. However, notice that if death *only led to evils* and loss of a leg *only led to evils*, but were not themselves evils, intending them might still be analogous behaviors. Hence, the permissibility of intending one might imply the permissibility of intending the other.

16. Thomas Nagel, a contemporary proponent of the DDE, agrees that a prohibition on intending harm may be overridden if it is for the greater good of the one who is harmed, but he still feels moral discomfort at its being overridden. (See p. 182 in *The View from Nowhere* (New York: Oxford University Press, 1986)).

17. I first presented this argument in *Creation and Abortion* (New York: Oxford University Press, 1992), pp. 33–35, and again in *Mortality, Mortality*, vol. 2 (New York: Oxford University Press, 1996), pp. 194–98.

18. Notice that this argument given for a duty differs from the following one: If the Three-Step Argument is correct, then, with patient consent, it is at least permissible to intend a patient's death when it is a lesser evil for the sake of a greater good. But if the doctor has a duty to relieve physical suffering, then she has a duty to do whatever is permissible in order to fulfill her duty. Hence, she has a duty to kill the patient, if death is the lesser evil, in order to produce the greater good of pain relief. This argument is unsatisfactory, since one does not have a duty to do whatever it would be permissible to do in order to carry out another duty. Sometimes, the permissible is still supererogatory. For example, it is permissible for a doctor to give up all his money to save his patient's life, and he has a duty to save his patient's life, but that does not mean he has a duty to give up all his money to save his patient's life. The Duty Argument is a better argument because it begins by pointing to giving morphine when one foresees it will cause death. This is an act that is, in some important respects, like the one that the Three-Step Argument says is permissible: giving morphine intending to cause death. It shows that one has a *duty* to do that analogous act, and shifts the burden of proof to showing why one does *not* also have a duty to intend the death if it is permissible to intend it.

19. To waive one's right to life and give a right to another a) to do what will kill one as a side effect, as well as b) to deliberately kill one, is not the same as alienating or giving up one's right to life. The latter would occur if slavery were permitted. For then, one cedes one's right over one's life to another, and one may be forever under another's power to decide whether one lives or dies. It is true that if one successfully waives one's right to live and is killed, one will never again exercise one's right to live, and this is also a consequence of alienating one's right. But only in the case of alienating does one give one's right away and live on under the control of another person.

20. For discussion of waivers, see Philippa Foot in "Euthanasia," *Philosophy & Public Affairs*

6 (2) (Winter 1977): 85–112, and Joel Feinberg in "Voluntary Euthanasia and the Inalienable Right to Life," *Philosophy & Public Affairs* 7 (2) (Winter 1978): 93–123. It is important to point out that when Foot argues for the permission to kill because a patient has waived his right to life and it is in his interest to die, she does not think there is any point in arguing separately for the permissibility of intending death rather than doing what one foresees will cause the death. The waiver plus the interests of the person in being killed give another permission to intend death and there is then no reason why it is impermissible for him to do so, she seems to think. It is possible, however, that a patient can only give permission for someone to do what foreseeably kills him but not what intentionally kills him, for reasons having nothing to do with an inability to waive his right to life or with his being unable to release others from a duty not to do what kills him.

21. Warren Quinn, "Actions, Intentions, and Consequences: The Doctrine of Double Effect," reprinted in his *Morality and Action* (New York: Cambridge University Press, 1993). For a discussion of his views, see my review in *The Journal of Philosophy* (November 1996).

22. Considering another case in which the lesser evil may be foreseen but not permissibly intended may help strengthen the case against intending death. It is permissible for me to lecture a class to give new knowledge, foreseeing that as a side effect, a few false beliefs will be formed by the class (e.g., by misunderstanding my lecture). I tolerate this as a lesser evil to the greater good. But suppose I had to deliberately instill a few false beliefs to transmit more knowledge. I might lie to do this, but I needn't. I might turn in a certain direction while lecturing, knowing that this will confuse students and lead to a false belief. It might be wrong to either do this or lie. Hence, it is not always permissible to intend the lesser evil for a person's own greater good though one may bring it about with mere foresight. In this classroom case, it could be said, I would be insulting the students by undermining their reason as a tool to the students' own greater good. If taking control over and destroying one's life is more like intentionally telling a lie than amputating a leg—a course of action intrinsically disrespectful of the nature of persons—then it could be a constraint on PAS or E. Of course, a prohibition on telling a lie could be overridden (by a greater good) or annulled (because the person we lie to has forfeited his right not to be lied to). The same may be true of intentionally destroying the person.

23. In E and PAS, we also terminate human life considered independently of whether it is the life of a rational being. It may seem harder to justify destroying a rational being than human life that lacks qualities which make for rationality e.g., a functioning complex brain. But I will assume that one could substitute "human life" for "rational being" 1) in an argument I will give *against* intentional killing, and 2) in an argument I will give to show it is *permissible* to intend to kill. Note also that some may think an entity is a "person" even if it is not a rational being but is more than mere human life. I wish the arguments to also apply to such a person, though my use of person in this paper equates person with rational being. For purposes of my discussion, I do not think it is necessary to deny that preserving human life per se is as or more important than preserving persons or rational humanity. However, we must also not ignore the fact that there is more than one way in which to destroy a person. One might lobotomize or drug someone so that they are permanently demented in order to eliminate pain. Then human life remains, but the person as rational being is destroyed. One might argue that killing the person is not so morally offensive a way to end pain as is destroying the person so that "he" lives on in these other ways. A complete argument for the permissibility of intentionally killing in PAS or E might have to distinguish these cases, and this will probably involve taking a stand on the worth of various forms of human life.

24. I have already noted that Quinn suggests we distinguish the idea of not treating persons as ends and treating them as mere means. I am focusing on the latter.

25. Because we have worth in ourselves it is important that our lives also be good for us. A Kantian might go so far as to claim that there is no value in pleasure or the absence of pain unless these occur in the life of a rational being. It is not that pain is not as unpleasant for a mouse as for us; it is that the nature of the negative qualia is not the reason it shouldn't exist. I cannot agree with this.

26. Or death would at least not harm me, if there were not intrinsic evils in my life, release from which would benefit me. This can be true when someone is unconscious.

27. Whether we would start life support or merely allow it to be kept in place, I think it is appropriate to use the term "force life support on the patient."

28. I do not here provide an argument to support this trumping, however.

29. Let us make this point in somewhat greater detail. Above (p. 3), I concluded that often when someone interferes with lifesaving aid that neither he nor something that belongs to him is providing to someone else, he kills that other person. He also kills if he induces death by introducing what I called an original cause of death, and if he interferes with the person who is receiving aid so as to remove him from the aid. By contrast, someone lets another die when he stops himself or something that belongs to him from providing life-sustaining aid to someone. He also lets another die when he refrains from beginning such aid. What happens when someone disconnects *himself* from life support that does not belong to him? Is he killing himself because he neither stops aid he is providing nor stops something that belongs to him? We said he let himself die—though he may intend his death and so commit suicide without killing himself—because he stops himself from receiving assistance. Suppose he wishes to stop himself from receiving aid but cannot do so, and I act as his agent. Do I *kill* him because I stop aid that neither I nor what belongs to me provides? I said no. If he would let himself die if he acted, and I act in his stead, I think I let him die. If this is so, then, in cases in which I stop aid he wishes me to stop, I let die and the alternative to my doing so is his having treatment imposed on him that he does not want. In all these cases, the alternative to letting die is forcing treatment. (Suppose I killed him if I stopped a machine that was not his when he asked me to do so. Then, some cases in which I *refrain from killing* would involve someone having treatment imposed on him against his will. It seems clear that not having treatment imposed is a crucial issue, and whether our terminating treatment is a killing or letting die is secondary. Then the moral necessity of not imposing treatment would not track the killing/letting die distinction.) It might happen that he is receiving lifesaving aid which he does not want and which cannot be disconnected. If I do not give him a lethal injection, he will receive treatment he does not want, but that does not mean that if I do not kill him, the treatment is imposed on him. This is because I neither start it against his will nor refuse to stop it *when I can.*

30. This last point was emphasized to me by Timothy Hall.

31. I owe this case to Timothy Hall.

32. But might the doctor permissibly refuse to give the morphine drip for pain relief once he finds out that his patient does not care about pain relief and intends his death? Consider the following alternative reasoning: I would like to avoid killing a person, but am willing to do so if death is the side effect of eliminating pain that the patient wants eliminated even at the cost of death. But when the patient does not care about the greater good, I refuse to produce the greater good if it means I will kill. If the doctor does not give the comparable argument in the Blindness Case, is this because causing death even when it is the lesser evil and not even intended by the doctor plays a different role from causing blindness? Or is it because the removal of pain that the patient does not care about is not a greater good; that is, does not caring about pain change the weight of the positive value of its removal in a way that not caring about life does not change the weight of its positive value? In any case, if the doctor could permissibly refuse in the Death Drip Case, this would show that the *patient's* intention does affect whether he has

a right to be invaded with pain relievers. It would also show that a doctor could point to the fact that he will be a killer as a reason for not acting (even when he would not intend death) *when this fact* is conjoined with another fact, namely the patient's *intending* death. Presumably, he could not refuse to give morphine when the patient wants it for pain relief. Also he could not refuse to *stop treatment* when a mentally competent patient's suicidal intention is known. This would mean that the killing and letting die distinction had renewed importance *on its own*, rather than because of what is involved in the alternatives to each (i.e., to not killing to leaving someone alone, and to not letting die, forcing treatment).

33. Thomas Hill makes this mistake in "Self-Regarding Suicide: A Modified Kantian View," in *Autonomy and Self-Respect* (New York: Cambridge University Press, 1991), pp. 85–103. He provides Kantian objections to some types of suicide by focusing on the claim that rational agency has worth in itself rather than being a mere means to other goods. But he fails to notice that we can lack the appropriate attitude to our lives, even when we merely do what we foresee will lead to our deaths, and therefore this inappropriate attitude does not suffice to distinguish between, for example, suicide and taking morphine to knock out pain when we foresee fatal results. In a sense, therefore, his discussion is beside the point in explaining the distinction Kant, I believe, thought existed between intending one's death (suicide) and merely foreseeing it.

34. For example, Tyler Burge, in conversation, and David Velleman in unpublished writing.

35. Suggested by David Kaplan.

36. Suggested to me by Barbara Herman.

37. Peter Singer, *Rethinking Life and Death* (New York: St. Martin's Press, 1994), p. 146.

38. Op. cit., pp. 147–48.

39. There is another type of *nonpropositional* attitude psychological suffering, e.g., clinical depression or schizophrenia. Here the primary cause of depression is not an evaluation of one's life but a chemical imbalance. I believe it can more clearly occupy the same role as physical suffering in the argument for PAS or E.

40. The Solicitor General's brief in the Supreme Court review of two lower-court judgments permitting PAS argued that we have a right to avoid physical pain and also psychological suffering brought on by awareness of our life condition. This is a liberal position. By contrast, Daniel Callahan insists that there is a moral distinction between seeking means to avoid physical pain and to avoid psychological suffering. But he seems not to separate propositional from nonpropositional psychological suffering, and so treats clinical depression the same as inability to cope with life. See his "When Self-Determination Runs Amok," *The Hastings Center Report*, March–April (1992), pp. 52–55.

41. The distinction between cases in which we may and may not give the drug that foreseeably causes death may bear on the different reasons that philosophers have isolated for wanting to die or to help someone die. One consideration is said to be mercy or charity, concerned with the patient's well-being. A broader consideration is referred to as the patient's critical interests. These essentially relate to his commitments, projects, and, in general, what he thinks is truly valuable. (See Ronald Dworkin, *Life's Dominion*, A. Knopf, 1993.) He may think the welfare of his family is more valuable than his own well-being. (The satisfaction of his desires for them is not necessarily followed by his own well-being.) Those who think it is permissible to be killed in order to preserve the finances of one's family may be giving much weight to critical interests. Nevertheless, if one thinks it is wrong to give the cheaper medicine in the case I described, one is denying the weight of the patient's critical interests. One may still think it is permissible to terminate the more expensive treatment at the patient's request, so as not to force treatment on him. But notice that a consequence of both not giving the cheaper drug *and* terminating the more expensive one is that, without *any* medication, the

patient may die even sooner than if he were given the cheap medicine that would shortly kill him.

42. The Finances Case is different: The cheaper treatment still provides some improvement and so gives some reason for action. The question is whether we should achieve this good if the drug causes death when the drug causing greater good causes financial drain.

43. Ronald Dworkin, "Assisted Suicide: The Philosophers' Brief," *New York Review of Books*, March 27, 1997. See also appendix B of this volume.

44. See my discussion in "A Right to Choose Death," *The Boston Review*, Summer 1997, pp. 20–23.

45. The Court did not, however, agree that Nancy Cruzan had clearly decided, before an automobile accident that left her in a persistent vegetative state, that she would refuse treatment.

46. Arguably, omissions cannot "cause" deaths at all, but I shall not dwell on this point.

47. Assisting suicide can also occur without an act (e.g., not giving sedation so that someone can shoot himself). Also, not providing life-saving treatment is not in direct contrast with acts of assisted suicide, for the latter are not sufficient to lead to death regardless of what the patient then does. For this reason, some may find assisting suicide even morally preferable.

48. Those who think that doctors should not only not violate their patient's rights but should promote their patient's autonomy may treat this case differently. For while not being given the experimental aid does not violate a positive right to aid, it does not heed a person's wishes for how his life should go. This shows that respect for rights is not the same as promoting autonomy. But, as Timothy Hall points out, even if we had to give the saving aid in accordance with the will of the patient and *against his interests* to promote autonomy, it hardly seems likely that we would have to—or even that it would be permissible to—kill him if he requests it when it is against his interests. This again indicates a difference between killing and letting die.

49. It seems to me that the Court in *Compassion in Dying* v. *Washington* also overlooked this point when they said that whether we assist killing or let die is not morally or legally crucial. For even that court was concerned to limit the doctor's right to assist in killing the patient to cases where the patient's life is going to end shortly anyway and when death is not against his interests. But the right to refuse treatment and have it terminated applies much more broadly. If killing and letting die make no moral or legal difference per se, refusing treatment should be permitted no more broadly than assisting killing.

50. 505 U.S. 833, 851 (1992).

51. Dan Brock, "Voluntary Active Euthanasia," in *Life and Death*, p. 211.

52. Op. cit., p. 230.

53. Op. cit., p. 204.

3

Physician–Assisted Suicide

Safe, Legal, Rare?

MARGARET P. BATTIN

Despite the vigor of the debate over physician-assisted suicide, both proponents and opponents of legalization appear to agree that if adequate pain control were available, requests for physician-assisted suicide would and should be rare, a last resort in those few cases in which pain control proves inadequate after all. This ubiquitous view treats concern with physician-assisted suicide as a "phenomenon of discrepant development," a symptom of the disparity between our capacities to prolong life and to control pain. However, interest in physician-assisted suicide can also be viewed as a symptom of far more substantial cultural, religious, and epidemiological changes, involving a shift towards self-directed dying: Death is no longer seen as "something that happens to you," but "something you do." In this essay I explore what might motivate such a shift, and how changes in a decisional perspective from an "enmeshed" to a distanced but still personal perspective may make physician-assisted suicide a societally preferred alternative.

∗   ∗   ∗

The Way It Looks Now

OBSERVE THE CURRENT DEBATE over physician-assisted suicide: On the one side, supporters of legalization appeal to the principle of autonomy, or self-determination, to insist that terminally ill patients have the right to extricate themselves from pain and suffering and to control as much as possible the ends of their lives. On the other, opponents resolutely insist on various religious, principled, or slippery-slope grounds that physician-assisted suicide cannot be allowed, whether because it is sacrilegious, immoral, or poses risks of abuse. As vociferous and politicized as these two sides of the debate have become, however, proponents and opponents (tacitly) agree on a core issue: that the patient may choose to avoid suffering and pain. They disagree, it seems, largely about the means the patient and his or her physician may use to do so.

They also disagree about the actualities of pain control. Proponents of legalization insist that currently available forms of pain and symptom control are grossly inadequate and unsatisfactory. Citing such data as the SUPPORT study, they point to high rates of reported pain among terminally ill patients, inadequately developed pain-control therapies, physicians' lack of training in pain-control techniques, and obstacles and limitations to delivery of pain-control treatment, including restrictions on narcotic and other drugs.[1] Pain and the suf-

fering associated with other symptoms just aren't adequately controlled, proponents of legalization insist, so the patient is surely entitled to avoid them—if he
or she so chooses—by turning to earlier, humanely assisted dying.

Opponents of legalization, on the other hand, insist that these claims are
uninformed. Effective methods of pain control include timely withholding and
withdrawal of treatment, sufficient use of morphine or other drugs for pain
(even at the risk of foreseen, through unintended, shortening of life), and the
discontinuation of artificial nutrition and hydration. When all other measures to
control pain and suffering fail, there is always the possibility of terminal sedation: the induction of coma with concomitant withholding of nutrition and
hydration, which, though it results in death, is not to be seen as killing.

Proponents laugh at this claim. Terminal sedation, they retort, like the
overuse of morphine, is functionally equivalent to *causing* death.

Despite these continuing disagreements about the effectiveness, availability,
and significance of current pain control, both proponents and opponents in the
debate appear to agree that *if* adequate pain control were available, there would
be far less call for physician-assisted suicide. This claim is both predictive and
normative. *If* adequate pain control were available, both sides argue, then physician-assisted suicide would be and should be quite infrequent—a "last resort,"
as Timothy Quill puts it, to be used only in exceptionally difficult cases when pain
control really does fail. Borrowing an expression used by President Clinton to
describe his view of abortion, proponents insist that physician-assisted suicide
should be "safe, legal, and rare." Opponents do not believe that it should be legal,
but they also think that if it cannot be suppressed altogether or if a few very difficult cases remain, it should be very, very rare. The only real disagreement
between opponents and proponents concerns those cases in which adequate pain
control cannot be achieved.

What accounts for the opposing sides' underlying agreement that physician-
assisted suicide should be rare is, I think, an unexamined assumption they share.
This assumption is the view that the call for physician-assisted suicide is what
might be called a *phenomenon of discrepant development:* a symptom of the disparity in development between two distinct capacities of modern medicine, the
capacity to extend or prolong life and the capacity to control pain. Research,
development, and delivery of technologies for the prolongation of life have raced
far ahead; those for control of pain lagged far behind. It is this situation of discrepant development that has triggered the current concern with physician-
assisted suicide and the volatile public debate over whether to legalize it or not.

The opposing sides both also hold in common the view that what would lead
to the resolution of the problem is whatever set of mechanisms would tend to
equalize the degree of development of medicine's capacities to prolong life and
to control pain. To achieve this equalization, two simultaneous strategies are recommended: cutting back on overzealous prolongation of life (as Dan Callahan,
for example, has long recommended), and at the same time (as Hospice and others have been insisting) accelerating the development of technologies, modes of

delivery, and physician training for more effective methods of pain control.[2] As life prolongation is held back a bit, pain control can catch up, and the current situation of discrepant development between the two can be alleviated. Thus calls for physician-assisted suicide can be expected to become rarer and rarer, and as medicine's capacities for pain control are finally equalized with its capacities for life prolongation, finally virtually to disappear. Almost no one imagines that there will not still be a few difficult situations in which life is prolonged beyond the point at which pain can be effectively controlled, but these will be increasingly infrequent, it is assumed, and in general, as the disparity between our capacities for life prolongation and for pain control shrinks, interest in and need for physician-assisted suicide will decrease and all but disappear.

Fortunately, this view continues, the public debate over physician-assisted suicide now so intense will not have been a waste, since it has both warned against the potential cruelty of overzealous prolongation of life and at the same time stimulated greater attention to imperatives of pain control. The current debate serves as social pressure for bringing equalization of the disparity about. Yet as useful as this debate is, this view holds, it will soon subside and disappear; we're just currently caught in a turbulent—but fleeting—little maelstrom.

The Longer View

That's how things look now. But I think we can also see our current concern with physician-assisted suicide in a longer-term, historically informed view. Consider just three of the many profound changes that affect matters of how we die. First, there has been a shift, beginning in the middle of the last century, in the ways in which human beings characteristically die. Termed the "epidemiological transition," this change involves a shift away from death due to parasitic and infectious disease (ubiquitous among humans in all parts of the globe prior to about 1850) to death in later life of degenerative disease-especially cancer and heart disease, which together account for almost two-thirds of deaths in the developed countries.[3] This means dramatically extended lifespans and also deaths from diseases with characteristically extended downhill terminal courses. Second, there have been changes in religious attitudes about death: People are less likely to see death as divine punishment for sin, or to see suffering as a prerequisite for the afterlife, or to see suicide as a highly stigmatized and serious sin rather than the product of mental illness or depression. Third among the major shifts in cultural attitudes that affect the way we die is the increasing emphasis on the notion of individual rights of self-determination, reinforced in the latter part of this century by the civil rights movement's attention to individuals in vulnerable groups. This shift has affected self-perceptions and attitudes towards the terminally ill, and patients, including dying patients, are now recognized to have a wide array of rights previously eclipsed by the paternalistic practices of medicine.

These three transitions, along with many other concomitant cultural changes, invite us to see our current concern with physician-assisted suicide in a quite different way-not just as a phenomenon resulting from the currently disparate development of life-prolonging and pain-controlling technologies, a temporary anomaly, but as a precursor, an early symptom of a much more substantial sea change in attitudes about death. We might call this shift in attitudes a shift towards "directed dying" or "self-directed dying," in which the individual who is dying plays a far more prominent, directive role than in earlier eras in determining how and when his or her death shall occur. In this changed view, dying is no longer *something that happens to you* but *something you do.*

To be sure, this shift—if it is one—can be seen as already well under way. Taking its legally visible start with the California Natural Death Act of 1976, terminally ill patients have already gained dramatically enlarged rights of self-determination in matters of guiding and controlling their own deaths, including rights to refuse treatment, discontinue treatment, stipulate treatment to be withheld at a later date, designate decisionmakers, and to negotiate with their physicians, or have their surrogates do so, such matters as DNR orders, withholding and withdrawal of ventilators, surgical procedures, nutrition and hydration, the use of opioids, and even terminal sedation. Some patients also negotiate, or attempt to negotiate, physician-assisted suicide or physician-performed euthanasia with their physicians. In all of this, we already see the patient playing a far more prominent role in determining the course of his or her dying process and its character and timing, and far more willingness on the part of physicians, family members, the law, and other parties to respect the patient's preferences and choices in these matters.

But this may be just the tip of a looming iceberg. For we may ask whether, much as we human beings have made dramatic gains in control over our own reproduction (particularly rapidly in very recent times—the birth control pill was introduced just thirty years ago), we human beings are beginning to make dramatic gains in control over our own dying, particularly rapidly in the last several decades. We cannot keep from dying altogether, of course. But by using directly caused death, as in physician-assisted suicide, it is possible to control many of dying's features: its timing in the downhill course of a terminal disease, its place, the exact agents which cause it, its observers, and so on. Indeed, as Robert Kastenbaum has argued, because it makes it possible to control the time, place, manner and people present at one's death, assisted suicide will become the *preferred* manner of dying.[4]

But this conjecture doesn't yet show what could actually motivate such substantial social change, away from a culture which sees dying primarily as *something that happens to you*, to a culture which sees it as *something you do*—a deliberate, planned activity, one's final and culminative activity. What might do this, I think, is a conceptual change, or, more exactly, a shift in decisional perspective in choice-making about pain, suffering, and other elements of dying. It is the kind of shift in decisional perspective that evolves on a society-wide scale as a populace gains understanding of and control over a matter, a shift in choicemaking perspective from a stance we might describe as immediately involved or "enmeshed," to one that is distanced and reflective. (I'll use two Latin names for these stances later.) This shift can occur for many features of human experience—it has already largely occurred in the developed world with respect to reproduction—but it has not yet occurred with respect to death and dying. It has not yet occurred—or rather, perhaps, it has just begun.

Take a patient, an average man. This particular man is so average that he just happens to have contracted that disease which is the usual diagnosis (as we know from the Netherlands) in cases of physician-assisted suicide—cancer—and he is also so average that this disease will kill him at just the average life-expectancy for males in the United States, 72.8 years.[5] Furthermore, he is also so average that if he does turn to physician-assisted suicide, he will choose to forgo just about the same amount of life that, on average, Dutch patients receiving euthanasia or physician-assisted suicide do, less than 3.3 weeks.[6] He has been considering physician-asssisted suicide since his illness was first diagnosed (since he is an average man, this was about 29.6 months ago), but now, as his condition deteriorates, he thinks more seriously about it. His motivation includes both pre-emptive elements, the desire to avoid some of the very worst things that terminal cancer might bring him, and reactive elements, the desire to relieve some of the symptoms and other suffering that he is already experiencing. *It's bad enough now*, he tells his doctor, *and it will probably get worse*. He asks his doctor for the pills. He is perfectly aware of what he may miss—a number of weeks of continued life, the possibility of an unexpected cure, the chance, even if it is a longshot, of spontaneous regression or remission, and—not to be overlooked—the possibility that that the worst is over, so to speak, and that the remainder of his downhill course in terminal cancer won't be so bad. He is also well aware that even a bad agonal phase may nevertheless include moments of great intimacy and importance with his family or friends. But he makes what he sees as a rational choice, seeking to balance the risks and possible benefits of easy death now, versus a little more continuing life with a greater possibility of a hard death. He is making his choice *in medias res*, in the middle of things, as the physical, social, and emotional realities of terminal illness engulf him. He is enmeshed in his situation, caught in it, trapped between what seem like two bad alternatives—suffering, or suicide.

But, of course, he might have done his deciding about how his life shall end and whether to elect physician-assisted suicide in preference to the final stages of terminal illness from a quite different, more distanced perspective, a secular version of the view *sub specie aeternitatis*. This is not just an objective, depersonalized view—anybody's view—but his own, distinctively personal view not confined to a specific timepoint.[7] Rather than assessing his prospects from the point of view he has at the time at which he would continue or discontinue his life—that point late in the course of his illness when things have already become "bad enough" and are likely to get worse—he might have done his deciding, albeit rather more hypothetically, from the perspective of a more generalized view of his life.

From this alternative perspective, what he would have seen is the overall shape of his life, and it is with respect to this that he would have made his choices about how it shall end. Of course, he could not know in advance whether he will contract cancer, or succumb to heart disease, or be hit by a bus—though he does know that he will die sometime or other. Consequently, his choices are necessarily conditional in form: "*If* I get cancer, I'll refuse agressive treatment and use hospice care"; "*If* I get AIDS, I'll ask for physician-assisted suicide"; "If I get Alzheimer's, I'll commit suicide on my own, since no physician besides Jack Kevorkian would help me," and so on. Although conditional in form and predicated on circumstances that may not occur, these may be real choices nonetheless, and, particularly because they are reiterated and repeated over the course of a lifetime, have real motive force.

The difference, then, between these two views is substantial. In the first, our average man with an average terminal cancer, doing his deciding *in medias res*, is deciding whether or not to take the pills his physician has given him now. It is his last possible couple of weeks or a month (on average, 3.3 weeks) that he is deciding about. Even if continuing life threatens pain and other suffering, it is still all he has left, and while it may be difficult to live this life—all he has left— it may also be very difficult to relinquish it.

In contrast, if our average man were doing his deciding *sub specie aeternitatis*, from a distanced though still personal viewpoint not tied to a specific moment in his life, he would have been deciding all along between two different conceptions of his own demise, between two possible lives for himself. One of his possible lives would, on average, be 72.8 years long, the average lifespan for a male in the United States, with the possibility of substantial suffering at the end—on average, as the SUPPORT study finds, a 50 percent chance of moderate to severe pain at least 50 percent of the time during the last three days before his death. The other of his possible lives would be about 72.7 years long, foreshortened on average 3.3 weeks by physician-assisted suicide, but with a markedly reduced possibility of substantial suffering at the end. (This shortening of the lifespan is not age-based but time-to-death based, planned for, on average, 3.3 weeks before an unassisted death would have occurred; it occurs in this example at age 72.7 just because our man is so average.) This latter, shortened life also offers our man the opportunity to control the timing, the place, the manner, and other features of his death in the way he likes. Viewed *sub specie aeternitatis*, at any or many earlier points in one's life or from a vantage point standing outside life, so to speak, the difference between 72.8 and 72.7 seems negligible: These are both lives of average length not interrupted by grossly premature death. Why not choose the one in which the risk of agonal pain—as high as 50/50, according to the SUPPORT study—is far, far less great, and the possibility of conscious, culminative experience, surrounded by family members, trusted friends, and permitting final prayers and goodbyes, is far, far greater?

It may seem difficult to distinguish these two choices in practice. This is because we typically make our decisions about death and dying *in medias res*, not *sub specie aeternitatis*, and our medical practices, our bioethics discussions, and our background culture strongly encourage this. The call for assisted dying, like other patient pleas, is seen as a reaction to the circumstances of dying, not a settled, longer term, preemptive preference.[8] True, some independently minded individuals consider these issues in a kind of background, hypothetical way throughout their lives, but this is certainly not the practical norm. We can only really understand this view as involving a substantial cultural shift from our current perspective.

But if this shift occurs, a slightly abbreviated lifespan in which there is dramatically reduced risk of pain and suffering will not only seem to be preferable to one which is negligibly longer but carries substantial risk of pain and suffering in its agonal phase, it will also be seen as rational and normal to plan for this abbreviated lifespan and to plan the means of bringing it about. The way to ensure it, of course, is to plan for direct termination of life. After all, one cannot count on being able to discontinue some life-prolonging treatment or other—refusing antibiotics, disconnecting a respirator—to hasten death and thus avoid what might be the worst weeks at the end. This most likely means planning for physician-assisted suicide. From this distanced perspective, a 72.7-year life with a virtually assured good end looks much, much better than a 72.8-year life that has an even chance of coming to a bad end. Arguably, it would be rational for any individual, except those for whom religious commitments or other scruples rule out suicide altogether, to plan to ensure this. But if it looks this way to one individual, it will look this way to many; and it is thus plausible to imagine that physician-assisted suicide would not be rare but rather a choice viewed as rational and preemptively prudent by many or most members of the culture. Thus it can come to be seen as a normal course of action, not a rarity or a "last resort." To be sure, there are other ways of abbreviating a lifespan to avoid terminal suffering—withdrawing or withholding treatment, overusing of morphine or other pain-relieving drugs, discontinuing artificial nutrition and hydration, and terminal sedation—but these cannot be used unless the patient's condition has already worsened and is thus likely to involve that pain or suffering the person might choose to avoid. Thus these other modalities function primarily reactively; it is assisted suicide that can function preemptively.

But, as soon as planning for a normal, slight abbreviation in the lifespan by means of assisted suicide becomes conceptually possible not just for our average man but for actual persons in general, it also becomes possible to imagine a wide range of context-specific cultural practices which might emerge surrounding physician-assisted suicide. After all, that a person understands and expects his lifespan to be one which will end in an assisted death a few weeks before he might otherwise have died, while he is still conscious, alert, and capable of deciding what location he wants it to take place in, what family members, caregivers, clergy, or others he wants to have present, what ceremonies, religious or symbolic, he wants conducted, etc., suggests that more general social practices would grow up around these possibilities. After all, our average man sees his life this way; but it is possible for him to do this partly because the others in his society see their lives this way as well. Attitudes about death are heavily socially conditioned, and so are the perspectives from which choice-making about death is seen.

This is the precondition for the development of a whole range of social practices supporting such choices. These might include various kinds of practical supports, such as legal, insurance, and other policies that treat assisted dying as acceptable and normal; various sorts of cultural and religious practices that similarly treat assisted dying as acceptable and normal (for instance by developing rituals and rites concerning the forthcoming death); familial supports within the family, including family gatherings, preparing for the death, and sharing reminiscences and goodbyes; pre-death dispositions of wills and life insurance (we already recognize viaticums, pre-death payoffs of life insurance for terminally ill patients); and even such now-inconceivable practices as pre-death funerals, understood as ceremonies of leavetaking and farewell, expressions of both celebration of a life complete and grief at its loss. In turn, such social practices come to function as positive reasons for choosing a somewhat earlier, elective death—formerly and rudely called "physician-assisted suicide," even when pain control is no longer the issue at all—and the new social pattern, so different from our current one—reinforces itself. This has nothing to do with a *Soylent Green* sort of view, in which people are forced into choices they do not genuinely make (this film can be understood only from our current, *in medias res* view); but a world in which their normal choices have genuinely changed, and changed for reasons which seem to them good.

Furthermore, if the culture-wide view of choice making about death and dying were more fully held *sub specie aeternitatis* in this distanced, less enmeshed and less merely reactive way, in which earlier, elective death becomes the norm, we could also expect the more frequent practice of "setting a date," as people who have contracted predictably terminal illnesses carry out the plans they had been developing all along for their own demises. Setting a date for one's own death—presumably, a couple of weeks or so before the date it might naturally have been, revisable of course in the light of any changes in the diagnosis or prognosis—would still be both preemptive and reactive in character, but far more preemptive than choices made *in medias res*, where choices will be highly reactive to the then-current circumstances the patient finds himself or herself in. The timing of such choices might always be revised in consultation with the physician; but what would be culturally reinforced would be the general commitment to advance planning for one's own death as well as a commitment to assuming a comparatively autonomist, directive role in it. Self-directed dying would be the norm, though of course different people would direct their deaths in quite different ways.

If profound changes affecting matters of how we die are already underway—the epidemiological transition, shifting from parasitic and infectious disease deaths to deaths of predictably degenerative disease; the changes in religious conceptions of suicide so that it is not understood primarily as sin; and the steadily increasing attention to patients' and terminally ill patients' rights of self-determination—it is an open conjecture whether this is where we may be going.

Are we in fact experiencing just a temporary aberration in our basic cultural patterns of death and dying, an aberration which is a function of the discrepant development of technologies for life prolongation and for pain control? Or are we seeing the first breaking waves of a sea-change from one perspective on death and dying to another, a far more autonomist and directive one much as we have seen changes in reproduction?

Obviously, I can't say. But I can say that if this is what is happening, the assumption that physician-assisted suicide would or should be rare, an assumption still held by both sides in the current debate, will collapse. We would have no reason to assume that assisted dying should be rare, whatever the relationship between capacities for life prolongation and pain control. Of course, such a picture is very difficult to envision, since we do not think that way about death and dying now. But if we can at least see what is different about viewing personal choices about one's own death *sub specie aeternitatis* and in our current way, *in medias res*, enmeshed in particular circumstances, we can understand why it might occur.

Would it be a good thing, or a bad thing? I can hardly answer that question here, but let me close with a story I heard somewhere in the Netherlands several years ago. I do not remember the exact source of the story nor the specific dates or names, and it is certainly not representative of current practice in Holland. But it was told to me as a true story, and it went something like this:

> Two friends, old sailing buddies, are planning a sailing trip in the North Sea in the summer. It is late February now, and they are discussing possible dates.
>
> "How about July 21?" says Willem. "The North Sea will be calm, the moon bright, and there's a music festival on the southern coast of Denmark we could visit."
>
> "Sounds great," answers Joost. "I'd love to get to the music festival. But I can't be gone then; the twenty-first is the date of my father's death."
>
> "Oh, I'm so sorry, Joost," Willem replies. "I knew your father was ill. Very ill, with cancer. But I didn't realize he had died."
>
> "He hasn't," Joost replies. "That's the day he will be dying. He's picked a date and made up his mind, and we all want to be there with him."

Such a story seems just that, a story, a fiction, somehow horrifying and also somehow liberating, but in any case virtually inconceivable to us. But it was not told to me as a fiction, but as a true story. I've tried to explore the conceptual assumptions that might lie behind such a story, and to consider whether in the future such stories might become more and more the norm. I have not tried to say whether this would be good or bad, but only that this might well be where we are going. In fact, I think it would be good—just as I think increasing personal control over reproduction is good—but I haven't argued for that view here.

In this respect, what the Supreme Court has done in its 1997 *Washington* v. *Glucksberg* and *Vacco* v. *Quill* decision may make a substantial difference. To ban physician-assisted suicide altogether would have been to reinforce the conception that physician-assisted suicide, if it occurs at all, should be rare; to recognize it as a constitutionally based right would have been to begin to create the psychological and legal space within which individuals could reflect in a longer term way about their own future choices when they come to dying, perhaps making physician-assisted suicide an eventual part of their plans, and indeed planning whatever family gatherings, ceremonies, and religious observances they might wish—not as a desperate last resort or reactive escape from bad circumstances, but as a preemptively prudent, significant, culminative experience. To leave the matter with the states, as the Supreme Court in fact did, will be somewhere in between, depending on whether most individual states respond by reinforcing prohibitions or permitting legalization; here, only time will tell.

Notes

1. According to the SUPPORT study, about 50 percent of dying hospitalized patients were reported to have experienced moderate to severe pain at least 50 percent of the time in their last three days of life. The Support Principal Investigators, "A Controlled Trial to Improve Care for Seriously Ill Hospitalized Patients," *Journal of the American Medical Association* 274 (20) (1995): 1951–98.
2. See, e.g., Daniel Callahan, *Setting Limits: Medical Goals in an Aging Society* (New York: Simon and Schuster, 1987), *What Kind of Life? The Limits of Medical Progress* (New York: Simon and Schuster, 1990), and *The Troubled Dream of Life: Living with Mortality* (New York: Simon and Schuster, 1993). On acceleration of pain-control development, see especially the work of Kathleen Foley, "Pain, physician-assisted suicide, and euthanasia," *Pain Forum* 4 (3) (1995) and other works.
3. The term originates with A. R. Omran, "The Epidemiologic Transition: A Theory of the Epidemiology of Population Change," *Milbank Memorial Fund Quarterly* 49 (4): 509–38 (1971); and the theory is augmented in A. Jay Olshansky and A. Brian Ault, "The Fourth Stage of the Epidemiologic Transition: The Age of Delayed Degenerative Disease," in Timothy M. Smeeding et al., eds., *Should Medical Care Be Rationed By Age?* (Totowa, NJ: Rowman and Littlefield, 1987, pp. 11–43.
4. Robert Kastenbaum, "Suicide as the Preferred Way of Death," in Edwin S. Shneidman, ed. *Suicidology: Contemporary Developments* (New York: Grune and Stratton, 1976), pp. 425–41.
5. Data on physician-assisted suicide and euthanasia in the Netherlands is provided by what is called the "Remmelink Commission Report." Paul J. van der Maas, Johannes J. M. van Delden, and Loes Pijnenborg, "Euthanasia and Other Medical Decisions Concerning the End of Life," published in full in English as a special issue of *Health Policy* 22, nos. 1 and 2 (1992); and, with Caspar W. M. Looman, in summary in *The Lancet* 338 (Sept. 14, 1991): 669–74; and the five-year update in Paul J. van der Maas, et al., "Euthanasia, Physician-Assisted Suicide, and Other Medical Practices involving the End of Life in the Netherlands, 1990–1995," *New England Journal of Medicine* 335 (22): 1699–1705 (1996).
6. See Ezekiel J. Emanuel and Margaret P. Battin, "The Economics of Euthanasia: What are the Potential Cost Savings from Legalizing Physician-Assisted Suicide?" MSS in progress, citing data from the Netherlands.
7. The distinction I am drawing here between personal views *in medias res* and *sub specie aeternitatis* is thus not quite the same as that drawn by Thomas Nagel between subjective and objective views, though it has much in common with Nagel's distinction in contexts concerning death. See Nagel, *The View from Nowhere* (New York: Oxford University Press, 1986), especially chapter XI, section 3, on death.
8. See C. G. Prado, *The Last Choice: Preemptive Suicide in Advanced Age* (Westport, Conn.: Greenwood Press, 1990).

Part Two

Considering Those at Risk

SOME PEOPLE THINK they would rather end their lives artificially than endure a prolonged painful natural death. Should the state prohibit physicians (and other medical personnel) from offering their services to citizens who prefer to hasten their own deaths? One of the most dramatic arguments against physician-assisted suicide portrays policies permitting such assistance as too dangerous, if not for all citizens, then at least for certain classes of people whom the state has a heightened duty to protect.

This line of argument identifies people who are very old, or are severely or terminally ill, or have serious disabilities, or are members of other subordinated or marginalized groups, as especially susceptible to manipulation or coercion. Regardless of what legalizing physician-assisted suicide offers competent individuals, the argument goes, there are classes of people so likely to be devalued or to devalue themselves that their lives inevitably will be at risk if suicide is made easy for them. Seeing themselves as having little to live for, they may be more disposed than other people to want to die. And, conceivably, their situations might be interpreted as so burdensome to themselves and others that they would be expected, or even urged, to die, whether or not they really wanted to do so.

In this section, contributors examine various aspects of the claim that weak or socially marginalized people will unfairly bear a heightened risk unless the state works aggressively to prevent suicides. From a public policy perspective, the collective obligation to safeguard powerless people (especially those identified as belonging to vulnerable groups) takes precedence over individuals' preferences for more comfortable deaths. But is whatever public good we achieve by protecting especially vulnerable populations incompatible with the personal good sought by individuals who want to end their agony? How sure must we be that community welfare would otherwise be threatened before we invoke the public good to justify demands that individuals prolong their suffering? The challenge of acknowledging both communitarian and individualistic perspectives has become a crucial feature of the discussion about permitting physicians to assist patients who want to die.

Leslie Francis's essay considers whether to relax, or to raise, the standard of protection for elderly people. Should the relatively limited extent of their future lives make us more or less vigilant in permitting them access to the means to end their lives? And what vigilance must we exercise to safeguard the classes usually protected against discrimination from misuses of the mechanisms meant to assist in suicide? Patricia King explores whether physician-assisted suicide poses a special threat to the African-American community. Dena Davis weighs assertions that legalizing physician-assisted suicide would place women at special risk. To the contrary, she finds, banning such assistance jeopardizes women by prolonging the kind of oppression that curtails their authority over their own bodies.

The next essays in this section examine the danger in which severely ill people or people with disabilities might be placed if physicians are allowed to help those who say they wish to do so terminate their lives. Jerome Bickenback believes that the relentless social devaluation experienced by people with disabilities induces everyone to undervalue their existence. Thus, persons with disabilities who want to die are propelled, not by self-determination, but by discriminatory social influences. In contrast Anita Silvers urges that describing people with disabilities as easily coerced or manipulated into killing themselves characterizes them as less capable of self-determination than other people are. Making physician-assisted suicide seem dangerous to them by devaluing their competence of judgment and strength of character reiterates the familiar patterns of disability discrimination. Finally, Felicia Ackerman argues that a policy for assisting the suicides of terminally ill and severely disabled individuals but not others cannot be defended morally. A morally acceptable policy rationale will justify making such aid available to all citizens or to none, but not just to terminally ill or incurably disabled ones.

4

Assisted Suicide

Are the Elderly a Special Case?

LESLIE PICKERING FRANCIS

Many elder advocates worry that if legalization of physician aid-in-dying becomes widespread, the elderly may be particularly subject to abuse and coercion. Other elder advocates view aid-in-dying as an important way for the elderly to maintain autonomy in the manner of their deaths. In this chapter I explore whether the elderly are a special case with respect to aid-in-dying. I argue that all of the theoretical reasons for thinking that the elderly have a special interest in aid-in-dying are contingent and do not support treating the elderly differently as a group. The theories do, however, give us good reason for insisting on strong safeguards before PAS is contemplated by any patient, including assessments of competence, examination for depression, and full understanding of the medical situation and the available options for palliative care. The theories also suggest public policy that limits PAS to patients who are terminally ill, if PAS is to be available at all.

*　　*　　*

A ID-IN-DYING is a deeply troubling issue for groups devoted to protecting the interests of the elderly. Elder advocates worry that the elderly would be particularly subject to abuse and coercion should legalized aid-in-dying become widespread. The American Bar Association's Commission on the Legal Problems of the Elderly, for example, has voiced considerable concern about the impact on vulnerable populations should physician-assisted suicide (PAS) become more widely accepted, legally or morally. The Commission successfully sponsored a resolution at the 1997 annual meeting of the ABA that read:

> RESOLVED, That any consideration of the matter of physician-assisted suicide which involves personal, religious, emotional, medical, legal and ethical considerations and considerations of appropriate care alternatives, supportive services, pain relief, potential for abuse, legal protection, competency and needed research in many fields, should be left to be resolved by state legislatures and their electorates after extensive and informed public discussion.
>
> FURTHER RESOLVED, That in the event that any state or territory chooses to adopt legislation permitting physician-assisted suicide, it should ensure that information and reporting systems are established to achieve close monitoring of the impact of such practices, especially with respect to vulnerable populations who may be particularly at risk if such practices are authorized.[1]

The conditions in the first paragraph of the resolution are so stringent that they may not realistically be achievable; if they are not, the resolution's real target may seem to be opposition to the legalization of PAS under any conditions.

Indeed, many advocates of good healthcare for the elderly regard PAS with trepidation.[2] The American Geriatrics Society, for example, has issued a statement opposing both PAS and voluntary active euthanasia. Their concerns are that expanded reliance on aid-in-dying will reduce pressures for adequate palliative care and for the improvement of care for the dying. In the Society's estimate, most requests for aid-in-dying arise from fear of inadequate palliation, a fear that can be allayed by improved treatment modalities. The Society is also deeply concerned about risks of coercion, and recommends that it should be illegal for caregivers to receive compensation for assisting in suicide.[3] In the recent PAS litigation before the United States Supreme Court, moreover, the Society recommended reversal of the Ninth and the Second Circuit decisions, arguing that PAS should not be constitutionalized but should be left to reasoned public debate and policy-making at the state level. The Brief for the Society described the potential moral difficulties raised for geriatricians by legalization of PAS: How should a physician act to further the interests of his/her patients, when PAS appears to be a desirable alternative because of the inadequacies of care or the lack of resources devoted to healthcare and social services for the elderly?[4]

At the same time, other elder advocates express deep adherence to patient autonomy, and defenders of the legalization of aid-in-dying believe its availability is a crucial aspect of autonomy. The AARP has taken a position of official neutrality on aid-in-dying: "After careful consideration, our National Legislative Council recommends to the Board of Directors that it not take a position on physician-assisted suicide. The NLC concluded that this intensely personal issue is one about which each individual should make his or her own decision."[5]

The interest of the ABA Commission, the American Geriatrics Society, the AARP, and other elder advocate groups in aid-in-dying suggests that it is at least an issue of special concern for the elderly. In this paper, I take up the question of whether the elderly are in any theoretical sense a special case with respect to aid-in-dying. I argue that all of the reasons for thinking that the elderly have a special interest in this issue are contingent; they do not support a conclusion that the elderly should be treated differently as a group. These reasons do, however, provide us with important insights into the role of presumptions in our public policies about decision making at the end of life.

Presumptions define what I call the "default" position—the position that will be assumed to operate unless there is evidence at some specified level to the contrary. For example, in emergency medicine the default position is that treatment should be undertaken; the presumption is that people want to avoid mortality or morbidity to the extent possible. Only if there is evidence (most likely, clear and convincing evidence) that limitations on interventions would be preferred is treatment withheld. Some states now offer a formal DNR procedure for patients dying at home as a way to override the presumption that resuscitation is preferred when paramedics are called.[6]

Presumptions about three issues in particular will be my focus here. First are presumptions about competence; depending on what these are, aid-in-dying proposals will take different positions about whether affirmative evidence of competence is required. Second are presumptions about depression; depending on whether there are presumptions that patients contemplating suicide are depressed, aid-in-dying proposals will adopt different strategies for requiring mental health consultation. Finally are presumptions about typical preferences—whether, for example, elderly people who are terminally ill and in pain would typically prefer availability of the option of aid-in-dying. These presumptions function in discussions about whether to look behind preferences for PAS to scrutinize their rationality with special care, and might function as well in determinations of what level of proof might be required for an advance directive for aid-in-dying, although that is not my topic here. They also function in the decision to limit aid-in-dying to the terminally ill. I will argue that there is no reason to think presumptions should be different for the elderly as a group, although examining issues about the elderly suggests what our presumptions should be more generally in developing aid-in-dying policies.

Autonomy, Cognitive Capacities, and Competence

The elderly, especially elderly white males, commit suicide at a higher rate than other groups in the population, two to three times even the rate for teenagers.[7] When elderly people attempt suicide, moreover, they are far more likely to use lethal weapons such as guns, and to succeed; suicide among the elderly appears to be a resolution, not a cry for help. Over the last two decades, after a long decline attributed by commentators to improved healthcare, suicide rates among the elderly have been rising. Speculation is that reported rates underestimate the actual incidence of suicide among the elderly, with treatment refusals and accidents masking actual suicides.[8] What should be made of these facts, however, is unclear. Perhaps the data reveal that suicide is the last rational act of many autonomous elders. Or perhaps they reveal that the elderly on the whole are more likely to be subject to tragedy of all kinds, including the increased incidence of untimely death among incompetent or otherwise vulnerable populations.

Advocates of the availability of PAS defend it as an important aspect of patient autonomy at the end of life. The exercise of autonomy involves reasoned choice among a reasonable range of alternatives; if a preferred alternative is legally prohibited, and so generally absent from the range, autonomy is correspondingly impaired. If patients in a certain category (say, patients in a persistent vegetative state) are not and cannot be capable of reasoned choice, then respect for their autonomy is not a principal moral value in treating them. If there were grounds for believing the elderly are not capable of reasoned decision-making—or even grounds for believing that capacity for reasoned decision-making is especially problematic among the elderly—then there would be grounds for regarding the elderly as a special case with respect to PAS. The autonomy argument would not support the availability of PAS for the elderly, although it might for other age groups. But there are no such grounds for believing age itself clouds reason. There are, however, grounds for believing the capacity for reasoned decision-making is a special concern whenever PAS is considered, for the elderly or otherwise.

Understanding these grounds requires laying out some basics of an account of reasoned choice, the capacity for reasoned decision-making, and its relationship to judgments of competence.[9] For a choice to be reasoned, a person must be able to identify his/her values, have and understand relevant information about the consequences of available alternatives for the realization of these values, and choose among alternatives based on some linkage between these values and these consequences. Reasoned decision-making thus calls on a complex set of capacities, of identification, understanding, and connecting. An optimally reasoned decision would be the one which maximizes the realization of the person's values based on full understanding of the consequences of available alternatives. Many—indeed very many—reasoned decisions fall short of optimality in this sense.

In contrast, the judgment that a person is competent expresses the legal conclusion that he or she has the power to act for him or herself. A competent person need not always reason optimally; judgments of competence reflect the conclusion that a person's capacities for reasoned decision-making meet a minimum level such that interference with them is not warranted. The conclusion that a person is competent and that his/her decisions should thus be respected is put in question when one or more of the capacities involved in reasoned decisionmaking is significantly impaired. If a person cannot describe his or her values, or if there is some reason for questioning the person's process of identifying values, competence would be put into question. Likewise, competence would be at issue if a person cannot understand and use relevant information in assessing alternatives. Finally, competence might be put at issue if there is an inexplicable lack of fit between a person's actual choices and the choices that would realize his or her values, or if there is some reason to question how the person goes about fitting values to alternatives. Whether the elderly are a special case with respect to competence, then, would involve whether there is reason to question, on the basis of age alone, a person's possession of the capacities involved in reasoned decision-making.

Now, there surely are grounds for believing judgments of competence are of special concern whenever PAS is considered. PAS, like any suicide, is an irrevocable and momentous choice. When the stakes are so high, it might be argued, it is especially important to insure that the decision was the result of reasoned choice. Along these lines, Buchanan and Brock have argued for a sliding scale standard of competence, with insistence on a heightened standard when the stakes are high.[10] That is, Buchanan and Brock would require more developed abilities to articulate values, assimilate information, and relate the two, when life itself is on the line. An alternative conclusion to Buchanan and Brock's, short of adopting a shifting standard of competence, is insistence that special care be taken in determining that the standard of competence is met when the stakes are high.

Even so, it is less clear that the possession of the capacities involved in reasoned decision-making is a special problem among the elderly. There are, to be sure, issues about each of these capacities that arise with frequency in populations of older people. The focus of the remainder of this section will be cognitive capacities; the focus of the next section will be vulnerabilities. In general, cognitive capacities decline somewhat with age. Diseases of impaired cognition, such as the variety of dementias, occur with increasing frequency with age. So do losses of cognitive capacity associated with other physical conditions—dyspnea, for example, or compromised nutritional status.[11] Fluctuations in competence due to physical debility or medications also are more common among the elderly, and it may be difficult to treat elderly patients so as to enable them to engage in reasoned decision-making. These are all just frequency judgments, however; there is no reason to believe losses of cognitive capacity are necessarily tied to age per se, especially at the level required for judgments of incompetence and consequent legal disability. People at all ages suffer cognitive losses comparable to those found with dementias. The import of more gradual decline in capacities for judgments of competence depends on how quickly the decline occurs and what the person's capacities were to begin with.[12] These frequencies suggest at most that there is reason to take a careful look at capacities when questions of competence are raised among the elderly. Such a careful look does not require treating the elderly as a special case, but can be established through evidentiary standards, such as the requirement that there be specific findings of competence, especially in a decision such as PAS where life is at stake.

Comparison with our judgments about competence at the other side of the age range—in the young—are instructive in considering why evidentiary standards are preferable to treating the elderly as a special case. For the young, we do use age to presume incompetence; with limited exceptions, those under the age of eighteen are unable to make legal decisions for themselves. In general, the law does not look behind chronology to scrutinize capacities in individual cases, although there are exceptions.[13] The law simply selects the age of eighteen as the magic moment of competence, assuming that it corresponds relatively well in most cases with the actual acquisition of minimal levels of the capacity for reasoned decision-making. Imagine the analogous strategy for competency determinations in the old: we would select an age that roughly corresponds to the diminution of capacities below a minimum level, and presume incompetence after that point. Driven by symmetry, we might select eighty-two as the magic moment; it is, after all, one hundred minus eighteen. (We could set the level higher; the point is to ask whether we should set any level at all, based on estimates of when the loss of capacities has reached the level to warrant a presumption of incompetence.) There might be advantages to such a cutoff in contrast to case-by-case determinations, akin to the advantages of mandatory retirement:

we save the costs and the considerable personal trauma associated with the judgment that someone's cherished capacities have diminished significantly. Like retirement celebrations at age sixty-five, and celebrations of majority at age eighteen, there might even be celebrations of incapacity at age eighty-two.

This image of an age of second childhood is chilling, perhaps too chilling ever to be defended seriously. But it challenges us to justify the asymmetry in current public policy of an age cutoff for competence in the young but not in the old. (We might, of course, drop any use of an age cutoff for the young, perhaps a worthy target but not mine here.) One answer is empirical: The asymmetry reflects asymmetries in the facts about capacities; declines in capacities among the elderly do not cluster around an age in the way we assume acquisitions of capacity cluster around an age in the young. Another answer is normative: A mistake of presuming incompetence in the face of adequate decision-making capacities is worse at one end of the life cycle than the other. The sixteen-year-old who is legally incompetent despite finely honed capacities for decision-making will in the normal course of events acquire competence at age eighteen. In contrast, the eighty-three-year-old's time will never recur, despite a lifetime of developed values and reasoned choice. Both of these answers support rejecting an age-related presumption of incompetence, but neither undermines the case for careful scrutiny of competence when PAS is contemplated at any age.

At most, therefore, concerns about cognitive capacities in the elderly suggest the need for close scrutiny when judgments of competence are made. Such scrutiny might be effected by the requirement of an assessment of decision-making capacity for a decision such as PAS. Or it might be effected by a required assessment whenever there is reason to question decision-making processes. Examples of such reasons might be a relatively significant and apparently inexplicable shift in values, an inability to demonstrate understanding of the consequences of available alternatives, or a sizeable and apparently inexplicable discontinuity between the alternative selected and the alternative that would maximize values. Because such discontinuities are frequently linked to vulnerabilities, it is to the relevance of vulnerabilities to decision-making capacity in the elderly that I now turn.

Autonomy and Vulnerabilities

The ABA Commission resolution assumes that there are vulnerable populations (presumably children, minorities, and people with disabilities), and that the elderly are among them. The putative vulnerabilities of the elderly are indeed legion: physical debility, depression, loss of loved ones, and economic insecurity, among others. If any of these vulnerabilities raise questions about the capacity of the elderly for reasoned decision-making, they too would be reason for concern about the applicability of the autonomy paradigm to the elderly as a group.

Studies of suicide among the elderly do find correlations between physical debility and increased incidence of suicide.[14] There is some evidence that chronic dyspnea, for example, is a risk factor both for depression and for suicide among the elderly.[15] Physical debility can lead to significant dependency on others to meet basic needs of life: shopping for food; cooking; transportation to social occasions, church, or even to doctor's appointments, cleaning, and the ability to continue to live at home. Loss of bodily function, such as incontinence, can be the source of humiliation and self-disgust. Declining vision or hearing can make cherished pastimes such as reading, sewing, or listening to music no longer possible. Physical losses thus may result in other losses, of pleasures or of independent living.[16]

Beyond the physical, elders are more likely to be subject to other kinds of losses. They are more likely than other age cohorts to experience the deaths of family members or friends. Despite the legal end of mandatory retirement, age at retirement has been falling and the elderly are more likely to experience job loss and resulting loss of activity and identity. Remaining family members may be physically or emotionally remote, particularly in the face of apparently increasing needs and demands. Even the loss of pets, due to death or the inability to care for them physically or in reduced surroundings, is more significant in the elderly. Moves—for family proximity, for ease of physical maintenance, or for nursing care—represent the loss of perhaps a lifetime of familiar and cherished surroundings. All of these losses appear to increase suicide risks among the elderly.[17]

One vulnerability the elderly do not suffer from disproportionately as a group is poverty. This is not to say that there are not significant numbers of the elderly living in poverty; it is just to say that the percentages of the elderly in poverty are lower than percentages in other age cohorts. Access to medical care through Medicare and Medicaid, and to other social services, moreover, is also higher among the elderly than among other social groups. The elderly—12.5 percent of the population—receive 60 percent of federal social spending.[18] Elderly immigrants dependent on Medicaid or SSI, however, recently received a bitter reminder of the uncertain foundation of such social safety net spending. Speculations about the insecurity of Social Security and Medicare more generally are much in the public eye. Although the voting elderly as a political force remain virtually untouchable, intergenerational strife may put increasing pressure on expenditures on the elderly in more or less subtle ways, such as the vast expansion in the efforts to reduce Medicare spending. And although the current elderly are relatively well off in comparison to other age cohorts, they still have many unmet needs—for example, for social services that support continued independent living or appropriate levels of long-term care.[19] Indeed, social service spending on the elderly often fails to be directed towards amelioration of the losses of independence that appear to be associated with increased risks of suicide. Suicide in nursing homes, for example, appears to be associated with such factors as lack of privacy in living design, staff turnover, and limited staff education.[20]

The link between all of these losses and suicide among the elderly is depression. Physical debility, the death of loved ones, reduced independence, and economic instability, all contribute to depression among the elderly. What we should conclude from these facts about competence and the rationality of suicide among the elderly is controversial. Suicide prevention specialists conclude that "suicide in the elderly is treatable and preventable," and that prevention starts with treatment of depression.[21] The conclusion that suicide in the elderly always results from treatable depression, however, would appear to be an assertion that is neither empirical nor based in a clear distinction between depression and reasoned evaluation of problematic life circumstances. Richman, for example, contends that the vulnerabilities of the elderly, particularly depression, mean that suicide is virtually never freely chosen: "The so-called free choice of death is rarely free because of the complex of forces impinging upon the suicidal person. If the right to live is disregarded, then the right to die may become a compulsion to die. The choice of not committing suicide is an affirmation of life, but we hear too little of that for the elderly."[22] Other commentators regard depression among the elderly as grounds for rejecting insistence on paradigms of autonomy for them: "It is at least arguable that the pure autonomy model often used in bioethics and the law is a too-abstract, rationalistic myth that does not square with or explain the concrete situations such as those involving the depressed elderly. No one is ever truly and completely autonomous. Autonomy is, rather, a matter of degree."[23]

Careful attention to the nature of depression, and its relationship to capacities for reasoned decision-making, suggests instead renewed scrutiny of the evidence we require for judgments of competence. In the mental health literature, major depression is defined as a combination of a persistent dysphoric mood with symptoms such as loss of appetite, insomnia, decreased energy and increased fatigue, restlessness, loss of interest or pleasure, self-reproach, diminished ability to concentrate, preoccupation with bodily functions, and suicidal ideations.[24] It is not simply grief from a loss, disappointment in the inability to enjoy former valued activities, or worry about economic security. In some cases, depression is secondary to physical conditions that occur with greater frequency among the elderly: parkinsonism, dyspnea, or anti-hypertensive therapy, for example. When depression is secondary, the possibility at least exists that it can be alleviated by adjustment of therapy. For primary depression, or for secondary depression that cannot otherwise be remedied, treatment options range from psychotropic medication to psychotherapy to a variety of nursing and other therapeutic interventions. In either case—treatable or not—the issue of relevance to PAS and the elderly is whether the frequency of depression among the elderly reflects special issues about the capacity of the elderly for reasoned decision-making, or, in turn, special reasons to question the competence of the elderly. My contention is that, like the prevalence of cognitive decline, the frequency of depression suggests careful attention to evidence about competence generally, rather than the judgment that the elderly are special with regard to PAS.

Depression can impair capacities for reasoned decision-making in several major ways. First, the process for identifying values can be affected. Sufferers from major depression may lose interest in anything, or cease to find pleasure in once-cherished activities. Such extensive losses of the ability to enjoy anything are quite different from the recognition that one can no longer engage in the activities that gave life pleasure, be they playing the violin (because arthritis has compromised dexterity), attending concerts (because physical weakness makes it very difficult), or simply listening to music (because deafness has become profound and irremediable). Sufferers from depression may also experience reduced cognitive capacities; indeed, one of the difficulties in diagnosing depression among the elderly apparently consists in sorting out whether cognitive deficits are symptomatic of depression or of associated physical ailments.[25] Yet another problem associated with depression is the ability to link information to outcomes that will realize values, either because of cognitive decline or because of loss of interest and unwillingness to perform reasoning tasks. Decisions that apparently rest on a loss of values or an abrupt change of values, or on inadequately understood information, would, then, raise questions about loss of capacities for reasoned decision-making due to depression. So would decisions that apparently mismatched values and chosen alternatives, without proffered explanation. If serious enough, such impairments might trigger judgments of incompetence.

Although the elderly experience depression with some frequency, it is not a condition that is confined to them. Similar apparent difficulties in reasoned decision-making ought to trigger inquiries about capacities and competence at any age. Indeed, as I have suggested earlier, where life is at stake as in PAS there is reason to seek evidence of competence whatever the apparent capacity for reasoned decision-making. My conclusion would therefore be a required psychological consultation in any policy permitting PAS, whether for the elderly or for other age groups.

Impaired decision-making capacity is not the only way in which vulnerability and loss might affect the autonomy of the elderly. Autonomy requires not only the capacity for reasoned decision-making, but a reasonable range of alternatives among which to choose. For the elderly, economic insecurity, family rejection or pressures, or availability of social services such as home care may significantly reduce the range of available options. Such limits in options are viewed by the ABA Commission as a major obstacle to the desirability of legalizing assisted suicide. So they are. But they do not show the elderly are a special case; indeed, the elderly may be better off in some of these respects than other age cohorts. What they do show is the need for great caution, and nowhere is this more apparent than in the availability of medical services.

Access to Healthcare and Support

Another concern about the vulnerability of the elderly raised with respect to PAS is access to healthcare. The American Geriatrics Society's opposition to PAS rests on the dilemma for the physician who seeks to serve the interests of patients in a context of inadequate resources. Inadequacies may range from unwillingness to fund aggressive care aimed at cure, to perceived legal barriers to adequate palliation, to the inadequacies in nursing home staffing that correlate with higher suicide rates. Concerns about the availability of good palliative care in the United States are well known. In the wake of the passage and repassage of the Oregon

Death with Dignity Act, healthcare providers at the Oregon Health Sciences University have concentrated on improving good palliative care and access to hospice care in the state so that patients are not coerced by pain to select PAS.[26]

These concerns are all very real and are grounds for significant caution in any move towards legalization of PAS. In addition, the need for such services correlates with being older. Issues of access to palliative and other forms of care are not, however, in any way unique to the elderly. Once again, the conclusion to be drawn is that concerns about access are grounds for careful scrutiny of any individual decision to undertake PAS. This would suggest a required medical consultation in any PAS decision, both as to whether available care modalities have been explored and as to whether palliative care has been adequate—as well as whether its potentialities have been adequately explained to the patient.

The Moral Significance of Being Old

To this point, I have argued that cognitive declines, vulnerabilities, and inadequate access to healthcare are reasons for careful scrutiny of any decision involving PAS—in particular, of competence, absence of major depression, and understanding of available therapeutic alternatives. My argument has been based on the observation that although all these are issues that arise with frequency in the elderly, they are not issues that arise specifically with being old. What is unique to the elderly, however, is the fact of being old itself. In this section, I take up two reasons why age itself might be thought relevant to PAS. First, the elderly, by being old, have lived longer and experienced more of the good of life. Second, the elderly, by being closer to death, have less to lose in PAS. I argue that neither is a reason for thinking the default position about the reasonableness of PAS should be set differently for the elderly than for other age groups. Critical assessment of each of these reasons, however, suggests that we should not easily assume PAS is the rational decision for members of any age cohort. One public policy this assessment suggests is a limitation of PAS, at least for the near future, to patients who are terminally ill.

The elderly, to be sure, have lived longer than the young. This fact might be thought to have important distributive justice consequences. Because the elderly have experienced more of the good of life, an egalitarian might argue, there is reason to skew distribution of scarce goods to the young. This point was defended a number of years ago by Veatch.[27] It was also perhaps Governor Lamm's point in advocating rationing after a certain age. In seeking to prevent a future of gloom, Lamm hurled dire prophesies for the year 2000. For healthcare, the prophesy was a proposal not to fund organ transplants, artificial organs, or any extraordinary procedures for anyone over the age of sixty-five. Lamm's ironic fantasy defense of such a policy, aimed to get public policy makers to consider rationing seriously, was perhaps not meant to be taken literally: "We should spend our money intelligently where it will buy the greatest amount of American health. That would clearly not be on artificial organs for the few but on preventive healthcare for the many."[28]

Such rather straightforward egalitarianism assumes that having lived longer is a rough correlate for having had more of the goods of life. But those who have not been particularly fortunate in distribution of the goods of life—the poor, or perhaps women who have spent their lives in caring for others—might quite reasonably object that age alone is no indicator of distributive privilege. Norman Daniels's well-known defense of a more sophisticated egalitarian argument for age-rationing in healthcare avoids this objection. Daniels's argument is that rational individuals who do not know their ages but who have access to a fair share of resources for healthcare would choose to allocate those resources differentially over the life-span. At younger ages, they would prefer to spend resources to maximize their chances of living a normal life-span; at older ages, they would prefer to spend resources on comfort care. At all ages, spending would be directed to efforts to achieve the normal opportunity range for that age.[29] Thus against a background of the just distribution of social goods, there might be reason to skew the distribution of scarce and expensive life-extending care to the young; if so, the elderly, faced with more limited therapeutic options although hopefully not more limited palliative options (assuming palliation is relatively cheap), might rationally prefer the availability of PAS.

Daniels's argument, however, does not show that the elderly would have special reason to want PAS. It shows at most that they might want it more frequently. For there will be cases among the young, too, where life-extending care might not be expected to work, where palliation is problematic, or where control of the shape of death is a paramount value. In such cases, whether for an older person or for a younger person, PAS might be a desired option, and so availability of PAS might be important to the range of choices needed for autonomy.

On the other hand, on Daniels's view, there is an important reason for being careful about whether PAS is the desired option for anyone. Daniels argues that people would allocate resources over the life cycle with regard to the normal opportunity range at each stage of life. The notion of a "normal opportunity range" is defined as "the array of life plans reasonable persons are likely to construct for themselves. The normal range is thus dependent on key features of the society—its stage of historical development, its level of material wealth and technological development, and even important cultural facts about it."[30] This definition of the normal opportunity range raises the possibility that cultural attitudes might shift, due for example to economic pressures, and that such shifts might in turn be experienced as coercive by those faced with the choice. Indeed, such shifts might be based on stereotypical assumptions about what people want when they are old, which bear tenuous relationships to what people actually want. Indeed, there is some empirical data to suggest just such stereotypes might be operative; both younger people and even older people themselves overestimate significantly the actual self-reported rates of loneliness and ill-health among the elderly.[31] If, for example, PAS became more common, even offered as one of the range of medical options, it might come to be seen as part of the normal opportunity range or even as the option older people really ought to take. It is the possibility of such subtle or not-so-subtle cultural shifts, with attendent risks that people will be encouraged or pressured into the option, that groups such as the ABA Commission fear when they recommend extreme caution in the legalization of PAS. The point that there are reasons based in distributive justice for differential allocations across the life-span, then, should not be confused with the assumption that people are characteristically less likely to want potentially life-extending therapy at one point in the life-cycle than at another.[32] Indeed, if we do think that life-cycle rationing is to some extent justified, we should be especially careful not to confuse that allocative decision within a single life, with pressure on one generation (that, say, born in the 1920s) to make way for a later generation (that, say, born in the 1960s). The conclusion to be drawn from the idea of life-cycle rationing is thus that we should be especially careful not to sacrifice one generation to the next through stereotyping or covert economic pressure. Far from presuming that PAS is a rational option for the elderly, we should instead be careful to examine whether it is a reasoned choice in any circumstances—that is, whether the choice really stems from the patient's understanding of his or her values and options, or whether it results from subtle forms of coercion.

Another characteristic of the elderly qua elderly is that they are closer to the end of a standard life span. This proximity, it might be argued, changes the understanding of the extent to which death is an evil for the elderly. A considerable amount of recent philosophical attention has been devoted to what is bad about death itself, for the person who dies (not what is painful or otherwise problematic about the dying process—what is bad about death itself). On an experience-based account, what is bad about death is that it involves bad experiences, or at least the bad experience of not having good experiences. If there is no experiencing subject after death, however, it would seem that there are no bad experiences postmortem, either. Assuming the absence of an experiencing subject, what then is bad about death? One nonexperiential account is that death is bad because it results in there being less intrinsic value in the world: Someone who dies has fewer of the actively experienced goods of life than s/he otherwise would have had.[33] On this view, for the elderly, death might then be less bad than for the young, since there is presumably a shorter strand of lost goods of life in the one case than in the other. (Of course, if the ongoing stream would have contained actively experienced evils rather than goods, the person who dies sooner suffers a lesser evil than the person who dies later.) Frances Kamm points out that we may think death is bad not just because the person who dies has fewer of the goods of life, but because the person's having goods is all over.[34] On this account, what is different about the old is that they are closer to the standard time at which their having of the goods of life will be all over. Another similar account of the evil of death, offered by Bernard Williams, is that it interferes with categorical plans—plans a person has that are not contingent on whether s/he goes on living. On this account, being old might be a special case if the old have characteristically fewer or different categorical plans—if, for example, they are at a place in the life-cycle where closure rather than new beginnings tends to be typical.[35] Finally, Frances Kamm suggests that an explanation of the asymmetry of our judgments about birth and death—death seems worse than not having been born, declines worse than inclines—is that we are deeply concerned about the shape of our ending because people tend to be remembered for what happens last.[36] This, too, might suggest increased interest among the elderly in control over the manner of their dying.

If these accounts suggest that death is differently evil for the elderly, they might be grounds for drawing different conclusions about whether PAS is generally reasonable in that age group. Do the elderly, in short, have less to lose (and perhaps more to gain) through PAS? To the contrary, these accounts of what is bad about death arguably suggest that being terminally ill, rather than being old, is what might support a judgment that PAS is reasonable. If a terminally ill person dies earlier, the lost stream of valued experiences that s/he might have had extends only over the time s/he would have had before death. Sad but true, the time at which it will be all over is near. The categorical plans that are cut off by a suicide instead of by a slightly later death may be relatively few. And the moment of decline may be at hand, indeed a moment of decline that is etched more starkly in the memories of survivors for having come untimely soon. Thus accounts of the evil of death suggest, sadly but surely, that it is terminal illness rather than age itself that may be connected to the reasonableness of PAS. This is not to argue for a stereotyped view about terminal illness—that PAS is in fact reasonable in such cases. Perhaps particularly for the terminally ill there may be a great deal to lose with PAS: life's most precious, because fleeting, moments. It is to argue that on some contemporary nonexperiential accounts of the evil of death, being near to death, not being old, is the factor that would matter with respect to the reasonableness of PAS.

Background presumptions about reasonableness, it seems to me, play a role in deciding regulatory limits as well as in specifying evidentiary standards. The judgment that PAS is highly likely to be unreasonable in a particular group may be grounds for keeping the barriers to its exercise in that group quite high indeed. I have just argued that on some contemporary accounts of the evil of death, age itself is not a relevant factor to the reasonableness of PAS. Slightly earlier timing, especially in light of unwanted and expected evils in the dying process, may be relevant instead. What this suggests for public policy is that if there are grounds for lowering the barriers to PAS, for example through legalization, terminal illness rather than age is a more relevant starting point.

Conclusion

Background presumptions about reasonableness determine the "default" position—the position that will be assumed to operate unless there is evidence at some specified level to the contrary. With respect to PAS, I have argued, being old does not suggest a shift in the default position and a presumption against PAS. The successful carrying out of PAS is a momentous decision from which there is no return. The default position with respect to PAS, therefore, recommends that we should insist on evidence of competence, absence of major depression, and understanding of medical (including palliative) alternatives, before the choice is undertaken. Translated into public policy, this default position would recommend safeguards that include a competence assessment, a psychological consultation, and at least a second medical opinion, regardless of the age of the patient contemplating PAS.

Background presumptions about reasonableness may also lead us to erect regulatory barriers against certain behavior, on the basis that it is highly unlikely to be reasonable. I have examined and rejected arguments that, because the elderly have lived longer or because they are closer to the end of a normal life span, PAS is more likely to be reasonable for them. If there is any connection between the nearness of death and the reasonableness of PAS, it is for the terminally ill, not the old. This perhaps is the best explanation for a public policy choice to make an exception for the terminally ill, if indeed we are going to lower the barriers to PAS in any case. At the same time, ironically for the same reasons, it is especially important to be sure that PAS is a genuinely autonomous choice in this group of patients. If we think PAS may be more reasonable for the terminally ill than for others, there is all the more reason to be certain it is genuinely chosen in any particular case.

Notes

1. American Bar Association, Commission on the Legal Problems of the Elderly, Report to the House of Delegates, May 21, 1997.
2. G. A. Sachs, J. C. Aronheim, J. A. Rhymes, L. Volicer, and J. Lynn, "Good Care of Dying Patients: the Alternatives to Physician-Assisted Suicide and Euthanasia," *Journal of the American Geriatrics Society* 43: 553–62 (1995). Sounding a theme similar to that of the ABA, a recent editorial in *Geriatrics* observed, "Americans may soon be in the peculiar position of having the legal right to secure physicians' help in committing suicide before they have the universal right to healthcare." Robert Butler, "The Dangers of Physician-Assisted Suicide," *Geriatrics* 51: 14–15 (1996).
3. American Geriatrics Society Ethics Committee, "Position Statement: Physician-Assisted Suicide and Voluntary Active Euthanasia," *Journal of the American Geriatrics Society* 43: 579–80 (1995).
4. Brief of the American Geriatrics Society as Amicus Curiae, *Vacco* v. *Quill*, *Washington* v. *Glucksberg*, Nos. 95–1858 and 96–110 (Nov. 12, 1996).
5. *Modern Maturity*, Nov./Dec. 1997, p. 91.
6. For example, Utah Code Ann. § 75–2–1105.5 (1997). That the Utah procedure is quite cumbersome reflects the strength of the presumption that people would prefer aggressive intervention when paramedics are called.
7. Roberta Richardson, Steven Lowenstein, and Michael Weissberg, "Coping With the Suicidal Elderly: A Physician's Guide," *Geriatrics* 44: 43–51 (1989). Richard Posner points out, however, that aggregate data may conceal important differences, for example in the rates of suicide when state of health is held constant. Richard Posner, *Aging and Old Age* (Chicago: University of Chicago Press, 1995), p. 236.
8. Nancy J. Osgood, Barbara A. Brant, and Aaron Lipman, *Suicide Among the Elderly in Long-Term Care Facilities* (New York: Greenwood Press), 1991, pp. 1–2.
9. See Susan Parry, "Rationality, Competence, and Informed Consent," M.A. Thesis, University of Utah, 1997 (on file at the University of Utah Marriott Library).
10. Allen Buchanan and Dan Brock, *Deciding for Others: The Ethics of Surrogate Decision-making* (New York: Cambridge University Press, 1989). "Competence" expresses the

conclusion that a person's decisions ought to be respected—that, for example, the person is regarded as a legal decision-maker in his or her own right.

11. See, e.g., Sara Horton-Deutsch, David Clark, and Carol Ferrin, "Chronic Dyspnea and Suicide in Elderly Men," *Hospital and Community Psychiatry* 43: 1198–1203 (1992), p. 1202.

12. Richard Posner, *Aging and Old Age* (Chicago: University of Chicago Press, 1995), p. 20.

13. Some courts have applied the "mature minor" doctrine to allow near-eighteen-year-olds to refuse medical treatment. For example, the Illinois Supreme Court affirmed a decision that a seventeen-and-a-half-year-old Jehovah's Witness should be allowed to refuse blood transfusions in connection with treatment for leukemia: "In the matter before us, E. G. was a minor, but one who was just months shy of her eighteenth birthday, and an individual that the record indicates was mature for her age. Although the age of majority in Illinois is eighteen, that age is not an impenetrable barrier that magically precludes a minor from possessing and exercising certain rights normally associated with adulthood." In *re E.G.*, 549 N.E.2d 322 (Ill. 1989).

14. See, e.g., Larry Strasburger and Sue Welpton, "Elderly Suicide: Minimizing Risk for Patient and Professional," *Journal of Geriatric Psychiatry* 24: 235–59 (1991), p. 239.

15. Sara L. Horton-Deutsch, David Clark, and Carol J. Farran, "Chronic Dyspnea and Suicide in Elderly Men," *Hospital and Community Psychiatry* 43: 1198–1203 (1992).

16. See, e.g., Nancy J. Osgood, Barbara A. Brant, and Aaron Lipman, *Suicide Among the Elderly in Long-Term Care Facilities* (New York: Greenwood Press, 1991), pp. 95–98.

17. See, e.g., Larry Strasburger and Sue Welpton, "Elderly Suicide: Minimizing Risk for Patient and Professional," *Journal of Geriatric Psychiatry* 24: 235–59 (1991).

18. Samuel Issacharoff and Erica Worth Harris, "Is Age Discrimination Really Age Discrimination?: The ADEA's Unnatural Solution," *New York University Law Review* 72: 780–837 (1997), p. 811.

19. Norman Daniels, *Am I My Parents' Keeper?* (New York: Oxford University Press, 1988).

20. Osgood et al., chapter 8.

21. E.g., Joseph Richman, *Preventing Elderly Suicide* (New York: Springer Publishing Co., 1993), p. vii.

22. Richman, p. xii.

23. Adil E. Shamoo and Dianne N. Irving, "The PSDA and the Depressed Elderly: "Intermittent Competency" Revisited," *The Journal of Clinical Ethics* 4: 74–80 (1993).

24. See, e.g., Osgood et al., p. 109.

25. Roberta Richardson, Steven Lowenstein, and Michael Weissberg, "Coping With the Suicidal Elderly: A Physician's Guide," *Geriatrics* 44: 43–51 (1989).

26. Susan Tolle made this point in a 1997 posting on Bioethics Network.

27. Robert Veatch, ed., *Life Span: Values and Life-Extending Technologies* (New York: Harper and Row, 1979).

28. Governor Richard Lamm, *Megatraumas* (Boston: Houghton-Mifflin, 1985), p. 46. Governor Lamm might have added that the probabilities are that a life-saving procedure in a sixty-five-year-old will buy fewer years of lives lived than a life-saving procedure in a thirty-five-year-old.

29. Norman Daniels, *Am I My Parents' Keeper?* (New York: Oxford University Press, 1988). Daniels' argument is that age-rationing in healthcare should be viewed as a problem in allocation across the life-cycle, rather than as a conflict between age cohorts. Particularly because different generations experience different starting levels, and because public policy changes as they go along, it is not clear that actual public policy making can avoid inter-cohort conflicts. The abolition of mandatory retirement is a good example; while it may in fact appear reasonable from the point of view of intra-cohort justice to abandon mandatory retirement in favor of liberty of choice about how long one will work, there is evidence that this choice for the current age cohort is having potentially serious consequences for the age cohorts that follow. Samuel Issacharoff and Erica Worth Harris, "Is Age Discrimination Really Age Discrimination?: The ADEA's Unnatural Solution," *New York University Law Review* 72: 780–836 (1997).

30. Norman Daniels, *Am I My Parents' Keeper?* (New York: Oxford University Press, 1988), p. 69.

31. Roberta Richardson, Steven Lowenstein, and Michael Weissberg, "Suicide in the Elderly: An Image Problem." *Geriatrics* 44: 47 (1989). The authors suggest that mistaken beliefs that rates of poor health and depression are very high among the elderly may contribute to judgments that suicide would be rational in this age group—for example, that "the elder "has every reason to be depressed," or that "if I were in his place I would want to die, too," or "It's his right to die if he wishes.' "

32. This point parallels Daniels's observation that allocation over the life span of a given generation should not be confused with allocation among generations.

33. Thomas Nagel, *Mortal Questions* (Cambridge: Cambridge University Press, 1979). Fred Feldman defends a similar non-experience based account of the evil of death for the one who dies—that the life of one who dies young contains less intrinsically-based value for him than the live of one who lives on. *Conversations with the Reaper* (New York: Oxford University Press, 1992), p. 139.

34. F. M. Kamm, *Morality, Mortality*, vol. 1, *Death and Whom to Save from It* (New York: Oxford University Press, 1993), p. 20.

35. See Bernard Williams, "The Makropoulos Case, or the Tedium of Immortality," in James Rachels, ed., *Moral Problems*, 1st ed. (New York: Harper and Row, 1971).

36. F. M. Kamm. *Morality, Mortality*, vol. 1, *Death and Whom to Save from It* (New York: Oxford University Press, 1993), pp. 67–71.

5

Lessons for Physician–Assisted Suicide from the African–American Experience

PATRICIA A. KING AND LESLIE E. WOLF

This chapter is premised on the view that this society has an insufficient understanding of how and why competent individuals are rendered vulnerable near the end-of-life. Specifically, inadequate attention has been given to the socio-historical and cultural contexts in which individuals function and the import such contexts have for end-of-life decision-making. It explores the African-American experience with medicine for the insights that such scrutiny offers for protecting persons from coercion, stigma, and societal indifference. Historical interactions between African-Americans and medicine and persistent health disparities between blacks and whites have implications for the relationship between African-Americans and the healthcare system. African-Americans reasonably worry that their lives are not as highly valued as whites and that their preferences for end-of-life care are neither understood nor respected. It concludes that with greater appreciation and knowledge of the realities of African-Americans as well as other patients' lives, it should be possible to modify existing institutional arrangements and practices in the healthcare system in ways that will empower and protect all patients. Only then should physician-assisted suicide be made available as an option for dying patients.

*   *   *

> While we were watching round her bed,
> She turned her eyes and looked away,
> She saw what we couldn't see;
> She saw Old Death. She saw Old Death.
> Coming like a falling star.
> But Death didn't frighten Sister Caroline;
> He looked to her like a welcome friend.
> And she whispered to us: I'm going home,
> And she smiled and closed, her eyes.
>
> —James Weldon Johnson,
> *Go Down Death—A Funeral Sermon*

THE INCREASING MEDICALIZATION of death has led to widespread fear that death is unnecessarily prolonged, painful, expensive, and without dignity. This fear has given momentum to the desire of patients to have more control over their dying and to the movement to legalize physician-assisted suicide (PAS) and active voluntary euthanasia (AVE). Others may have a different fear.

They may be concerned that their lives are not highly valued in this society and thus fear that they will not have access to life-prolonging treatment or palliative care that for them represents death with dignity. Moreover, many others may not share either of these fears, considering death a "welcome friend" to be greeted with family or, in any event, a process that is beyond their control. Making sure that all of these voices are heard in the PAS debate is a challenge.

When the Supreme Court held unanimously in *Washington* v. *Glucksberg* and *Quill* v. *Vacco* that state laws prohibiting assisted suicides did not violate the due process or equal protection clauses of the Fourteenth Amendment, the opinions of the Justices reflected concern that the interests of all patients should be protected.[1] For example, the majority opinion in *Glucksberg* recognized that states have an interest "in protecting vulnerable groups—including the poor, the elderly, and disabled persons—from abuse, neglect, and mistakes."[2] Citing the work of the New York State Task Force on Life and the Law (New York Task Force), the majority opinion stated that "[t]he risk of harm is greatest for the many individuals in our society whose autonomy and well-being are already compromised by poverty, lack of access to good medical care, advanced age or membership in a stigmatized social group."[3] Significantly, the opinion pointed out that "[t]he state's interest [in protecting the interests of all patients] . . . goes beyond protecting the vulnerable from coercion; it extends to protecting disabled and terminally ill people from prejudice, negative and inaccurate stereotypes and societal indifference."[4]

As a result of these rulings, the states will have the responsibility for insuring that the interests of all patients near the end-of-life are not imperiled. Whether it is possible for the states to make available a compassionate option of last resort for some competent, terminally ill patients, without, as a practical matter, making it harder for other patients to exercise their preferences for life prolonging treatment or palliative care is a vexing public policy matter. As the New York Task Force has pointed out, "[f]or purposes of public debate, one can describe cases of assisted suicide in which all recommended safeguards would be satisfied. But positing an 'ideal' or 'good' case is not sufficient for public policy, if it bears little relation to prevalent social and medical practices."[5] Moreover, the medical context is inextricably linked with the social and economic inequities existing in the broader society. Again, as the New York Task Force persuasively notes, "no matter how carefully any guidelines are framed, assisted suicide and euthanasia will be practiced through the prism of social inequality and bias that characterizes the delivery of services in all segments of our society, including healthcare."[6]

While we share many of the concerns and values espoused by proponents of PAS and AVE, we believe that existing prohibitions on PAS and AVE should be maintained for the foreseeable future. Central to our argument is the view that this society does not have a sufficient understanding of how and why competent individuals are rendered vulnerable near the end-of-life. We are especially concerned that inadequate attention has been given to the socio-historical and cultural contexts in which competent individuals function. If we do not fully appreciate the multiple ways in which an individual's autonomy and well-being can be compromised, we cannot modify existing institutional arrangements and practices in the healthcare system in ways that will empower and protect *all* patients. It is important to empower patients so that their decisions will be respected, while at the same time protecting them from abuse and exploitation.

The African-American Experience Illuminates the PAS Debate

In a real sense all patients near the end-of-life are at risk of having their autonomy and well-being compromised. It is commonly accepted, however, that members of certain groups are at special risk and perhaps in need of protection. The term "vulnerable" which is applied to a broad spectrum of groups reflects this concern. What makes group members vulnerable, or how their vulnerability is the same or different across groups, however, is neither well defined nor understood.

There is broad consensus that groups whose members lack capacity altogether or have impaired capacity should be viewed as vulnerable. There is less agreement on whether groups whose members are primarily competent adults, such as prisoners or physically disabled persons, should be considered vulnerable to coercion. Even if we can agree that these groups are deserving of special attention, controversy may remain about what circumstances, conditions, or social practices should trigger closer scrutiny of decisions made by members of the group.[7]

Whether particular group members, in contrast to groups themselves, are at special risk of coercion is even more difficult to unravel. Individuals may belong to multiple groups and thus are potentially vulnerable for many different reasons. Alternatively, individual members of a group that is regarded as vulnerable may not be susceptible to coercion or undue influence. Here the danger is that appeal to a shared experience may obscure the heterogeneity of group members.[8]

Our dilemma is this. There is general agreement that with competent adults paternalism or interference with self-determination should be avoided. At the same time there is fear that the institutional and social context will constrain competent patients' choices in such a way as to suggest that their choices are coerced. We seem to have only two options.

One approach is to protect vulnerable persons through increased vigilance or special procedural safeguards. Frequently however, there is disagreement about what restrictions promote and respect self-determination or where there is so little protection that exploitation results. Moreover, restrictions may not offer needed protection. And if adequate protection is afforded, safeguards may result in denying desired benefits to individuals who are members of the group we are seeking to protect.

An alternative approach permits competent persons to make choices. This approach ignores the conditions that make for vulnerability and emphasizes the potential and undesirability of paternalism, leaving vulnerable persons to look after themselves and to secure benefits they desire. The Ninth Circuit opinion in *Compassion in Dying* v. *Washington* is instructive in this regard. The majority opinion reasoned:

[t]his rationale [prohibiting PAS in order to protect the poor and minorities from exploitation] simply recycles one of the more disingenuous and fallacious arguments raised in opposition to the legalization of abortion. It is equally meretricious here. . . . [A]s with abortion, there is far more reason to raise the opposite concern: the concern that the poor and the minorities, who have historically received the least adequate healthcare, will not be afforded a fair opportunity to obtain the medical assistance to which they are entitled—the assistance that would allow them to end their lives with a measure of dignity. The argument that disadvantaged persons will receive *more* medical services than the remainder of the population . . . is ludicrous on its face. So too, is the argument that the poor and the minorities will rush to volunteer for physician-assisted suicide because of their inability to secure adequate medical treatment.[9]

The court ignores the fact that historically minorities and the poor have been abused and have had their preferences ignored, if indeed, their preferences were solicited at all. While it correctly points out that some minority group members may be denied a benefit that they seek, the court overlooks the fact that minorities might prefer benefits that promote health and well-being in view of existing inequities in health status, healthcare coverage, and the delivery of healthcare services rather than access to PAS. Even if minority individuals desired access to PAS, they are not necessarily able to secure this or other benefits because they lack power in the society. Thus, neither approach is optimal because it is necessary both to provide access to benefits and at the same time avoid harms.

It is therefore important to assess carefully the conditions of inclusion or access to benefits. For example, an empowered patient may need fewer protections from society because the ability to protect oneself may have increased. The starting point is to develop thick descriptions of patients in order to learn why, if at all, they are vulnerable. We need to know patients not merely in terms of abnormalities in the structure and function of their body organs and systems, but also as persons situated in broader social, economic, historical, and cultural contexts.[10] In actual encounters with healthcare professionals, the patient's understanding of illness and how the patient communicates about his or her health problems is shaped by these factors. We also need to understand who the physician is, the dynamics of the relationship between professional and patient, and the impact of societal structures on that relationship. It is only by understanding these matters that we will be able to identify and modify the structural inequities in medicine that compromise the interests of competent persons when making end-of-life decisions.

An examination of the African-American patient will expand the array of portraits of patients who face death and worry about dying with dignity. In expanding the images of patients faced with end-of-life decision-making, we enhance our understanding of patients' cultural, religious, and family values and the complexity of decision-making with respect to PAS. Some of these patients will prefer life-prolonging treatment or palliative care. Other patients will not seek access to PAS and AVE because they mistrust healthcare professionals and medical institutions.

Yale Kamisar points out that, "[m]any people, understandably, are greatly affected by the heart-wrenching facts of individual cases."[13] There is no doubt that the suffering and anguish of some patients is compelling. Many people identify with these patients and worry that they will find themselves in the same position. We are understandably reluctant to deny interventions that would relieve suffering and bring about desired relief through death. There are also moving stories that point out the dangers of too quickly acceding to requests for physician-assisted suicide and euthanasia. Yet, the portraits of potential victims of PAS and euthanasia have attracted less public attention. John Arras, a philosopher and bioethicist, writes:

> The victims of the current policy are easy to identify: they are on the news, the talk shows, the documentaries, and often on Dr. Kevorkian's roster of so-called "patients." The victims of legalization, by contrast, will be largely hidden from view: they will include the clinically depressed 80-year-old man who could have lived for another year of good quality if only he had been treated; the 50-year-old woman who asks for death because doctors in her financially stretched HMO cannot/will not effectively treat her unrelenting but mysterious pelvic pain; and perhaps eventually, if we slide far enough down the slope, the uncommunicative stroke victim whose distant children deem an earlier death a better death. Unlike Dr. Kevorkian's "patients," these victims will not get their pictures in the paper, but they will have faces and they will all be cheated of good months or perhaps even years.[12]

Most descriptions of potential victims of legalizing PAS, however, fail to include images of members of stigmatized minority groups.[13]

There is evidence that members of groups considered vulnerable have different attitudes about end-of-life treatment than the majority of Americans who support assisting the terminally ill to die. Disparities are greatest, however, in attitudes, values, and beliefs about end-of-life decision-making with racial and ethnic minorities. Studies show that blacks are substantially less likely than whites to support legalization of physician-assisted suicide.[14] Although the support for legalization has increased over time in both groups, the gap in support between blacks and whites persists.[15] There is also evidence that these differences arise in attitudes towards other end-of-life issues such as use of life-prolonging treatment, advance directives and living wills.[16]

Why these substantial gaps in attitudes about end-of-life decision-making exist is not clear. The available evidence indicates that these differences persist even when researchers control for education, age, and socioeconomic status. Possible reasons for this difference in attitude include religious preferences, blacks' distrust of physicians, medical institutions and the healthcare system generally, and cultural characteristics such as trusting families more than physicians.[17]

Specifically, these differences in attitude towards PAS may reflect differences in black expression of health and illness as well as concerns about death. Not only have African-Americans experienced disrespect for their autonomy, they have suffered injustice in medicine as well as in the broader society. As a group, blacks have been abused, neglected and exploited. They have reason to believe that their lives are not valued in the same way as whites' and rationally perceive that, in their encounters with the healthcare system, they are frequently treated differently solely because of their race.[18] African-Americans have reason to be suspicious of physicians and rightly worry about giving them too much authority. In the medical context, physician paternalism builds on and reinforces ubiquitous race differentials in power and authority. In short, historical and current experiences with American medicine have made African-Americans acutely aware of the difficulty of looking after their own interests because they lack power in the society and in the healthcare system, and in their relationships with physicians.

Ordinary practices, norms, and habits of well-intentioned institutions and professions can result in unjust practices for some groups.[19] Those with power in the society are able to impose their norms, values, and beliefs on those who lack power. The dominant group's ideas, beliefs, and judgments serve to stigmatize and mark other groups as different and deficient. Behaviors and practices of the stigmatized group are often considered unworthy of study or respect.

The myth of white superiority persists and has profoundly affected both whites and blacks. As Professor Charles Lawrence notes, "[w]e do not recognize the ways in which our [shared] cultural experience has influenced our beliefs about race or the occasions on which those beliefs affect our actions."[20] Stereotypes that capture and reflect negative attitudes towards African-Americans flourish and become embedded in the culture to the point where they may not be consciously noticed. Thus, injury frequently is inflicted on blacks without the actors being consciously aware of racial motivation.[21]

It is not only the dominant group, however, that is affected. Negative messages are also absorbed by blacks themselves. Feelings of inferiority and unworthiness are among the psychic injuries inflicted on blacks. As a result, they carry the additional burden of not always appreciating their own worth as human beings. As Herbert Nickens points out, "such stigma is never far from consciousness for minorities and is one of the lenses through which life is perceived."[22]

Although other racial and ethnic groups have separate and distinct experiences with American medicine, an additional reason for examining the African-American experience is that African-Americans are the paradigmatic minority group in this country. They constitute approximately 12 percent of the population. Although they were not willing immigrants and endured slavery and its aftermath of rigid segregation, as people of color they have not been easily assimilated and do not share the Western European heritage and culture of some immigrants. Features of black health experience such as persistent poverty, limited access to healthcare, poorer health status, and low numbers of healthcare professionals are common to other minorities as well.

It is important to reflect on the African-American experience because it offers insights into the nature of society's responsibilities for those who are competent but whose autonomy and well-being may be compromised by historical, social, and cultural forces at work in society itself. Sadly, some individuals are in need of protection because they have been rendered vulnerable by their own society.

An Inherent Distrust of Medicine

The relationship between blacks and medicine has in the main not been beneficial for blacks. Medicine played a critical role in the development of racial differences that stamped blacks as an inherently inferior people.[23] It provided much of the theory and data that supported beliefs about biological differences observed in differences in skin color, hair appearance, and behavior between blacks and whites and confirmed the superiority of whites.[24]

The assumption that blacks were biologically inferior to whites paved the way for abuse and exploitation of blacks in medical research, education, and experimentation. Racial ideology posed obstacles to the development of adequate healthcare for blacks. Biological explanations were sometimes invoked to explain black-white differences in health. Indeed, race is still used, without appropriate explanation, along with age and gender, as a key variable in medical and epidemiological research because of the assumption that race conveys important health information. Medicine's interest in black health status historically was motivated by the self-interest of whites rather than the needs of African-Americans. This legacy of suspicion of medical professionals and institutions explains why African-Americans are likely to approach PAS with caution.

A Means to Achieve the Ends of Others

The rise of medical institutions in the nineteenth century affected blacks in at least two ways: 1) blacks were used as specimens for clinical instruction and public display and 2) blacks were disproportionately involved in research and experimentation.[25] And, although there was widespread public sentiment opposed to dissection and autopsy, black bodies were used because blacks were in no position to protect their dead.[26] Professor Todd Savitt notes that "[s]outhern medical schools could and did boast that their cities' large black populations provided ample supplies of clinical and anatomical material. And white physicians trained at these institutions carried with them into their own careers this idea of the medical usefulness of blacks."[27]

Use of black bodies for dissection and autopsy is just one example in a long history of blacks being exploited or used as a means to achieve the ends of others in medical research and experimentation.[28] During slavery blacks were subject to experimental procedures that were exploitive.[29] After slavery, the extent to which blacks were experimental subjects without their consent has not been documented. Professor Vanessa Northington Gamble's examination of folklore in the late nineteenth and early twentieth centuries, however, makes clear that blacks believed that these practices persisted.[30] Concerns about such abuse and exploitation of blacks in medical experimentation were used to press for the creation of black-controlled hospitals in the early twentieth century.[31]

The best known twentieth-century example of the use of blacks as unconsenting experimental subjects is the Tuskegee Syphilis Study. It illustrates the nature of the relationship between medicine and blacks that evolved during slavery, continued during the postemancipation period, and in some aspects is still prevalent today.

The United States Public Health Service (PHS) sponsored the Tuskegee Syphilis Study, which began in 1932 and lasted forty years. It involved 399 black men who lived in Macon County, Alabama.[32] The study was intended to observe the effects of untreated syphilis on blacks and thus held out no promise of benefit to the subjects. The subjects never consented. They were misled and never given important information about the study. When effective treatment for syphilis became available, the subjects were not provided with penicillin. Indeed, measures were taken to prevent their being treated.

Assumptions about biologically based differences in disease between blacks and whites and negative stereotypes about blacks played an important role in the creation and implementation of the Tuskegee Study. For example, the investigators accepted the medical view prevailing in the United States that syphilis affected blacks differently than whites. The PHS doctors believed that blacks had different sexual natures than whites and that blacks were more promiscuous. They also wrongly believed that blacks would not seek medical care.[33]

The PHS investigators took advantage of the subjects' bleak social and economic situation. These men were poor and lived in a rural and segregated county in the deep South. They were accustomed to responding to the authority of whites. Offers of free healthcare and payment of burial expenses were powerful incentives for participation in the Tuskegee Study. In sum, although these men were capable of making rational decisions for themselves in terms of their own interests and preferences, they were vulnerable to exploitation because of conditions in their environment. They were powerless and in no position to protect themselves from those who would take advantage of them. They understood the limitations of their lives and environment and were powerless to change it.

The lesson of Tuskegee is not only that vulnerable people can be easily exploited, but also that healthcare professionals do not always act in the best interests of their patients. It shows how scientific objectivity can be infected with bias. It suggests that abstract concepts like autonomy, self-determination, and informed consent have little meaning in circumstances where an individual's ability to protect himself or herself is blunted by persons and forces that are authoritative and powerful.

Black experience with being used as objects in medical research and experimentation has left a legacy of distrust that continues to affect the behavior and beliefs of blacks.[34] There is concern that, despite reforms in the conduct of human experimentation, blacks are still devalued in the modern research context.[35] Distrust is also evident in organ donation. Historically, blacks have been less likely than whites to agree to organ donation. Blacks have consistently linked their reluctance to the concern that if they were potential organ donors they might not be given adequate care.[36] Nation of Islam minister Louis Farrakhan's statement in a 1994 speech that whites do not stop black-on-black violence because it provides a source of organs for whites, while controversial, echoes the fear expressed by many blacks that their lives are valued less than the lives of white recipients.[37]

This distrust of the medical profession and the feeling that black lives are devalued in our society is also reflected in the allegations of genocide that are frequently voiced within the African-American community. The Tuskegee Syphilis Study left its mark in the widespread and often repeated (mis)understanding that the men of Tuskegee were deliberately infected with syphilis. The allegation of genocide also arose in connection with efforts to establish sickle cell anemia screening programs and birth control programs. More recently, the allegation has arisen in connection with the AIDS epidemic. Professor Gamble cites surveys indicating that up to one-third of African-Americans believe either that the AIDS virus was created to infect African-Americans or that it could have been created for that purpose.[38]

In short, African-Americans with reason believe that they are not always viewed as persons of unconditioned worth who are deserving of respect. These beliefs are reinforced because so little progress has been made in improving the health status of African-Americans.

The Absence of Equal Opportunity in Healthcare Access and Distribution

From the time blacks were first brought to America, one fact has been overwhelming. Blacks by any measure have been sicker and died younger than whites. Initially medical theories affirmed race-based explanations, as opposed to social and economic ones, for the difference in health status between blacks and whites. For example, during the post emancipation period, census reports, insurance statistics, and military data all indicated high mortality and morbidity rates among blacks. It was believed that the peculiar susceptibility of blacks to disease, vice, and crime were responsible for these differences.

At times, belief in the inherent differences between blacks and whites even posed obstacles to sorting through the complexities of disease such as tuberculosis and syphilis.[39] It was reassuring for whites to believe that diseases affected whites and blacks differently (and blacks more harshly) or that close observation confirmed the presence of two diseases rather than one. Negative stereotypes about blacks were frequently employed to justify perceived disease or health status disparities between blacks and whites. Often these stereotypes involved sexual promiscuity, intellectual performance, or susceptibility of blacks to disease and vice.

Explicit discrimination against African-Americans in all areas of medicine was the norm until the mid-1960s. As P. Preston Reynolds notes, "African-American students were denied admission to most medical and nursing schools, African-American physicians were rejected from membership to state and national medical societies, and African-Americans were refused care at most hospitals in this country."[40] Moreover, the Hospital Survey and Construction Act (Hill-

Burton Act) passed in 1946 contained a provision that required hospital facilities of equal quality to be built for minorities, thus introducing "separate but equal" into healthcare. As Justice Harlan points out in his dissent in *Plessey* v. *Ferguson*, the "real meaning" of segregation is "that colored citizens are so inferior and degraded that they cannot be allowed to sit in public coaches [or to share hospital wards and doctors' waiting rooms] occupied by white citizens."[41]

This explicit segregation in healthcare did not begin to change until the passage of the Civil Rights Act of 1964, which prohibited provision of federal funds to programs and institutions that discriminated on the basis of race. The creation of the Medicare program in 1965 virtually assured that every hospital in the nation would be subject to the act.

Although hospitals, unlike public schools, were required by the federal government to comply immediately with federal guidelines promulgated to achieve integration, resistance was strong. Eventually progress towards integration of facilities providing healthcare services was achieved. Yet, there is little reason to believe, in the health domain any more than in public education, that desegregation brought about equal access or equal quality of healthcare for blacks.[42] There is evidence to suggest that contemporary changes in the United States healthcare system is causing a further decline in an admittedly small pool of African-American physicians. In 1890 there were fourteen black medical schools. Today there are only four predominantly black schools training African-American physicians. Moreover, the persistent disparities in healthcare status between blacks and whites suggests that equal opportunity in health access and distribution remains an illusive goal.

African-Americans perceive that they are treated differently within the healthcare system and are more likely than whites to report difficulties in obtaining access to the healthcare system and, once they obtain care, dissatisfaction with the care they receive, including their communications with healthcare providers.[43] This perception of racial disparities in the healthcare system is supported by a host of studies demonstrating racial differences in health status, access to healthcare and quality of health across a variety of conditions and healthcare settings. While the majority of African-Americans may not be familiar with these studies, reports about them in the media reinforce the perception that African-American lives are devalued in our society.[44] The results of a recent study of Medicare beneficiaries, combined with other studies of racial disparities in health which persist after controlling for other factors thought to influence health, such as age, sex, insurance status, income, disease severity, other health conditions, and underlying incidence and prevalence rates, led one commentator to conclude that: "although both race and income have effects, race was the overriding determinant of disparities in care" and that "[h]igher incomes for blacks had a modifying—but never an equalizing—effect on black-white ratios for" certain types of care.[45]

Evidence of the racial disparities in health and healthcare comes in a number of different forms. For example, the United States mortality statistics have provided dramatic evidence of the racial difference in health status year after year. These statistics reveal that African-Americans have an overall mortality rate that is approximately 70 percent higher than that of whites.[46] The mortality differences exist across disease categories, so that the 1995 age-adjusted death rates for blacks were higher for most of the leading causes of death.[47] Indeed, a recent study reported that declines in breast cancer mortality were found only among white, not black, women.[48]

African-Americans also experience higher morbidity with respect to various disease categories, including diabetes, high blood pressure, and AIDS.[49] Similarly, numerous studies have demonstrated that African-Americans, when they are given care, receive different care than whites for the same conditions. For example, a number of studies have shown that blacks are less likely to receive angiography or to undergo coronary artery bypass surgery or angioplasty than whites.[50] Some of these differences in health status, but not all, may be explained by the fact that blacks are less likely than whites to have access to healthcare. For example, blacks are less likely than whites to have insurance and they make fewer visits to office-based physicians than whites.[51]

Recent studies suggest that these disparities in access to treatment remain, even when blacks gain access to the healthcare system.[52] For example, a number of studies have shown that blacks still have fewer physician visits and receive different treatments than whites, even within the Medicare or Veteran's Affairs populations where disparities in access have been minimized or eliminated.[53] Not only have studies shown that blacks are less likely than whites to receive certain, more common treatments, but that blacks were more likely than whites to receive certain, less common treatments. For example, blacks were more than 3.5 times more likely than whites to undergo amputation of all or part of the lower limb, even though diabetes mellitus (the most common reason for the amputation)is only 1.7 times as prevalent in elderly blacks as in whites.[54] In addition, there is evidence that, among patients seen in similar hospitals, blacks receive poorer quality of treatment than whites.[55]

While the racial disparities in treatment decisions cannot be denied, the reasons for the disparities are harder to identify. Because race is often used as a proxy for socioeconomic status, the racial disparities seen in health and healthcare could reflect socioeconomic or class differences, rather than racial differences.[56] However, racial differences in health and healthcare persist in studies that control or adjust for indicators of socioeconomic status, such as income, educational level, and insurance status. For example, a recent study which compared mortality rates among blacks and among whites living in comparable areas demonstrated that, although both poor blacks and poor whites experienced mortality rates higher than nationwide rates, poor blacks had lower survival rates than poor whites in all but one location.[57] This and other studies indicate that socioeconomic status alone cannot account for all of the documented racial differences in health and healthcare.

If racial disparities in health and healthcare access persist, as they do, among populations in which access issues have been equalized or minimized and among populations which face similar economic difficulties and barriers, we must look beyond access to explain the continuing disparities. Are there differences in the clinical encounter itself that might explain the disparities in health status between blacks and whites?

In addressing this question, some commentators have suggested that blacks and whites may differ in their treatment preferences.[58] Some evidence supports this hypothesis. For example, the Coronary Artery Surgery Study (CASS) found that whites were more likely than blacks to elect bypass surgery, even when some other, less invasive therapy was recommended and that blacks were 10 percent more likely than whites to decline an invasive treatment.[59] Differences by race have also been documented with respect to preferences for using life-sustaining treatments.[60] However, blacks still are treated differently, even when their preferences are the same.[61]

Cultural differences in the clinical encounter may account for some of these disparities. Clinical decision-making takes place within the context of a clinical relationship. Accordingly, clinical decisions are necessarily influenced by the social structure and context in which they are made. The "sociologic influences" on the clinical decision include the social characteristics of patients and physicians, the patterns of social interaction and authority in clinical settings, and the structure of healthcare organizations.[62] For example, cultural differences can result in medical advice that does not "fit" the patient's values and conceptions. They can also result in a physician's ignoring the patient's values and conceptions. In neither case will optimum health be achieved. To the extent that medicine's approach to a problem does not coincide with a patient's beliefs, patient noncompliance and dissatisfaction with healthcare become more likely.[63]

Cultural differences also give rise to communication problems between patient and healthcare provider. Studies have documented that white and black patients express themselves differently within the medical encounter.[64] To the extent that black patients downplay or fail to discuss their symptoms, their healthcare is likely to suffer.[65] More importantly, to the extent that African-American patients use different language or frame their decisions differently from that of their physicians, they are at greater risk of having their decisions ignored or overridden. One study of physician-patient encounters found that

> the person who hears a vernacular [e.g., Black English] dialect spoken tends to devalue the speaker of that dialect. Consciously or unconsciously, dialect speakers tend to get worse treatment, wait longer for service, are considered ignorant, and are told what to do rather than asked what they would like to do. Therefore, the effect of the patient's vernacular dialect in the medical interview is a potential source of interference to the effective exchange of information.[66]

Cultural differences may create difficulties not only in communication, but also because they may make health providers less comfortable in their dealings with their patients. This discomfort may hinder effective communication or preclude some communication altogether.[67] For example, at least two studies have suggested that blacks are less likely to be approached for organ donation by predominately white medical teams.[68]

Finally, physicians' unconscious stereotypes and biases, generally influenced by cultural differences, although sometimes influenced by views of biological differences,[69] may affect healthcare decision-making.[70] Some have suggested that the medical criteria used in clinical decision-making may reflect or incorporate unconscious biases.[71] Others have suggested that perceptions of the patient's support system, which may reflect the physician's racial and cultural biases, may influence the decision-making process.[72] Anecdotes of African-American patients support this view. In a recent article, Vanessa Northington Gamble relates two powerful examples of racial stereotyping experienced in the emergency room. In one, an African-American professor of nursing describes how her symptoms of severe abdominal pain were met immediately with questions regarding the number of sexual partners she had, recalling persistent stereotypes of black women as sexually promiscuous. The other (reported in the *Los Angeles Times*) describes the experience of an African-American medical school administrator with a broken arm who was assumed to be a welfare mother and told to hold her arm as if she were holding a can of beer.[73] In a similar vein, Herbert Nickens refers to his own experience in comparing the ways in which white healthcare workers treat those with cystic fibrosis (affects primarily whites) and sickle cell anemia (affects primarily blacks). He opines that healthcare workers often question whether those with sickle cell disease are having real pain or are exhibiting analgesic drug-seeking behavior.[74] Finally, physicians' racial and cultural biases can be inferred from their behavior. For example, the Coronary Artery Surgery Study demonstrated that providers are more likely to recommend whites for bypass surgery than blacks, "despite similar clinical and angiographic characteristics."[75] In a similar vein, researchers found that physicians in one Florida county were almost ten times as likely to report a black woman for substance abuse during pregnancy than a white woman, even though rates of drug use were similar.[76] In addition, a 1987 review of cases of court-ordered cesarean section demonstrated that 81 percent of the women were women of color (specifically, African-American, Asian, or Latina), 25 percent of the women did not speak English as their primary language, and all of the women were being treated at a teaching hospital clinic or were receiving public assistance.[77]

The enduring disparities in health status between blacks and whites perpetuate the legacy of mistrust of medicine. African-Americans rightly wonder what sort of society would allow such disparities to continue unchecked. They are understandably suspicious, therefore, of those who express concern that blacks will not be given a fair opportunity to assistance in ending their lives.

Conclusion

What lessons does the African-American experience with medicine and the healthcare system have for efforts to ensure that the interests and preferences of all patients will be respected should PAS be legalized? What does it mean to be rendered vulnerable because of poverty, prejudice, negative stereotypes, societal indifferences, or membership in a stigmatized group?

Given the general distrust of medical institutions and the medical profession and the belief that their lives are undervalued, African-Americans are likely to view the legalization of physician-assisted suicide with suspicion. Rather than see it as an opportunity to exercise their autonomy at the end of life, African-Americans may sense that this is yet another way through which less valued African-American lives can be eliminated. This distrust makes it less likely that African-Americans will be easily manipulated in making their end-of-life decisions. African-Americans may question more vigorously the judgments of their healthcare providers and be noncompliant with the medical regimes recommended to them. While mistrust serves to protect blacks in their contacts with the healthcare system, it also presents obstacles for them. The distrusting patient may have limited his or her access to desirable services. It is important that patients trust their healthcare providers, especially in end-of-life decision-making. If patients are to participate in managing and controlling their illnesses, patients and their families need to have confidence in the information they have received about diagnosis, prognosis, and options for care. If the patient's mistrust motivates him or her to ignore these recommendations, the patient may have lost an important opportunity to manage his or her dying. Conflicts between patients and families on the one hand and healthcare providers on the other can severely compromise patients' desires to die with dignity.[78]

Difficulties that exist in the clinical encounter also have significant implications for PAS. Assuming the very best intentions, cultural differences between African-American patients and their healthcare providers may give rise to communication difficulties, either because of differences in values or because of differences in communication styles. However, those cultural differences may create a barrier that prevents even the attempt at communication regarding such important and personal issues as end-of-life care. In a worst-case scenario, cultural differences may cause a physician to discount his African-American patient's values and wishes to such an extent that those wishes are not honored.

The African-American experience with medicine also cautions against placing too much confidence in the ability of physicians and other healthcare providers to insure that patient preferences are honored and respected. In the context of the patient-physician relationship, physicians have power. This power derives from several sources. The physician has superior knowledge and skill. The physician has broad discretion and is not easily held accountable for actions by patients or society. Dying patients and their families are disadvantaged in terms of questioning physicians by virtue of the crisis that they find themselves in. They may also be disadvantaged by a sense of helplessness that results from low socioeconomic status or low self-esteem. In the face of the power inequities in this relationship and the historical instances of misuse of power, African-Americans appreciate that making PAS available as an option for terminally ill patients does not necessarily empower those who have been disadvantaged. Thus, an important implication of the power inequities in physician-patient relationships is that greater equality for the seriously disadvantaged may be a precondition for the meaningful exercise of autonomy.

Moreover, physicians do not exist in isolation from the social milieu in which they find themselves any more than patients do. Both physicians and patients absorb the prevailing norms, values, and beliefs of the society. Physicians may have assimilated the negative messages about some groups. For example, physicians may be too quick to interpret ambivalent statements made by patients as being pleas to die, because at an unconscious level they perceive the patient as not deserving of money, resources, or other efforts that might be needed for care. Alternatively, patients may have absorbed the negative messages that society has heaped upon them and perceive themselves to be unworthy of the efforts that might be needed to prolong their treatment or provide them with palliative treatment. These patients might be easily coerced into believing that it would be easier for them and for others if their lives ended sooner. As a consequence these patients will not be able to effectively manage end-of-life care decisions. They may not be willing to discuss their medical problems with healthcare professionals. Still others may be unwilling to risk the contempt and lack of respect that they have encountered with health professionals in the past. In neither scenario will the patient receive optimum care. Thus, requirements for concurring physician diagnoses or that patients make repeated requests for PAS may not provide meaningful protection.[79] The essential point is that physicians have broad discretion and power. Unless there is confidence in physician objectivity and lack of unconscious bias, such cynicism is valid.

A commentator perceptively notes, "[h]ow in the world . . . is a white, middle class, twenty-five year old male doctor, who wants to perform his role in the most intelligent and beneficent way, to approach a poor, aging, folk-educated, black, female patient?"[80] At a minimum, before healthcare providers can maximize the participation of African-American patients in end-of-life decisions, they must know and appreciate the realities of their patients lives. Essentially, however, the appeal to develop thick descriptions of patients as persons situated in broader social, historical, and cultural contexts is really an invitation to conversation before PAS becomes an option in our healthcare system. This conversation should be about the changes and modifications that are required in the training of healthcare providers and the delivery of healthcare services before we can be confident that all patients will have the opportunity to die with dignity.

Notes

A version of this paper, "Empowering and Protecting Patients: Lessons for Physician-Assisted Suicide from the African-American Experience," was published in the *Minnesota Law Review* 82 (1998): 1015–43.

1. *Washington v. Glucksberg*, 117 Sup. Ct. 2258 (1997). *Vacco v. Quill*, 117 Sup. Ct. 2293 (1997).
2. *Washington v. Glucksberg*, 2273.

3. Ibid., at 2273.
4. Ibid., 2273.
5. The New York State Task Force on Life and the Law, *When Death Is Sought: Assisted Suicide and Euthanasia in the Medical Context*, xiii (1994).
6. Ibid., at 125.
7. For a general consideration of these issues see Alan Wertheimer, *Coercion* (Princeton: Princeton University Press, 1987).
8. See generally, Elizabeth Spelman, *Inessential Woman* (Boston: Beacon Press, 1988).
9. 79 F. 3d 790, 825 (1996).
10. See, generally, Arthur Kleinman, et al., "Culture, Illness, and Care: Clinical Lessons from Anthropologic and Cross-Cultural Research," *Annals of Internal Medicine* 88 (February 1978): 251–58; Dorothy E. Roberts, "Reconstructing the Patient: Starting with Women of Color," in Susan M. Wolf, ed., *Feminism and Bioethics* (New York: Oxford University Press, 1996), pp. 116–43.
11. Yale Kamisar, "The Reasons So Many People Support Physician-Assisted Suicide—And Why These Reasons Are Not Convincing," *Issues in Law and Medicine* 12 (Fall 1996): 113–31.
12. John Arras, "News from the Circuit Courts: How Not to Think About Physician-Assisted Suicide," *BioLaw* 2 (July-August 1996): S:171–188, S:184–185.
13. An exception is a composite description of an elderly black woman in Annette Dula, "The Life and Death of Miss Mildred," *Clinical Ethics* 10 (1994): 419–30. Sister Mildred says at one point,

    > [L]ook like every time I turn on the TV somebody's talking about euthanasia and doctors helping kill off old and sick folks. Well I ain't seen them ask nary a elderly black on none of them TV shows and news programs what they thought about euthanasia. I believe the Lord will take me away when it's time to go" (424–25).

    For a literary exploration of the black experience of health and illness see, Marion Gray Secundy ed., *Trials, Tribulations, and Celebrations: African-American Perspectives on Health, Illness, Aging and Loss* (Yarmouth: Intercultural Press, 1992).
14. Richard L. Lichtenstein, et al., "Black/White Differences in Attitudes Toward Physician-Assisted Suicide," *Journal of the National Medical Association* 89 (2) (1997): 125–33; Harold G. Koenig, et al., "Attitudes of Elderly Patients and Their Families Toward Physician-Assisted Suicide," *Archives of Internal Medicine* 156 (1996): 2240–48; P. V. Caralis, et al., "The Influence of Ethnicity and Race on Attitudes toward Advance Directives, Life-Prolonging Treatments, and Euthanasia," *Journal of Clinical Ethics* 4 (1993): 155–65; Robert J. Blendon and Ulrike S. Szalay, "The American Public and the Future of the Right-To-Die Debate," in Robert J. Blendon and T. S. Hyams, eds., *Reforming the System: Containing Health Care Costs in an Era of Universal Coverage* (New York: Faulkner and Gray Inc., 1992): 223–42; V. V. Prakasa Rao, et al., "Racial Differences in Attitudes Toward Euthanasia," *Euthanasia Review* 2 (Winter 1988): 260–77.
15. Richard L. Lichtenstein, et al., "Black/White Differences in Attitudes Toward Physician-Assisted Suicide," at 126.
16. Joshua M. Hauser, et al., "Minority Populations and Advance Directives: Insights from a Focus Group Methodology," *Cambridge Quarterly of Healthcare Ethics* 6 (1997): 58–71; Sheila T. Murphy, et al., "Ethnicity and Advance Care Directives," *Journal of Law, Medicine and Ethics* 24 (1996): 108–17.
17. In one study, religion seemed both to assist a patient's recovery and to constrain the physician's authority. Joshua M. Hauser, et. al., "Minority Populations and Advance Directives: Insights from a Focus Group Methodology," *Cambridge Quarterly of Healthcare Ethics* 6 (1997): 58–71, 65.
18. See Annette Dula, "African-American Suspicion of the Healthcare System Is Justified: What Do We Do About It?" *Cambridge Quarterly of Healthcare Ethics* 3 (1994): 347–57.
19. For a more complete account of this aspect of justice see Iris Marion Young, *Justice and the Politics of Difference* (Princeton: Princeton University Press, 1990).

20. Charles Lawrence, "The Epidemiology of Color-Blindness: Learning to Think and Talk About Race, Again," *Boston College Third World Law Journal* 15 (1995): 1–18, 4.

21. See Charles R. Lawrence, III, "The Id, the Ego and Equal Protection: Reckoning with Unconscious Racism," Stanford Law Review 39 (1987): 317–88.

22. Herbert Nickens, "The Genome Project and Health Services for Minority Populations," in Thomas H. Murray, et al., eds., *The Human Genome Project and the Future of Health Care* (Bloomington and Indianapolis: Indiana University Press, 1996): 58–78. A particularly chilling example of internalization of negative stereotypes by African-American children is recounted in Marc Elrich, "The Stereotype Within: Why Students Don't Buy Black History Month," *Washington Post*, (February 13, 1994), p. C1.

23. See, Atwood Gaines, "Race and Racism," in Warren T. Reich, ed., *Encyclopedia of Bioethics*, 2nd ed., vol. 4 (New York: Simon and Schuster Macmillan, 1995), pp. 2189–2201; Todd L. Savitt, *Medicine and Slavery: The Diseases and Health Care of Blacks in Antebellum Virginia* (Urbana: University of Illinois Press, 1978).

    Race is an imprecise concept used to explain differences between humans. The major theoretical issue is whether race is a matter of nature or of culture. Gamble and Blustein explain the two approaches as follows:

    > Biological constructionists hold that races are genetic entities that are fixed, immutable and genetically determined. . . . The social construction model holds that race is a social, historical, and political entity without any essential biological coherence. It is not a natural, fixed category; rather it has been created by society to recognize difference and establish social relationships. . . . [I]t cannot be understood outside of its historical and social context.

    Vanessa Nothington Gamble and Bonnie Ellen Blustein, "Racial Differentials in Medical Care: Implications for Research on Women," in Anna C. Mastroianni, et al., eds., *Women and Health Research: Ethical and Legal Issues of Including Women in Clinical Studies*, vol. 2 (Washington, D.C.: National Academy Press, 1994), pp. 174–91, 175.

    Moreover, the relationship between the terms "race" and "ethnicity" is not well understood. In general, ethnicity pertains to characteristics of a group of people who share a culture, religion, language or the like. In healthcare and health research classifying patients and subjects in terms of ethnic group identity may provide valuable information about lifestyle, diet, or values that relate to health outcomes. See Anna C. Mastroianni, et al., *Women and Health Research: Ethics and Legal Issues of Including Women in Clinical Studies*, vol. 1 (Washington, D.C.: National Academy Press, 1994), pp. 115–119.

24. John S. Haller, Jr., "The Physician Versus the Negro: Medical and Anthropological Concepts of Race in the Late Nineteenth Century," *Bulletin of the History of Medicine* 44 (1970): 154–67, 157.

25. Todd Savitt, "The Use of Blacks for Medical Experimentation and Demonstration in the Old South," *Journal of Southern History* 48 (August 1982): 331–48, 333.

26. David C. Humphrey, "Dissection and Discrimination: The Social Origins of Cadavers in America, 1970–1915," *Bulletin of the New York Academy of Medicine* 49 (1973): 819–27, 820.

27. Todd L. Savitt, "The Use of Blacks for Medical Experimentation and Demonstration in the Old South," *Journal of Southern History* 48 (August 1982): 331–48, 341.

28. For an exploration of the involvement of African-Americans in medical research see Patricia A. King, "Race, Justice and Research," in Jeffrey P. Kahn, Anna Mastroianni, and Jeremy Sugarman, eds., *Beyond Consent* (New York: Oxford University Press, forthcoming).

29. For example, Dr. Marion Sims, considered by medical historians to be the "father of American gynecology" and a former president of the American Medical Association, used slave women in developing surgical procedures to repair vesico-vaginal fistulas or tears in the vaginal wall that resulted in chronic leakage from the bladder. Dr. Sims operated repeatedly on three slave women, without the benefit of anesthesia, and only

sought white volunteers for the procedure after its success was demonstrated in the slave women. Diane E. Axelson, "Women as Victims of Medical Experimentation: J. Marion Sims' Surgery on Slave Women, 1845–1850," *Sage* 2 (Fall 1985):10–13, 10–11; David A. Richardson, "Ethics in Gynecological Surgical Innovation," *American Journal of Obstetrics and Gynecology* 170 (January 1994): 1–6.

30. Vanessa Northington Gamble, "Under the Shadow of Tuskegee: African Americans and Health Care," *American Journal of Public Health* 87 (November 1997): 1773–78, 1774.

31. Vanessa Northington Gamble, *Making A Place for Ourselves: The Black Hospital Movement 1900–1945* (New York: Oxford University Press, 1995), p. 13.

32. The seminal account of the Tuskegee syphilis experiment is found in James H. Jones, *Bad Blood: The Tuskegee Syphilis Experiment*, new and expanded ed. (New York: The Free Press, 1993).

33. Allen M. Brandt, "Racism and Research: The Case of the Tuskegee Syphilis Study," *Hastings Center Report* 8 (December 1978): 21–29, 23. Brandt provides a detailed account of the many negative stereotypes about blacks that influenced the physicians who formulated the study.

34. See Annette Dula, "African-American Suspicion of the Health Care System Is Justified: What Do We Do About It?" *Cambridge Quarterly of Healthcare Ethics* 3 (1994): 347–59. Vanessa Northington Gamble, "A Legacy of Distrust: African-Americans and Medical Research," *American Journal of Preventive Medicine* 9 (6 Suppl.) (November-December 1993): 35–38; James H. Jones, "The Tuskegee Legacy: AIDS and the Black Community," *Hastings Center Report* 22 (November-December 1992): 38–40.

35. In a recent government-sponsored measles vaccine study in which a large proportion of the subjects were African-Americans and other minorities, parents were not informed that the vaccine was experimental and not licensed for use in the United States or that it was associated with an increase in death rates in other countries. The Food and Drug Administration's recent adoption of regulations allowing waiver of informed consent of research subjects in emergency room research has also raised concern that minorities are likely to be disproportionately the subjects of the research. See Charles Marwick, "Questions Raised about Measles Vaccine Trial," *Journal of the American Medical Association* 276 (October 1996): 1288–89; Vanessa Northington Gamble, "Under the Shadow of Tuskegee: African Americans and Health Care," *American Journal of Public Health* 87 (November 1997): 1773–78, 1776–77.

36. See Clive O. Callender, et al., "Attitudes among Blacks toward Donating Kidneys for Transplantation: A Pilot Project," *Journal of the National Medical Association* 74 (1982): 807–9; Clive O. Callender, et al., "Organ Donations and Blacks: A Critical Frontier," *New England Journal of Medicine* 325 (1991): 442–44; Robert F. Creecy and Roosevelt Wright, "Correlates of Willingness to Consider Organ Donation Among Blacks," *Social Science and Medicine* 31 (1990): 1229–32.

37. "Farrakhan Links Race to Transplants," *New York Times*, May 2, 1994, p. A18.

38. Vanessa Northington Gamble, "Under the Shadow of Tuskegee: African Americans and Health Care," *American Journal of Public Health* 87 (1997): 1773–78, 1775.

39. For a good example of this phenomenon see Vanessa Northington Gamble and Bonnie Ellen Blustein, "Racial Differentials in Medical Care: Implications for Research on Women," in Mastroianni, et al., eds., *Women and Health Research*, pp. 174–91, at pp. 180–82.

40. P. Preston Reynolds, "The Federal Government's Use of Title VI and Medicare to Racially Integrate Hospitals in the United States, 1963 through 1967," *American Journal of Public Health* 87 (November 1997): 1850–58, 1850.

41. 163 U.S. 537, 560 (1896) (Harlan, J., dissenting).

42. For a thoughtful series of essays on the difficulty of eliminating separate but equal in public education see *Shades of Brown: New Perspectives On School Desegregation*, ed. Derrick Bell, (New York: New York Teachers College Press, Columbia University, 1980).

43. See for example, Council on Ethical and Judicial Affairs, "Black-White Disparities in Health Care," *Journal of the American Medical Association* 263 (1990): 2344–46; Sally

Trude and David C. Colby, "Monitoring the Impact of the Medicare Fee Schedule on Access to Care for Vulnerable Populations," *Journal of Health Politics, Policy and Law* 22 (February 1997): 49–71, 55.

44. For example, the preliminary results of a study looking at differences in life expectancies within different communities in the United States was reported on the front page of the Washington Post under the headline "Death Knocks Sooner for D.C.'s Black Men." "Death Knocks Sooner for D.C.'s Black Men," *Washington Post*, December 4, 1997, p. A1.

45. H. Jack Geiger, "Race and Health Care—An American Dilemma?" *New England Journal of Medicine* 335 (September 1996): 815–16, 816.

46. The racial difference in overall mortality rates (a ratio of 1.7) has persisted since 1987 and represents an increase from the 1960–1986 time period, when the death rate was approximately 1.5. Robert N. Anderson, et al., "Report of Final Mortality Statistics, 1995," *Monthly Vital Statistics Report* 45 (June 12, 1997): 1–80, 4.

47. Robert N. Anderson, et al., "Report of Final Mortality Statistics, 1995," *Monthly Vital Statistics Report* 45 (June 12, 1997): 2, 8.

48. Frances Chevarley and Emily White, "Recent Trends in Breast Cancer Mortality among White and Black U.S. Women," *American Journal of Public Health* 87 (May 1997): 775–81, 777.

49. U.S. Department of Health and Human Services, Pub. No. (PHS) 91–50212, *Healthy People 2000: National Health Promotion and Disease Prevention Objectives* (Full Report, With Commentary) (Washington, D.C.: Government Printing Office, 1991) p. 33. Diabetes is a third more common in blacks than whites; severe high blood pressure is four times more common in black men than white men; AIDS is three times more common in blacks than in whites, and between ten and fifteen times more common in black women than white women.

50. See, e.g., H. Jack Geiger, "Race and Health Care—An American Dilemma?" *New England Journal of Medicine* 335 (September 1996): 815–16; Council on Ethical and Judicial Affairs, "Black-White Disparities in Health Care," *Journal of the American Medical Association* 263 (1990): 2344–45; Marie A. Bernard, "The Health Status of African-American Elderly," *Journal of the National Medical Association* 85 (July 1993): 521–28. Treatment differences have also been demonstrated for pneumonia, cesarean sections, and kidney disease (Council on Ethical and Judicial Affairs, at 2344–45, and studies cited therein), as well as breast cancer (John Z. Ayanian and Edward Guadagnoli, "Variations in Breast Cancer Treatment by Patient and Provider Characteristics," *Breast Cancer Research and Treatment* 40 (1996): 65–74, 72).

51. United States Department of Commerce, "Health Insurance Coverage Status, by Selected Characteristics: 1987–1994 (No. 173)" and "Visits to Office Based Physicians: 1994 (No. 183)," in *Statistical Abstract of the United States 1996*, 116th ed. (Washington, D.C.: Government Printing Office, 1996), pp. 120, 125.

52. Council on Ethical and Judicial Affairs, "Black-White Disparities in Health Care," *Journal of the American Medical Association* 263 (1990): 2344–46.

53. See, e.g., Marian E. Gornick, et al., "Effects of Race and Income on Mortality and Use of Services among Medicare Beneficiaries," *New England Journal of Medicine* 335 (1996): 791–99, 793 (7.2 office visits for black Medicare patients compared to 8.1 visits for white Medicare patients); Sally Trude and David C. Colby, "Monitoring the Impact of the Medicare Fee Schedule on Access to Care for Vulnerable Populations," *Journal of Health Politics, Policy and Law* 22 (1997): 49–71, 56–57 (black Medicare beneficiaries more likely than whites and other beneficiaries to report access problems, delay in medical care, and lack of a usual source of care); Eric D. Peterson, et al., "Racial Variation in Cardiac Procedure Use and Survival Following Acute Myocardial Infarction in the Department of Veterans Affairs," *Journal of the American Medical Association* 271 (April 1994): 1175–80, 1178 (blacks in Veterans Affairs system less likely than whites to undergo coronary artery bypass grafting, angioplasty, and coronary revascularization); P. J. Held, "Access to Kidney Transplantation: Has the United States Eliminated Income and Racial Difference?" *Archive of Internal Medicine* 148 (1988): 2594–2600 (black Medicare

beneficiaries less likely than whites to receive a kidney transplant); and Katherine L. Kahn, et al., "Health Care for Black and Poor Hospitalized Medicare Patients," *Journal of the American Medical Association* 271 (1994): 1169–74 (black Medicare patients less likely than whites to receive mammograms).

Medicare minimizes the inequalities in access to healthcare by providing premium-free hospital benefits to people over age sixty-five with qualifying work history, permitting those resident citizens without qualifying work history to purchase this insurance, and providing *all* resident citizens the opportunity to purchase supplemental medical insurance (e.g., for outpatient services). David Calkins, et al., *Health Care Policy* (Cambridge: Blackwell Science, 1995), pp. 105–6, 112. Although some gaps in coverage remain, Medicare has improved access to care among previously underserved populations. José J. Escarce, "Racial Differences in the Elderly's Use of Medical Procedures and Diagnostic Tests," *American Journal of Public Health* 83 (1993): 948–54, 948. The Veterans Health Administration system provides medical care to all veterans who are disabled or financially disadvantaged without regard to patient's ability to pay. Patients within the Veteran's Affairs system are more likely than patients in the private sector to share the same socioeconomic status (middle to low income). Eric D. Peterson, et al., "Racial Variation in Cardiac Procedure Use and Survival Following Acute Myocardial Infarction in the Department of Veterans Affairs," *Journal of the American Medical Association* 271 (1994): 1175–80, 1178.

54. Marian E. Gornick, et al., "Effects of Race and Income on Mortality and Use of Services among Medicare Beneficiaries," *New England Journal of Medicine* 355 (1996): 791–99.

55. Katherine L. Kahn, et al., "Health Care for Black and Poor Hospitalized Medicare Patients," *Journal of the American Medical Association* 271 (1994): 1169–74 (finding differences in care in similar hospitals for black Medicare patients hospitalized with congestive heart failure, acute myocardial infarction, pneumonia, and cerebrovascular accident compared to other beneficiaries).

56. See, e.g., David R. Williams, "Socioeconomic Differentials in Health: A Review and Redirection," *Social Psychology Quarterly* 53 (1990): 81–91, 83.

57. Arline T. Geronimus, et al., "Excess Mortality among Blacks and Whites in the United States," *New England Journal of Medicine* 335 (November 1996): 1552–58, 1555.

58. Council on Ethical and Judicial Affairs, "Black-White Disparities in Health Care" at 2346.

59. Charles Maynard, et al., "Blacks in the Coronary Artery Surgery Study (CASS): Race and Clinical Decision Making," *American Journal of Public Health* 76 (December 1986): 1446–48, 1446. However, the small percentage of black enrollees in the study may limit the generalizability of this observation.

60. In one study, black patients were almost three times as likely as white patients to indicate they wanted more treatment, while whites were almost two-and-a-half-times more likely then blacks to indicate they wanted less treatment. Joanne Mills Garrett, et al., "Life-sustaining Treatments during Terminal Illness: Who Wants What?" *Journal of General Internal Medicine* 8 (July 1993): 361–68, 364.

61. For example, physicians treating AIDS patients were less likely to have conversations about resuscitation with patients of color even though their interest in having such a discussion was similar to that of whites. Jennifer S. Haas, et al., "Discussion of Preferences for Life-Sustaining Care by Persons with AIDS," *Archives of Internal Medicine* 153 (1993): 1241–48, 1246.

62. Jack A. Clark, Deborah A. Potter, and John B. McKinlay, "Bringing Social Structure Back into Clinical Decision Making," *Social Science and Medicine* 32 (1991): 853–866, 854.

63. Arthur Kleinman, Leon Eisenberg, and Byron Good, "Culture, Illness, and Care: Clinical Lessons from Anthropologic and Cross-Cultural Research," *Annals of Internal Medicine* 88 (1978): 251–58, 252.

64. See, e.g., Rayna Rapp, "Constructing Amniocentesis: Maternal and Medical Dis-

courses," in Faye Ginsburg and Anna Lowenhaupt Tsing, eds., *Uncertain Terms: Negotiating Gender in American Culture* (Boston: Beacon Press 1993), pp. 28–42, 31–32 (black women were less likely than white women to use medical language in responding to an offer of amniocentesis); James M. Raczynski, et al., "Diagnoses, Symptoms, and Attribution of Symptoms among Black and White Inpatients Admitted for Coronary Artery Disease," *American Journal of Public Health* 84 (June 1994): 951–56, 955 (blacks reported fewer painful symptoms and were more likely to attribute their symptoms to noncardiac origins); Sybil L. Crawford, et al., "Do Blacks and Whites Differ in Their Use of Health Care for Symptoms of Coronary Heart Disease," *American Journal of Public Health* 84 (June 1994): 957–64.

65. See, e.g., James M. Raczynski, et al., "Diagnoses, Symptoms, and Attribution of Symptoms among Black and White Inpatients Admitted for Coronary Artery Disease," *American Journal of Public Health* 84 (June 1994): 951–56, 955 (offering the difference in reporting symptoms as an explanation for the differences in coronary care treatment).

66. Roger W. Shuy, "Three Types of Interference to an Effective Exchange of Information in the Medical Interview," in Alexandra Dundas Todd and Sue Fisher, eds., *The Social Organization of Doctor-Patient Communication* (Norwood: Ablex Publishing Corp., 1983), pp. 17–30, 20. See, also, Alexandra Dundas Todd, *Intimate Adversaries: Cultural Conflict Between Doctors and Women Patients* (Philadelphia: University of Pennsylvania Press, 1989), p. 77 (observing a trend in a qualitative study of physician-patient encounters on reproductive issues that "the darker a woman's skin and/or the lower her place on the economic scale, the poorer the care and efforts at explanation she received.")

67. Based on her review of the literature and her own experience and research, Jennifer Daley concluded that "[p]atients of a different cultural, ethnic and socioeconomic background from their physicians are ... less likely to receive information from their doctors." Jennifer Daley, "Overcoming the Barrier of Words," in Margaret Gerteis, et al., eds., *Through the Patients Eyes* (San Francisco: Jossey-Bass Publishers, 1993), p. 83.

68. Mary S. Hartwig, et al., "Effect of Organ Donor Race on Health Team Procurement Efforts," *Archive Surgery* 128 (December 1993): 1331–35, 1334 (race had a strong influence on identifying organ donors and on actually requesting donation); Alice A. Mitchell and William E. Sedlacek, "Ethnically Sensitive Messengers: An Exploration of Racial Attitudes of Health-Care Workers and Organ Procurement Officers," *Journal of the National Medical Association* 88 (June 1996): 349–52, 351–52 (concluding that organ procurement employees may experience cognitive dissonance when dealing with donors of color).

69. In a study of racial differences in cardiac treatment in the Veteran's Affairs system, researchers pointed out that it had been believed that blacks had worse outcomes than whites following coronary artery bypass surgery, although that belief has not been born out in the literature. Eric D. Peterson, et al., "Racial Variation in Cardiac Procedure Use and Survival Following Acute Myocardial Infarction in the Department of Veterans Affairs," *Journal of the American Medical Association* 271 (1994): 1175–80, 1179.

70. See, e.g., Council on Ethical and Judicial Affairs, "Black-White Disparities in Health Care," *Journal of the American Medical Association* 263 (1990): 2346, "Disparities in treatment decisions may reflect the existence of subconscious bias." José J. Escarce, et al., "Racial Differences in the Elderly's Use of Medical Procedures and Diagnostic Tests," *American Journal of Public Health* 83 (1993): 948–54, 953 (suggesting that "[t]he effect of patient race on physician and institutional decision making" may be the cause of persistent racial differences in treatment).

71. See, e.g., Michael Lowe, et al., "These Sorts of People Don't Do Very Well": Race and Allocation of Health Care Resources," *Journal of Medical Ethics* 21 (December 1995): 356–60, 358 (suggesting that seemingly objective outcome criteria such as likely graft survival, patient survival, quality-of-style measures, and presence of significant comorbidity or disability used to identify recipients who are most likely to benefit from kidney transplantation may incorporate subtle racial discrimination, e.g., when prevalence of certain comorbidities is higher in a minority population).

72. Eric D. Peterson, Steven M. Wright, Jennifer Daley, and George E. Thibault, "Racial Variation in Cardiac Procedure Use and Survival Following Acute Myocardial Infarction in the Department of Veterans Affairs," *Journal of the American Medical Association* 271 (1994): 1175–80, 1179.

73. Vanessa Northington Gamble, "Under the Shadow of Tuskegee: African Americans and Health Care," *American Journal of Public Health* 87 (November 1997): 1773–78, 1776.

74. Herbert Nickens, "The Genome Project and Health Services for Minority Populations," in Thomas H. Murray, et al., eds., *The Human Genome Project and the Future of Health Care* (Indianapolis and Bloomington: Indiana University Press, 1996): 58–78, 67.

75. Charles Maynard, "Blacks in the Coronary Artery Surgery Study (CASS): Race and Clinical Decision Making," *American Journal of Public Health* 76 (1996): 1446–48, 1446.

76. Ira J. Chasnoff, et al., "The Prevalence of Illicit-Drug or Alcohol Use during Pregnancy and Discrepancies in Mandatory Reporting in Pinellas County, Florida," *New England Journal of Medicine* 322 (1990): 1202–6, 1203.

77. Veronika E. B. Kolder, et al., "Court-Ordered Obstetrical Interventions," *New England Journal of Medicine* 316 (May 1987): 1192–96 (1987). Commentators reviewing the court proceedings in these cases have indicated that the women's positions were discounted and viewed as inadequate and the women themselves were characterized negatively. See, e.g., Susan Irwin and Brigitte Jordan, "Knowledge, Practice and Power: Court-Ordered Cesarean Sections," *Medical Anthropology Quarterly* 1 (September 1987): 319–4, 329; and Lisa C. Ikemoto, "Furthering the Inquiry: Race, Class and Culture in the Forced Medical Treatment of Pregnant Women," *Tennessee Law Review* 59 (1992): 487–517, 502.

78. See for example, "Case Study: Mistrust, Racism and End-of-Life Treatment," *Hastings Center Report* (May-June, 1997): 23–25.

79. One commentator makes the point that features of the Oregon Death with Dignity Act (the only state law that permits PAS) are likely to enhance the coercive features of the physician-patient relationship. He writes:

> The doctor informs the patient of her diagnosis and prognosis, determining whether the patient is capable or in need of counseling, and ensures and records that all the required procedural steps have been taken. . . . Although the requirement that a second doctor confirm the diagnosis may in theory help to alleviate this problem, in practice a doctor called to confirm a colleague's diagnosis or prognosis is unlikely to disagree with her assessment.

See Patrick Curran, "Regulating the Unregulatable: Oregon's Death with Dignity Act and the Legalization of Physician-Assisted Suicide," *Georgetown Law Journal* 86 (1998).

80. Joanne Trautman Banks, "Foreword," in Marion Gray Secundy, ed., *Trials, Tribulations and Celebrations* (Yarmouth: Intercultural Press, 1992), pp. xv–xviii, xvii.

6

Why Suicide
Is Like Contraception

A Woman-Centered View

DENA S. DAVIS

A feminist view of contraception suggests an argument for a feminist view of rational suicide. To use contraception or sterilization is to view one's fertility as contingent rather than given, and to limit one's fertility as a way of maximizing one's interests and goals. To resort to rational suicide when faced with terminal illness or impending dementia is to view one's body's continued ability to pump blood and oxygen as contingent, and no longer a good for one's life but rather a threat to one's values and interests in how the final chapter of that life is written.

*　　*　　*

DESPITE THE FLOOD OF WRITING on assisted suicide in the last few years, relatively little has been written about suicide itself.[1] There are certainly important reasons to distinguish these two subjects. One could, for example, argue that suicide can be a good decision in some situations, but still acknowledge powerful reasons why *medical* people should not blur their mission by taking on this task. However, it is important, before tackling the issue of physician-assisted suicide, to think about suicide *simpliciter*. If one believes that suicide is sometimes a rational, even an admirable, decision, one is at least more sympathetic to the notion of assistance. Whereas someone who believes that virtually all suicides are really "cries for help," responses to social situations that could be ameliorated, or the product of clinical depression is likely to be much more suspicious of any steps society might take to make it easier. In the following pages, let me offer one feminist view of rational suicide.

Women live in a critique relationship with our bodies. Sometimes that is a negative thing, as when we judge ourselves by the "norm" of the tall, skinny model on the cover of *Vogue* and find ourselves wanting, or when we buy into male myths about how women ought to make love and experience orgasm. But it is also a positive thing. Women (at least in the West) learn in adolescence that we must take control of our fertility. We need to view that fertility as *contingent* rather than *given*; we need to evaluate our capacity for procreation with a critical eye, asking how and when that capacity fits into our plans for our lives. To use contraception is to say, "*Despite the fact that my body retains its capacity to be fertile from, say, age eleven to fifty-one, that capacity is not (now) a good for my life but rather a threat to my goals and plans; therefore, I will choose to limit my fertility."* To choose sterilization is to say, *"My fertility has permanently out-run its usefulness for my life and is now a danger, and, therefore, I will exert con-trol by bringing my body's physical capacities into line with my plans for the rest of my life."*

Thus, an important piece of the feminist project has been to argue that biol-ogy is not destiny. To decide how to deal with one's fertility—whether by celibacy, pregnancy, contraception, or sterilization—is to exercise choice and will over against the passive acceptance of what would otherwise happen to one's life because of one's bodily proclivities.[2] Sometimes, of course, these are very tragic choices, as when a woman longs for another child but knows that pregnancy will risk her health or the well-being of children already born.[3]

To choose suicide, when one is facing a diagnosis of dementia or the last stages of a terminal illness, is to say, *"My body's continued capacity to pump blood and oxygen is no longer a good for my life but rather a threat to my values and interests in how the final chapter of my life is written; therefore, I will exert control by com-mitting suicide."* These interests might include preserving my assets to use in ways consonant with my values (for example, to endow a scholarship or pay for my children's education); sparing family members the experience of coping with protracted dementia and death; preserving friends' and family's memories of me as a vital and competent person; ending my life with a final chapter that is a fit-ting capstone to the narrative as a whole.

Some religious ethicists, and those with natural law fidelities, will argue that it is arrogant and delusional, "autonomy run amok" as the current phrase has it, to imagine that one can control the course of one's life. In an article tellingly enti-tled, "Embracing Mystery, Losing Control," William F. May speaks of "a pur-poseful willing and waiting in the course of letting be and letting go."[4] David Novak mocks autonomy arguments for suicide when he says this:

> We want to die just as we have lived—autonomously. Since we have believed in life that our dignity is to be self-sufficient, we now believe that we must die with that same dignity. Death is no longer the ultimate horizon that teaches us that our essence in this world is not to be in control but to make our peace with an order greater than anything of our own making.[5]

Certainly, there is much that one simply has to accept—such as having terminal cancer or Alzheimer's Disease in the first place. Thus, the decision whether or not to commit suicide is often made in the context of tragedy; one would hugely pre-fer not to have gotten cancer, or not to live in a society where a nursing home stay will destroy one's assets, or not to be at the mercy of a medical system in which half of dying patients report severe or moderate pain at the end-of-life.[6]

Embracing the idea of suicide as one possible choice among others aligns us on the feminist side of two important divides that are present in the debate over contraception as well: *passive versus active,* and *natural (or "given") versus chosen.*[7]

Passive Versus Active

Not to use contraception, or rather not to include contraception as an active possibility in one's life, is to be passive, to be at the mercy of one's body. Indeed, one of the reasons "moralists" pushed for laws against contraceptives was that they "encouraged" immorality by allowing people to "escape" the consequences of their acts. To be fertile and sexually active without employing contraceptives (or abortion) is to be governed by the vicissitudes of fertility and fate. Given the impact of childbearing and motherhood on women's lives, the consequences for one's health, economic status, and career are enormous.

Conservatives opposed to contraception, especially Christian conservatives, would speak of "openness" rather than passivity, as in this illuminating quote from a woman pro-life activist interviewed by sociologist Kristin Luker:

> Because most pro-life people have a deep faith in God, they also believe in the rightness of His plan for the world. They are therefore skeptical about the ability of individual humans to understand, much less control, events that unfold according to a divine, rather than human, blueprint. From their point of view, human attempts at control are simply arrogance, an unwillingness to admit that larger forces than human will determine human fate. One woman made the point clearly: "God is the Creator of life, and I think all sexual activity should be open to that [creation]. That does not mean that you have to have a certain number of children or anything, but it should be open to Him and His will. The contraceptive mentality denies his will. "It's my will, not your will." And here again, the selfishness comes in.[8]

The idea of life as a "gift" also is common to those who argue for openness and against control. Sydney Callahan, for example, a pro-life feminist who also argues against assisted suicide, says that, "Having received the gift of life and social identity, one has a moral obligation to preserve and respect each human life and refrain from suppressing, killing, or destroying self or others."[9] This notion of the self as the receiver of a gift that one is then stuck with, and yet does not own, casts the self as receptive and passive.

By the same token, to allow oneself to be taken over by Alzheimer's Disease or cancer, past the point of possible cure or treatment, is to be passive. With regard to dementia, it is to be the object of others' concern, to be led by the hand, to be unable to drive a car or control one's finances—in short, to return to the infantilized notion of women that prevailed in the West in earlier times (and that still reigns in cultures such as Saudi Arabia). On the other hand, to seize control of one's destiny, perhaps especially under circumstances of great tragedy and limits, is to be active and dominant.

U.S. District Court Judge Barbara J. Rothstein and the Ninth Circuit Court of Appeals expressed the same point when they relied heavily on the U.S. Supreme Court's abortion decisions to ground the right of terminally ill persons to receive physician assistance in determining the time and manner of their deaths (an argument the Supreme Court ultimately rejected).[10] In *Compassion in Dying*, the

Ninth Circuit quoted *Planned Parenthood* v. *Casey*, a 1992 decision upholding women's rights to abortion, as saying that:

> At the heart of liberty is the right to define one's own concept of existence, of meaning, of the universe, and of the mystery of human life.[11]

Commenting on the string of contraception and abortion cases that began with *Griswold* v. *Connecticut* in 1965, the Ninth Circuit noted that:

> A common thread running through these cases is that they involve decisions that are highly personal and intimate, as well as of great importance to the individual. Certainly, few decisions are more personal, intimate, or important than the decision to end one's life, especially when the reason for doing so is to avoid excessive and protracted pain.[12]

Most (not all) feminists have long argued that, in the context of abortion, their right to control over their bodies and over the shape of their future lives is supreme. Although the decision whether or not to have an abortion is fraught with moral issues, most feminists have consistently resisted mandatory counseling, waiting periods, spousal notification, and other state interference. If we insist that we can and must be trusted with the power to decide whether or not to destroy a potential human life, how can we not insist on the right to be trusted with the decision whether or not to end our own?

Natural Versus Chosen

One of the principal ways in which women have been oppressed in our society is the identification of women with that which is "natural," and the demand that women simply accept rather than control their fertility. "Biology is destiny." Women are "made" for childbearing and childrearing. Birth control is "unnatural" (and will lead to immorality to boot!) Thus, Pope Pius XI, in the 1930 encyclical *Casti Connubii*, wrote:

> It is a divinely appointed law that whatsoever things are constituted by God, the author of nature, these we find the most useful and salutary, the more they remain in their natural state, unimpaired and unchanged, inasmuch as God, the Creator of all things, intimately knows what is suited to the constitution and the preservation of each, and by his will and mind has so ordained all things that each may duly achieve its purpose. . . .
>
> The conjugal act is of its very nature designed for the procreation of offspring; and therefore those who in performing it deliberately deprive it of its natural power and efficacy, act against nature and do something which is shameful and intrinsically immoral.

Other arguments that rely on a divinely constructed world order are equally pernicious to women, as in the notion of male-female "complementarity" which is so often used to support a "separate but equal" argument against women's full participation in public life.[13] Natural order arguments are also frequently associated with what Charles Curran terms a "negative dualism," in which women are identified with the bodily, the emotional, and the material, while men are identified with spirit and rationality. In this tradition, men are the "head" of the family and women are the "heart."[14]

Until the advent of reasonably dependable birth control in the middle of this century, most women faced the unenviable choice of uncontrolled fertility (often associated with poverty and ill health) or some form of celibacy. For too many poor and Third World women, that description still applies. Today, most feminists believe that access to contraception and sterilization is the *sine qua non* of women's self-determination. And, while long-acting contraceptives (such as Norplant) and the shameful history of forced sterilization of poor and minority women remind us of the problems associated with contraception when it is *forced* upon women, the potential for abuse does not tempt us to give up our support for the principle of contraception itself and women's control over their own fertility.[15] This feminist commitment to a "non-natural," *controlled* approach to our fertility suggests what ought to be our approach to end-of-life decisions as well. To quote Mary Rose Barrington, past chair of EXIT, the London-based Society for the Right to Die with Dignity:

> Very little is "natural" about our present-day existence, and least natural of all is the prolonged period of dying that is suffered by so many incurable patients solicitously kept alive to be killed by their disease.... If I seem to be suggesting that in a civilized society suicide ought to be considered a quite proper way for a well-brought-up person to end his life (unless he has the good luck to die suddenly and without warning), that is indeed the tenor of my argument; if it is received with astonishment and incredulity, the reader is referred to the reception of recommendations made earlier in the century that birth control should be practiced and encouraged. The idea is no more extraordinary and would be equally calculated to diminish the sum total of suffering among humankind.[16]

Physician-Assisted Suicide

It is tempting to carry my analogy to the next step and to argue that, just as medical assistance is the *sine qua non* of access to birth control and the "right" to contraception would be empty without it, the "right" to suicide is empty without the specialized assistance of a healthcare professional to prescribe the drugs and, preferably, to be present to smooth the way and ensure success.[17] Although I am a proponent of rational suicide, I am less convinced that the legalization of physician assistance is a good policy. The many concerns expressed about the effect on the medical profession, and the move to HMOs, with their tendency to look to the cheapest solution to any problem, give me pause. I am also influenced by Joanne Lynn's point about the "routinization" of medical procedures (for example, the routine use of ultrasound and amniocentesis during pregnancy, and the difficulty many pregnant women experience in resisting that expectation).[18] One can imagine that, rather than being an option people have to ask for, even fight for a little, physician-assisted suicide becomes one more track onto which certain patients are shunted.

Thus, we may have to settle for a compromise in which certain compassionate physicians continue to break the law. A better approach would be to look for creative solutions that do not involve the medical profession, for example, lay support groups, end-of-life "midwives," and so on. But this approach assumes a robust and public debate that can shake off the taboo of suicide in the same fashion that we are shaking off the taboo of contraception. Now that the Supreme Court has declined to find a constitutionally protected liberty interest in assisted suicide and left this question up to the political process in the several states, the time for such debate has certainly begun.[19] However, it is worth noting that, although there is widespread debate at the level of public policy and legislative action, the taboo against discussing suicide still holds in many other areas, including much of medical discourse. For example, when suicide as a response to a probable diagnosis of Huntington or Alzheimer's Disease is mentioned in the medical literature, it is characterized as an "adverse reaction,"[20]or as a "catastrophe."[21] Suicide is always described negatively as a "risk," rather than as a "response" or an "option."[22] Thus, discussions of the usefulness of certain kinds of genetic tests are truncated by the refusal to speak openly about the possibility that some people might use genetic testing to make a rational choice to commit suicide.

To date, the distinctly feminist voices in the debate have been opposed to assisted suicide. Sydney Callahan is one example; Susan M. Wolf is another. Wolf, in common with Callahan, is concerned that women will be particularly threatened by the legitimation of physician-assisted suicide.[23] Together, they note that women are more likely to live long lives, to outlive their spouses, to be poor and underinsured, and to be undermedicated for pain. The historic power inequality between (male) doctors and (female) patients makes it doubly difficult for women to assert themselves to get the medical care they need. Wolf notes that men are statistically more likely to complete acts of suicide, but women are more likely to attempt them. She hypothesizes that women may be more likely to use suicide attempts to effect changes in their environment; but, if a request for assistance in suicide becomes something to which a doctor can easily answer, "Yes," many women might commit suicide who really did not want to.[24] Both Callahan and Wolf find it significant that the majority of Kevorkian's clients have been women (including many who faced diseases, such as Alzheimer's or multiple sclerosis, that made them increasingly dependent, but not close to death).

Wolf's essay has a number of objectives and arguments. The argument I want to take issue with here is her concern that women's decisions to commit suicide, and society's acceptance of those decisions as appropriate, may be skewed by "a long history of cultural images revering women's sacrifice and self-sacrifice."[25] She worries, in other words, that women are asking (and receiving) suicide assistance for the "wrong" reasons, based on historical and cultural roles that feminists now reject.

Of course, Wolf is correct that self-sacrifice and womanhood have all too easily been considered a natural configuration. But I want to suggest a different way of looking at the content of self-sacrifice. My point is not to denigrate Wolf's picture of the historical and cultural assumptions about women that may play into suicide, but to show that these are actually multifaceted and cut in more than one direction.

Self-sacrifice can be seen, culturally speaking, along a number of different axes. The axis Wolf contemplates is that of resource use. On one end of this axis is the stereotypical mother who doesn't want resources used on her. On the other end is the person who is comfortable having time, money, and resources spent on her, even out of a limited family pool. Wolf argues that women have historically been consigned to the self-sacrificial end. Because women were traditionally expected to fulfill themselves through their families while their husbands pursued success in more public ways, women could all too easily be expected—and expect themselves—to put everyone else's needs first. But there is another sense in which, perhaps unwittingly, the opponents of rational suicide fall into another understanding of self-sacrifice. Here, the self-sacrifice expected is to undergo long periods of pain and disability, perhaps even dementia, rather than to do something as dramatic and unconventional as to put an end to one's life. The ill or dying person is being asked to forgo acting on her own interests in order to (1) avoid making her relatives look like selfish, uncaring brutes in the eyes of the more conventional world; (2) refrain from challenging the comfortable belief that life is always worth living; and (3) avoid giving society at large a push down the slippery slope in the direction of callousness toward those sick and disabled persons who do *not* wish to end their lives. Thus, one could argue that those who oppose rational suicide are asking women to shoulder yet another traditional female burden: the preservation of society's moral and religious values. The stereotypical virtues assigned to Victorian women of "piety, purity, submissiveness, and domesticity," which rightly disturb Wolf, can as easily be harnessed by traditionalists to argue against suicide as for it.[26]

Here again, we see a parallel with enforced motherhood. As Beverly Harrison points out, "We live in a world in which many, perhaps most, of the voluntary sacrifices on behalf of human well-being are made by women, but the assumption of a special obligation to self-giving or sacrifice is male-generated ideology."[27] It is, of course, often a valid argument that the interests of the individual must give way to the good of society as a whole. Although I am not yet persuaded by these arguments, we should certainly consider the concerns of, for example, the New York State Task Force on Life and the Law, which concluded that the probability of "mistake and abuse" was too high to countenance the legalization of physician-assisted suicide,[28] an argument the Supreme Court took very seriously when deciding that assistance in suicide was not a constitutionally protected liberty interest.[29] (We should also consider the accounts of observers in Oregon that the possibility of physician-assisted suicide has actually been *better* for patients, as doctors interpreted Measure 16 as a "wake-up call for medicine" and have been motivated to step up efforts in pain control and hospice care.)[30] But, if we are to make this sort of argument, then let us be honest about it: People are being required to forgo their own interests (and individual values) for the good of society as a whole. Women, who historically have suffered the brunt of that sort of reasoning, and who have special reasons for avoiding the indignity and dependence of being demented, pain-wracked, and bedridden, may decide that it is not worth the price.

Conclusion

There are many different ways in which women's experience can illuminate the complex debate over rational suicide. Some facets of this experience rightly suggest great caution, as women reflect on their greater vulnerability due to age, poverty, and historic oppression. My goal in this essay, by drawing an analogy between contraception and rational suicide, is to highlight one area in which women's experience can argue in favor of support for rational suicide.

Notes

I am grateful to colleagues Patricia Falk and David Forte for the opportunity to discuss these ideas (but neither of them can be held responsible for the contents of this essay, as they disagree with me completely). The writing of this essay was supported by a grant from the Cleveland-Marshall Fund.

1. One exception is M. Pabst Battin, *Ethical Issues in Suicide* (Englewood Cliffs, NJ: Prentice-Hall, 1982).
2. Of course, it would be highly preferable for men to take an equal interest in controlling *their* fertility, but women have far more to lose from unplanned pregnancy than do men and, therefore, a much greater interest in contraception.
3. *Infertility* can also challenge women to make very difficult choices. Feminists are divided about whether innovative reproductive technologies give women more choice or less. See, for example, Janice G. Raymond, *Women as Wombs: Reproductive Technologies and the Battle Over Women's Freedom* (San Francisco: Harper, 1993).
4. William F. May, "Embracing Mystery. Losing Control," *The Park Ridge Center Bulletin* 1: 15 (1997).
5. David Novak, "Suicide Is Not a Private Choice," *First Things* 75: 31–34 (1997).
6. The SUPPORT Principal Investigators, "A Controlled Trial to Improve Care for Seriously Ill Hospitalized Patients: The Study to Understand Prognoses and Preferences for Outcomes and Risks of Treatments (SUPPORT)," *Journal of the American Medical Association* 274: 1591–98 (1996); Joan Stephenson, "Experts Say AIDS Pain 'Dramatically Undertreated,'" *Journal of the American Medical Association* 276: 1369–1370 (1996).
7. I am keenly aware that there is tremendous diversity and controversy in feminist philosophy, and to speak of "the" feminist side is a kind of arrogance. Many feminist philosophers, e.g., Rosemarie Tong, have done a superb job of delineating the many different types of feminist thought and their implications for issues in bioethics. For me, being a feminist means always asking "the woman question," always being alert, as it were, for the impact upon women of a particular policy or perspective. As a liberal feminist, I take equality, justice, and respect for individual autonomy as crucial principles which I seek to extend to women (and to other historically oppressed groups) equally with men. While I agree that equal attention to women's experience will change our

notions of how those principles are applied (the abortion issue is an obvious example of this point), I reject the "relational" or "difference" feminism of Carol Gilligan, Robin West, and others.

8. Kristin Luker, *Abortion and the Politics of Motherhood* (Berkeley: University of California Press, 1984), p. 186.

9. Sydney Callahan, "A Feminist Case Against Euthanasia," Health Progress, November-December 1996, pp. 21–29, at p. 23.

10. For an argument against the assertion that the constitutionally protected interest in abortion and treatment refusal embraces a parallel interest in assisted suicide, see Susan M. Wolf, "Physician-Assisted Suicide, Abortion, and Treatment Refusal: Using Gender to Analyze the Difference," in Robert F. Weir, ed., Physician-Assisted Suicide (Bloomington: Indiana University Press, 1997), pp. 167–201.

11. *Compassion in Dying* v. *State of Washington*, 79 F. 3d (9th Cir. 1996), p. 813.

12. Ibid.

13. Margaret A. Farley, "Feminist Theology and Bioethics," in Lois K. Daly, ed., *Feminist Theological Ethics: A Reader* (Louisville, KY: Westminster John Knox Press, 1994), p. 198.

14. Charles Curran, "Sexual Ethics in the Roman Catholic Tradition," in Ronald M. Green, ed., *Religion and Sexual Health: Ethical, Theological and Clinical Perspectives* (Dordrecht, Kluwer Academic Publishers, 1992), pp. 17–36. See also Margaret Farley, "Feminist Theology and Bioethics," in Lois K. Daly, ed., *Feminist Theological Ethics: A Reader* (Louisville, KY: Westminster John Knox Press, 1994), pp. 192–212.

15. Ellen Moscowitz and Bruce Jennings, eds., *Coerced Contraception? Moral and Policy Challenges of Long-Acting Birth Control* (Washington, DC: Georgetown University Press, 1996).

16. Mary Rose Barrington, "Apologia for Suicide," in M. Pabst Battin and David J. Mayo, eds., *Suicide, The Philosophical Issues* (New York: St. Martin's Press, 1980), pp. 90–103.

17. It is interesting to note that the Supreme Court cases dealing with contraception are not directly about the right of persons to use contraception, but about the criminalization of physicians' and pharmacists' prescription and distribution of contraceptives.

18. Joanne Lynn, "What You Can Do for Your Dying Patient," Presentation at the Cleveland Clinic Foundation, October 10, 1996.

19. *Washington* v. *Glucksberg*, 117 S. Ct. 2258, 2274 (1997).

20. Medical and Scientific Advisory Committee, Alzheimer's Disease International, "Consensus Statement on Predictive Testing for Alzheimer's Disease," *Alzheimer's Disease and Associated Disorders* 9 (4) (1995): 182–87.

21. Sandi Wiggins, et al., "The Psychological Consequences of Predictive Testing for Huntington's Disease," *New England Journal of Medicine* 327 (20): 1401–1405 (Nov. 12, 1992).

22. Miriam Schoenfeld, et al., "Increased rate of suicide among patients with Huntington's disease," *Journal of Neurology, Neurosurgery, and Psychiatry* 47: 1283–87 (1984).

23. Susan M. Wolf, "Gender, Feminism, and Death: Physician-Assisted Suicide and Euthanasia," in Susan M. Wolf, ed., *Feminism and Bioethics: Beyond Reproduction* (New York: Oxford University Press, 1996).

24. On the other hand, if assisted suicide became open and legal, perhaps women who otherwise would use a suicide attempt as a "cry for help," will be forced to confront and articulate their real needs. To continue to play a societal game in which women "attempt" suicides they don't really intend, perpetuates a situation in which women are rewarded for communicating one thing and meaning another. This makes it more difficult for women to command respect for their real beliefs and wishes, as documented by Steven H. Miles and Allison August in "Courts, Gender and the "'Right to Die,'" *Law, Medicine and Health Care* 18: 85–95 (1990). I make a similar argument with respect to Jehovah's Witnesses and refusal of life-saving treatment in "Does 'No' Mean 'Yes'? The Continuing Problem of Jehovah's Witnesses and Refusal of Blood Products," *Second Opinion* 19: 35–43 (1994). (I am indebted for this point to Paul Finkelman.)

25. Ibid., p. 283.

26. Ibid., p. 298.

27. Beverly Wildung Harrison, *Our Right to Choose: Toward a New Ethic of Abortion*, quoted in Janice Raymond, "Reproductive Gifts and Gift-Giving: The Altruistic Woman," in Lois K. Daly, ed., *Feminist Theological Ethics, A Reader* (Louisville, KY: Westminster John Knox Press, 1994), p. 236.

28. The New York State Task Force on Life and the Law, *When Death Is Sought: Assisted Suicide and Euthanasia in the Medical Context* (New York: The New York State Task Force on Life and the Law, 1994).

29. *Washington v. Glucksberg*, 117 Sup. Ct. 2258, 2272–73 (1997).

30. Susan W. Tolle, "How Oregon's Physician-Assisted Suicide Law Spurs Improvements in End-of-Life Care," *Issues and Resources on Dying* (New York: Grantmakers Concerned with Care at the End of Life, 1977) pp. 3–4.

7

Disability and Life-Ending Decisions

JEROME E. BICKENBACH

The debate over physician-assisted suicide is usually carried out in terms of the rights to autonomy and self-determination. The submissions of two disability advocacy groups, in the United States decisions of *Washington* v. *Gluckman* and *Vacco* v. *Quill* and the Canadian decision in *Rodriguez* v. *British Columbia*, suggest that this approach is too facile. The fact of the social devaluation of the life of persons with disabilities, as a matter of both attitude and practice, demands that the governing moral principle ought to be equality, and in particular equality of autonomy. In a world in which physical and mental disability are systematically understood as decreasing the quality of life, the decision of a person with a severe disability to commit suicide, or seek assistance to do so, is morally coerced by the fact of socially limited options. There may be exceptional cases in which this is not so, but the law must be designed for the unexceptional and typical case, even if doing so limits the autonomy of the exceptional few.

*   *   *

Physician–Assisted Suicide and Equality

SUE RODRIGUEZ was a forty-two-year-old woman living in British Columbia, Canada. She was married and the mother of an eight-year-old son. She suffered from amyotrophic lateral sclerosis, better known as Lou Gehrig's disease. Her condition was rapidly deteriorating, and doctors told her she had between two and fourteen months to live. She was told that soon she would lose the ability to swallow, speak, walk, and move her body without assistance, and not long after that she would lose her capacity to breathe without a respirator or eat without a gastrotomy. A well-educated, articulate, and strong-willed woman, Sue Rodriguez decided that she wished to determine the time and manner of her death. As long as she had the capacity to enjoy life, she did not wish to die. But when her quality of life slipped below what was tolerable for her, she wished to terminate her life. But at that point, she realized, she would be physically unable to commit suicide without assistance.

Section 241(b) of Canada's *Criminal Code* prohibits anyone from counseling, aiding or abetting a person to commit suicide.[1] In 1993, Sue Rodriguez petitioned the British Columbia Supreme Court that section 241(b) violated the Canadian Charter of Rights and Freedoms and sought a court order allowing a qualified medical practitioner to set up the technological means by which she might, by her own hand and at the time of her choosing, end her life.[2] She argued that she had the constitutionally guaranteed right to the inherent dignity of a human person, the right to control her body, and the right to be free from government interference in making fundamental personal decisions concerning the final stages of her life. She lost at trial and on appeal. But, buoyed by a powerful dissent at the Court of Appeal, Sue Rodriguez brought her case before the Supreme Court of Canada. In due course, that court also dismissed her appeal in a five-to-four decision.[3] A few months later, a physician illegally assisted Ms. Rodriguez to end her life.

Like the United States Supreme Court decision in *Washington* v. *Glucksberg*, the Rodriguez case raises the legal issue of whether the prohibition of physician-assisted suicide impinges upon the liberty interests of individuals who wish to commit suicide, but cannot do so.[4] And on that question, the majority judgments are very similar: The state has legitimate interests in prohibiting assisted suicide, and doing so accords with, in Chief Justice Rehnquist's words, "a consistent and almost universal tradition that has long rejected the asserted right." The state also has an unqualified interest in the preservation of human life, in protecting integrity and ethics of the medical profession, in protecting vulnerable groups, and, finally, in prohibiting a practice which, if allowed, might lead first to voluntary and perhaps also involuntary euthanasia. Finally, the majority in *Rodriguez* agreed with the United States Supreme Court in *Quill* v. *Vacco*, that assisting in the termination of life is categorically different from withholding life-sustaining treatment for which consent has been refused.[5]

Still, the *Rodriguez* judgment differs from the two United States judgments in one crucial respect: Sue Rodriguez did not rest her case on liberty alone; she also argued that the ban against physician-assisted suicide violated her right to equality by discriminating against her on the basis of her disabilities. Her argument—which was developed in a long and carefully written dissent by Chief Justice Lamer—came to this: Persons with disabilities who are or will become unable to end their lives without assistance are discriminated against by the prohibition of assisted suicide since, unlike persons capable of causing their own deaths, they are deprived of the option of choosing suicide. In neither country is suicide illegal, and public attitudes on the practice are mixed. There is, therefore, a case to be made that being legally prevented from pursuing a legal option, on the basis of physical disability, is discriminatory.

Rodriguez was joined in this argument by the country's largest disability advocacy group, then known as the Coalition of Provincial Organizations of the Handicap (COPOH).[6] COPOH argued that disabled persons have been historically victimized by stereotypical attitudes about their abilities and worth, coupled with a paternalism that has undercut their right to self-determination. Denying people with disabilities the option of suicide is an example of this unequal treatment, and must be resisted as demeaning and discriminatory. It is also true, the COPOH submission quickly added, that persons with disabilities are vulnerable to abuse. Indeed the same social attitudes that deny them full autonomy also devalue their lives. In such a hostile social environment, persons with disabilities may come to believe that their lives are worthless and burdensome to others and, as a result, contemplate suicide. While this is certainly possible, COPOH argued that clear legal safeguards for physician-assisted suicide can protect the vulnerable while reinforcing the right of persons with disabilities to control over their bodies.

In the United States, by contrast, the amici curiae brief of the disability advocacy group Not Dead Yet argued that assisted suicide is the most lethal form of discrimination against people with disabilities, inasmuch as it is the "ultimate expression of society's fear and revulsion regarding disability."[7] Given the pervasive prejudice against people with disabilities and their devaluation by prevailing practices such as the denial of adequate healthcare and suicide-prevention services, safeguards are not the answer. "[S]afeguards cannot be established to prevent abuses resulting in the wrongful death of numerous disabled persons, old and young." Indeed, the only true safeguard against abuse "is that assisted suicide remain illegal and socially condemned for all citizens equally."

That COPOH and Not Dead Yet should come to such different conclusions is noteworthy, since they were in perfect agreement about everything else. Both groups chose to center their legal argument on equality. They agreed about the entrenched social inequality of persons with disabilities. They agreed that a history of neglect, stigmatization, and paternalism, especially among medical professionals, has robbed persons with disabilities of their dignity, self-respect, and autonomy. They agreed that the lives of persons with disability have been systematically devalued. Yet, for these two advocacy organizations, the demand for equality drove them in diametrically opposite directions.

In fact, this opposition is more apparent than real, or rather more strategic than substantial. As an advocacy group representing the interests of persons with disabilities, COPOH was in an awkward position. In its factum it argued that there is a real danger that "negative stereotypes and attitudes which exist about the lack of value and quality inherent in the life of a person with disability" may be the primary cause of the suicidal wish. Yet, in light of Sue Rodriguez's self-confident and single-minded determination to exert control over her own death, COPOH would have lost credibility if it had argued that she had succumbed to these subtle pressures or that she was a victim of social devaluation. Not Dead Yet was not similarly constrained and could argue, more powerfully and more consistently, that for people with disabilities as a group, the "lethal discrimination" of assisted suicide represents a social evil far more serious than the denial of unfettered autonomy in end-of-life decisions.

At the same time, Not Dead Yet can be taken to task for its paternalistic overemphasis of the vulnerability of persons with disabilities. The group's brief marshals evidence that the prevailing view of persons with disabilities is that they have a low quality of life; so low in certain instances that the life is simply not worth living. This view informs policies for allocating medical resources (including suicide-prevention services) and court decisions concerning withholding treatment and other end-of-life decisions. In this environment, they argued, when a person with a disability expresses the decision to die, it is too readily accepted by nondisabled people who are quick to believe that the request is rational. Indeed, social attitudes and practices have such a powerful influence over their decisions that, even absent outright coercion and manipulation, the decision by a person with a disability to die will not be autonomous: "as long as people with disabilities are treated as unwelcome and costly burdens on society, assisted suicide is not voluntary but is a forced 'choice.'"

The deterministic excesses of the Not Dead Yet argument should also be discounted as strategic. It was important to put to rest the simplistic view that people can make life-or-death decisions wholly unaffected by background social beliefs and practices about the value of their lives. Nonetheless, it is surely true that even in a cultural medium in which ill health and disability are assumed always to lower quality of life, and in which this is reflected in social attitudes, policies, and laws, one can still imagine a person with a disability making the autonomous decision to commit suicide. And Sue Rodriguez had the qualities of such an individual. She had been able to secure her sense of self and develop her self-esteem long before becoming ill. Her disease was rapidly and tragically debilitating, though it had no effect on her mental capacity. Most of all, she had support from relatives and friends who, throughout her ordeal, saw her not as a "disabled person," but as Sue Rodriguez taking control over her life.

That being said, even if Sue Rodriguez herself was neither vulnerable nor the victim of social attitudes about the low value of her life, her case is arguably exceptional. The weight of the evidence warrants caution about generalizing from her case. In any event, the law must be written for everyone, not just the exceptional person. It is a commonplace in political theory that an institutional constraint on autonomy may well be justified if, in general and in the long run, it protects people who are vulnerable, though on occasion it produces undesirable, even right-infringing, results for the exceptional few. Ignoring this point is the principal flaw in COPOH's position. Once that obstacle is removed, the submissions of COPOH and Not Dead Yet converge to produce a single, equality-based argument against physician-assisted suicide, an argument which takes seriously the concerns of persons with disabilities.

Inequality of Autonomy

Recentering the debate over physician-assisted suicide in terms of equality reveals issues that are of special concern to persons with disabilities. What the equality focus reveals is that, setting aside debates about the moral difference between physician-assisted suicide and "passive" practices such as the consensual removal of life-sustaining treatment, or general concerns about what the practice might do to the profession of medicine, the central question is whether the practice should be legalized in a social context characterized by *inequality of autonomy*.[8]

The common argument made by COPOH and Not Dead Yet is that persons with disabilities are vulnerable and lack full autonomy in end-of-life decision-making because of the prevailing view that their lives are not truly livable. To sustain this argument, however, what needs to be shown is that, as a rule (and exceptions like Sue Rodriguez notwithstanding), it is more likely than not that for a person with disabilities the decision to kill oneself, or seek assistance to do so, is a coerced, manipulated, or forced decision.

At this juncture, an important distinction has to be drawn. There are two, very different, ways of making out the claim that a decision has been forced or coerced.[9] The first of these gathers evidence of direct or indirect psychological pressures that come to bear on the decision-maker and argues that the nature and extent of the pressure was such that the person's will was overborne, and the "decision" was forced. Much of the evidence provided by both advocacy groups was of this sort. There is also a body of research on social attitudes about disability and its adverse psychological impact that adds some support to this view.[10] In short, this first approach characterizes coercion as a purely psychological phenomenon (an overborne will or psychological compulsion), a phenomenon that, given the variety of human natures and circumstances, would have to be plausibly demonstrated in each case.

Despite its initial plausibility, in this context the psychological approach to coercion is flawed because it miscasts the significance of the social attitudes and practices it cites as evidence of psychological pressure. This approach to coercion views adverse social attitudes and practices as neutral and immutable forces that, though causally linked to the psychological pressure, cannot be held morally accountable for it. It ignores the fact that there were morally responsible, human decisions that brought about the pressure in the first place.

In other words, the prevailing social attitude that a life with disabilities is devalued itself devalues life. The life is devalued by the social perception of disability and the social consequences of that perception. Whatever the effect of disabilities on quality of life—and there is no reason to assume it is inevitably adverse—it remains true that prejudicial social responses to disability also lower quality of life. And for this reason, a just legal system would respond to the injustice of a person suffering from disadvantages that flow, not from disabilities, but from attitudes about them.

But social attitudes also translate into social practice. To take one kind of example, quality-of-life assessment tools used in health outcome research and planning presume that the existence of a severe disability compromises quality of life.[11] International epidemiological measures of disease burden, such as the Quality of Life Adjusted Year (QALY) and Disability-Adjusted Life Year (DALY), are used by agencies like the World Bank and the World Health Organization to assess the cost-effectiveness of health interventions, in terms of the cost per unit of disease burden averted.[12] These and other quasi-scientific measures also incorporate the view that disease and its consequences lower quality of life, not as a matter of social attitude, but of purported fact. In a political environment in which economic considerations are dominant, these instruments create policy consequences that directly affect the resources available to persons with disabilities. They are also invoked to support economic judgments that it is not cost-effective to provide resources to those whose quality of life is, and will likely remain, too low.[13]

The first point, then, is that attitudes and practices that devalue the lives of persons with disabilities constitute far more than psychological pressure; they themselves lower quality of life. Consider as well the findings of psychologist Carol Gill that the desire among terminal patients to die may be motivated by the realization that death is the only escape from an intolerable institutional setting, or inadequate medical or palliative care. Her research also suggests that the suicidal urge may be viewed as the only effective means at the individual's disposal of sparing the family the financial and emotional strain of a lingering illness.[14] These are real pressures, and the decisions that are made in light of them are rational enough. But these pressures arise from discriminatory social responses to disabilities, not from the disabilities themselves.

And this leads to the second point. When an individual chooses death as the only way of escaping from an intolerable situation, it is perverse and unfair to say that this is an expression of self-determination or autonomy. Such a choice is voluntary in the sense that the person made the choice, consciously and knowingly. We would be concerned if the individual made the choice unconsciously, or unknowingly. But we should also be concerned if the choice was made only because there were no other viable options.

The second sense of "coercion," therefore, applies to choices that are forced by the artificial absence of viable alternatives and options, choices constrained as a result of social attitudes and practices. The distinction between the psychological and what might be called the moral sense of "coercion" is reflected in the domain of law. In legal terms, coercion as a defense to criminal or civil liability can be understood either as an excuse (in which an overborne and nonculpable will is said to have produced an involuntary, pseudochoice) or as a justification (in which unfair circumstances have limited options and forced a unwanted choice). [15] Of course, the constraints on options directly produced by human mortality and the limits of human knowledge or skill are not the constraints that characterize a coerced decision in this second sense. What is salient to the moral conception of coercion is that the range of options has been unfairly, arbitrarily, or unjustifiably limited, not by hard facts and physical laws, but by human beliefs, decisions, actions, and policies.

In this sense of coercion, the constraint of choice created by social attitudes and practices concerning disability is appropriately characterized as an infringement on equality of respect and concern. If, because of a mental or physical disability, one individual is confronted by a more limited range of options concerning his or her remaining life than another, then the decision setting is discriminatory. Straightforwardly, one person has a different set of opportunities than another, and that difference is neither immutable nor morally justifiable.

In this sense of "coercion," we can say with far more confidence that the unexceptional people with disability are vulnerable to forced decisions about wishing their own death or seeking assistance to die. Sue Rodriguez may still be an exception. She may have been immune from moral coercion, and her opportunities constrained only by the functional limitations of her disabilities, the prognosis of the disease, and limitations of human knowledge and skill. If so, then her autonomy is infringed by the prohibition against assisted suicide. But if hers is the rare case, the exception, then violating her autonomy may well be the price that must be paid to secure the legitimate state interest of protecting those persons with disabilities who are coerced by unfair limitations imposed on their options.

Viewed in this way, as an issue of equality in the first instance, the three cases take on another dimension. Recasting the evidence presented by COPOH and Not Dead Yet as evidence of moral rather than psychological coercion and conceptualizing vulnerability as an unjustifiable limitation of options available to a person with disabilities in a decision setting in which suicide is one option, the equality argument in favor of a ban on physician-assisted suicide falls into place. Using the framework provided by the Americans with Disabilities Act of 1990[16] (which has direct analogues in Canadian equality jurisprudence),[17] the laws banning physician-assisted suicide constitute a "reasonable accommodation" to the social devaluation of the lives of persons with disabilities.

In antidiscrimination jurisprudence, an accommodation is any adjustment to social practices that eliminates or lessens the adverse effect on persons with disabilities of the way the social world is organized and structured. Providing a ramp for the benefit of persons in wheelchairs is an accommodation to the constructed environment inasmuch as it makes possible equal access to buildings. Similarly, a flexible work schedule for a person with chronic fatigue syndrome is an accommodation to the conditions of employment that make it possible for the person to work during those periods when the health condition has abated and the person has enough energy to do the job.

An accommodation is "reasonable" when it does not cause an "undue hardship" to whomever is required to implement the change. There are various reasons why an accommodation might be unreasonable in this sense. If an employer cannot afford it, or if health and safety regulations would be violated, then the alternation may be judged to cause undue hardship. If the rights of others, those with and those without disabilities, are infringed or limited by the accommodation, that too may make the accommodation unreasonable.

Is the limitation of Sue Rodriguez's autonomy an undue hardship? This is not an easy question to answer. Accommodations invariably infringe someone's autonomy, so the issue is not whether there is infringement, but whether it is justifiable. Doubtless, the degree of hardship experienced by Ms. Rodriguez, and, indeed, (if this were measurable) the diminution of her quality of life that resulted, were considerable. But how is that commensurable with the legitimate state interest of protecting vulnerable individuals against moral coercion?

Undoubtedly, it was this difficult question that persuaded COPOH, and at least one member of the Canadian Supreme Court, to seek the apparent compromise of a liberalized law constrained by safeguards. What is typically meant by safeguards in the case of physician-assisted suicide are procedural techniques for ensuring that the potential suicide is competent, has made the decision freely and voluntarily, is in a terminal state or in great and unrelievable pain, is physically incapable of performing the act of suicide, and has adequate opportunity to change his or her mind. COPOH argued that perhaps as well the law should require a mandatory visit from a trained advocate who would inform the person of his or her rights and entitlements. As we saw, Not Dead Yet in its submissions finessed the question of safeguards entirely by making the sweeping claim that, in the cultural environment in which people with disabilities live, autonomy for end-of-life decisions is simply not possible.

Though safeguards are a tempting compromise, Not Dead Yet was probably wise not to enter into a discussion of them. If the point of safeguards is to ensure that exceptional cases, the Sue Rodriguezes of the world, are not denied autonomy, then the only relevant safeguard would be a reliable determination of competency and a free and voluntary decision. It is wholly irrelevant what a person's physical condition is. If autonomy is to be preserved even in the face of a life-ending decision, then there is no reason, indeed we have no right, to inquire into the motivation for the decision. Why should the right to physician-assisted suicide depend on whether one is physically able to perform the act? Why does it matter that one is in pain, or in a terminal state, or has any medical condition whatsoever? We learn from John Stuart Mill that the value and importance of self-determination is not contingent on what is decided or done. Respecting autonomy does not mean respecting the right of people to arrive at correct decisions that are in their self-interest and consistent with their welfare; it means respecting their right to make whatever decision they wish.

To its credit, Not Dead Yet realizes this, and makes the point, as a final submission, that if the court ignores all of its preceding arguments and finds a constitutional right to assisted suicide, then it should apply that right to "every citizen, regardless of their health status. . . ." Though a rhetorical flourish, the submission is not without a point. It is telling that in all of the hundreds of pages in these three courts decisions, there is never any suggestion that the right to physician-assisted suicide should extend to people who do not have a severe disability. Implicit in the judgments themselves, in other words, is precisely the prevailing prejudicial social attitude that having a disability is a sensible reason for committing suicide.

Perhaps proponents of physician-assisted suicide would be steadfast in their view even if it meant that qualified doctors could patrol school grounds waiting for despondent but mentally competent seventeen-year-olds who, having failed geography or been unable to find a date for the prom, might want to use their assisted-suicide services. Why indeed do we have the right to demand that the seventeen-year-olds continue to live; are we not forcing them to die later of accident, disease, or old age? We have no less an authority than Ronald Dworkin who, in an often quoted passage, claims that "making someone die in a way that others approve, but he believes a horrifying contradiction of his life, is a devastating, odious form tyranny."[18]

But if proponents refuse to embrace autonomy in this blunt and unalloyed form, then the argument for physician-assisted suicide shifts its center of gravity. If respecting autonomy itself is not enough, then proponents must return to the view that some lives are not worth living; that is, that people can be justified in wanting to have themselves killed. This move constitutes the first, sliding step down a slope that Not Dead Yet describes in its submission: If some lives, because of their low quality, are justifiably ended by means of assisted suicide, what point is there in insisting upon mental competency?

We already have legal evidence of how the slide will proceed. In an English case, *Airedale N.H.S. Trust* v. *Bland*, the father of a seventeen-year-old who sustained massive head injuries in an accident asked the court to allow physicians to discontinue life-sustaining treatment.[19] The court agreed, arguing that being in persistent vegetative state the boy had no further interest in being kept alive. The father said he was convinced that his son, were he competent, would not "want to be left like that."[20] And in Canada, Mr. Latimer killed his twelve-year-old daughter because cystic fibrosis had left her impaired, not only severely mentally and physically disabled, but also in a constant state of pain. The case is still making its way through the courts, but both at trial and before the Court of Appeal, Mr. Latimer argued in defense that he was merely assisting his daughter in relieving her pain, something she would have requested were she competent.[21]

If anything, the equality-based argument against physician-assisted suicide is stronger in the case of people who are not mentally competent. It is common to argue that, quite independently of the presence of pain, physical debilitation, or shortened lifespan, the most profound assault on quality to life is the diminution of autonomy itself, brought about by the mental incapacity to recognize and appreciate options and choices.[22] As a result, the social devaluation of life is far more evident among people with developmental disabilities and other forms of mental and psychiatric impairments than those who, like Ms. Rodriguez, are mentally unaffected by illness or disability. When autonomy itself is disabled, surrogate decision-makers like Mr. Bland and Mr. Latimer can more easily make the argument that continued life is "not in the best interest of the patient." The options thought available to a person who is mentally incompetent are, as a consequence, far more constrained; indeed, often the choice is not even theirs to make.

Conclusion

The debate over physician-assisted suicide has typically been carried out in terms of the rights to autonomy and self-determination. What the disability community has argued, time and again, is that this approach is too facile. The fact of the social devaluation of the life of persons with disabilities, as a matter of both attitude and practice, demands that the governing moral principle ought to be equality, and in particular equality of autonomy. In a world in which physical and mental disability were not systematically viewed as grounds for judging a life to be of less value, or indeed of no value, and in which the decisions about life and death did not have to be made in the context of moral coercion, then we might judge physician-assisted suicide entirely on the grounds of autonomy and self-determination. But ours is not that world.

Notes

1. *Revised Statutes of Canada*, 1985, c. C-46.
2. Part B, *Constitution Act*, 1982.
3. *Rodriguez* v. *British Columbia (Attorney General)* 107 D.L.R. (4th) 342 (1993). All subsequent quotes from this case come from this report.
4. See appendix A at the end of this volume.
5. See appendix A at the end of this volume.
6. This and all subsequent references to COPOH's arguments come from COPOH's Intervener Factum (Court File No. 23476) and the affidavit of Francine Arsenault, submitted 10 May 1993.
7. This and all subsequent references to the arguments of Not Dead Yet come from the Amici Curiae Brief of Not Dead Yet and American Disabled for Attendant Programs Today in Support of Petitioners in *Vacco* v. *Quill*, the Supreme Court of the United States, No. 95–1858, October Term, 1995. *Vacco* v. *Quill*, 117 Sup. Ct 2293 (1997).
8. See the review of standard arguments pro and con in Robert F. Weir, "The Morality of Physician-Assisted Suicide," *Law, Medicine and Health Care* 20: 116–126 (1992).
9. I am following a distinction developed in considerable detail in Alan Wertheimer's book *Coercion* (Princeton, NJ: Princeton University Press, 1989).
10. I discuss this literature in my *Physical Disability and Social Policy* (Toronto: University of Toronto Press, 1993).
11. See Ian McDowell and Claire Newell, *Measuring Health* (New York: Oxford University Press, 1987), chapter 6; and Dan Brock's review of the notion and the standard measuring instruments in "Quality of Life Measures in Health Care and Medical Ethics' in Martha C. Nussbaum and Amartya Sen, eds., *The Quality of Life* (Oxford: Clarendon Press, 1993), pp. 94–132.
12. For a discussion of QALYs see Alan Williams, "The Value of QALYS," *Health and Social Service Journal* (1985): 3–15. For DALYs, their development and use internationally, see Christopher J. L. Murray and Alan D. Lopez, eds., *The Global Burden of Disease* (Boston, MA: Harvard University Press, 1996).
13. For a general discussion of this and related points see David Orentlicher "Destructuring Disability: Rationing of Health Care and Unfair Discrimination against the Sick" *Harvard Civil Rights/Civil Liberties Law Review* 13: 49–89 (1996).
14. C. J. Gill "Suicide Intervention for People With Disabilities: A Lesson in Inequality," *Issues in Law and Medicine* 8: 37–56 (1992).
15. See Paul H. Robinson, *Criminal Law Defenses*, vol. 1, (St. Paul, MN: West Publishing Co., 1984) chapter 2.
16. 42 U.S.C. section 12111.
17. See *Law Society of British Columbia et al.* v. *Andrews* 1 S.C.R. 143 (1989).
18. Ronald Dworkin, *Life's Dominion* (New York: Knopf, 1993), p. 217.
19. 1 All ER 821 (1992).
20. On the clinical side, G. R. Scofield has argued that consent for ending life-sustaining treatment ought not to be necessary if the quality of life is too low. See "Is Consent Useful When Resuscitation Isn't?" *Hastings Center Report* 21: 28–30 (1991).
21. *R.* v. *Latimer* 128 Sask. R. 19 (1995) (Saskatchewan Court of Appeal).
22. See the discussion by Brock, *supra* note 11, 105–16.

8

Protecting the Innocents from Physician–Assisted Suicide

Disability Discrimination and the Duty to Protect Otherwise Vulnerable Groups

ANITA SILVERS

An increasingly influential line of thought in the debate about physician-assisted suicide urges us to sacrifice any interests individuals have to the common good. Because physician-assisted suicide is thought to place vulnerable groups like people with disabilities at unconscionable risk, it is supposed to defile the community. Consequently, the argument goes, in the common interest the state must prohibit this practice.

In this essay I examine the reasons people with disabilities are thought to be so vulnerable as to be at special risk from the practice of physician-assisted suicide. This claim stereotypes the disabled as a definitively weak class. The Supreme Court amici briefs offer analogies and anecdotes, but no data, to establish the special vulnerability of people with disabilities. Characterizing people with disabilities as incompetent, easily coerced, and inclined to end their lives places them in the roles to which they have been confined by disability discrimination. And the question of disability discrimination also arises when, as the Supreme Court does, ways of living that depend on mechanical devices are assigned a status different from those that do not.

There is no doubt that people with disabilities are a minority who suffer because the dominant class's social organization fails to accommodate and include them. Unfortunately, the movement to remedy these social ills seems to have been distracted, if not derailed, by the debate about physician-assisted suicide. This debate obscures disability by, among other things, conflating it with illness. Invoking our protective feelings toward the weakest among us almost always is an effective political appeal. But it is difficult to see why a campaign to replace real goods for individuals with abstract appeals to idealized community interest should be interpreted as respectful of people with disabilities.

*   *   *

Introduction

IN AN AMICUS BRIEF filed with the Supreme Court in support of the lower court judgments in *State of Washington et al.* v. *Glucksberg et al.* and *Vacco et al.* v. *Quill et al.*, six influential moral philosophers (Ronald Dworkin, Thomas Nagel, Robert Nozick, John Rawls, Thomas Scanlon, and Judith Jarvis Thomson) argue that decisions to continue or to end one's life are matters of profound, principled personal conviction. The philosophers write:

Denying that opportunity to terminally ill patients who are in agonizing pain or otherwise doomed to an existence they regard as intolerable could only be justified on the basis of a religious or ethical conviction about the value or meaning of life itself. Our Constitution forbids government to impose such convictions on its citizens.[1]

By framing the issue in this way, the philosophers propose that in respect to the disposal of one's life, the principle of self-determination takes precedence. But there are, they acknowledge, several considerations which constrain this principle. First, "states have a constitutionally legitimate interest in protecting individuals from irrational, ill-informed, pressured, or unstable decisions to hasten their own death." Second, "in some circumstances a state has the constitutional power ... to prevent assisted suicide by people who—it is plausible to think—would later be grateful if they were prevented from dying."[2]

This is to say that the principle of self-determination is defeated in circumstances in which the individual in question is incompetent or coerced. And its preeminence erodes in circumstances where the individual mistakenly believes her future life to be void of plausible possibilities that would make it worth her living. What the philosophers seem unprepared for is the claim that there are many cases where these circumstances obtain but where, nevertheless, suicides would be facilitated were it not for the existing state sanctions. If this is the case, then on the philosophers' own qualification of their principle, state sanctions against assisting suicide should remain in place.

This argument, built on the state's obligation to protect especially vulnerable classes, is increasingly influential. Society now treats members of these classes with deplorable disregard, it is argued, and their inferior social status would place them in even greater jeopardy if physicians no longer faced punishment for assisting them to die. The argument supposes that a society in which the everyday existence of these classes' members is made so perilous is hardly likely to recognize how bias and exclusion compromise their competence and made them more coercible. Moreover, the argument continues, the public's inability to conceive any future in which people like these would be grateful for life will make their dying seem rationally self-determined when it is not so.

As John Arras and Bonnie Steinbock point out in the introduction to *Ethical Issues in Modern Medicine*, in the framework of communitarian ethics such considerations weigh against allowing anyone to have access to physician-assisted suicide:

One could argue ... that even though individuals have a powerful claim of self-determination in this matter, the social costs of allowing ... assisted suicide in a society distinguished by ... discrimination against vulnerable minority groups would be prohibitive.[3]

That is to say, in a flawed society like our own, individuals' goods may need to be sacrificed for the sake of a good community.

That this line of argument exercises considerable influence is suggested by the weight placed on it in the majority opinion written by Supreme Court Chief Justice Rehnquist: "All admit that suicide is a serious public health problem," he observes, and then emphasizes, "especially among persons in otherwise vulnerable groups.... The state has an interest in protecting vulnerable groups ... against abuse, neglect, and mistakes."[4] The decision continues:

> "An insidious bias against the handicapped ... makes them especially in need of ... statutory protection." The state's interest here goes beyond protecting the vulnerable from coercion; it extends to protecting disabled and terminally ill people from prejudice, negative and inaccurate stereotypes, and societal indifference.[5]

As a matter of public interest and policy, then, the other-regarding principle requiring protection of these "innocents" trumps the self-regarding principle of self-determination so decisively that the former justifies restricting opportunity to exercise the latter. At least, such a view seems to impel the Court's thinking:

> The State's assisted suicide ban reflects and reinforces its policy that the lives of terminally ill, disabled, and elderly people must be no less valued than the young and the healthy, and that a seriously disabled person's suicidal impulses should be interpreted and treated the same way as anyone else's.[6]

Protection or Paternalism?

The commitment to protect those who are more vulnerable than most is civilized and admirable. But a fairly thin line separates such a benign disposition from a malignantly paternalistic one. For the history of marking marginalized groups as needing special protection is replete with instances in which to characterize a class of persons as weak is to deprive them of the power of self-determination. For instance, it was not so long ago that women were treated as a "weak" class for whom special protective measures were not just warranted but mandated. Until 1913 "the desirability of special protection for the weaker members of the working community had never been questioned [even though this policy placed women] in an inferior economic position."[7]

Characterizing a group as vulnerable further isolates its members from others in society. Doing so emphasizes their supposed fragility, which becomes a reason to deny that they are capable, and therefore deserving, of full social participation. So we must carefully avoid stereotyping and bias in depicting them as especially vulnerable. We should not proclaim the group's members to be unusually vulnerable or at special risk without good evidence that they are so. For to make any group subject to special protective measures because they are exceedingly vulnerable is to decree them to be disempowered.

We should not condescend to protect them unless they demonstrably need protection, even if they request protection. Even if they seem likely to be vulnerable, we must be sure the activities which we propose to ban "for their own good" actually are hazardous for them. There is no benefit in iterating discriminatory effects like those occasioned by the worker's protection laws which, earlier in the century, kept women from well-remunerated full-time work and, consequently, from a living wage, on the insidiously paternalistic hypothesis that they were too fragile to bear the jeopardy of greater responsibility and its concomitant stress.

Disability and Vulnerability

This essay's purpose is to consider whether the increasingly influential view that physician-assisted suicide poses a special danger to "weak" classes, especially to the disabled, is similarly paternalistic. Two assertions of fact are typically advanced to urge that permitting physicians to facilitate suicides poses a significant threat to people with disabilities, whom the state has a special duty to make secure. The first is that society's disregard of them makes people with disabilities more likely than other people to commit suicide. The second is that society's disregard of them makes medical personnel more likely to agree in their cases than in other people's to hasten their deaths.

The first assertion emerges from the view that society makes so little place for individuals with disabilities, and their isolation is so global, as to destroy their opportunity for the connectedness with other people that makes our lives as social beings worth living. Under conditions such as they are made to endure, it is supposed, individuals with disabilities who seek to end their life can hardly be self-determining: They understandably feel too depressed to be competent, so worthless and without hope of well-being in future that they are motivated chiefly by others' complaints that they are burdensome.

Writing in a recent *San Francisco Examiner* column, Mark O'Brien, who describes himself as quadriplegic and is the subject of the Academy Award–winning documentary *Breathing Lessons: The Life and Work of Mark O'Brien*, judges such individuals as helpless victims: "There's a killer on the loose. . . . He kills disabled people. . . . Kevorkian's main interest . . . is killing disabled people or people who say they are disabled. This mostly cashes out to mean depressed middle-aged women."[8]

Having so stigmatized people with disabilities as to place them in special jeopardy, this thinking goes, society is at least obligated to make it as difficult as possible for them to be further victimized. Under the circumstances, they must not have access to the means of ending their lives. It is from this perspective that Justice Rehnquist praises the state's banning assisted suicide as a public expression of the belief that the lives of people with disabilities are of as much value as other people's.

As for the second assertion, the dismissive doctor is a figure all too familiar in the experience of people with disabilities. Jenny Morris, a successful British politician and university lecturer who has been a wheelchair user since a fall injured her spinal cord, invokes the image of the arrogant physician Karl Brandt as an emblem of how the medical profession disregards the value of disabled people's lives. Brandt was designated by the Nazi government to diagnose people with disabilities as incurable and to euthanize them. He explained at Nuremberg that his actions were informed by "pity for the victim and . . . a desire to free the family and loved ones from a lifetime of needless sacrifice." He defended himself by insisting that his practice expressed the best judgment of the medical profession in other countries.[9]

In the same vein, former U.S. Equal Employment Opportunities Commission Chairman Evan Kemp Jr. writes that when he was diagnosed with Kugelburg Weylander syndrome nearly fifty years ago, his prognosis then was for less than ten years more of life. In an article entitled "Could You Please Die Now?", Kemp proposes that such pessimism on the part of physicians about disabled people's prospects disposes them against opposing the deaths of people with disabilities. He writes: "I believe the right-to-die option will inevitably be transformed into a means for rationing healthcare."[10]

These are powerfully disquieting convictions. But it is important to assess them in the context of the facts about how society's disregard affects people with disabilities. One matter that bears consideration is whether physician-assisted suicide can plausibly be construed as discriminating on the basis of disability under the 1990 Americans With Disabilities Act (ADA), which revolutionizes the understanding of disability in American jurisprudence and policy. Although the Court remained silent on this point, several of the amici briefs suggest that physician-assisted suicide is a form of disability discrimination as defined by the ADA. As I will show, however, it is not physician-assisted suicide but rather the insistence that, as a class, people with disabilities need special protection from it that controverts the ADA's strategy for liberating people with disabilities from their historical oppression.

What Is Disability?

First, though, it will be useful to understand what disability is. Who is designated as disabled has commonly been determined by the eligibility criteria for programs that offer charitable treatment, special benefits, or exemptions from obligations to members of specific groups that the different charitable policies are designed to serve. Programs vary in how they draw the definition. However, the definitions established by such entitlement programs are of less relevance, because narrower, than the one designed to identify disability discrimination in the 1990 Americans With Disabilities Act, legislation that extends our conception of civil rights.

In this legislation disability means the substantial limitation of one or more major life activities due to a physical or mental impairment, or having a history of such, or being regarded as such. To illustrate, neither retinal damage nor being in pain are, on this understanding, disabilities. Conditions such as these are relevant to disability just to the extent that they substantially limit such major life activities as walking or seeing.

The ADA establishes a generally applicable civil right rather than a group differentiated right. It assigns all individuals the right to be protected against disability discrimination. But only some individuals can claim group differentiated disability rights to benefits, entitlements, insurance, and compensation. Unlike the definitions of disability created for entitlement programs, all of which reflect prior agreements regarding the ultimate size and scope of the clientele to be served, the ADA contains no notion of eligibility other than the demonstration that an individual has been discriminated against on the basis of supposed incompetence attendant on an actual or imagined impairment rather than disadvantaged for some other reason.[11]

As I have explained elsewhere, unlike protection from disability discrimination, group differentiated disability entitlements are not corollaries of the principles or values of democratic political morality, which focuses on the achievement of equality.[12] Rather, they derive from an older notion of charity owed to the weak and unfortunate. While these entitlements focus on compensating individuals for what they can't do, the ADA secures their opportunity for demonstrating how they are competent. This equalizing strategy is adopted because disability discrimination is the denial of opportunity based on the misperception that being limited in performing major activities also limits competence. Consequently, whether a practice is biased by disability discrimination is gauged by whether it assumes that individuals whose physical or mental impairment substantially limits one or more major life activities are less competent than they in fact are, or whether the practice otherwise prevents them from demonstrating their competence.

The ADA is thoroughly informed by the belief that disability is socially constructed. The analysis of disability that grounds this legislation merges a line of thought drawn from Hegel, Marx, and Foucault with the classical liberal theory of the American civil rights movement. The thrust of the resulting view is that disability is not a "natural kind," nor is disadvantage attendant on it an immutable fact of nature.

Problematizing disability this way emerged nearly two decades ago as a result of crossovers from radical philosophy to the disability movement in Britain. Subsequently, American disability activists adopted the model because it illuminated and gave a direction to social reform. The model explains the isolation of people with disabilities not as the unavoidable outcome of impairment, but rather as the correctable product of how such individuals interact with stigmatizing social values and debilitating social arrangements. But neither the model, nor the legislation which introduces it into United States public policy, discounts impairment.

Thus, for instance, neither expects impairments to be ignored or overcome. What is at issue is whether the social and built environment is so arranged as to make individuals with physical or mental impairments dysfunctional when they would not be so in a more accommodating environment. The distinction between impairment and dysfunction is an important one to preserve in assessing whether we should construe the hostile environment that oppresses people with disabilities as precluding them from self-determination. For now, we should notice that some impairments clearly do more than limit cognitive activity. They obstruct cognition to such an extent that no environmental change or adaptation could raise it to the level required for competent self-determination.

This is not the place to analyze what degree of cognitive competence is presupposed by the principle of self-determination. But for the purposes of this discussion, we should notice that the principle of self-determination itself rules out individuals with dementia, retardation, or other impairments that substantially limit their relevant cognitive functioning from being assisted in suicide. Moreover, on the reading of disability the social model makes, there is no disability discrimination in safeguarding individuals from being assisted in suicide if their cognitive impairments demonstrably preclude their functioning at the requisite level for self-determination.

Disability and Despair

What of individuals with other than cognitive disabilities? Does society's rejection so mislead them into thinking of themselves as worthless and burdensome that they are no longer competent to judge the worth of their lives? Noticeably absent from the current discussion about assisted suicide are data showing that people with disabilities are more apt to end their lives than other classes of people.

Although Chief Justice Rehnquist asserts that suicide is an "especially serious public health problem . . . for otherwise vulnerable groups," the reference he cites is not to individuals with disabilities but instead to the young and the elderly. The amicus brief filed by the American Suicide Foundation admits that "there is little evidence that chronic or terminal illness is a risk factor outside the context of depression or other mental illness."[13] In fact, the American Suicide Foundation brief states that problems associated with physical illness play a role in only one in four suicides, and that studies of elderly individuals who attributed their suicides to physical illness showed that more than half of these did not have the illness which they claimed as the reason for their suicides.

Persons without disabilities often imagine that the experience of disability is one of hopelessness, limit, and loss. Permitting such suppositions to influence public policy clearly has its dangers. The State of Oregon's 1992 attempt to ration healthcare by disallowing or diminishing medical treatment with reference to whether the patient would be left with a disability illustrates how the unwarranted presumption of dysfunction is discriminatory. Oregon's policies grew out of a telephone survey of able-bodied individuals who surmised, for example, that if they were confined to a wheelchair, they would rather be dead."[14]

The Oregon telephone survey tapped the fearful fantasies the general public entertains about being disabled.[15] But to formulate public policy using such a source of judgment about the lives of people with disabilities illustrates the bias described in the Congressional Findings that preface the ADA:

[I]ndividuals with disabilities are a discrete and insular minority who have been . . . subjected to a history of purposeful unequal treatment . . . resulting from . . .

assumptions not truly indicative of the . . . ability of such individuals to participate in, and contribute to society.[16]

Because this bias was embedded in Oregon's proposed ranking system, the federal government did not permit Oregon to implement this element of its policy.

The amicus briefs supply no data showing individuals with disabilities to be
at special risk of suicide. (Parenthetically, ADA case law suggests that it is discriminatory to deny people with disabilities opportunity because they might be
at "elevated" risk; "substantial" risk must be demonstrated.) Instead, some of
the briefs present anecdotal information regarding the depression that disability
often occasions. Because the public believes that impairment must be experienced as irrevocable loss, the proposal that individuals with disabilities are likely
to be despondent and depressed seems plausible to people without disabilities.
Even if this is admitted, however, it does not follow that individuals whose experience is pervaded by hopelessness are suicidal. Nor does it follow that the dire-
ness of their personal or social circumstances puts them in need of special
psychological treatment or medication to prevent their suicide.

Depression is the absence of that hopefulness that initiates functioning. But
such hopelessness cannot be simply a pathological condition resulting from
imbalance, for there are circumstances in which an individual's familiar life activities and options really have become so narrowed as to be not worth initiating.
Granted the benefits that accrue when individuals in difficult circumstances,
especially terminally ill individuals, are so capable of hope they can find meaningful opportunity for positive action. But such possibilities as engaging in
enriched personal relations or creating psychosocial and material legacies are
options whoever is hopeless is likely to find fatuous, trivial or unconsoling.

Furthermore, to be hopeless is not always to be in deficit, needing a cure.
Hopelessness surely is appropriate and even productive where it deters someone
from pursuing a futile option. Within people's lives, hopelessness can be an effective stimulus or trigger for revising unrealistic goals and initiating change.

For instance, the hopelessness engendered by an oppressive government
inspires activity aimed at revolutionary change. Similarly, while the hopelessness
that is the realistic response to permanent impairment may be depressing, it is
also a helpful incentive to recognizing that having fewer or different options may
still mean having satisfying ones. Those who insist that all depression should be
medicated step onto a slope as theoretically slippery as any other. For there is a
clear danger that the same drugs that make individuals accommodate to chronic
suffering also make them accepting of intolerable or oppressive environments
and unlikely to protest against these.

Consider the case of Larry McAfee, a respirator-dependent quadriplegic
warehoused by the Georgia social service system. McAfee was sent out of state
and placed in a series of rigidly managed nursing homes, although it would have
been less expensive to place him in an independent-living situation close to his
family. As published and broadcast interviews with Georgia social service officials

made clear, by wanting to be in an independent-living environment rather than an institution, McAfee challenged the authority of their system. When he went to court to obtain immunity for whoever would manufacture the assistive device he had designed to permit him to shut his own ventilator off, McAfee, no victim, very effectively catapulted himself out of the healthcare system in which he was mere property, a source of income for a nursing home, into the legal system which gave him standing as a person.[17]

For although the social service system premised his incompetence to determine his life, the justice system premised his competence to do so. He sometimes is misrepresented as contending that if one must live with a disability, it is more rational to die. But in fact his claim was otherwise, namely that the state's interest in continuing his suffering did not take precedence over his own interest in discontinuing his suffering. In upholding him, the court agreed that his disability placed him under no obligation to the state, to his friends and family, even to himself, to suffer without complaint or escape.

By winning recognition of his competence to control his dying, he also gained the power to control his living, a paramount issue in the lives of the many disabled people who struggle to control machines and other people, to achieve what their own hands or legs or eyes or ears or voices cannot execute. McAfee never used the option he had gained in court, because public opinion forced Georgia authorities to permit him to reside in an independent-living situation. To have medicated him so that he was accepting of his lack of control clearly would have compromised his ability to address what he identified as the cause of his suffering, which was that nursing home regimes had stripped him of self-determination in the intimate details of his daily life.

The cases of McAfee, David Rivlin, Kenneth Bergstedt, and Elizabeth Bouvia, all quadriplegics, often are cited as evidence that individuals with disabilities who seek to die are not afforded the same suicide prevention measures as those without disabilities. The first three, all respirator-dependent, sought court authorization to turn off the machine; the last sought an order prohibiting a hospital from nourishing her artificially. However, it was not their disabilities but the procedure they requested that made suicide prevention measures inappropriate. For the Supreme Court has been (in *Cruzan*) and continues to be (in *Quill*) explicit in distinguishing the refusal of life-preserving treatment from suicide. The courts framed all these cases not as potential suicides but as cases in which death would result from underlying causes if life-supporting machines were turned off and invasive therapies terminated.

Intolerable Suffering: Eliminating the Problem

The cases of these four individuals are often mentioned as evidence of how people with serious disabilities are deprived of suicide-prevention counseling. All four told the courts they wished to die because their isolation and insecurity, and their lack of control of the most intimate details of their daily lives, were too much to endure. There were two alternatives for relieving their suffering, either to change their personal circumstance by dying, or to change the undeniable source of their suffering, namely, their social situation. A political climate that makes obtaining the latter change more difficult than the former is, of course, deplorable. But there is no reason to believe that changing the degree of difficulty in implementing one alternative either eases or hinders obtaining the other. Avoiding the question of social justice by medicating or counseling such individuals to accept their social situations is appalling.

Some argue that such palliative measures are warranted because aversion to people with disabilities runs so deep as to make improvements to their social status improbable. Groups that oppose physician-assisted suicide in the name of protecting the vulnerable disabled maintain that society is so aversive to them as to be more inclined to facilitate their deaths than to improve their living situations. Consequently, it is maintained, public policy must focus on preserving their lives regardless of what they themselves claim to desire.

Some individuals with disabilities who require a high level of personal care appear convinced that facilitating their dying will prevail over supporting their living where it is less burdensome on caregivers. Thus, they maintain there is continued need for state sanctions that increase the burdensomeness of the former choice. As the law is at present, they argue, society can sustain people with serious disabilities in misery or, alternatively, so that they thrive. Of these two options, suffering or flourishing, the latter is desirable and humane. But changing the law to open a third alternative—the possibility of not sustaining persons with disabilities at all—changes the options, weakening the "flourishing" position with which people with serious disabilities leverage a higher level of care.

The third option diffuses responsibility for sustaining the disabled. The need to care for people with disabilities can be discharged by one of two means: Nondisabled people may help disabled people live independently, or, if the former course is rejected as too difficult, disabled people may "volunteer" to erase their very presence. Which choice will seem preferable to people without disabilities?

Earlier, we considered, but found no statistical evidence nor experiential basis for suggesting that, as a group, people with disabilities are pathologically disposed to suicide. There was no reason to accept the claim that the judgment of individuals with disabilities is so incapacitated by the exclusion and isolation they face as to make them incompetent and incapable of self-determination. Moreover, despite acknowledging the systematic marginalization that people with disabilities endure, it seems wrong to think that having any kind of disability means being cognitively or psychologically disabled by society. To do so is to equate being disabled in any way with being globally debilitated.

But here a new claim has emerged, namely, that regardless of whether individuals with disabilities are competent to decide if their suffering should be prolonged, no one of them may do so in order to safeguard other members of their class from nondisabled people who desire their suicides. This position disallows justifying ending people's lives to relieve their suffering, even in instances in which individuals propose to exercise self-determination by ending their own suffering. Several reasons are typically advanced in support of this idea.

First, there is the force of horrid examples: the Nazis who claimed that their euthanasia program was to relieve its victims of their intolerable suffering, even though very few were in pain and many were incapable of the level of reflection needed to understand such a possibility; the cases in which Dutch physicians are said to have acted on their negative feelings about disability rather than on the self-determination of the patient; and the notorious instances of so-called mercy killings in which the victim clearly was incapable of or shamed into assenting to dying. Second, there is concern about future threats, of which the most compelling is the contention that economic arrangements, such as the capitation scheme for healthcare payment, will make it attractive to end rather than continue the lives of those who incur prolonged high medical costs.

There should be no doubt, I think, that we have created a healthcare system that prefers to ignore rather than address how vulnerable populations are threatened. No one should discount the increasing peril in which our healthcare system appears to place those who want to live but must depend upon others for help in such fundamentals as eating, moving, or even breathing. Nevertheless, we should ask whether sanctions against suicide effectively oppose this trend and other social forces that imperil people with disabilities, or whether they merely distract us into imagining that in forbidding anyone to assist their suicides we safeguard them from broad social harm.

A theme that pervades both the Supreme Court's majority opinion, and the discussion of public policy in which it is embedded, is the suggestion that a public commitment to the intrinsic value of life is itself a protection against the aversions and exclusions that jeopardize especially vulnerable populations. So Chief Justice Rehnquist writes: "The laws of almost every Western democracy express a commitment to the protection and preservation of all human life equally."[18] The Chief Justice goes on to detail how taking one's own life was once a criminal transgression of this state-endorsed principle. But history suggests it is a mistake to imagine that the early prohibitions against suicide, though much stronger than those we have today, contributed to an environment securing the well-being of people with disabilities.

To the contrary, if it shows anything, the historical record suggests an inverse correlation between the existence of strong sanctions against suicide and the existence of strong efforts to preserve and enhance the lives of people with disabilities. Consequently, the faith that public recognition of the intrinsic value of life stretches into a commitment to maintain a decent quality of life for people with disabilities appears to be an illusion. The evidence is more compatible with the remark made by Justice Stevens in his concurring opinion to the effect that our system of law has never valued all lives equally.[19]

The laws that punish the abrogation of responsibility by those remunerated to care for people with disabilities suggest that a lower value is attached to their lives. To illustrate, in state after state, nursing homes bear very little burden if their employees' negligence or abuse leads to patients' deaths: In California, for instance, the fine is as little as $5,000; nevertheless, nursing homes have gone to court to insist that they should not be held to account at all for their employees' mortally irresponsible actions. Recall that Larry McAfee sought control over his own death precisely to escape from a nursing home system in which he believed his life to be at least at much at risk from others' negligence as from his own self-determination.

A system of law that excuses negligence in caregiving precisely because its victims are vulnerable does not value all human life equally. Moreover, the risk to those dependent on being cared for is exacerbated in a system where a victim's vulnerability lessens the responsibility of those whose actions or omissions lead to his death just because an underlying cause contributes significantly to it. It is precisely this devaluing of the care owed to fragile individuals that jeopardises people with disabilities and encourages an environment hostile to them. Ironically, then, the Supreme Court's attempt to find a natural way of permitting physicians to end lives dependent on machines or medication, while prohibiting them from assisting in doing so otherwise, suggests an unintended bias against the former group of individuals.

That persons are substantially limited in performing major life activities so as to affect the performance of such functions as breathing, eating, and eliminating wastes, and that those individuals consequently rely on adaptive interventions (machines or medications) to perform these functions, should make no difference in the strength of the state's interest in whether they live or die. To imagine that the state has a greater interest in continuing the lives of individuals who do not rely on these devices than it does in the lives of those who do seems to express that bias identified by the ADA as disability discrimination. For such a distinction in the strength of the state's interest in preserving lives appears to suppose that people with these kinds of disabilities are, as a class, less able to contribute to the community than others, a demonstrable misperception of their competence.

In sum, to enforce a commitment to the intrinsic value of life, state interest would have to override personal interest by prohibiting any policy in which ending life is facilitated to relieve suffering. To suppose that this commitment is consistent with facilitating the life endings of those dependent on machines or medication, as the Court reiterates in *Quill*, cannot help but weaken the claim that such lives have intrinsic value. In this light, it appears as if framing the issue so that state interest is more significant than personal interest devalues rather than defends people on the basis of their disabilities.

Moreover, substituting public judgment about their well-being for their own personal assessments of the worth of their lives is disrespectful of people who are seriously limited in the major life activities they can perform unaided. In his concurring opinion Justice Stevens observes: "Allowing the individual, rather than the state, to make judgments about the 'quality' of a life that a particular individual may enjoy does not mean that the lives of terminally ill, disabled people have less value than the lives of those who are healthy."[20] Though the state owes maximum protection to every individual's interests in remaining alive, he says, "properly viewed, however, this interest is not a collective interest that should always outweigh the interests of a person who ... finds her life intolerable but, rather, an aspect of individual freedom."[21]

This approach to weighing the competing principles of personal self-determination and public interest is more respectful of the competence of individuals with disabilities than the majority opinion. In striking a fairer balance between self-determination and the paternalism of the state, Justice Stevens's account better respects the fact that individuals with disabilities are the best judges of their personal potential for participating in and contributing to the community.

Parenthetically, in October 1997, the Supreme Court let stand a March 1997 appeals court ruling that Oregon's assisted-suicide provision did not discriminate against or place in special danger a woman with muscular dystrophy. The appeals court ruled there was no proof the woman's condition or that of others in similar situations caused "depression severe enough to prevent them from making an informed decision."[22] As another report of the event states: "Right to Life lawyers argued ... these patients, but not others, are not shielded from subtle pressures to end their lives. Leaders of the Right To Life Committee condemned the Supreme Court for failing to protect "our most vulnerable citizens."[23]

On reflection, this October 1997 decision raises a question about Justice Rehnquist's earlier declaration that the state has an overriding duty to protect vulnerable classes. For the patient who brought the Oregon action appears to fully satisfy the familiar description of an individual so vulnerable as to be in jeopardy should the state condone physician-assisted suicide. This plaintiff was an often depressed individual with a progressively crippling condition, one which in the long-run often is so debilitating as to leave no defense against life-ending illness.

Yet the Supreme Court agreed that such an individual suffers no special threat from Oregon's procedure for permitting physicians to assist in suicide. Who, if not such persons as the plaintiff in the Oregon case, are the vulnerable disabled people to whom Justice Rehnquist refers in *Washington* v. *Glucksberg*? One cannot help but wonder whether this is a class that has been constructed as the occasion for articulating a policy that surely is an ornament of a good and caring community, namely, the commitment to protect incompetents from those who would take advantage of them. Despite the virtue of promoting such a policy, however, designating any group of people as being in heightened need of protection should not be undertaken unsystematically nor in the absence of affirmative provisions to keep from isolating them.

Conflating Vulnerable Classes

So far, I have argued that construing people with disabilities as a class so vulnerable as to warrant substituting the state's protective judgment for their self-determination so misperceives their competence as to exacerbate the bias which already contracts their opportunity for social participation. While not all indi-viduals with disabilities are qualified to self-determine, this is also the case for classes considered to be not so vulnerable, such as the proverbially "strong" class of young white males.

Our conceptual tools for determining competence are reasonably reliable if carefully applied. They should not be warped by magnifying what is true of some members of a class into a characterization of the entire class. To suggest that the hardship and bias imposed on a class categorically compromises its members' confidence debilitates the idea of self-determination. Ironically, liberating such an oppressed class itself depends on the strength of public commitment to pro-moting self-determination for everyone.

While the disabled are the so-called vulnerable class whose situation I have examined here, the points regarding respect for their competence apply as well to the elderly and the ill. Nevertheless, because people with impairments fear they will be counted as incurably ill, especially if they depend on machines or medication to perform major life activities, it is useful to emphasize the distinc-tion here.

We speak of suffering an illness, but of having or living with a disability. We cannot be both well and ill at the same time, but we can be both perfectly well and yet disabled, as are the competitors in the Para-Olympics. When we are ill we take medication to relieve pain, discomfort, weakness, loss of appetite, but there are no medications for disability.

The distinction can be sharpened by noticing what shifts when illness (or acci-dent) eventuates in disability. Although illness is traceable to specific physiolog-ical sites, its effects are diffused and so are manifested not just in the pathology of the site but in such conditions as pain, discomfort, weakness, lassitude, absence of appetite, and disorientation. Illness defeats performances not asso-ciated with or originating at the impaired site(s), and this global debilitation invites the individual who is ill to assume the sick role.

Disabilities, on the other hand, rarely involve any such diffused manifesta-tions. Thus, we describe someone who cannot see as being visually disabled, meaning she is unable to engage in performances that necessitate vision (although she may successfully execute functions such as reading that are typi-cally performed by seeing, by adopting alternative performance modes). Or we call the group of people who cannot manipulate text (because they cannot see it, cannot interpret it, or cannot hold the pages or papers on which it is inscribed) "print disabled." In contrast, an individual who is ill usually is more globally and diffusely incapacitated.

None of this is to deny that illness can be the preceding or chronic cause of dis-ability (although traumatic accident is equally a cause of disability). As Susan Wendell points out, people often are disabled by chronic diseases such as diabetes that cause a variety of impairments such as loss of limbs and blindness.[24] And the hostility of the environments people with disabilities must endure sometimes causes them to become ill. Of course, that it is informative to say diseases cause disabilities, or to present evidence that being disabled in our built environment increases one's exposure to becoming diseased, indicates that there is no analytic, definitive, or conceptual connection or identity between the two conditions.

Wendell fears that "some of the initial opposition in disability rights groups to including people with illnesses in the category of people with disabilities may have come from an understandable desire to avoid the additional stigma of illness." Her point is well-taken, and it is important to emphasize again that the distinction as I draw it does not deny that illness can result in disability. Nor is there a justification for excluding people from being identified as disabled because they are ill.

It is important as well to understand that, as with disability, it is the way society stigmatizes being ill or being elderly that exaggerates the weakness and vulnerability of members of these classes. Ron Amundson points out that the "sick" role is a kind of social stepping or stopping out inappropriate for someone with no illness but only a disability.

> [T]he "sick role" ... relieves a person of normal responsibilities, but carries other obligations with it. The sick person is expected to ... regard his or her condition as undesirable.... One interesting correlation is that able bodied people are often offended by disabled people who appear satisfied or happy with their condition. A mood of regret and sadness is socially expected.[25]

Because physician-assisted suicide is cast as an outcome of the "stepping out" process that is definitive of the sick role, classes of individuals (primarily, the disabled and the elderly) who are compelled for lack of more propitious adaptive social arrangements to assume this role may fear that they will be especially vulnerable to its misuse. But a coherent political strategy for protecting disabled, elderly and nonterminally, chronically ill individuals from being consigned to the "sick role" and being expected to "step out" appears preferable to paternalistic approaches that portray them as incapable, incompetent, weak, and vulnerable. Such a strategy is additionally beneficial because it would increase these groups' opportunity for social participation and contribution. Unfortunately, the movement to achieve these social goals seems to have been distracted and undercut by the debate about physician-assisted suicide. What has been substituted is a campaign to replace real goods for individuals with an abstract contribution to an idealized community interest.

Undoubtedly, there will continue to be individuals with disabilities who think about killing themselves because the isolating built and social environment has not been reformed and renovated to accommodate and include them. One disquieting theme that has become increasingly prominent in the debate about physician-assisted suicide has been to belittle such persons because their reasons are too individualistic and consequently are incompatible with communitarian ideals. But despite the attention addressed during the debate over physician-assisted suicide to deplorable social conditions that could incline such people to want to die, almost nothing has been accomplished that will alleviate their suffering. To refuse suffering people the social change that would bring them optimal relief, but also to bar other avenues of relief on the ground such relief is less than optimal for the community at large, burdens those already suffering by imposing more real suffering on them in the name of an abstract and idealized community which still sets them apart.

Notes

This paper grew out of a talk I gave at a September 1996 conference on physician-assisted suicide sponsored by the Stanford University Center for Biomedical Ethics. A longer version of that talk was published in *The Western Journal of Medicine*, June, 1997. This paper takes up the philosophical analysis needed to support the original talk. I would like to thank Margaret Battin, Leslie Francis, Anne Hallum, Ellen Moskowitz, Rosamond Rhodes, and Mary Rorty for making me aware of a variety of considerations that must be given weight. I also benefited from the work on vulnerable groups by the fine scholars who were my colleagues during a year at Stanford's Institute for Research on Women and Gender.

1. Ronald Dworkin, "Introduction to The Philosophers' Brief," *New York Review of Books*, March 27, 1997, p. 41.

2. Ronald Dworkin, et al., "Assisted Suicide: The Philosophers' Brief," *New York Review of Books*, March 27, 1997, pp. 46–47

3. John Arras and Bonnie Steinbock, *Ethical Issues in Modern Medicine*. (Mountain View, CA: Mayfield Publishing Company, 1995), p. 28.

4. *Washington* v. *Glucksberg*, 117 Sup. Ct. 2258 (1997).

5. *Washington* v. *Glucksberg*, 117 Sup. Ct. 2258 (1997).

6. *Washington* v. *Glucksberg*, 117 Sup. Ct. 2258 (1997).

7. International Labor Office, "The International Protection of Women Workers." Studies and Reports, series I, no. 1 (Geneva: International Labor Office, 1921), p. 4.

8. Mark O'Brien, "A High Quad Answers Dr. Kevorkian's 'Quality of Life' Theory," *San Francisco Examiner*, Wednesday, October 9, 1996, p. A-19.

9. Jenny Morris, "Tyrannies of Perfection," *The New Internationalist*, July 1, 1992. pp. 16–17.

10. Evan Kemp Jr., "Could You Please Die Now?" *Washington Post*, January 5, 1997.

11. Section 3, Definitions (2) of Public Law 101–336 (1990).

12. Anita Silvers, "Disability Rights," *The Encyclopaedia of Applied Ethics*, ed. Ruth Chadwick (San Diego: Academic Press, in press, 1988).

13. *Washington* v. *Glucksberg*, 117 Sup. Ct. 2258 (1997).

14. See Anita Silvers, "(In)Equality, (Ab)Normality, and the "Americans With Disabilities' Act," *The Journal of Medicine and Philosophy* 21: 209–224 (1996), and " 'Defective" Agents: Equality, Difference and the Tyranny of the Normal," *The Journal of Social Philosophy*, June 1994, special twenty-fifth anniversary issue, pp. 154–75.

15. Anita Silvers, "Reconciling Equality To Difference: Caring (F)or Justice for People With Disabilities," *Hypatia*, 10 (1): 30–55 (Winter 1995).

16. Section 2 of Public Law 101–336 (1990).

17. Anita Silvers, "Protecting the Innocents: People With Disabilities and Physician-Assisted Dying," *The Western Journal of Medicine*, June 1997.

18. *Washington* v. *Glucksberg*, 117 Sup. Ct. 2258 (1997).

19. *Vacco* v. *Quill*, 117 Sup. Ct. 2293 (1997).

20. *Washington* v. *Glucksberg*, 117 Sup. Ct. 2258 (1997).

21. *Washington* v. *Glucksberg*, 117 Sup. Ct. 2258 (1997).

22. Richard Carelli, "Top Court Rejects Suit Challenging Assisted Suicide," *San Francisco Examiner*, Tuesday, October 14, 1997, p. A–11

23. David Savage, "High Court Lets Oregon Legalize Assisted Suicide," *San Francisco Chronicle*, Wednesday, October 15, 1997, pp. A-1, A-5.

24. Susan Wendell, *The Rejected Body* (London: Routledge, 1996), pp. 20–21.

25. Ron Amundson, "Disability, Handicap, and the Environment," *Journal of Social Philosophy* 23 (1): 114, 118.

9

Assisted Suicide, Terminal Illness, Severe Disability, and the Double Standard

FELICIA ACKERMAN

This essay aims to reorient the debate over physician-assisted suicide. For the most part, the debate is currently between legalizing physician-assisted suicide just for the terminally ill (or possibly just for the terminally ill and the severely and permanently disabled) and keeping physician-assisted suicide illegal for everyone. This essay argues that it would be morally unacceptable to legalize physician-assisted suicide just for the terminally ill or just for the terminally ill and the severely and permanently disabled, and that the debate should be between keeping physician-assisted suicide illegal for everyone and legalizing it for all competent adults.

*   *   *

> For all the while a prisoner may have his health of
> body he may endure under the mercy of God and in
> hope of good deliverance; but when sickness
> toucheth a prisoner's body, then may a prisoner say
> all wealth is him bereft, and then he hath cause to
> wail and to weep. Right so did Sir Tristram when
> sickness had undertake him, for then he took such
> sorrow that he had almost slain himself.
>
> —Sir Thomas Malory, *Le Morte D'Arthur*

Here are three positions about assisted suicide.

1. Physician-assisted suicide should be legally available to all competent adults.
2. Physician-assisted suicide should be legally available just to the terminally ill, or possibly just to the terminally ill and to the severely and permanently disabled. (Note that positions 1 and 2 hold that the law should *allow* doctors to provide suicide assistance, not that the law should *require* them to do so.)
3. Physician-assisted suicide should be legally available to no one.

For the most part, the current debate over physician-assisted suicide is between positions 2 and 3.[1] This essay aims to reorient the debate. I think it should be between positions 1 and 3. Positions 1 and 3 both embody reasonable, although opposing, outlooks, and this essay will not try to decide between them. What it will argue is that position 2, although popular with "death with dignity" advocates and many liberals, is morally untenable.

Although assisted-suicide advocates do not characteristically endorse position 1, they often give arguments that can be used to support it. For example, on the very day I am writing this, the *New York Times* has a news story saying that

> In Florida, [AIDS patient Charles E.] Hall's legal arguments for assisted suicide [for the terminally ill] hinge on a state constitutional amendment ... that asserts a stronger right of privacy than that offered in the United States Constitution. With few exceptions, the amendment says, "every natural person has the right to be let alone and free from government intrusion into his private life."[2]

Appeals to privacy and autonomy are characteristic of assisted-suicide advocates. They have filtered into popular culture in the form of slogans like "Whose life is it, anyway?" These appeals have intuitive force. But why not apply them to all competent adults? If the issues are really autonomy and privacy, then why legalize suicide assistance only for the terminally ill?[3] Why not grant this right of privacy equally to the young and healthy—the very people our society values most—if they come to decide, for whatever reason, that they do not want to go on living? Such people could doubtless use suicide assistance in the form of prescriptions for lethal drugs, advice about administration, etc. What factors could justify granting this right of privacy only to the terminally ill?

Extreme Pain

Assisted-suicide advocates frequently paint a picture of the terminally ill in extreme and unrelievable pain, begging to die, and frustrated in this desperate wish by religious fanatics and reactionaries who insist each human life is sacred, regardless of how much the bearer of that life wants to end it. Some terminally ill people do suffer great unrelievable pain. But as a reason for legalizing physician-assisted suicide for only the terminally ill, this rationale is a failure. First, it is obviously false that all and only the terminally ill have severe and unrelievable pain. Many non–life-threatening illnesses, such as rheumatoid arthritis, cause severe unrelievable pain, and many terminal illnesses do not. In fact, a recent study found that "severe, uncontrolled pain or the fear of it" was a less influential factor than (treatable) clinical depression in terminally ill patients who requested suicide assistance.[4] Second, as Yale Kamisar points out, where extreme and unrelievable pain is present, there is a stronger rationale for allowing suicide assistance in cases where the pain will *not* soon be ended by death.[5] For people who find that severe pain makes their life an intolerable burden, surely thirty years of such life is a greater burden than six months. A possible reply is that, the longer the projected lifespan, the more likely that some cure or new form of pain relief may eventually be found. But respect for privacy and autonomy would seem to require that it be each pain-wracked patient, rather than his government, who gets to decide in his own case whether it is worth going for such a long shot.

Finally, if severe and intractable pain, rather than terminal illness, is made the condition for legalizing suicide assistance, we have the problem that this revised condition is still out of accord with the rhetoric of privacy and autonomy. True privacy and autonomy would allow each person to determine for himself what conditions would justify suicide.

Loss of "Dignity" and Other "Quality of Life" Considerations

Even aside from the question of pain, assisted-suicide advocate Dr. Timothy Quill has suggested that "suicide could be appropriate for patients if they did not want to linger comatose, demented, or incontinent."[6] Arguments of this sort are common among assisted-suicide advocates, often involving recourse to patients' right to "die with dignity," rather than linger in the "undignified" conditions just mentioned. For example, the Philosophers' Brief in favor of legalizing assisted suicide for the terminally ill holds that "it is intolerable for government to dictate that doctors may never, under any circumstances, help someone to die who believes that further life means only degradation."[7]

This sort of thinking invites a flip reply: Haven't Dr. Quill and his ilk ever heard of Depend?[8] To put the matter less flippantly, I think we need to question our society's bigoted and superficial view of human dignity, which holds that the old, ill, and disabled have less human dignity than the young and strong. Does Dr. Quill really want to endorse the view that human dignity resides in the bladder and the rectum? If being unable to control the discharge of one's urine and feces deprives one of human dignity, then what about being unable to control the discharge of one's menstrual blood? Should physician-assisted suicide also be legalized for all premenopausal women who believe that the milder "remedy" of a hysterectomy would also undermine their dignity?

Of course, the autonomy reply can be invoked here. The point is not what Dr. Quill or the signatories to the Philosophers' Brief or I believe is inimical to human dignity, but what each individual person believes about his own dignity. And of course, this is the position of mainstream assisted-suicide advocates, who do not endorse the "indignity" of incontinence as a reason for suicide except for patients who themselves want to die for this reason. To be consistent, however, such a position would also have to endorse legalizing assisted suicide for people who believe their menstruation, or their irremediable stuttering, clumsiness, or foolishness deprives them of human dignity. It was not so long ago in American history that most white Americans had difficulty recognizing the human dignity of black Americans. If there are black Americans nowadays who buy into this, would Dr. Quill want suicide assistance to be legalized for them? If not, why legalize assisted suicide for people who believe it is their incontinence, rather than their skin color, that deprives them of human dignity? A similar point applies to people who believe it is their "dependence," rather than their skin color, that deprives them of human dignity.[9] In all these cases, it seems clear that the supposed lack of dignity is a social construct arising from the low value our society places on people of a certain sort, rather than from anything inherent in the person's condition itself. The case of a person's becoming comatose or demented is in some ways different, as being comatose or demented directly and intrinsically undermines one's personality. But whether this would undermine one's human dignity more than incontinence, menstruation, stuttering, or the "wrong" skin color should be each person's own decision if we truly accept each person's "right to make momentous personal decisions which invoke fundamental religious or philosophical convictions about life's value for himself."[10]

The most general of all "quality of life" considerations is unhappiness. Although the National Hospice Organization opposes the legalization of assisted suicide,[11] its "philosophy of hospice" includes a statement that "[p]sychological and spiritual pain are as significant as physical pain."[12] But "psychological and spiritual pain" (the contemporary psychobabble for unhappiness and despair) are hardly limited to the terminally ill. So if "psychological and spiritual pain" are really as "significant" as physical pain, why not allow suicide assistance to every competent adult in these conditions who requests it?[13]

Negligible Prospects for Improvement

The standard reply is that many cases of unhappiness and despair are transient and/or can be alleviated. For example, the introduction to the Philosophers' Brief holds that "[s]tates may be allowed to prevent assisted suicide by people who—it is plausible to think—would later be grateful if they were prevented from dying,"[14] such as "a sixteen-year-old suffering from a severe case of unrequited love."[15] Putting the condition this way skews the criterion in favor of limiting suicide assistance to people with little time left to live. The less time people have left to live, the less likely they are to change their minds about *anything* during the time they have left. But not all people with predictably little time left to live are terminally ill. Would the authors of the Philosophers' Brief endorse the legalization of assisted suicide for Death Row inmates who have used up all their appeals, whose executions are due to occur in less than six months, and whose chance of a reprieve is no greater than a terminal patient's chance of a miracle cure?

The reasoning of the Philosophers' Brief can also be applied to actions other than assisted suicide. Selling one's kidney is illegal in the United States. But suppose a Death Row inmate in the above-mentioned situation or a terminally ill person has a strong and stable desire to sell his kidney. Such a person seems unlikely ever to be grateful if he is prevented from doing this—as unlikely as he would ever be to be grateful for having been denied suicide assistance. Why not let him make this "momentous personal [decision] which invoke[s] fundamental religious or philosophical convictions about life's value for himself"?[16]

Another problem, of course, is that it is not just people with predictably little time left to live who are unlikely ever to be grateful for having been denied suicide assistance. Suppose Barnes and Starnes both have the same strong, stable, and longstanding reason for finding life unbearable and wanting suicide assistance (being paralyzed from the neck down, for example, a condition many suicide advocates readily accept as a reasonable ground for wanting to die). Then, as I have suggested, it may be argued that if Barnes is terminally ill but Starnes is not, giving Barnes but not Starnes suicide assistance may well prevent less misery than would the reverse decision.

I do not know how the authors of the Philosophers' Brief would handle the cases about Death Row inmates and selling kidneys. But the introduction to the brief does consider the third sort of case. The introduction suggests that "if the [Supreme] Court adopted [the brief's] argument, the federal courts would no doubt be faced with a succession of cases in years to come testing whether, for example, it is plausible to assume that a desperately crippled patient in constant pain but with years to live, who has formed a settled and repeatedly stated wish to die, would one day be glad he was forced to stay alive."[17] The brief itself grants that "[a] state might assert ... that people who are not terminally ill, but who have formed a desire to die are, as a group, very likely later to be grateful if they are prevented from taking their own lives. It might then claim that it is legitimate" to deny all such people suicide assistance.[18] But on what grounds would the state make this claim about likelihood? And why does the example involve a "desperately crippled" (does that mean "severely crippled"?) person, rather than a young, healthy, and able-bodied person who is serving a life sentence without possibility of parole or who is desperately poor, unskilled, and stupid, and able to earn a living only by working at drudge work he detests? Such people may be just as unlikely as the "desperately crippled" person to have their lives improve to the point where they are ever glad they were forced to stay alive. How would Ronald Dworkin, author of the introduction to the Philosophers' Brief, feel about such cases?

I do not know, but one possible rationale for treating the "desperately crippled" case differently from the other two would be to say that the misery of the "desperately crippled" person arises directly from the medical facts of his situation, while the misery in the latter two cases arises from correctable social injustices. Prisons need not be unbearable places, and poverty can be alleviated. Such a rationale would face two objections. First, if unbearable misery arises from a social injustice that is not being corrected, it is hard to see how justice is served by forcing the victims to live with it, rather than by correcting the injustice or by allowing the victims suicide assistance if the injustice is not corrected. Second, it is implausible that the poor "quality of life" of even a severely disabled person in constant pain arises solely from his physical condition. In the Malory quotation at the beginning of this essay, Tristram "had almost slain himself," not just because he was sick, but because he was "a prisoner."[19] In real life, Stephen Hawking is about as "desperately crippled" as a man can be, but by all accounts he is happy. Nor does one have to be a scientific genius to be happy although "desperately" paralyzed. The local paper of the city where I live has an editor who, like Hawking, is almost completely paralyzed by Lou Gehrig's disease. This editor lives happily at home, aided by a family eager to help him stay alive—as eager as many families nowadays are to help their terminally ill loved ones die.

He also has an accommodating employer who is "pledged to supply him with whatever he [needs] to write from home"[20] and who has spent thousands of dollars on an eye-activated computer. The fact that he produces, not great works of physics, but hackneyed prose like "[w]e can gaze at a spectacular sunset, listen with rapture to a Beethoven symphony, or smile at the face of a loved one, and the experience leaves us transformed and enlarged" seems not to dim his happiness one bit.[21] Since there are severely disabled and terminally ill people who can live so happily, however, it is worth considering whether those who want to die are, like Tristram, prisoners—not prisoners in actual dungeons, but prisoners of inadequate support and backup services, a result of the low value our society places on the lives of the severely disabled and/or terminally ill.

Arguments of this sort can be found in the disability-rights movement,[22] a source of progressive opinion that seems to have had no effect on the Philosophers' Brief.[23] But an obvious reply here is that even given excellent backup services, some people will find life with Lou Gehrig's disease bearable (and even enjoyable) and some will not. This is plausible, but it is also plausible that some people will prefer death to a life sentence in even a humane prison, and even that some widows and widowers will prefer death to living without their beloved spouses.[24] Some disability-rights activists hold that the only drawbacks of disability result from prejudice and discrimination, and that, inherently, "it is . . . good to be disabled."[25] But one does not have to hold such extreme views in order to recognize that allowing assisted suicide for the terminally ill or for the terminally ill and for the severely and permanently disabled, but not for people facing other severe and irremediable misfortunes, involves a systematic devaluation of the lives of the terminally ill or of the terminally ill and the severely and permanently disabled.

Desire Not to Be a "Burden"

A popular figure in popular culture, as well as in contemporary medical ethics, is the terminally ill person who would rather die quickly than linger to be a burden to his family.[26] Although some writers oppose legalizing assisted suicide on the grounds that legalization may lead to pressure to bow out quickly, others of course disagree. The most prominent grounds for such disagreement fall into two categories.

First, some writers hold that, as Marcia Angell puts it, "Admittedly, overburdened families or cost-conscious doctors might pressure vulnerable patients to request suicide, but similar wrongdoing is at least as likely in the case of withdrawing life-sustaining treatment. . . . Yet there is no evidence of widespread abuse" of the latter sort.[27] But this overlooks the evidence disability-rights groups and other sources offer.[28] Moreover, as David Velleman points out, having the option of ending one's life can harm the patient even if no one is actively pressuring him to use it. The option may create a generally pressured climate where patients feel the need to justify their decisions to go on living.[29] I will not try to settle here whether, given existing healthcare conditions, legalizing physician-assisted suicide would be likely to do patients overall more harm than good. As I have indicated, this essay has the limited scope of arguing that if physician-assisted suicide is to be legalized, it should be legalized for all competent adults, not just for the terminally ill or for the terminally ill and the severely and permanently disabled. And clearly, the danger of pressure toward suicide is apt to be much greater with the terminally ill and the severely and permanently disabled than with the able-bodied and healthy.

But there is another response to the claim that legalizing suicide assistance might lead to pressure on patients to request it in order to avoid being a burden to their families. This is the view that such a motivation would not be a bad thing—or, at least, would not be something that the state should interfere with. Here is how the Philosophers' Brief disposes of the risk " that a patient will be unduly influenced [to request suicide assistance] by considerations that the state might deem it not in his best interests to be swayed by, for example, the feelings and views of close family members."[30]

> [W]hat a patient regards as proper grounds for [deciding to request suicide assis-tance] ... reflects ... the judgments of personal ethics—of why his life is impor-tant and what affects its value—that patients have a crucial liberty interest in deciding for themselves. Even people who are dying have a right to ... if they wish, act on what others might wish to tell or suggest or even hint to them, and it would be dangerous to suppose that a state may prevent this on the ground that it knows better than its citizens when they should ... yield to particular advice or suggestions .... It is not a good reply that some people may not decide as they really wish—as they would decide, for example, if free from the "pressure" of others. That possibility could hardly justify the most serious pressure of all—the criminal law which tells them that they may not decide for death if they need the help of a doctor in dying, no matter how firmly they wish it.[31]

This overlooks Velleman's sort of point that, even on the nonpaternalistic assumption that patients will always make the right decision, they may be made worse off simply by having the option of physician-assisted suicide. The pres-ence of this option may cause families to treat patients differently, and in any case, this option deprives patients of the option of staying alive *without* ex-plicitly choosing to do so and being seen as choosing to do so, and thus with-out having to justify their decisions to stay alive.[32] Whether losing this latter option would be worse on the whole for patients than lacking the option of physician-assisted suicide needs far more discussion, both philosophical and empirical, than the Philosophers' Brief provides. The Philosophers' Brief claims that the number of terminally ill people who correctly believe it would be in their best interest to die but who could not get suicide assistance under a blanket prohibition against it "would undoubtedly be ... vastly greater" than the number of people who would "mistakenly" get suicide assistance under the system the brief advocates.[33] But the brief gives no good reason to believe this far-from-obvious claim.

The Philosophers' Brief's view about patients' lives and families' burdens is, by current standards, relatively mild. John Hardwig holds a harsher view, that sometimes sick people have a *duty* to die (including a duty to commit suicide) in order to avoid burdening their families. Such a view would not automatically preclude Velleman's sorts of concerns. One might fear that the legalization of assisted suicide would lead to pressure on patients to end their lives even when the burden on their families was not great enough to "justify" this. But Hardwig's conception of what constitutes an intolerable family burden seems amazingly weak. He mentions living "with a spouse who is increasingly distant, uncommunicative, unresponsive, foreign, and unreachable," as well as that "[f]or a young person, the chance to go to college may be lost to the attempt to pay debts due to an illness in the family," and that "there is no opportunity to go out to see friends and the home is no longer a place suitable for having friends in."[34] He also offers a detailed discussion of the question of whether a person with a duty to die should carry out his own suicide or solicit suicide assistance from his loving family or from doctors.[35]

Hardwig's views invite obvious objections. Should being distant, uncommunicative, and unresponsive really be a capital offense anywhere, let alone in a "loving" family? Does a loving family really welcome a beloved member's suicide in order to keep a young person from having to work (and borrow) his way through college? Hardwig's views also illustrate how communitarianism, a movement that bills itself as humane, can have ruthless implications for the old and ill. Rather than recognizing the old and ill as citizens with a right to healthcare, communitarianism can be used to argue that the costs of keeping such people alive are not worth it to the "family" or "community" (i.e., to its younger and/or healthier members). Paradoxically, this would give communitarianism just the sort of brutal consequence for which individualism is often condemned—the consequence that the weak get winnowed out. Hardwig says that "[w]e fear death too much."[36] But to the extent that his views are widespread, I think that what we fear too much is the possibility of being burdened by the dependence of our sick and disabled loved ones—loved ones who are accordingly apt to be endangered if assisted suicide is made legal.

Both the views of Hardwig and of the Philosophers' Brief also raise a problem that elsewhere I have called "the paradox of the selfless invalid."[37] That is, either the patient's loved ones want him to die quickly in order to save money or otherwise make their lives easier, or they do not. If they do not, the patient does them no favor by ending his life for their sake. If they do, why is the patient sacrificing what would otherwise be left of his life for people who love him so little that they value his life less than money or freedom from encumbrance? Wouldn't a truly loving family find such a sacrifice appalling? Of course, families can have mixed feelings, which include both the desire to have the patient stay alive and the self-interested desire to get it all over with and to keep expenses down.[38] But the basic point remains. Decent and loving families, as part of their decency and lovingness, will recognize the latter desire as ignoble and, on balance, will not want patients to pander to it.

A possible exception here, pointed out by Donna Harvey in discussion, might be a case involving an old couple, both of whom have medical problems, but only one of whom is terminally ill, and where the couple's life's savings would be exhausted by medical care for the terminal one, leaving nothing for the ongoing medical needs of the other. But this is a far cry from a case involving a "loving" wife who would welcome her "beloved" husband's suicide in order to spare her the burden of living with a spouse who is distant, uncommunicative, and unresponsive.

Another objection, offered by Joseph Goldfarb in discussion, is as follows. Suppose that the motivation of the selfless invalid is paternalistic; i.e., suppose the invalid is choosing suicide in order to promote what he takes to be his family's long-term welfare, even though he knows that such a sacrifice goes against his family's wishes. Goldfarb offers the case of a terminally ill patriarch whose whole adult life has been dedicated to providing for his family and insuring their financial security and position in the community. Such a patriarch may think he is benefiting his family by forgoing an extra month of life that would use up his family's savings, even if he is aware that his family disagrees. But this case invites the question of when it is appropriate to override other people's wishes because of what you take to be their own good. Clearly, such paternalism can be justified with respect to the irrational or unwise desires of one's own small children. It may also at times be justifiable when dealing with grossly irrational desires of adults with impaired judgment. But there is nothing inherently irrational about loving one's husband or father enough to value his life above money and social standing. There is nothing inherently irrational about being appalled at the prospect of financial security and social position that are bought at the price of an extra month of a beloved husband or father's life. A truly loving (or even minimally decent) family values each member as an end in himself, not as a means to money and social position. A man who paternalistically overrides his loving family's wishes in this regard insults them by showing a lack of respect for their love for him—as a beloved family member, not as a meal ticket—and for the role this love plays in their life.

Of course, this argument cuts both ways. The family that opposes the patriarch's beneficent desire to end his life is also behaving paternalistically toward him. It is tempting to say, once again, that the point is not what any medical ethicist thinks is a good reason to end one's life, but what each patient thinks. But what would the authors of the Philosophers' Brief say about a healthy young man who has a strong, stable, and longstanding desire to kill himself because he thinks his life insurance will be more valuable to his family than he is?[39] People who endorse legalizing assisted suicide in this case because they regard this decision about "why [one's] life is important and what affects its value" as being on a par with the decision of a terminally ill or severely and permanently disabled person who requests suicide assistance in order to avoid burdening his family are genuinely advocating autonomy. Those who favor legalizing suicide assistance only in the latter case, however, are using a double standard that devalues the lives of the severely and permanently disabled and/or terminally ill.

So far, the thrust of this essay has been to argue that position 2 that I sketched at the beginning is morally untenable. But I have not tried to decide between positions 1 and 3. Each has a respectable philosophical outlook behind it. Many ethicists have defended position 3.[40] Position 1, however, deserves more consideration than it has received. Position 1 is the true expression of the notions of privacy and autonomy. After all, our society allows its adult members to engage in all sorts of risky and potentially lethal activities: race-car driving, jumping across the Snake River canyon on a motorcycle, hang-gliding.[41] We allow people to assist others who engage in such activities. We do not require the participants to undergo counseling or psychological assessment to prove their rationality.[42] Why not treat suicide the same way?

Daniel Callahan offers one possible answer, the answer that there is something inherently wrong with an individual's seeking that much control over his own death.[43] But this invites an obvious reply. If you are not supposed to control your own death, who or what is? God? This answer cannot be a basis for law in a secular society. The vicissitudes of nature? Then why take antibiotics or get yourself vaccinated? Other people? Well, whose life is it, anyway? Callahan's lack of respect for individual choice about one's own life and death makes his views unsuitable as a basis for law in a pluralistic society, although the considerations stressed by Velleman, Kamisar and disability-rights groups make me wary of position 1 as well. My aim in this essay, however, has been simply to undermine position 2.[44]

Notes

1. Although Yale Kamisar and some disability-rights groups seem more sympathetic to position 1 than to position 2, the thrust of their arguments is to oppose any legalization of assisted suicide, rather than to offer position 1 as a serious contender. See the amicus brief of Not Dead Yet and ADAPT (*Vacco* v. *Quill*, and *State of Washington* v. *Glucksberg*, October 1995). See also Yale Kamisar, "Against Assisted Suicide—Even a Very Limited Form," *University of Detroit Mercy Law Review* 72 (4) (1995): 735–69; "Physician-Assisted Suicide: The Last Bridge to Active Voluntary Euthanasia," in John Keown, ed., *Euthanasia Examined* (Cambridge: Cambridge University Press, 1995), pp. 225–60; "The Reasons So Many People Support Physician-Assisted Suicide—And Why These Reasons Are Not Convincing," *Issues in Law and Medicine* 12 (2) (1996): 113–31, and "The 'Right to Die': On Drawing (and Erasing) Lines," *Duquesne Law Review* 35 (1) (1996): 481–521.
2. Mireya Navarro, "Assisted Suicide Decision Looms in Florida," *New York Times*, July 3, 1997, A14.
3. All the references cited in note 1 raise this question. See also Leon Kass and Nelson Lund, "Courting Death: Assisted Suicide, Doctors, and the Law," *Commentary* 100 (December 1996): 23.
4. Jane Brody, "Personal Health" column, *New York Times*, June 18, 1997. See also H. M. Chochinov, et al., "Desire for Death in the Terminally Ill," *American Journal of Psychiatry* 152 (8) (1995): 1185–91.

5. Kamisar, "Against Assisted Suicide—Even a Very Limited Form," 740–41.

6. Jane Gross, "Quiet Doctor Finds a Mission in Assisted Suicide Case," *New York Times,* January 2, 1997, p. B1.

7. R. Dworkin, et al., "Assisted Suicide: The Philosophers' Brief," *New York Review of Books,* March 27, 1997, p. 44. See also appendix B in this volume.

8. Incontinence underpants, available in any drug store.

9. For criticisms of the view that human dignity requires youth, health, able-bodiedness, and independence, see my "No, Thanks, I Don't Want to Die With Dignity," op-ed, *Providence Journal-Bulletin,* April 19, 1990; and "Goldilocks and Mrs. Ilych: A Critical Look at the 'Philosophy of Hospice,' " *Cambridge Quarterly of Healthcare Ethics* 6 (1997): 318; as well as J. David Velleman, "Against the Right to Die," *The Journal of Medicine and Philosophy* 17 (1992): 666–67.

10. Dworkin, introduction to "Assisted Suicide: The Philosophers' Brief," p. 41.

11. See Linda Greenhouse, "Before the Court, the Sanctity of Life and Death," *New York Times,* January 5, 1997, p. 5. As I have argued elsewhere, since hospices also eschew life-prolonging treatment for the terminally ill, the National Hospice Organization seems committed to an arbitrary "Goldilocks Principle" for the terminally ill, holding that "death by assisted suicide is too soon, death after high-tech life-prolonging treatment is too late, [but] 'natural' death is just right, [even though] hospices do not eschew intervention through technology or other forms of human ingenuity in other areas" ("Goldilocks and Mrs. Ilych: A Critical Look at the 'Philosophy of Hospice,' " 317). For further critical treatment of the hospice approach to death and dying, see my short story, "Flourish Your Heart in This World," in M. Nussbaum and C. Sunstein, eds., *Clones and Clones: Facts and Fantasies About Human Cloning* (New York: Norton, 1998), pp. 312–33.

12. B. Menard and C. Perrone, *Hospice Care: An Introduction and Review of the Evidence* (Arlington, VA: National Hospice Organization, 1994), p. 4. The term "philosophy of hospice" is theirs.

13. Yale Kamisar stresses this sort of point in "Against Assisted Suicide—Even a Very Limited Form," 744–45.

14. R. Dworkin, introduction to "Assisted Suicide: The Philosophers' Brief," *New York Review of Books,* March 27, 1997, p. 41.

15. Ibid.

16. Ibid.

17. Ibid.

18. Dworkin, et al., "Assisted Suicide: The Philosopher's Brief," pp. 46–47 (see also appendix B of this volume). Note that the formulations in these two quoted passages need improvement. The crucial issue can hardly be simply whether "one day" or "later" (for how long?) the patient would be glad he was forced to stay alive. What if he is glad for only one day out of thousands—or for only five minutes?

19. While we are on the subject of quality of life, let me suggest that the reader's own quality of life will be immeasurably increased if he reads *Le Morte D'Arthur.*

20. Gerald S. Goldstein, "How to Live," *Brown Alumni Monthly,* March 1996, p. 32.

21. Ibid.

22. For example, psychologist and disability-rights activist Carol Gill claims that, "In the vast majority of cases, when a severely disabled person persists in wanting to die, there is an identifiable problem in the support system" (Mary Johnson, "Unanswered Questions," *The Disability Rag,* September/October 1990, p. 17). See also the ADAPT/Not Dead Yet brief. Surprisingly, however, some (although definitely not all) disability-rights activists do not apply such considerations to the terminally ill, but instead write as though suicide can be reasonable for the terminally ill, but not for the severely and permanently disabled. For examples, see Anne Peters, "A Misunderstood Case," *The Disability Rag,* February/March 1984, pp. 9–10 and Kathi Wolfe, "Death—Take a Holiday," *The Disability Rag,* January/February 1994. For criticisms of this double standard for the severely and permanently disabled and the terminally ill, see my letter

to the editor, ibid. (July/August 1994), as well as the letter from Wesley J. Smith, ibid. (March/April 1995).

23. This oversight is also found in *Life's Dominion*, by Ronald Dworkin, one of the signatories to the Philosophers' Brief and the author of its introduction. Although he respects people like Stephen Hawking, who live happily with severe disability, Dworkin approvingly cites the case of quadriplegic Nancy B., who successfully sued to have her respirator turned off because, as she put it, "The only thing I have is television and looking at the walls. It's enough. It's been two and a half years. . . ." (Ronald Dworkin, *Life's Dominion*, (New York: Knopf, 1993), p. 184. It is remarkable that this prominent liberal does not even mention that Nancy B.'s having nothing to do but look at the walls or watch television is a result not of her disability but of her lacking the sort of backup services readily available to Stephen Hawking. Nor does Dworkin's book suggest the life-ending option for people whose poverty makes life unbearable by their standards. His book's use of the word "vegetable" for comatose people further betrays his readiness to devalue the lives of the ill and disabled. Even more surprisingly, Yale Kamisar, who generally shows great respect for the lives of the terminally ill and/or severely disabled, approvingly quotes Jed Rubenfields's claim that denying patients the right to terminate life supports would force them into "a particular, all-consuming, totally dependent, and indeed rigidly standardized life: the life of one confined to a hospital bed" (Kamisar, "The Reasons So Many People Support Physician-Assisted Suicide—And Why These Reasons Are Not Convincing," p. 126). This grim description does not fit the life of Stephen Hawking, the Providence editor described above, or many other severely disabled respirator-users who have adequate backup services. But I am not claiming that a ban on physician assistance in removing life supports would be as defensible as a ban on physician-assisted suicide. For some relevant differences, see Ibid., 120–28.

24. The example about widows and widowers echoes a question from the ADAPT/Not Dead Yet Brief.

25. Disability-rights activist Cyndi Jones, as quoted in Joseph Shapiro, *No Pity* (New York: Times Books, 1993), p. 12.

26. For example, see Steven Erlanger, "A Scholar's Suicide: Trying to Spare a Family Anguish," *New York Times*, October 26, 1987, p. B1, which admiringly recounts the suicide of seventy-five-year-old Richard Schlatter, who committed suicide because he wanted to spare his family the burden of coping with his terminal illness. See also my letter to the editor, November 4, 1987.

27. Marcia Angell, "The Supreme Court and Physician-Assisted Suicide—The Ultimate Right," *New England Journal of Medicine*, 336 (January 2, 1997): 52. See also The Philosophers' Brief, pp. 45–46 [Appendix B], as well as Bioethicists' Brief Supporting Respondents, *Vacco* v. *Quill* and State of *Washington* v. *Glucksberg*.

28. See the ADAPT/Not Dead Yet Brief, as well as the references in my "Goldilocks and Mrs. Ilych: A Critical Look at the 'Philosophy of Hospice,'" notes 21, 61, and 62. See also Ann Hood, "Rage Against the Dying of the Light," op-ed, *New York Times*, August 2, 1997.

29. See Velleman, "Against the Right to Die." (His view have some complexities that I am not addressing.)

30. Dworkin, et al., "The Philosophers' Brief," p. 46. See also appendix B in this volume.

31. Ibid. Note that the first occurrence of the word "pressure" in this passage is in double quotes, suggesting remarkably, that such pressure is always merely alleged rather than real. (But see ibid., pp. 44 and 45, where the brief does mention the possibility of pressure from relatives.)

32. See Velleman, "Against the Right to Die."

33. Dworkin, et al., "The Philosophers' Brief," p. 46.

34. John Hardwig, "Is There a Duty to Die?" *Hastings Center Report* 27 (2) (March/April 1997): 36.

35. John Hardwig, "Dying at the Right Time: Reflections on (Un)assisted Suicide," in H. LaFollette (ed.), *Ethics in Practice* (Cambridge, MA: Blackwell, 1997), pp. 53–65.

36. Hardwig, "Is There a Duty to Die?" p. 40.
37. Ackerman, "Goldilocks and Mrs. Ilych: A Critical Look at the 'Philosophy of Hospice,'" p. 318. See also my "The Forecasting Game," in W. Abrahams, ed., *Prize Stories 1990: The O. Henry Awards* (New York: Doubleday, 1990), pp. 318–19, and my letter to the editor, *New York Times*, November 4, 1987.
38. I owe this point to Sara Ann Ketchum.
39. Yale Kamisar offers another possibility, the case of "a healthy septuagenarian, who has struggled to overcome the hardships of poverty all his life [and] wants to assure that his two grandchildren have a better life than he did. So he decides he will sell his heart for $500,000 and arrange to have a trust fund established for his grandchildren" ("The Reasons So Many People Support Physician-Assisted Suicide—And Why These Reasons Are Not Convincing," 114). "But would 'society' allow this transaction to take place?" Kamisar asks, answering, "I think not." (Ibid.) While I think he is correct, I consider the case less clear-cut than the one I offer. There is so much ageism in our society that I suspect there are people who would object to sacrificial suicide in my case of a healthy young person but who would admire it in Kamisar's case of the septuagenarian grandfather. See also Kamisar, "The 'Right to Die'—On Drawing and Erasing Lines," note 116, p. 507–508.
40. For example, see the Kamisar references in note 1 here, as well as Daniel Callahan, *What Kind of Life?* (New York: Simon and Shuster, 1990), and Kass and Lund, "Courting Death: Assisted Suicide, Doctors, and the Law."
41. See Dworkin, *Life's Dominion*, p. 222–24.
42. Positions 1 and 2 have variants, depending on whether such safeguards as counseling, waiting periods, proof of rationality, etc. would be required of those seeking suicide assistance from physicians. Space limitations prevent me from discussing these issues in detail here. But it is worth noting two objections to requiring counseling or even certification of rationality by a therapist, beyond such basic competence tests as giving consistent answers to questions like "Do you want suicide assistance?" and "Do you want to stay alive?" First, such a requirement would give therapists enormous power over people's lives. Second, judgments of rationality in this context seem particularly subject to therapists' own ideologies about suicide. Is it really likely that disability-rights psychologist Carol Gill (quoted in note 22, above) and a therapist who favors assisted suicide will agree about a severely and permanently disabled person's underlying rationality in requesting suicide assistance?
43. Callahan, *What Kind of Life?*, chapter 8.
44. I thank James Dreier, Joseph Goldfarb, Donna Harvey, Sara Ann Ketchum, Thomasine Kushner, Lynn Pasquerella, and James Van Cleve for helpful discussions of this material.

Part Three

Considering the Practice of Medicine

THE PHYSICIAN'S ROLE is an especially controversial feature in the debate over the legalization of physician-assisted suicide. We find a wide range of strongly held views on this aspect of the issue. Some who believe that assisted suicide should be forbidden see physician involvement as significantly more immoral or more dangerous than cooperation from a non-physician. Some who believe that legalizing assisted suicide could be permissible might still have strong feelings about its being something that doctors should never do. Some believe that, in certain circumstances, assistance with suicide is actually part of a physician's obligation. And some believe that there are some particular death-hastening acts that physicians should perform, others that physicians should not perform.

Trust is a key component of the contention over the role of doctors. Some maintain that patients' trust will be enhanced by their knowing that doctors will not make them suffer for nothing. They also expect that patients will feel free to accept therapeutic efforts if they know that they will be helped to die when things do not go well. Some expect that patient trust would be undermined by the legalization of physician-assisted suicide because the physicians' commitment to preserve life would be contaminated by a license to kill.

The chapters in this section present the range of views on the place of assisted suicide in the practice of medicine. Rosamond Rhodes's "Physicians, Assisted Suicide, and the Right to Live or Die" presents an argument for seeing assisted suicide as a special obligation for physicians. Bernard Baumrin's "Physician, Stay Thy Hand!" argues for the opposite view, that assisted suicide is completely forbidden for physicians. Then there are two intermediate positions. Michael Teitelman, recognizing that the character of an act is influenced by its setting, presents reasons for keeping physician-assisted suicide out of the hospital setting. In his essay "Not in the House: Arguments for a Policy of Excluding Physician-Assisted Suicide From the Practice of Hospital Medicine," he argues for treating hospital medicine as a special case with special policies that might be different in other healthcare environments. In "An Alternative to Physician-Assisted Suicide," Bernard Gert, Charles Culver, and K. Danner Clouser offer another sort of compromise. They argue for allowing some death-hastening acts under certain circumstances and forbidding others under other circumstances. They also make a case for carefully choosing our words: The language we use to describe these acts makes a significant difference.

10

Physicians, Assisted Suicide, and the Right To Live or Die

ROSAMOND RHODES

When we are confronted with compelling individual cases that incline us toward accepting the legalization of physician-assisted suicide, we are moved. The humane response to the suffering of others is to want to help alleviate their pain. And so, compassion and empathy are typically invoked as our justification for wanting to remove some of the sanctions against assisting others to die. This essay presents a discussion in a different voice. It offers an analysis of some of the concepts that are central to the discussion of physician-assisted suicide: the nature of rights in general, the right to life and its relation to the right to die, the moral principles of respect and beneficence, and a conception of physician duty. By weaving these ideas together I present an argument for concluding that some acts of euthanasia, assisted suicide, and withholding treatment can be ethical and that assisted suicide can sometimes be part of a doctor's duty.

*   *   *

MANY DISCUSSIONS of the possibility of ending life invoke rights. Some arguments appeal to the right to life while others refer to the right to die. These concepts have infused public discussion to such an extent that we find certain social action groups identified as "Right-to-Lifers," and there has even been a "Society for the Right to Die." Yet, there has been no explication of these rights in the philosophic literature which also employs rights language in discussions of life ending.[1] Rather, the subject of choosing to end one's own life is usually analyzed from the perspective of autonomy, utility, or theology.

One aim of this essay is to show the role of rights in understanding the morality of choosing death.[2] Arguments in *Washington v. Glucksberg* and *Vacco v. Quill* and in the Supreme Court decisions on these cases all address and acknowledge the importance of the right to die in confronting the issue of physician-assisted suicide. So, I will begin with some preliminary remarks about the nature of rights in general and then proceed to discuss the right to life and its relation to the right to die. I shall attempt to illuminate the nature and relation of these rights so that the concepts can serve as useful tools in confronting the serious issue of people choosing death for themselves or others.

Another aim is to show how the concept of a right to life actually supports the case for physician-assisted suicide. Here I will introduce the well-established moral principles of respect and beneficence along with a general conception of physician responsibility. I will try to show how weaving these strands together with the concept of a right to life leads to the conclusion that, under certain circumstances, physicians have a moral responsibility to assist a patient in hastening death. In short, I will try to make a case for the moral acceptability of withholding treatment, assisting suicide, or even euthanasia, and attempt to show that sometimes these acts may be morally required of physicians.

A Conceptual Framework

Everyone agrees that murder is wrong. But, is euthanasia murder? Is assisting another in suicide murder? Is withholding treatment murder? If they are murder then, surely, such actions are immoral. If, however, euthanasia, assisting suicide, or withholding treatment can be distinguished from murder, they would not necessarily be immoral. In certain cases committing such acts might then be permissible, and in some situations they might even be morally required.

An analogy here may help to illustrate the conceptual framework for answering these questions. Many actions which may be described as "taking what is not yours" are morally permissible. Accepting a gift and quoting lines from a poem with attribution are acts of taking what is not yours, and they can certainly be acceptable. Theft, however, is wrongful taking, and so is plagiarism. Theft is immoral because it violates property rights, while accepting a gift and quoting (with attribution) do not.

Perhaps murder, which is wrongful killing, can be distinguished from other acts of killing. Perhaps murder is wrong because it, too, violates a right—the right to life—while other kinds of killing may not violate that right. If this analogy holds, the right to life could be the basis for distinguishing moral from immoral killing.

The Right to Life

A right to life is acknowledged by nearly every moral tradition. In the natural rights tradition, the right to life is universally recognized as the most basic of all natural rights and as the foundation for many other natural rights. The right to life is also implicitly accepted as a fundamental given by every system of legal rights. Divine rights theories typically consider life to be a God-given quality which amounts to a right to life that must not be breached without divine authority. And contractarian theories derive the right to life as the most basic guarantee of either a social contract or a rational personal commitment. But what is a right to life and what does having such a right suggest?

Rights

For the purpose of this discussion we need only appeal to the weakest and most comprehensive sense of right as liberty.[3] Thomas Hobbes, the seventeenth-century British philosopher who was the first to explicitly define the concept of a right, relied upon this liberty sense. For him a right is a moral freedom to do something—or not do it. So, for example, if someone has the right to speak, she is free to either speak or not speak. If someone has a property right to some thing, she is free to either use it or let it lie fallow.

Now, moral rights are usually held to be correlative with moral duties. In other words, (typically) when someone has a right, another has a duty.[4] According to this correlativity thesis, morality is primarily concerned with relations between parties.[5] Whenever we encounter a moral relationship, it can be defined by the assignment of rights and duties to the parties. So, if someone has a right, someone (else) has a duty. When someone has a right to speak, that person is free to speak or not to speak, while whoever has the correlative duty *must*, *should*, is *obliged*, *bound*, *required*, or *constrained* to allow the one with the right to either speak or to remain silent. The party with the duty *owes* the one with the right the respect of his liberty to talk or not. And the one who is bound is constrained from either coercing the one with the right to make any utterance or silencing him. Similarly, with property rights, when someone has a right to use or not use something, others owe the correlative duty to allow the property owner to wield or not wield, to exploit or not exploit the thing.

The Right to Die

What does this analysis of rights imply for those who admit that people have a right to life? It suggests that someone with a right to life would have the liberty to live and also the liberty to not live, the freedom to act to preserve life and also the freedom to end it. In other words, in the case of the right to life, having that right implies having the right to die.[6]

This may seem like a strange or counter-intuitive conclusion. Yet, unless we have some reason to believe that the concept of rights should be conceived in a different sense when applied to life itself, we have to accept the conclusion that whoever has a right to live also has a right to die. And, if the right to life is something a person always has, then she also always has the right to die.[7] Certainly the moribund person has it, but so does the disabled one, the one who is in pain, and even the one who has no pain. They each have a right to die whenever they choose because we agree that they have a right to life and that involves having the choice of whether to live or not.

This is not, however, to suggest that a person will always be doing the right thing by acting on either of these rights. Exercising the right to life or the right to die could conflict with some other overriding duty which an individual might have. When all of a person's duties are reckoned together, some duty or combination of duties may conflict with and outweigh either their right to live or their right to die.[8] For example, someone's right to life could be limited by the duty to respect another's similar right. One cannot, for instance, take another's life jacket to save oneself. Similarly, a right to die could be outweighed by some duty. A parent's right to die could be limited by the duty to care for, nurture, and protect dependent children.

Although we give serious moral weight to other people's right to life, we also recognize that even the right to life can be overridden. We can be justified in killing an armed attacker in order to preserve our own lives. But, just as we need serious moral reasons to justify overriding another's right to life, the symmetry of our analysis suggests that overriding another's right to die also requires significant justification. People who have a right to live, therefore, also have a *prima facie* right to commit suicide, and, within the medical environment, they have the right to refuse (or discontinue) life prolonging therapy.

Killing and Letting Die

To make this last inference clear we need to examine the relationship between killing and letting die. In the philosophic literature and the domain of medical practice, it has seemed morally permissible to allow someone to die from the natural course of her disease even though her life could be prolonged somewhat by a therapeutic intervention. However, the deliberate act of hastening (another's) death, i.e., killing, has seemed immoral to many people inside and outside of the medical professions.

In an influential article, "Active and Passive Euthanasia," philosopher James Rachels discusses this intuitively appealing distinction between killing and letting die and argues that the concepts are morally equivalent.

Rachels presented the cases of Smith and Jones. Smith drowns his young cousin in the bath by holding his head under water. Jones, on the other hand, has the same intentions relative to his own cousin, but "merely" watches as his cousin "drowns all by himself." Rachels frames the issue in a question.

> Now Smith killed the child, whereas Jones "merely" let the child die. That is the only difference between them. Did either man behave better, from a moral point of view?[9]

Since our moral intuition finds Smith and Jones to be equally bad and their actions equally culpable, Rachels suggests that there is no moral distinction between killing and letting die. In the cases of Smith and Jones, both of their actions count as murder because they accomplish the same thing (the wrongful death of their cousins) and the means used were sufficient to achieve the desired result. (Killing by drowning, by shooting, by stabbing, by choking, or by doing nothing when one could interfere with the process could each be expected to be sufficient means for killing.) If killing and letting die can be equally wrong when we know that the active performance would be wrong, then killing and letting die can be equally right when we know that the passive performance would be right.

Applying this insight to the subjects of suicide and the refusal of treatment shows that when we find one's refusal of the initiation or continuance of treatment (i.e., passive suicide) to be justified by the right to die, active suicide (i.e., killing oneself) is thus equally justified. Conversely, since killing and letting die are morally equivalent, if choosing to withhold treatment is wrong, then suicide must be wrong as well.

Having established grounds for the right to die and for thinking that there is no moral difference between killing and letting die, we can now move on to considering whether killing is ever morally required. Our analysis of rights only told us that we must allow others to try to sustain themselves or to try to kill themselves. Aside from self-defense, can killing another ever be the right thing for us to do?

The word, "euthanasia," derived from *eu-thanatos*, "a good death," suggests that there are situations in which some people consider killing another to be a good thing for the one who is killed. But, what can make such killings right and can such euthanasia killings ever be morally required? If they were required, who would have the responsibility for performing the deeds?

Our rights analysis tells us nothing about what we must actively do. It merely explains "negative rights," the choices we must allow others to make for themselves. It gives us the duty not to interfere. But a duty to try to help another save or end a life would have to come from another source. Our understanding of the right to life leaves us no understanding, for example, of why Smith should have pulled his young cousin to safety and instituted resuscitative measures. Our understanding of the right to die does not explain why anyone should help another in committing suicide nor does it explain why anyone should ever actually kill another.

To complete the argument we need an account of the "positive rights" that bear on this issue. To explain these positive rights, we must invoke the principles of respect and beneficence. Both are moral duties; and, like the right to life, both are endorsed in some form by most moral theories.[10]

Respect

Respect for another individual's autonomy is the most fundamental of all moral principles. It derives from the recognition that what distinguishes moral beings from other creatures and what entitles persons to special treatment are 1) the ability to conceive of moral principles or rules; 2) the ability to choose actions to conform with moral rules; and 3) the ability to limit action to conform with those principles. Having these three abilities, which amount to the ability to be moral, is essential to being an autonomous agent. Autonomy, therefore, deserves ultimate respect because it is taken as the ground for both moral treatment and moral responsibility.

While it is clear that everyone is not fully autonomous, respect for autonomy requires that we presume that individuals are autonomous and allow people to make their own choices even when it seems that they are not doing what is best for them. Respect for autonomy and the symmetrical force of the rights to live and to die require that we allow everyone who we can presume to be autonomous (i.e., those people whom we have no good reason to consider lacking in autonomy) to act on decisions about their own lives and deaths.[11] So, while the explication of the right to life accounts for people's right to make decisions about their own deaths, the duty of respect for others' autonomy provides a fuller perspective for appreciating why others should not interfere with those choices.

Beneficence

Beneficence is the duty to get involved, the duty to do good for another. It requires that we try to do what we can to help others meet their needs.[12] The

general duty of beneficence falls on the shoulder of every person, although it
may require different actions from different individuals in similar situations in
order to achieve the good for the other. In similar situations the difference in
what precisely is required of different people varies according to the relationship between the beneficiary and the benefactor, and it also depends on what
the benefactor actually can do.[13] And what a person can do is directly related to
having the relevant knowledge and ability. If good Cousin Gold comes upon his
young cousin drowning in the bathtub, Gold must do what he can to try to save
his cousin, because we usually presume that life is a good and because the
floundering child needs help to save himself. Gold pulls the now unresponsive
child out of the tub and does not know what to do besides calling 911 for help.
Doing what he can satisfies his duty. Good Cousin Green, the doctor, in the
same situation but knowing more about possible interventions, would be
obliged to do more.

Physician Responsibility

In medicine, the duty of beneficence is explicitly expressed in the codes and oaths
of the profession as the duty to act for the good of one's patients.[14] Beneficence
morally binds healthcare providers because everyone (them included) must try
to help others in need and because physicians have assumed special obligations
of acting for the good of their patients by joining their profession.[15]

Respect for patients is also an important feature of physician responsibility.
Again, respect is a general obligation for all people (including doctors) and it is
also a feature of physicians' professional responsibility. In the tradition of medicine, the duty to respect patients is expressed in the Oath of Maimonides's commitment, "May I never consider the patient merely a vessel of disease." And the
much more recent American Medical Association's Principles of Ethics explicitly
proclaim that "A physician shall be dedicated to providing competent medical
service with compassion and respect for human dignity."[16]

We also know that different people may have different views of what is good
or best in a particular situation. Sometimes a doctor's view of what is best can be
at odds with a patient's view. Once that much is acknowledged it is easy to appreciate that accepting the patient's view of what is good or best as a guide to treatment can be a significant value to that patient. People like having their own way,
and, when the decisions are intimately concerned with a person's own body and
life, the differences between alternatives can be tremendously important. In this
way the patient's ranking of goods becomes incorporated into the physician's
duty. When a doctor recognizes a professional obligation of beneficence (the duty
to act for the patient's good), the patient's perspective on that good has to be fac-
tored into the scope of that professional responsibility. In some circumstances a
patient will consider the doctor's choice to be no good at all. Therefore, identifying the place of the patient's choice in meeting the doctor's duty of beneficence
illuminates the significance of respect for autonomy to medicine and provides
insight into the link between these two central obligations.

Life-Ending Decisions and Physician Responsibility

If everyone has the duty to act from beneficence when confronted by a needy person, then who has the right to beneficent care? Obviously, whoever has a need which can be met by the other within the constraints of their other obligations.[17] And again, as with the rights and duties relating to life and death, the rights and duties related to beneficence can be outweighed by conflicting moral claims. When there are no overriding duties, however, beneficence makes a strong claim on the one in a position to provide aid, and the person in need seems entitled to the assistance.

The more assistance a needy person requires, the greater the amount of assistance that must be given. In standard medical care this proportionality is clearly the governing principle. When a patient requiring medication is able to obtain it and administer it himself he is handed a prescription slip and sent on his way. When the patient needs more and is unable, because of disability or lack of the requisite skill, to care for himself, he is provided, according to his need, with home health aid, hospital treatment, or surgery.

Now, if alleviation of suffering (both mental and physical) is a need, or if preservation of dignity is a need, or if respect for self-determination (autonomy) is a need, then there certainly may be times when beneficence requires assisting others in meeting their needs. Therefore, when some need can only (or best) be met by ending life, the duty of beneficence provides a ground both for assisting in suicide and for euthanasia. The more assistance that is required, the more that must be provided. Because of one's relationship with the other, one's knowledge and one's ability, that duty may fall more heavily on some than on others. A doctor's commitment to acting for patients' good creates a clear obligation to help a patient avoid an agonizing, protracted death. Allowing a patient to suffer when the suffering could be ended is an obvious violation of the duty of beneficence.

If a person needs to alleviate suffering, preserve dignity, or continue to act from his own choices, and if he also requests the assistance of another in doing what he cannot do for himself, then beneficence binds the one who can to aid the one who cannot. The doctor, in particular, may have a greater obligation than others to provide help in hastening death. One significant reason is that, by professional training, doctors should know how to hasten death with minimum discomfort or violence, and another is that, because of their access to medical technology and pharmacology, they are in a position to implement their choice of best means.[18]

The physician who also may have a special caring relationship with the patient also incurs greater obligation, just because of that relationship. A history of the doctor and patient caring for and about one another can increase the responsibilities to one another. The patient's trust in the doctor's being there and meeting his life- and health-related needs creates an expectation that his doctor will continue to be there and meet such needs. When health fails and life is no longer a good in the patient's eyes, it is not unreasonable for a patient to continue to expect his doctor to care about his well-being and for a patient to rely upon his doctor to continue to provide for his related needs.

Furthermore, the doctor's place in our society makes the doctor the most fitting person to assist patients in their life-ending decisions. We are legitimately concerned that a patient's declared wish to die may not be the expression of an autonomous choice or that it may express a choice made without awareness of all of the relevant alternatives. Doctors are well situated to make this assessment. Often the doctor has known the patient over a period of time and may also know, if she has taken care to enquire, whether the patient's long-held beliefs support the present decision. However, when a doctor is asked to cooperate with a patient's decision to end life, because the choice involves a deviation from the usual life-preserving physician activities, she is entitled to verbally challenge the patient's decision. Doing so gives the patient the opportunity to again examine the reasons for choosing death and consider whether the decision to hasten death is, in fact, the only or best means of achieving his ends (e.g., the patient may be concerned about avoiding pain or abandonment and may, therefore, want to die as a means to achieving those ends, which, perhaps, could be achieved by other means).[19] The physician is also the one who is able to improve the patient's pain management and who has access to our society's means for addressing other issues that may be troubling the patient. For example, the physician has contact with social workers, home health services, nursing homes, and hospice care facilities. Furthermore, by training, a physician ought to be especially able to assess whether or not the patient is clinically depressed or otherwise lacking in the capacity for making a life-ending decision, and a physician is able to initiate the appropriate intervention.

These considerations are especially significant because assisting in suicide and practicing euthanasia are exceptions to the standard requirements of morality which forbid killing and demand that we thwart suicide attempts. Our default assumption is that life is a benefit and most people want to live. But we know this is not always true.

A final and telling consideration for doctors being the ones to assist patients with their life-ending choices is that doctors already do it. For years doctors have been legally required to comply with patient refusals of life-preserving treatment and with patient requests for discontinuing life-prolonging treatment. For years doctors have even been legally required to abide by patient advance directives and surrogate decisions about these matters. For years doctors' actions in these matters have largely followed the legal requirements and our society has largely been satisfied with their performance.

Our society broadly recognizes the necessity and appropriateness of allowing doctors to do what others are forbidden from doing. Physicians are expected to administer potentially lethal drugs that would be counted as poisons in less trusted hands. Surgeons are asked to plunge their knives into bodies and sometimes to remove limbs and vital organs. Others committing similar violence would be charged with assault and battery or murder. Psychiatrists are required to restrain and confine people who are likely to harm themselves or others. Non-physicians would be accused of unlawful imprisonment or kidnapping. We don't even find that the words "poisoning," "assult," or "kidnapping" are appropriate when applied to what the physician does. All of these special physician authorizations suggest three understandings: These life-threatening actions are potentially dangerous, so they should be forbidden; sometimes it is important to do what is usually forbidden; doctors should be the ones who are trusted to act in the domain of health (life and death) and to do those actions which are prohibitted for non-physicians. In light of the many ways in which we already trust doctors to make decisions about life-threatening palliation and initiating or discontinuing life-preserving treatment, it seems reasonable to remove the (unreasonable) prohibition on doctors assisting in their patients' suicides.

Doctors, and more specifically doctors in the hospital setting, have developed institutional practices and support (e.g., institutional procedures, in-service education, ethics committees) for making and implementing life-ending decisions. Most typically, decisions to cooperate with hastening patients' deaths are discussed in the semipublic arena of team decision-making and unit conferences, thereby giving physicians the opportunity to reexamine cases, to justify their decisions to their peers, to raise additional considerations, and to voice objections. This ongoing practice has allowed doctors and their institutions to accumulate substantial experience in managing life-ending decisions. And because of the generally satisfactory results, our society has come to trust doctors to cooperate with patient decisions, to act for the right reasons, and to do the job well.

None of this is to say that there is no room for improvement. There certainly is. But it does argue that doctors should be the ones to assist patients in dying. Doctors already have experience with life ending, they have developed institutional practices and supports that help to insure that life-ending choices are carefully examined, and society already has historical reasons to trust its doctors with morally critical life and death decisions. If we openly acknowledge physician life-ending responsibilities we can also demand that medical education pay special attention to preparing our doctors to do the job well. We can assure that our physicians be prepared to fulfill this aspect of their obligations by training (or retraining) them to acquire information about patient life-ending decisions, to adequately assess and treat depression, to treat pain, and to end life.

Conclusions

These complex considerations provide reasons for accepting the moral insights that (a) there is a right to die; (b) there is no ethical difference between killing and letting die; and (c) beneficence can require that we assist another in ending his life. Taken together they point to conclusions about suicide, assisted suicide, and physician-assisted suicide.

ⓘ We have a duty to interfere with suicide when we cannot comprehend it as the choice of a rational agent. Since the consequences are so serious and since we know that suicide is sometimes the expression of irrationality or transient emotions, when we do not know the person or the circumstances and reasons for the choice we must act to prevent the suicide when we can. Beneficence requires us to intervene, presuming that life is a good to the person in question. Duty requires temporarily overriding the person's autonomy and right to die until we can know more about the choice.

2. We have a duty *not* to interfere with a suicide when we know enough about the person and the choice to appreciate that the action clearly is autonomous (rational).

3. Assisting in suicide or performing euthanasia is permissible if someone is choosing to die *and* we can appreciate the rationality of the person's choice to die *and* the person needing assistance requests help that we are able to provide. As Phillipa Foot explains, we need to see that life is no longer a basic good to such persons and that for them life has become an evil.[20]

4. Sometimes, because of special features of the need, or because of the special relationship, or because of the uniqueness of the knowledge involved, a physician may have a professional obligation to assist in a suicide or perform euthanasia.

5. When choosing death seems rational to us, but the person in question is unable to communicate, it would be permissible to practice euthanasia at the request of a formally designated proxy or in compliance with a formal advanced directive. Surrogate's decisions can be verbally challenged in much the same way that one could ask an individual to justify any choice that requires the cooperation of others. Even when an advance directive allows no possibility for challenge, respect for autonomy can justify compliance with such decisions.

6. Without previous direction from the patient, euthanasia could *not* be justified on the grounds discussed above. The right to die would not provide grounds for ending life. In such cases the right to die would not be on equal footing with the right to life because most of the time most people want to live. Invoking the principle of autonomy for killing someone who had never indicated that dying would be a good for them in these circumstances would require a specious analogy to one's own autonomous choice. There may be valid grounds for euthanasia in such cases, but additional arguments would need to be provided.

Law and Morality

The conclusions above attempt to reflect what should be done from the moral perspective. As is well known, however, morality and the law do not always coincide. If my arguments are sound, then today we live with a disparity between the law and the conclusions of ethical reasoning.

The enactment of proxy laws and the Patient Self-Determination Act and the acceptance of living wills reflect the acceptance of passive suicide in our society. Withholding and withdrawing treatment have been allowed for some time. Yet, assisting in suicide and active euthanasia are still prohibited by law. The complex argument I have offered suggests, however, that they should be legally allowed and that doctors should consider assisted suicide and even euthanasia as sometimes part of their job.

When we are confronted with compelling individual cases that incline us toward accepting the legalization of physician-assisted suicide, we are moved. The humane response to the suffering of others is to want to help alleviate their pain. And so, compassion and empathy are typically invoked as our justification for wanting to remove some of the sanctions against assisting others to die. Stopping there, at the acknowledgement of powerful emotions, is stopping short of an argument. It invites others who are inclined the other way, by powerful feelings of repulsion at the thought of killing innocents, to wage a battle of emotions on equal footing. This paper has presented a discussion in a different voice. It offered an analysis of key terms and a formal argument for the moral acceptability of physician-assisted suicide. Its conclusion suggests that the appropriate position will conform with reason and that an understanding of the arguments can inform our emotions. It also suggests that opponents of this view address these points and put forward a response grounded in moral reasoning.

Notes

1. E.g., a recent title on the subject, J. P. Moreland and Norman L. Geisler, *The Life and Death Debate: Moral Issues of Our Time* (New York: Praeger, 1990), offers a survey of the arguments mustered for and against euthanasia and suicide (among other issues). While they review and summarize a good deal of the philosophic literature and mention the right to life they fail to give an analysis of its function within the debate. Similarly, the collection of essays edited by John Donnelly, *Suicide: Right or Wrong?* (Buffalo: Prometheus, 1990) has no sustained discussion of the right to life or the right to die and the survey article included in that text ("Theistic and Nontheistic Arguments" Milton A. Gonsalves, pp. 179–83; reprinted from Fagothey's *Right and Reason: Ethics in Theory and Practice* [Columbus: Merrill, 1989]) again mentions rights but offers no rights argument in its list.

2. Because my focus is limited to the right to life and the right to die, in this essay I will not be discussing the extensive literature on the sanctity of life.

3. There are certainly many different conceptions of rights. For example, according to Hohfeld, rights can be explicated as four distinct classes of moral entities: liberties, claims, powers, and entitlement. The liberty sense in which I am using the concept, however, is sufficiently weak to be recognized and accepted, at least in part, by most rights theorists. It also goes beyond the scope of this paper to discuss the differences and their implication. Most rights theories embrace the substantive assertions I make about rights i.e., correlativity.

   The rights theories I concern myself with are deontological. Although consequentialist theorists sometimes use rights language, they have no commitment to the existence of rights. For them rights talk amounts to no more than useful jargon or a pragmatic schema for representing their version of morality. In this essay I shall not be discussing such approaches to rights.

4. Here duties to oneself are the notable exception.

5. Virtue theory might be an exception.

6. Here, the apparent exception would be a theological position that takes G-d to hold the right to each individual's life. This view, however, conforms with the general pattern of the right to life entailing the right to end life. Those who see decisions about human lives as belonging to G-d would grant that He can choose whether a person will continue to live or not.

Theological positions of this sort are, however, beyond the scope of my discussion because they would deny that individuals have a right to life. Such theological views can only accord individuals more limited rights, perhaps as agents for G-d, the proper right-holder. This essay is not aimed at a discussion of theology, but at arguments for policy within a society that accepts a separation of church from state.

7. Notice that I am *not* claiming that the person who claims a right to die has alienated the right to life. I am asserting the opposite, that it is because the person holds fast to the right to life that the person has the right to choose not to live.

8. E.g., a Rossian analysis of weighing those respects in which an action would be *prima facie* right against those respects in which it would be *prima facie* wrong would reveal my *prima facie* duty. Sir W. David Ross, *Foundations of Ethics* (Oxford: Oxford University Press, 1939).

9. James Rachels, "Active and Passive Euthanasia," *The New England Journal of Medicine*, vol. 292, No. 2 (Jan. 9, 1975), pp. 78–80. While other authors have attempted to refute Rachel's claim (e.g., Tom L. Beauchamp, "A Reply to Rachels on Active and Passive Euthanasia," in *Contemporary Issues in Bioethics*, 3rd ed. [Belmont, CA: Wadsworth, 1990] 248–55; Thomas D. Sullivan, "Active and Passive Euthanasia: An Impertinent Distinction," *Human Life Review*, Summer 1977, pp. 40–46), I find Rachels' main point, that killing and letting die *can be* morally equivalent, is left unaffected by their remarks.

10. Focusing on the moral features of action that are endorsed by most moral theories has come to be called principlism. Tom L. Beauchamp and James F. Childress, *Principles of Biomedical Ethics*, 4th ed. (New York: Oxford University Press, 1994).

11. Rosamond Rhodes, "Debatable Donors: When Can We Count Their Consent?" *The Mount Sinai Journal of Medicine* 60 (1) (1993): 45–50.

12. Kant, for example, gives such an account of beneficence. Immanuel Kant, *Foundation of the Metaphysics of Morals*, trans. by Lewis White Beck (Indianapolis: The Library of Liberal Arts, 1959), p. 424.

13. The obliging nature of a particular relationship may be either a matter of chance involving a general obligation (e.g., being there—walking into the bathroom as the child slips under the water) or a matter of the ongoing nature of a special obligation (e.g., parenthood).

14. E.g., the Hippocratic Oath, the Code of Maimonides, the Code for Nurses, the American Medical Association Principles of Medical Ethics.

15. Defining the parameters of "everyone" and "other" is beyond the scope of this paper. Obvious inclusionary/exclusionary categories might be: persons, humans, potential members of the moral community, sentient beings, those with a future like ours.

16. In her paper on physician obligation Margaret Battin argues in a similar vein from the principles of beneficence and autonomy. Margaret P. Battin, "Physician-Assisted Suicide and Opt-Out Conscience Clauses: Is a Physician Ever Obligated to Help?" forthcoming in Linda Emanuel, ed. *Physician-Assisted Suicide* (Cambridge, MA: Harvard University Press, 1998).

17. The issue of whether rights based on needs create duties (e.g., Gewirth) or whether the assumption of duties create rights (e.g., Nozick) is important to moral theory but beyond the scope of this paper. The point here, that there is an obligation to meet another's needs, is neutral on the question of the source of the obligation.

18. "Knowledge of how to do the job well" is a crucial consideration. People who decide to end their lives are legitimately concerned with failing and instead only making themselves worse off. Indeed, in the early experience with euthanasia in the Netherlands, physicians lacked the knowledge of how to do the job well and frequently failed to achieve death for their patients. Again, a choice of the "best" means for a particular patient would have to reflect the patient's choice and ranking of considerations.

19. Dan W. Brock makes this point in *Deciding for Others: The Ethics of Surrogate Decision-making* (Cambridge: Cambridge University Press, 1989).

20. Phillipa Foot, "Euthanasia," *Philosophy and Public Affairs* 6 (2) (1977).

11

Physician, Stay Thy Hand!

BERNARD BAUMRIN

In this brief note I argue that physicians, under no circumstances, should be parties in assisting patients in ending their lives. The argument, in its bare bones, is that physicians alive today are the beneficiaries of a two-and-a-half-millennia-old tradition that abjured assisting patients in suicide and killing people at the behest of others. None alive today has the right to betray the public trust that that tradition has endowed them with and, furthermore, there is no need for them to participate. Others can do what is required, and physicians should stay out of the business altogether.

*　　*　　*

SUICIDE MAY OR MAY NOT BE A NATURAL RIGHT, that depends on whether there are natural rights and whether one owns one's own being to dispose of as the owner sees fit. Suicide is only a legal right where it has been established by law, customary or explicit. States, in general, prohibit suicide rather than facilitate it. Further, aiding suicide is so fraught with the possibility of serving merely to disguise murder that there is a tendency to legislate against it even more vigorously than against suicide itself.

Enlisting someone to aid in one's suicide endangers the confederate. However clear the one dying might make to posterity that the person aiding was dragooned into the role, suspicions might still linger and, where aiding in a suicide is illegal, the costs might be very great. Can we readily distinguish Pindarus stabbing Cassius at Cassius's insistence from Strato holding the sword that Brutus runs upon? Do we really know that Pindarus and Strato aided in the suicides of Cassius and Brutus rather than that they killed them, perhaps to be free, perhaps to run from the battlefield, perhaps to escape Anthony and Augustus's slaughtering troops? Where are Cassius and Brutus to testify that Pindarus and Strato aided in their deaths at their commands or entreaties? Where is the testimony that they are now to be free? Who is left in danger when the suicide is successful?

That Cassius and Brutus did not wish to face the fate that defeat destined them to (dragged to their place of execution in public humiliation) is quite understandable (neither did Hitler, nor Goering) and that may justify their belief that suicide was a more desirable way to die. And so it may have always seemed—if one must die and, if the time between knowing that and it occurring promises to be one of maximal psychic or physical discomfort, then suicide seems a quite reasonable alternative. Probably the best way to go is quickly and painlessly, but people have chosen to drown, to starve, and to eviscerate themselves. Those who have chosen painless exits, at least relative to the obviously painful ones, have tended to favor poison—it doesn't maim, it can be taken in comfort, and one can preserve one's vision of oneself intact, just merely dead. So, if you want to die by your own hand, peacefully, painlessly, and relatively quickly, you go to an expert in poisons. One versed in the properties of poisons should be able to provide the perfect solution. Such a person, one with knowledge of the various properties of poisons, will be able to provide a quick-acting, hopefully painless potion that one can take at one's leisure.

In the Greek world such persons, ones with knowledge of the properties of potions, poisonous and otherwise, included physicians. And one may imagine that they were called upon often to provide such potions both for murder and suicide. So, with good reason, as an article of their craft, as part of their undertaking among themselves, they forswore providing poisons to patients, presumably regardless of the entreaties they might be subjected to. The Hippocratic Oath included that solemn undertaking, and it implied that physicians were not in the business of ending lives, whether of fetuses or of the distraught.

When Socrates took hemlock, he drank it himself, and it was provided by the prison guard. We might take this case as the paradigm of the good suicide—a drug which causes no pain, which causes a creeping numbness, which permits one to be in control of ones faculties until the last moment, and which one takes oneself. All that remains to be settled is procuring the poison. Effective poisons are readily available today without it being required that physicians prepare them. Moreover, the effects (and side effects) of various drugs and their lethal doses are well known and, in any case, can be readily found in the *Physician's Desk Reference*. The physician as pharmacist is no longer required and need have no role to play in aiding a suicide. If the state wished to legitimize suicide and take a favorable attitude toward drug-facilitated death, it could set up a special pharmacy to dispense suicide drugs (upon proper proof that it was intended for self-use, and of identification). If that idea sounds strange, it is at least partly because we immediately see avenues for abuse, and partly because we can foresee the possibility that lethal potions would lie about unused for some time.

But, in principle, there is no pressing need for physician assistance in the normal case of suicide, and there is a long standing tradition amongst physicians that they do not aid in (and surely do not abet) the suicide of others. I do not extend this tradition to other healthcare workers; first, because they do not have long traditions (except perhaps for nuns who have maintained hospitals for at least several hundred years) and, second, there is as yet no suggestion that persons have a right to their aid in dying (though surely many a nurse has engaged in both involuntary as well as voluntary euthanasia, and one can be sure that many would readily volunteer).

My argument is only about physicians and their duties. Anyone claiming a right to physician assistance in dying must show that some physician has a duty to satisfy that right . Were a legal right to physician assistance in dying created, the physician might still be duty bound to reject the legal claim on several grounds, the most salient of which is his professional obligation not to aid in suicide. This might be founded on an oath, or simply on the assumption that the doctoring tradition he or she has joined does not do that sort of thing. The scientific tradition assumes truth in reporting, and there is justifiable public outrage when there is a breach. The teaching tradition assumes that grades and examinations will be dealt with as objectively as possible, and there is justifiable outrage at trading grades for favors, or passing exams that are clearly failures. The doctoring tradition assumes that the physician will do his or her utmost to heal the sick and to preserve and extend life. That is the "reason to be" for physicians, just as truth is the reason to be for scientists. The doctor trades on an aura developed in antiquity and extended through the centuries by a continuous line of physicians, summed up, if crudely, as "Do no harm." Among the obvious implications of this commanding injunction is that the physician will not do anything that unnecessarily endangers the life of the patient. Only medical necessity, and the paucity of knowledge, permit the physician to endanger the patient's life. There are of course (and there always have been) numerous occasions when the physician does endanger the patient, but never knowingly or intentionally, unless some treatment promises to have a good outcome.

Every physician, I contend, trades on this aura that the present physician did not create. It is the product of his or her predecessors. Not one alive today has a right to abjure that aura without publicly and prominently labeling himself or herself a "physician" of a special sort, a doctor for hire who has no prior commitments to the principles of the physician's profession.

The reasoning behind the Hippocratic Oath is to us now merely guesswork, but the fact that it served well for so long suggests that it created a public perception and a public trust that benefited every adherent. From the itinerant Greek physicians in the Roman Empire to Doctors Without Borders, the public trust that physicians are partisans for life and health has opened doors, provided security in times of war, has created a perception of neutrality greater than the neutrality of the cloth. We can see in our mind's eye clerics—priests, ministers, rabbis, imams, etc.—leading their followers into holy battle, but we can not see that as part of the calling of physicians. The physicians' holy icon is life, not victory; the enemy is death and disease, not people and their states. This allegiance is not any physician's personal property to dispose of. The lesson of the Nazi doctors during World War II, and the outrage that greeted the disclosure of their behavior, is that physicians can not engage in activities that deliberately endanger the health and life of patients. It is absolutely forbidden, not merely undesirable; the prohibition attaches to them irrevocably in a way that can not be abjured.

It is not merely qua physician that one must not deliberately endanger others under the guise of doing medicine, but that a physician is to be always a champion of life and health in every context. That is the public perception, and the public perception binds the practitioner as tightly as an oath, as tightly as any obligation can bind.

The contemporary debate about physician-assisted suicide turns on two special kinds of cases that are cited as exceptions to the general principles set out above. I think that those principles are beyond reasonable dispute, but if there is an argument to be made that physicians don't have the duties cited above, then the rest of my argument will be irrelevant because it depends on those principles for its premises.

The two exceptions are the irreversibly comatose and the terminally ill. The cases are actually very different because in the latter there is a range of communication issues entirely absent from the former. In the former case, whether or not there are advance directives about the cessation of care or not commencing care, the cases that we have to deal with primarily are those where the patient is under care and can no longer communicate his or her present wishes about anything. Thus the first exception, the irreversibly comatose, can only metaphorically be considered physician-assisted suicide; rather, it is physician (or someone else) killing. The issue of physician-assisted suicide with the comatose (irreversible or not!) only arises when a patient has left such an explicit advance directive that called upon someone (physician or otherwise) to kill the patient when certain explicitly identified events occurred. Even in this restricted class of case, and one might imagine that there were fairly few, it is a stretch to consider killing that patient a case of suicide. If the patient's coma was possibly reversible then it is unlikely that the advance directive, however explicit, would be taken at its word.

The case of the terminally ill is not straight-forward because the range of complications and the elasticity of the relevant time frame make determining who is to count as terminally ill either too easy or too difficult—too easy because anyone who has an illness or condition which will result in death if not cured is terminally ill, and nevertheless there may be much life left, and life well worth living for anyone who is terminally ill. "Terminally ill" is only superficially a medical term; at base it is a catchall for such states as declining rapidly, irreversibly ill (i.e. incurable with a prognosis of imminent death—but then imminent has a wide range itself), prone to sudden heart attact, stroke, seizure, etc. For many in such condition there is realistic hope that the state they are in can be reversed or at least stabilized, and the threatened decline abated. Of course, for a great many that is not and will not be the case. We do all die, and our deaths are frequently preceded by periods of irreversible decline.

We can then isolate a class of noncontroversial cases: those who are facing the imminence of death, with conditions reliably predicted to be irreversible. It is irrelevant whatever they are or are not in pain; what matters is that they do not want to face whatever the future holds for them, brief as it may be. This desire may be entirely rational, though of course it is sometimes quite irrational. We can assume that there are cases that reasonable people would agree merited serious consideration for suicide. The question then, and the only question that I am addressing, is whether any physician should be involved in implementing that decision.

On the positive side, there are all the obvious issues of patient self-determination (patient autonomy), easing suffering (beneficence), reducing the dangers of unauthorized individuals volunteering, and largely eliminating the chance that things will go wrong and the patient will survive though more maimed than before.

On the negative side, the principal consideration is that aiding a suicide compromises the physician's professional persona. Trust is betrayed, and it is likely   ?
that it will be replaced by an image of the physician as "angel of death" (which was what Doctor Mengele was called in the camps). Should physician-assisted suicide be decriminalized, patients will routinely ask for such help and only the mean-spirited will decline. The physician who wishes to perpetuate the tradition of the doctor as the unflagging opponent of death will cease to be perceived as heroic but now as curmudgeonly. Those who see themselves as duty-bound not to aid in suicide will be castigated as old-fashioned and uncooperative.

Yet, nothing, absolutely nothing, requires that physicians be the instruments of suicide aid. Assuming the would-be suicide cannot muster the courage or get the appropriate drugs, some public-spirited nonprofit group, like the Society for the Right to Die or the Hemlock Society, can be called in to do the appropriate paperwork; obtain the relevant information from the physician or hospital; procure the relevant official government approvals; get the drugs; administer the drugs; and arrange to have the whole thing on videotape. Except for signing the death certificate, no physician needs to be involved and none should. The physician's task is to tell the patient (and relevant others when the patient is either a minor, under guardianship, or comatose) what's wrong, and to the best of the doctor's ability, what is going to happen. The physician's job is to heal the sick, to stave off death, and to say as best as he or she can what the future will be like for each particular patient. The physician gets to be the helpless person's medical guide because he or she is trusted to hold the patient's good uppermost, and the patient's good does not include death.   ← not necessarily

I have not strayed far from the beginning. Doctors must not engage in assisting suicide. They are inheritors of a valuable tradition that inspires public trust. None should be even partly responsible for the erosion of that trust. Nothing that is remotely beneficial to some particular patient in extremis is worth the damage that will be created by the perception that physicians sometimes aid and even abet people in taking their own lives.

Who knows if, after the legalization of physician-assisted suicide is publicly approved, doctors will also be entreated (by the state, or relatives, or HMOs), to end "lives that are not worth living."

12

An Alternative to Physician–Assisted Suicide

A Conceptual and Moral Analysis

BERNARD GERT, CHARLES M. CULVER,
AND K. DANNER CLOUSER

The standard ways of distinguishing between voluntary active euthanasia (VAE) and voluntary passive euthanasia (VPE) are shown to be inadequate. Nevertheless, a critical moral difference between them is revealed by emphasizing the distinction between patient requests and patient refusals. Using this latter distinction it is shown that patient refusal of food and fluids counts as VPE and thus provides an alternative to a request for physician-assisted suicide (PAS). This alternative has been largely overlooked in the ongoing debate concerning the legalization of PAS. This is partly due to the widespread false belief that going without food and fluids is painful for terminally ill patients. Educating patients and physicians about this alternative should lessen the demand for PAS. After analyses of the concepts of killing, suicide, and assisting suicide to determine their appropriate application we critically examine the Supreme Court decision concerning PAS. The article concludes with a model statute that requires patients to be informed of the alternative of refusing food and fluids and guarantees that physicians who provide appropriate pain medication during this refusal will not be regarded as assisting suicide.

*   *   *

TWO TASKS ARE NECESSARY in order to determine whether physician-assisted suicide should be legalized.[1] The first is to clarify the meaning of the phrase "physician-assisted suicide"(PAS) so that one can be precise about what procedures are correctly specified by that phrase. The second task is to inquire into the moral acceptability of doctors' carrying out those procedures that are appropriately labeled as PAS. It is essential to settle the conceptual task before deciding about PAS's moral acceptability. Once conceptual matters are clarified and the moral acceptability of PAS is determined, disagreements about the social consequences of legalizing PAS continue to make it an issue on which reasonable people can take either side. However, we shall show that awareness of an alternative to PAS, namely, the refusal of food and fluids, significantly weakens the arguments in favor of legalizing PAS.

It may seem odd to claim that there is a problem in clarifying what is meant by PAS. The prototypical example of PAS, and the way it is almost always practiced, is for a doctor to provide a lethal quantity of sedating medication to a patient who subsequently ingests it and dies. Everyone agrees that the doctor who carries out such an action has engaged in PAS. The conceptual problem arises not with the prototypical example but with the conceptual analyses that some philosophers and some courts have made in commenting on whether PAS is morally justified, or is legally sanctioned or forbidden. One philosopher, for example, has claimed that there is no morally significant difference between killing a patient (voluntary, active euthanasia; VAE) and helping a patient commit suicide (PAS).[2] One circuit court has argued that performing PAS is exactly the same as withdrawing life support and rendering palliative care as a patient dies.[3] Thus PAS has been identified both as the same as killing a patient (VAE) and the same as allowing a patient to die (voluntary, passive euthanasia; VPE). We believe that the three alternatives, 1) PAS; 2) killing a patient (VAE); and 3) allowing a patient to die (VPE), are quite distinct from one another conceptually and morally.

Active and Passive Euthanasia

To understand how PAS, VAE, and VPE differ, it is useful to begin with the distinction between VAE and VPE. A distinction between these two has traditionally been made and accepted both by clinicians and by philosophers. VAE is killing and, even if requested by a competent patient, is illegal and has been historically prohibited by the American Medical Association. VPE is "allowing to die" and, if requested by a competent patient, it is legally permitted and morally acceptable.

None of the standard attempts to describe the conceptual distinction between VAE and VPE have gained wide acceptance. These attempts have involved the following concepts and issues: 1) acts versus omissions, 2) stopping treatment (withdrawing) versus not starting treatment (withholding), 3) ordinary care versus extraordinary care, and 4) whether the patient's death is due to an underlying malady. However none of these four ways of making the distinction has any clear moral significance and all are inadequate because they all fail to appreciate the moral significance of the *kind of decision* the patient makes, in particular whether it is a request or a refusal.[4] It is this failure that leads to the mistaken conclusion that there is no morally significant distinction between VAE and VPE.

First, a terminological matter needs to be clarified. It is perfectly standard English to use the term "request" when talking about a refusal. Thus one can say that a patient requests that a treatment (such as ventilation) be stopped. The patient is, in fact, refusing continued use of the respirator. Unfortunately, this perfectly correct and common way of talking obscures the crucial moral distinction between patients' refusals and requests. When combined with the use of the terms "choice" and "decision," which also can be applied to both requests and refusals, the language fosters the false conclusion that all patient decisions or choices, whether refusals or requests, generate the same moral obligation for physicians.

This confusion is compounded because the most common use of the terms "decision" and "choice" with regard to a patient involves neither refusals nor requests, but rather the patient's picking one of the options that her physician has presented to her during the process of informed consent. However, when dealing with patients who want to die, this most common use of "decision" or "choice" is not relevant. Rather a patient is either 1) refusing life-sustaining treatment (VPE), or 2) requesting that the physician kill her (VAE), or 3) requesting that the physician provide the medical means for the patient to kill herself (PAS). Thus talking of a patient's decision or choice to die can be extremely ambiguous. Furthermore, refusals of treatment and requests for treatment, whether or not death is a foreseeable result, have very different moral and legal implications.[5]

The Duties of Physicians

Treating terminally ill patients often troubles physicians because they seem to have two irreconcilable duties, one to prolong the lives of their patients, and another to relieve their pain and suffering. Further, even if they do not believe that they always have a duty to prolong the lives of their patients, they still have a dilemma, for it seems to some physicians that the only way to relieve the pain and suffering of some of their patients is to kill them. Yet many of these physicians think that it is always inappropriate for physicians to kill their patients. In order to resolve this dilemma, the duties of physicians must first be determined. Then a morally significant way to make the distinction between VAE and VPE, or between killing and allowing to die, must be provided. Only after this is done can the moral acceptability of helping patients die (that is, PAS, a practice which is more than allowing to die, but less than killing) be determined.

Determining the duties of physicians is important because not doing what one has a duty to do is morally unacceptable unless one can justify the failure to perform that duty. How are physicians' duties determined? It is done partly by sociological investigation of the society in which the physicians are practicing their profession since duties are largely determined by the function of a particular job or profession in the society. The function of medicine is similar in every society, so one would expect physicians in all societies to have similar duties. Some differences in the relative importance of different duties, however, should also be expected; e.g., some societies place greater weight on duties to the individual patient while others place greater weight on duties to protect the health of the society as a whole.

However, the concept of duty is not completely equivalent to "what one is required to do by one's job or profession." Duties must be compatible with what is morally acceptable. An act is morally acceptable if and only if an impartial rational person would be willing for everyone to know that they are allowed to do that kind of act, i.e., that it be publicly allowed.[6] If no impartial rational person can advocate that a given kind of act be publicly allowed, having a job or belonging to a profession cannot provide a duty to perform that violation. A "professional" pickpocket does not have a duty to steal, even if he is being paid to do so by his employer. Indeed, it is hard even to imagine a profession in which there is a duty to do what is morally unacceptable, although there are some who mistakenly view lawyers as having a duty to act in a morally unacceptable way if it is necessary to defend their clients. Showing that a kind of action is morally unacceptable shows that no one can have a duty to do that kind of action. Thus it may be possible to rule out some mistaken claims about the duties of physicians without doing any sociological investigations.

Refusal of Treatment and the Duties of a Physician

Overruling a competent informed patient's rational refusal of treatment, including life preserving treatment, always involves depriving the patient of freedom, and usually involves causing him pain. No impartial rational person would publicly allow these kinds of paternalistic actions and so they are morally unacceptable. Since it is morally unacceptable to overrule the rational refusal of a competent informed patient, it cannot be the duty of a physician to do so. Theoretically, the situation does not change when lack of treatment will result in the patient's death, but as a practical matter, it does make a difference. Death is such a serious harm that it is never irrational to choose any other harm in order to prevent death. Even though it is sometimes rational to choose death over other harms, choosing death may be, and often is, irrational. Further, people are usually ambivalent about choosing death, often changing their minds several times, but death is permanent, and once it occurs, no further change of mind is possible.

The seriousness of death requires physicians to make certain that patients realize that death will result from failure to receive the life sustaining treatment. It also requires physicians to make sure a patient's desire to die is not due to suffering that can be relieved by palliative care. The physician also must make certain that a patient's desire to die and hence his request to die, is not primarily the result of a treatable depression and, more generally, that a patient's unavoidable suffering is sufficient to make it rational for him to prefer death to continuing to live. When patients have terminal diseases, however, it is generally the case that when they want to die, it is rational for them to choose death. Further, although there is often some ambivalence, in our experience, their desire to die usually remains their dominant desire. When an informed competent patient makes a rational decision to stop life prolonging treatment, a physician cannot have a duty to overrule his refusal of treatment, even though normally a physician has a duty to prevent death.

We have shown that physicians cannot have a duty to preserve the lives of their competent patients when those patients want to die and their desires are informed and rational. When prolonging a person's life requires unjustifiably depriving him of freedom, it is morally unacceptable to do so. We have thus established that physicians do not and cannot have a duty to prolong the lives of their patients when their patients have a rational desire to die. We are not suggesting that whenever a patient with a terminal disease makes any tentative suggestion that treatment be stopped, the physician should, with no question, immediately do so. It is part of the duty of a physician to make sure both that the refusal is rational and that it is the informed, considered, and noncoerced preference of the patient. When, however, it is clear that a patient really does want to die and the refusal is rational, then it is morally unacceptable for the physician to administer life prolonging treatment.

Killing Versus Allowing to Die

Having shown that a physician does not have a duty to prolong the lives of patients who rationally prefer to die, the next issue to be settled is whether not treating such patients counts as killing them. If it does count as killing them, then the conclusions of the previous section may have to be revised. In the previous section not treating was taken as simply not prolonging the life of a competent patient when he rationally refuses treatment. However, not treating is sometimes correctly regarded as killing. If a physician turns off the respirator of a competent patient who does not want to die, with the result that the patient dies, the physician has killed him. The same is true if the physician discontinues antibiotics, or food and fluids. It may even count as killing if the physician refuses to start any of these treatments for his patient when the patient wants the treatment started and there is no medical reason for not starting it. Just as parents whose children die because of not being fed can be regarded as having killed their children, physicians who have a duty to provide life-saving treatment for their patients can be regarded as killing them if they do not provide that treatment. However, we have shown that a physician does not have a duty to provide life-saving treatment when a competent patient rationally refuses such treatment. Not treating counts as killing only when there is a duty to treat; in the absence of such a duty, not treating does not count as killing.[7]

If the patient refuses treatment and there is no duty to treat, then it does not make any moral difference whether the physician stops treating by an act, e.g., turning off the respirator, or an omission, e.g., not giving antibiotics. It also makes no moral difference whether the physician stops some treatment that has already started, e.g., turning off the respirator or discontinuing antibiotics, or simply does not start such treatment. Granted that it may be psychologically easier to omit rather than to act, and not to start than to stop, nevertheless there is no moral difference between these different ways of abiding by a patient's refusal. Similarly, it makes no moral difference whether the treatment is extraordinary, e.g., involving some elaborate technology, or is quite ordinary, e.g., simply providing food and fluids, or whether or not the death is due to an underlying malady. If there is no duty to treat, not treating is not killing. If a competent patient rationally refuses treatment, there is no duty to treat. Therefore, if a competent patient rationally refuses treatment, abiding by that refusal is not killing. Further, since the refusal is rational, it is, in fact, morally prohibited to override the patient's refusal by treating, and to do so is an unjustified deprivation of the patient's freedom. Recognition that honoring the rational refusal of treatment or of food and fluids is not killing, but, at most, allowing to die, reveals the significant difference between VAE and VPE. There is no inconsistency in strongly supporting VPE and being against legalizing PAS or VAE.

Stopping Food and Fluids

It might be objected that the analysis given above does not apply to providing food and fluids because providing them is not medical treatment, and so failing to provide them is killing. As noted before, children who die because their parents did not feed them are correctly regarded as having been killed by their parents. Similarly, it may be objected, patients who die because their physicians do not provide them with food and fluids are killed by them. This objection is based on the mistaken view that anything at all in the above analysis turns upon the concept of treatment. It is because parents have a duty to feed their children that not feeding them counts as killing. Physicians have no duty to overrule rational refusals by competent patients, so their not providing them with food and fluids does not count as killing. When a patient wants not to be kept alive and it is rational to want not to be kept alive, then it is morally prohibited for his physician to force him to accept anything to keep him alive. On the other hand, his physician should continue to provide comfort and palliative care to such a patient.

Since the point of dying sooner is to avoid the pain and suffering of a terminal illness, stopping only food while continuing fluids is not a good method of dying because it takes a long time, often more than a month. However, when fluids are also stopped, dying is much quicker; usually unconsciousness occurs within a week and death less than a week later. Further, contrary to what is widely assumed, dying because of lack of food and fluids is not physically unpleasant or painful if there is even minimal nursing care.[8] When there is no medical treatment keeping the patient alive, stopping food and fluids may be the best way of allowing a patient to die. It is usually painless, it takes long enough for the patient to have the opportunity to change his mind, but is short enough that significant relief from pain and suffering is gained. However, because of the psychological difficulties involved in a longer dying process, some patients may still prefer PAS to discontinuing food and fluids.

Analysis of Killing

It may be thought that, if complying with a patient's refusal of treatment requires the physician to perform some identifiable act, e.g., turning off a respirator, which is the act that results in the patient's death, then regardless of what was said before, the doctor has killed the patient. This seems to have the support of the *Oxford English Dictionary* which says that to kill is simply to deprive of life. One may accept that a doctor is morally and legally required to turn off the respirator and thus is justified in killing her patient, but still maintain that she has killed him. Even those who accept the death penalty and hold that some prison official is morally and legally required to execute the prisoner do not deny that the official has killed the prisoner. Killing in self-defense is both morally and legally allowed, yet no one denies that it is killing. Similarly, one could agree that the doctor is doing nothing morally or legally unacceptable by turning off the respirator and even that the doctor is morally and legally required to do so, yet claim that in doing so the doctor is killing the patient.

If one accepts this analysis, then it might also seem plausible to say that an identifiable decision to omit a life-prolonging treatment, even if such an omission is morally and legally required, also counts as killing the patient. One could simply stipulate that doctors are sometimes morally and legally required to kill their patients, namely, when their action or omission is the result of a competent patient rationally refusing to start or to continue a life prolonging treatment. Thus it would seem that the important point is that the doctor is morally and legally required to act as she does, not whether what she does is appropriately called killing. However, it is still significant whether such an action should be regarded as killing because having a too simple account of killing can cause numerous problems.

Many doctors do not want to regard themselves as killing their patients, even justifiably killing them. More importantly, all killing requires a justification or an excuse. If all the morally relevant features are the same, the justification or excuse that is not adequate for one way of killing will not be adequate for all other ways of killing either.[9] Thus, if a justification is not publicly allowed for injecting a lethal dose of morphine, then it will not be publicly allowed for disconnecting the patient from the respirator. Since even advocates of VAE do not propose that doctors should ever be morally and legally required to kill their patients, even justifiably, doctors would not be required to comply with rational refusals of treatment by competent patients. It might even come to be thought justifiable to prohibit physicians from honoring the rational refusals of life-sustaining treatments of competent patients. Thus changing the way killing is understood (i.e., counting complying with a patient's rational refusal as killing him) would have unfortunate implications.

Those who favor legalizing VAE do not want to require doctors to kill their patients; they merely want to allow those doctors who are willing to kill, to do so. Similarly for PAS, no one has yet suggested that a doctor be required to comply with a patient's request for a lethal prescription. On the other hand, since doctors are morally and legally required to comply with a competent patient's rational refusal of life-sustaining treatment, complying with such a refusal has not been regarded as killing. Providing palliative care to a patient who refuses life-sustaining treatment is not morally controversial either. Killing a competent patient on his rational request or assisting him to commit suicide are morally controversial. No one claims that doctors are morally and legally required to do either. Thus it is clear that complying with a competent patient's rational refusal of treatment is not normally regarded as killing, nor does providing palliative care to such a patient count as assisting suicide.

Part of the problem is that insufficient attention is paid to the way in which the term "kill" is actually used. Killing is not as simple a concept as it is often taken to be. Killing is causing death, but what counts as causing death or any other harm is a complex matter.[10] If the harm that results from one's action, or omission, needs to be justified or excused, then one is regarded as having caused that harm. Of course, causing harm often can be completely justified or excused, so that one can cause a harm and be completely free of any unfavorable moral judgment. So killing, taken as causing death, may be completely justified, perhaps even morally required.

All acts that are done in order to bring about someone's death count as causing the person's death, or killing him, for all such intentional actions need justification. Also, if the act which results in death is the kind of act which is morally unacceptable such as deceiving, breaking a promise, cheating, breaking the law, or neglecting one's duty, knowingly performing the act or omission needs justification and so counts as killing. For example, if I lie to someone, telling him that a mushroom that I know to be intensely poisonous is safe to eat, then if he eats the mushroom and dies, I have caused his death. Or if a child dies because her parents did not feed her, they have killed her, because parents have a duty to feed their children. This analysis shows why it is important to make clear that doctors have no duty to treat, or even feed, patients who refuse treatment or food. However, if one does not intend, but only knows, that one's act will result in someone's death, and the act is the kind of act that is morally acceptable, (such as giving a patient sufficient analgesia to control her severe pain) then even though this act results in the person's death, it may not count as causing his death.[11]

When complying with the rational refusal of a competent patient, the doctor's intention is not to kill the patient, but rather to honor the patient's refusal even though she knows that the result will be that the patient dies. Even if the doctor agrees that it is best for the patient to die, her honoring that refusal does not count as intentionally causing his death. Of course, an individual doctor can want her patient to die, but her intention in these circumstances is not determined by whether she wants her patient to die. Rather, the intention is determined by what facts account for her deciding to act in one way rather than another. If she would cease treatment even if she did not want the patient to die and would not cease it if the patient had not refused such treatment, then her intention is not to kill the patient but to comply with the patient's refusal. Further, most doctors do not want to kill their patients, even if such actions were morally and legally justified, so clearly their intentions are simply to honor their patients' rational refusals.[12]

Whether an act or omission which does not involve doing some morally unacceptable kind of act such as deceiving and which knowingly, but not intentionally, results in someone's death, counts as killing depends on whether the society regards such acts as needing a justification or an excuse. Presently, in our society doctors do not need a justification or excuse to comply with a competent patient's rational refusal, even if everyone knows that such an act will result in the patient's death. It is sufficient for a doctor to say that he was complying with a competent patient's rational refusal. Thus it has never been considered killing for a doctor to comply with such a refusal.[13] It is now considered killing for a doctor to grant a competent patient's rational request that he do something that will immediately result in the patient's death. Few who favor VAE argue that such an action is not killing; rather many argue that VPE, i.e., complying with a patient's refusal, is also killing, and since it is allowed, VAE should also be allowed. Thus they claim that people are inconsistent in allowing, or even requiring VPE, but not allowing VAE or even PAS.[14]

That our society does not regard death resulting from complying with a competent patient's rational refusal, even a refusal of food and fluids, as killing, is shown by the fact that almost all states have advance directives that explicitly require a physician to stop treatment, even food and fluids, if the patient has the appropriate advance directive. They also allow a presently competent patient to refuse treatment and food and fluids. None of these states allow a physician to kill a patient, under any circumstances. Most of these states do not even allow physicians to assist suicide, which strongly suggests that turning off a respirator, is not regarded even as assisting suicide when doing so is required by the rational refusal of a competent patient.

Thus, complying with a competent patient's rational refusal of treatment is not killing or assisting suicide, and it may even be misleading to say that a physician is allowing the patient to die. To talk of a physician allowing the patient to die suggests that the physician has a choice, that it is up to her to decide whether or not to save the patient's life. When a competent patient has rationally refused treatment, however, a physician has no choice. It is morally and legally prohibited to overrule the patient's refusal. The physician allows her patient to die only in the sense that it is physically possible for her to save her patient and she does not. Complying with the rational refusal of life-saving treatment by a competent patient is not merely morally acceptable, it is morally required. Overruling such a refusal is itself a morally unacceptable deprivation of freedom. It does not make any moral difference whether complying with that refusal involves an act or an omission, stopping treatment or not starting it, whether the treatment is ordinary or extraordinary, or whether or not it results in a death from an underlying malady. If complying with a competent patient's rational refusal of treatment or of food and fluids were all that was involved there would be no further problems to resolve. However, it is normally the case that the doctor must also provide palliative care at the same time, and this creates a new problem.

Physician–Assisted Suicide (PAS)

Refusal of treatment, as well as refusal of food and fluids, is almost always accompanied by some pain and suffering if the patient is not given appropriate palliative care. Doctors are not morally and legally required to provide that palliation. If a doctor does not wish to provide palliative care to a patient who has refused life prolonging treatment, she may not be required to do so. This distinction between doctors being required to comply with a competent patient's refusal, but not being required to provide palliation, was made clear by one court in the Elizabeth Bouvier case. Bouvier, who was suffering from a severe case of cerebral palsy and crippling degenerative arthritis, wanted to stay in the hospital and be given palliative treatment while refusing food and fluids. Her doctors wanted to force her to take food and fluids. The court decided, correctly, that her doctors could not force her to take food and fluids, but only *recommended* that they provide palliative care while she was denying herself the food and fluids.

We believe that if the patient is competent and the request is rational, physicians should do what they can to ameliorate the pain and suffering of a patient who is refusing life-prolonging treatment. Providing such palliative care is neither killing nor even assisting suicide; rather it is achieving one of the primary goals of medicine, the relief of pain and suffering. Thus, we strongly support doctors providing psychological support and appropriate palliation to competent patients who have made rational decisions to discontinue life-prolonging treatment or to refuse food and fluids. However, if a patient's refusal of treatment and especially refusal of food and fluids were to count as suicide, then it would seem, at least initially, that providing palliation for this patient should count as assisting suicide.

There are two questions here. The first is whether a patient's refusal of treatment or of food and fluids counts as suicide. The second is whether a physician who provides palliative care for such a patient is assisting suicide. Indeed, usually a patient will not refuse treatment if the doctor will not provide the appropriate palliative care. If the answer to the first question is that the patient's refusal does not count as suicide, then there is no need to be concerned with the second question, for providing palliative care to such a patient cannot be assisting suicide. However, if the answer to the first question is that a patient's refusal does count as suicide, then it is still an open question whether providing palliative care to such a patient counts as assisting suicide.

Is the Refusal of Life-Sustaining Treatment Suicide?

If suicide is regarded simply as killing oneself, then the analysis of killing should apply to it in a fairly straightforward fashion. An action or an omission which is intended to result in the death of a patient and which does result in his death counts as killing. Therefore, one might argue that the refusal of treatment or of food and fluids that is intended by the patient to result in his own death and which does result in his death, should count as suicide. And if "assisting suicide" simply means doing those acts which help the person commit suicide, then physicians who provide palliative care to patients who are refusing life sustaining treatments are assisting suicide. Accepting this analysis would make providing palliative care to such patients a kind of assisted suicide.

However, it is not clear that the view that suicide is simply killing oneself should be accepted. Partly, this may be because "killing oneself" does not seem to need a justification or excuse as much as killing another person. This may be because our society, with some limitations, regards each person as allowed to do anything he wants to himself, as long as no one else is harmed. Indeed, it seems that any act which one does not intend but only knows will result in one's own death does not count as suicide. (It is only in an extended sense that someone who continues to smoke or drink or eat too much, when he knows that it may result in his death, could be said to be, slowly committing suicide.)[15] It also seems that our society does not count as suicide any death that results from omissions, at least omissions stemming from rational decisions to omit or to stop treatment. Rather only those positive acts that are done in order to bring about one's own death immediately count as suicide, since those acts so closely resemble the paradigms of killing. Patients who take some pills to bring about their own death are committing suicide, but those who have the respirator removed or who refuse food and fluids are usually not regarded as committing suicide.[16]

This more complex analysis of suicide explains why the law has never regarded providing palliative care to those who are refusing treatment as assisting suicide. Even those states which explicitly forbid assisting suicide do not prohibit providing palliative care to those who are refusing treatment or food and fluids. Of course those who support legalizing PAS favor the simpler account of suicide because they can then claim that some PAS is already allowed, and hence that it is simply inconsistent not to allow other quicker and less painful suicides. That our society does not count refusals of treatment as suicide and hence does not count palliative care for patients who refuse treatment as assisting suicide is not intended by us as an argument against legalizing PAS. However, it does show that one argument for legalizing PAS, namely, that PAS is already allowed in the provision of palliative care for those who are refusing life-prolonging treatment, is based on a misunderstanding of how our society regards providing such palliative care.

Our argument places PAS much closer to VPE than to VAE, and so allowing PAS, one could argue, need not lead to allowing VAE. It is compatible with our analyses so far that one can either be for or against legalizing PAS. However, we believe that recognition of the option of refusing treatment or food and fluids makes much stronger the major argument against legalizing PAS, namely, that doing so will not have sufficient benefits to compensate for the risks involved. But we are also aware that different people can rank and weigh these benefits and risks differently. How much pain and anxiety would be relieved by legalizing PAS? How many abuses and pressures to commit suicide would ensue? Even if one could answer these questions with any precision, which is extremely unlikely, it is still not clear that everyone would agree that the amount of pain and anxiety relieved outweighs the increase in the number of unwanted deaths, or vice versa.

Although our argument against PAS is not based on the use of the term "suicide," we are aware that calling a death a suicide has a negative connotation, even though suicide is no longer illegal. Misdescribing palliation as assisting suicide may discourage some physicians from providing it. We think physicians should be encouraged to provide palliative care so we oppose adopting terminology that may discourage them from doing so.

The Supreme Court Decision on Physician-Assisted Suicide

We are pleased that the Supreme Court reversed the rulings of the United States Court of Appeals for the Second Circuit and the Ninth Circuit, rulings which invalidated the New York and Washington state laws banning assisted suicide (see Appendix A of this volume). However, we are troubled by some of the Supreme Court's arguments. The majority opinion by Chief Justice Rehnquist is correct in denying the claim of the appeals court for the Second Circuit "that ending or refusing lifesaving medical treatment 'is nothing more than assisted suicide.' Unlike the Court of Appeals, we [the Supreme Court] think the distinction between assisting suicide and withdrawing life sustaining treatment, a distinction widely recognized and endorsed in the medical profession and in our legal traditions, is both important and logical; it is certainly rational."

The Supreme Court is also correct in claiming that none of the following are constitutionally established rights: "a right to 'determin[e] the time and manner of one's death,' the 'right to die,' a 'liberty to choose how to die,' a right to 'control one's final days,' 'the right to choose a humane, dignified death,' and 'the liberty to shape death.'" According to the opinion of the court, "the constitutionally protected right to refuse lifesaving nutrition and hydration that was discussed in *Cruzan*. . . . was not simply deduced from abstract concepts of personal autonomy, but was instead grounded in the Nation's history and traditions, given the common law rule that forced medication was a battery, and the long legal tradition protecting the decision to refuse unwanted medical treatment." The Court was also correct in pointing out the interests that support a law prohibiting PAS, including "protecting the poor, the elderly, disabled persons, the terminally ill, and persons in other vulnerable groups from indifference, prejudice, and psychological and financial pressure to end their lives; and avoiding a possible slide towards voluntary and perhaps even involuntary euthanasia."

However, some claims that are made in the course of these decisions are quite misleading. For example, Rehnquist says "when a patient refuses life sustaining medical treatment, he dies from an underlying fatal disease or pathology, but if a patient ingests lethal medication prescribed by a physician, he is killed by that medication . . . (when the feeding tube is removed, death 'result[s] . . . from [the patient's] underlying medical condition')." But by putting the matter in this way, Rehnquist, like too many other jurists and philosophers before him, simply overlooks a patient's refusal of food and fluids not being administered intravenously. Someone who is able to eat and drink in the normal way and refuses food and fluids may not even be suffering from a terminal disease, but rather from severe chronic pain or serious permanent disability. In such a case, the patient does not die from "an underlying fatal disease or pathology," but from an electrolyte imbalance caused by the lack of fluids.

Rehnquist is closer to the mark when he says "a physician who withdraws, or honors a patient's refusal to begin, life sustaining medical treatment purposefully intends, or may so intend, only to respect his patient's wishes and 'to cease doing useless and futile or degrading things to a patient when [the patient] no longer stands to benefit from them.' The same is true when a doctor provides aggressive palliative care; in some cases, painkilling drugs may hasten a patient's death, but the physician's purpose or intent is, or may be, only to ease his patient's pain. A doctor who assists a suicide, however, 'must necessarily and indubitably, intend primarily that the patient be made dead.'" But this way of putting it is misleading. It suggests that it is only what the doctor intends that is crucial. But as Justice Stevens points out in his concurring opinion, a doctor who assists a suicide may only intend to respect his patient's wishes to commit suicide. The crucial feature is that a physician is morally and legally required to comply with a patient's refusal of treatment, for not doing so is violating his freedom. There is, however, no similar moral and legal requirement to grant a patient's request for lethal medication, nor does any proponent of legalizing PAS even propose that physicians be required to grant such requests. By failing to note the morally crucial distinction between refusals and requests, Rehnquist is unable to explain why the right to refuse life-sustaining medication cannot be glossed simply as the right to die, etc. Nor is he able to support as well as he could his claim that "the distinction between assisting suicide and withdrawing life sustaining treatment . . . is certainly rational."

Further, by using the phrase "medical treatment," Rehnquist continues the misleading view that a person only has the right to refuse *artificial* life support, rather than a more general right to refuse even *natural* life support, such as food and fluids. The court notes that "nearly all states expressly disapprove of suicide and assisted suicide either in statutes dealing with durable powers of attorney in healthcare situations or in 'living will' statutes." Almost all state statutes make clear that a person has the right to refuse food and fluids. It is absurd to claim that providing nutrition and hydration to those who cannot eat in the normal way can be refused only because it is a medical treatment. As the Bouvier and other cases have consistently decided, patients have the right to refuse food and fluids whether they are capable of taking food and fluids in the normal way or only intravenously. Any competent patient is permitted to refuse food and fluids, and it is permitted to provide her with palliative care while she is refusing, whether or not she is on life support.[17] Consider the consequences of someone not being permitted to refuse taking food and fluids in the normal way while being permitted to refuse taking them intravenously. A patient who refused to eat and drink in the normal way could not be force fed intravenously, for supposedly she is permitted to refuse that method of feeding.

Stevens, in his concurring opinion, claims "that there are situations in which an interest in hastening death is legitimate," and even "that there are times when it is entitled to constitutional protection." But Stevens seems unaware that no one is even proposing a law that allows PAS without at least a two-week waiting period, so that legalizing PAS would not result in death coming earlier than by the refusal of food and fluids. Furthermore, the right to refuse food and fluids is already constitutionally protected. However, in other places Stevens is clear that he is not talking primarily about the hastening of death, but of how one dies. Stevens is correct that a person may have an interest in how she dies, e.g., "in determining the character of the memories that will survive long after her death." However, it seems to us that given that the time involved in dying by refusing food and fluids is as short or shorter than that provided by PAS, and that this way of dying can be as pain-free as PAS, the state interest in preventing suicide would not have to be very great in order to allow states to continue prohibiting PAS.

Stevens also agrees with Rehnquist's mistaken view "that the distinction between permitting death to ensue from an underlying fatal disease and causing it to occur by the administration of medication or other means provides a constitutionally sufficient basis for the State's classification." Our point in this context is that it is not what causes death that justifies the distinction between refusing treatment and PAS. Rather it is that there is a constitutionally protected liberty interest in preventing unauthorized touching or forcing anything into a person, and there is no similarly strong liberty interest in permitting someone to assist with a suicide. A patient who is suffering from severe chronic pain or serious permanent disability may refuse food and fluids and this refusal must be honored even though the patient will not die from an underlying fatal malady. It is the refusal, not the cause of death, that is important.

Other justices who concurred with Rehnquist's decisions also failed to take into account the option of refusing food and fluids. Justice O'Connor agrees that "a patient who is suffering from a terminal illness and who is experiencing great pain has no legal barriers to obtaining medication, from qualified physicians, to alleviate that suffering, even to the point of causing unconsciousness and hastening death." But O'Connor does not mention that all patients have the right to refuse food and fluids, taken normally or intravenously. Not only is it morally acceptable for physicians to provide them with appropriate pain medication for the week or less that they remain conscious, present standards of medical practice encourage them to do so.

Knowledge of the facts is crucial in making any moral or legal decision, and unfortunately it seems that the Supreme Court, like both of the appeals courts that it overruled, did not know all of the relevant facts about the refusal of food and fluids. We are pleased that the Supreme Court rejected many of the appeals courts' arguments and that they make some of the same distinctions that we provide in our discussion of these decisions.[18] However, we believe that by failing to uncover the real basis for the distinction between *refusing* treatment or food and fluids, and *requesting* physician assistance in suicide, they perpetuated the confusion that permeates this issue. In the final section of this article, we propose a model statute for states to adopt. This statute is primarily designed to publicize the legality of refusing food and fluids and to make clear to physicians that in providing pain medication to patients who are refusing food and fluids they are not assisting suicide.

Is Killing Patients Ever Justified?

Stopping food and fluids is often the best way of allowing a patient to die, but it may be claimed that killing is sometimes better. Given present knowledge and technology, one can kill a patient or allow a patient to kill herself absolutely painlessly within a matter of minutes. If patients have a rational desire to die, why wait several days or weeks for them to die; why not kill them or let them kill themselves quickly and painlessly in a matter of minutes? We have provided no argument against allowing patients to kill themselves or even killing patients who want to die that applies to an ideal world where there are never any misunderstandings between people and everyone is completely moral and trustworthy. In such a world, if one could provide a patient with pills or inject the patient with appropriate drugs so that the patient dies painlessly and almost instantaneously, there would be no need to worry about the distinction between refusals and requests, or between killing, assisting suicide, and allowing to die. But in the real world, there are misunderstandings and not everyone is completely moral and trustworthy. In the real world no one even proposes that PAS or VAE be allowed without elaborate procedural safeguards, which almost always require at least two weeks. So, on a practical level, legalizing PAS or VAE would not result in a quicker death than simply complying with a refusal of food and fluids.[19]

On our account, VPE is complying with the rational refusal of life-saving treatment or food and fluids by a competent patient. Since there is no duty to overrule a rational refusal by a competent patient, complying with this refusal does not count as killing. Further, failing to comply with such a refusal is itself morally prohibited, for it is an unjustified deprivation of the patient's freedom. Also, in some newer codes of medical ethics, e.g., that of The American College of Physicians, respecting patients' refusals is now listed as a duty. Physicians are not merely morally allowed to practice VPE, they are morally required to do so. VAE is killing; it is complying with the rational request of a competent patient to be killed. Although PAS is not killing, it does involve active intervention by the physician that is more than merely stopping treatment. It is not simply complying with a patient's desire to be left alone; it is providing the patient with some substance that causes his death, when one has no duty to do so.

VAE is killing and so needs to be justified. This contrasts quite sharply with VPE, and even with PAS, which may not even need to be morally justified. When a patient refuses treatment or food and fluids, it is not the complying with a patient's refusal but rather the overruling of the refusal that needs to be justified. But, as noted earlier, physicians may cause pain to their patients and be completely justified, because they do so at their patients' request, or at least with their consent, and do it in order to prevent what the patient takes to be a greater harm, e.g., disability or death. VAE could be regarded as no different than any other instance of a doctor being morally justified in doing a morally unacceptable *kind* *of act* with regard to a patient at the patient's request, in order to prevent what the patient takes to be a greater harm. In VAE the patient takes death to be a lesser harm than suffering pain and requests that the moral rule prohibiting killing be violated with regard to himself.

If causing pain can be justified, why is killing not justified when all of the other morally relevant features are the same? The answer is that killing needs a stronger justification because of a special feature of death that distinguishes it from all of the other serious harms. The special feature is that, after death, the person killed no longer exists and so cannot protest that he did not want to be killed. All impartial rational persons would advocate that violations against causing pain be publicly allowed when the person toward whom the rule is being violated rationally prefers to suffer that pain rather than suffer some other harm, e.g., disability or death. It is uncertain how many impartial rational persons would advocate that killing be publicly allowed when the person being killed rationally prefers to be killed rather than to continue to suffer pain. This uncertainty stems from taking seriously the two features that are essential to morality, the public character of morality and the fallibility of persons.

Causing pain with valid consent can be publicly allowed without any significant anxiety being caused thereby. Patients can usually correct a mistake rather quickly by ordering a stop to the painful treatment. Also physicians have a constant incentive to be careful not to cause pain by mistake, for patients will complain if they did not really want the pain caused. Killing, even with valid consent, being publicly allowed may create significant anxiety. Patients may fear that they will be mistakenly killed and that they will have no opportunity to correct that mistake. That a patient will not be around to complain if they are mistakenly killed removes a strong safeguard against mistaken violations. But it is not merely mistakes about which a patient would not be able to complain. If a physician tries to take advantage of legalized killing and intentionally kills a patient, complaint would not be possible. Taking advantage of causing pain being publicly allowed does not pose similar problems.

Legalizing PAS might prevent some pain and suffering that could not be prevented by greater education concerning refusing food and fluids, but it would also be likely to create significant anxiety and some unwanted deaths. Impartial rational persons can therefore disagree on whether they would advocate legalizing PAS. Once it is recognized that withholding food and fluids 1) can be painless; 2) usually results in unconsciousness in one week and death in two weeks; and 3) allows for patients to change their minds, the need for PAS significantly diminishes.

Unlike others who argue against legalizing PAS, we do not claim that PAS is in itself morally unacceptable, only that it may create a serious risk of unwanted deaths. Since impartial rational persons can rank these risks as outweighing the benefits of legalization, legalizing PAS is controversial. If the goal is to allow a patient to choose her own time of dying and also dying to be accomplished relatively painlessly, there seems to be little need for PAS. If patient refusal of treatment, including refusal of food and fluids, were not sufficient for a relatively quick and painless death for the overwhelming number of terminally ill patients, then we would favor PAS, although we would still have serious objections to VAE.[20] However, since VPE, especially when this includes refusing food and fluids, is available together with appropriate palliative care, it seems far more difficult to justify controversial methods like PAS. The harms prevented by PAS are no longer the long term suffering of patients who have no other way to die, they are only the one week of suffering that may be present while the patient is refusing food and fluids, and this suffering can be almost completely controlled by appropriate palliative care. This is an excellent example of why the presence of an alternative is a morally relevant feature.[21]

Given the alternative of refusing food and fluids, very little additional harm seems to be prevented by PAS. The presence of an alternative is a morally relevant feature and makes it questionable whether it has sufficient benefits to justify the risks involved in legalizing it.[22] There are good reasons for believing that the advantages of refusing food and fluids together with adequate palliative care make it preferable to legalizing PAS. This is especially true in a multicultural society where doctors and patients sometimes do not even speak the same language. There are a small number of cases in which refusal of food and fluids might be difficult, but it is necessary to weigh the benefit to this relatively small number of people against the harm that might be suffered by a great number of people by the legalizing of PAS.[23]

PAS has several morally significant disadvantages. Although it usually requires a two-week waiting period, it allows for almost instantaneous death. This makes it less likely that its legalization will support the use of palliative care. It may take a week before a patient who refuses food and fluids becomes unconscious, thus it is clear that palliative care must be practiced. The relative speed and ease with which PAS can bring about death makes it seem more likely that patients will be pressured to hasten their deaths when they would prefer not to do so. Because of the time it takes, it is much less likely that patients will be pressured to refuse food and fluids. This time also permits patients to change their mind, and for friends and family to know that the patient was firm in his decision to die. Indeed, for patients not on life-sustaining treatments, refusing food and fluids seems to have more overall benefits than any other method of hastening death.[24] Major drawbacks are 1) public and physician ignorance of the fact that it is not painful for terminal patients to do without food and fluids; 2) the association of feeding with caring; and 3) some patients' dislike of the idea and the process of refusing food and fluids.

Since PAS is morally controversial, physicians cannot be required to participate in it. This means that physicians would always have to take full personal responsibility for assisting suicide. Like physicians performing abortions, they are likely to be subject to criticism and abuse from those opposed to such practices. Since physicians are morally required to practice VPE (i.e., they are not allowed to overrule a competent patient's refusal of treatment), they do not have to bear this criticism and abuse. Patients cannot require someone to assist them in committing suicide; they can require others to leave them alone, even if that requires physicians to discontinue their treatment. Thus, from the point of view of physicians, providing their terminally ill patients with adequate palliative care and informing them that they can refuse any life preserving treatment, as well as food and fluids, together with assuring them that palliative care will continue for as long as necessary during their refusal, seems, on balance, a safer and more desirable option than the legalization of PAS.

Summary

PAS has been shown to be different from both VAE and VPE. It resembles VAE in that it is a request for the physician to do something, namely, to prescribe lethal drugs that will result in the patient's death, but it is not killing as VAE is. It is not VPE, for it is not based on a refusal of treatment, with which a physician is morally required to comply. However, PAS resembles providing palliative care for those who are refusing life-prolonging treatment or food and fluids. It differs from providing such palliative care in that those who refuse life-prolonging treatment or food and fluids are not committing suicide, while those for whom the lethal drugs are prescribed are committing suicide. Since PAS is not killing, the only moral argument against legalizing it is that it will lead to overall worse consequences. Whether or not this is true is an empirical matter. Since PAS is not killing, its legalization does not provide a reason for legalizing VAE, which is killing.

Morality thus makes clear the moral significance of the distinction between refusals and requests and allows for a meaningful distinction between VAE and VPE. There is no need to make an ad hoc distinction that applies only to dying patients, as the standard discussions do; rather the moral significance of a commonly used distinction in medical practice, between requests and refusals, is acknowledged and applied to the question of euthanasia. The medical fact about the consequences of refusing food and fluids, that it normally causes no additional suffering, makes clear that there is a viable alternative open to patients, whether or not they are on life support, to hasten their deaths. We have not only tried to show the inadequacy of accepting the standard ad hoc and unsystematic attempts to distinguish between VAE and VPE, we have also shown how the commonly applied medical distinction between requests and refusals can be used to make this distinction.

We believe that the strongest argument against PAS is that, given the alternatives available, it does not provide sufficient benefit to individual patients to justify the societal risks. Patients already have the alternative of refusing treatment and food and fluids, and of receiving palliative care while they are refusing that treatment. If physicians were to educate patients about these matters and to make clear that they will support their choices and continue to care for them if they choose to refuse treatment, there might be little, if any, call for PAS. Because of the time involved, patients seem far less likely to be pressured into refusing treatment or food and fluids than they are to avail themselves of PAS. There would also be far fewer opportunities for abuse. PAS provides less incentive to be concerned with palliative care. And finally, given the bureaucratic safeguards that most regard as necessary with PAS, death can come as soon or sooner with refusal of treatment or refusal of food and fluids than it would with PAS.[25]

A Practical Proposal for State Legislators

In order to avoid the serious societal risks of legalizing physician-assisted suicide, while still providing a method for allowing seriously ill patients to determine the timing of their deaths, we think that states should consider passing legislation based on language such as the following. This language is completely consistent with the statement of the United States Supreme Court that, "Just as a State may prohibit assisting suicide while permitting patients to refuse unwanted lifesaving treatment, it may permit palliative care related to that refusal, which may have the foreseen but unintended 'double effect' of hastening the patient's death."

> If a competent patient is terminally ill or suffering from a condition involving severe chronic pain or serious permanent disability, that patient's refusal of treatment, or refusal of food and fluids, shall not count as suicide, even though the patient knows that death will result from not starting or from stopping that treatment. All physicians and other healthcare workers shall be informed that they are legally prohibited from overruling any rational refusal of a competent patient, including refusal of food and fluids, even though it is known that death will result. All patients will be informed that they are allowed to refuse any treatment, or to refuse food and fluids, even though it is known that death will result, and that physicians and other healthcare workers are legally prohibited from overruling any such rational refusal by a competent patient.
>
> Further, there shall be no prohibition placed upon any physician who provides pain relief in any form, in order to relieve the pain and suffering of the patient who has refused treatment, or food and fluids. In particular, providing pain medication shall not be considered as assisting suicide, and there shall be no liability for the physician who provides such pain medication for the purpose of relieving pain and suffering. The physician shall not provide such medication for the purpose of hastening the time of death, but is not prohibited from providing medication which is consistent with adequate pain relief even if he knows that such medication will hasten the time of death. Physicians are required to rigorously follow the accepted standards of medical practice in determining the competence of patients who refuse any treatment, or who refuse food and fluids, when they know that death will result from complying with that refusal.

Notes

1. This article is derived from our book, *Bioethics: A Return to Fundamentals* (New York: Oxford University Press, 1997).
2. Dan W. Brock, "Voluntary Active Euthanasia," *Hastings Center Report* 22 (2): 10–22 (1992).
3. *Quill v. Vacco*, the U.S. Court of Appeals for the Second Circuit.

4. See James L. Bernat, Bernard Gert, and R. Peter Mogielnicki, "Patient Refusal of Hydration and Nutrition: An Alternative to Physician Assisted Suicide or Voluntary Euthanasia," *Archives of Internal Medicine* 153: 2723–28 (December 27, 1993).

5. See Bernard Gert, James L. Bernat, and R. Peter Mogielnicki, "Distinguishing between Patients' Refusals and Requests," *The Hastings Center Report* 24 (4): 13–15 (July–August 1994).

6. See Bernard Gert, *Morality: Its Nature and Justification* (New York: Oxford University Press, 1998), for detailed analyses of impartiality, rationality, duty, and publicly allowing.

7. See K. Danner Clouser, "Allowing or Causing: Another Look," *Annals of Internal Medicine* 87: 622–24 (1977).

8. See Kathleen M. Foley, M.D., "The Relationship of Pain and Symptom Management to Patient Requests for Physician-Assisted Suicide," *Journal of Pain and Symptom Management* 6 (5): 289–297 (July 1991). See also, James L. Bernat, Bernard Gert, and R. Peter Mogielnicki, op cit.

9. It may be that "killing" that is the result of abiding by a refusal never has the same morally relevant features as killing that is done at the request of a patient. However, killing is such a serious violation of a moral rule, that the morally relevant features would have to be dramatically different for one way of killing to be justified and the other not.

10. Contrary to one's initial inclination, what counts as "causing harm" is not determined by some scientific analysis, but rather by whether it is held that a justification or excuse is needed for such behavior. See Gert, *Morality*, op. cit.

11. But one can also kill a person unintentionally, even when one is not negligent, as when one's car skids on some black ice and hits a person resulting in his death. Such a killing may be completely excusable, but it is still killing.

12. Given that it is not only morally but also legally required to abide by a patient's rational refusal of treatment, legally abiding by such refusals cannot be treated as intentionally killing the patient.

13. However, in trying to change a long-standing practice, it is not uncommon for people, especially philosophers, to try to change the ways of extending the paradigms, so as to justify the change they are promoting. And sometime these efforts are successful and what counts as killing does change.

14. See Dan W. Brock, op. cit. People would be inconsistent if such concepts as "killing" were as simple as some philosophers claim them to be. However, philosophers often confuse complexity with inconsistency.

15. That this is an extended sense is shown by the fact that life insurance policies that exclude payment if death is due to suicide, cannot refuse to pay if death is due to these kinds of causes.

16. This view is not held by all. Some, especially those with religious views, regard refusing treatment and especially refusing food and fluids when treatment, or food and fluids would sustain life for a long time, as committing suicide. But this is not the prevailing view, nor is it the view that governs the legal classification of the act. However, a terminally ill patient who intentionally goes into the woods in order to stop eating and drinking, does so, and thereby dies, would be regarded by most as having committed suicide. For a sensitive analysis of the difficulty of formulating a precise definition of "suicide," see Tom L. Beauchamp, "Suicide" in Tom Regan, ed., *Matters of Life and Death*, 2nd ed. (New York: Random House, 1986), pp. 77–89.

17. See David Eddy's article about his mother refusing food and fluids. *Journal of the American Medical Association* 272: 179–81 (1994).

18. See Bernard Gert, Charles M. Culver, and K. Danner Clouser, *Bioethics: A Return to Fundamentals*, chapter 12, "Euthanasia."

19. This is not an argument against killing someone in an emergency situation, e.g., someone who has been captured by a sadistic enemy, or an unrescueable person in an accident who is about to be burned to death. This shows the importance of the morally

relevant feature concerning emergency situations. See Gert, *Morality* for further discussion of morally relevant features.

20. But Dan Brock, for example, has claimed that there is no more serious reservations about active euthanasia. See Brock, op. cit.

21. See Gert, *Morality*.

22. Many people claim to prefer physician-assisted suicide, or even active euthanasia, to discontinuing food and fluids. However, this may be due to their focus on their own particular cases, viz., they see only the ease and quickness of the former two methods, and fail to appreciate their far greater potential for abuse. Also, there is so much misinformation about the pain and suffering involved in discontinuing food and fluids, that it seems likely that their preferences often do not count as informed preferences. However, even with accurate information and the support of their physicians, some patients, because of the psychological difficulties involved in a longer dying process, may still prefer physician-assisted suicide to discontinuing food and fluids. How much importance should be given to these preferences is a matter of dispute, even among the authors of this article.

23. This is an argument against legalizing physician-assisted suicide. It is not an argument against using it if it were legalized.

24. However, for some the personal benefits of knowing that they can die quickly and painlessly may outweigh all of the benefits of discontinuing food and fluids. This is not an irrational ranking.

25. See K. Danner Clouser, "The Challenge for Future Debate on Euthanasia," *The Journal of Pain and Symptom Management* 6 (5): 306–311 (July 1991).

13

Not in the House

Arguments for a Policy of Excluding Physician-Assisted Suicide from the Practice of Hospital Medicine

MICHAEL TEITELMAN

In the debate concerning the legalization of physician-assisted suicide, it has been implicitly assumed that if legal prohibitions are lifted, patients with progressive, terminal diseases will request and, under appropriate conditions, should receive suicide assistance from their physicians while they are being care for in the hospital. In this essay, the basis for this assumption is examined. Even if PAS is legalized, there are reasons for not introducing it into the practice of hospital medicine. Four arguments for excluding PAS from hospital practice describe moral and social costs of PAS in the hospital that ought to concern advocates as well as opponents of PAS.

*   *   *

ONE LIKELY CONSEQUENCE of the Supreme Court's decision on assisted suicide is that the social debate about physician-assisted suicide of the last ten years will give way to political efforts to legalize physician-assisted suicide (PAS). In states in which advocates of PAS are numerous and strong enough, the debate will be carried on in state legislatures or in campaigns to change the law through electoral referenda, as has already occurred in Oregon and California.

While the large issues of individual freedom, the morality of physician assistance, and the potential for abuse of PAS will continue to be discussed, the debate will become more focused on specific sets of rules to regulate the practice of PAS if the decision is made to permit it. Legislative debate is necessarily concerned with the details of law and regulation, because a legislature can decide to permit PAS only by adopting a specific set of rules regulating the practice.[1]

This makes it timely to raise an issue concerning the social regulation of PAS which has been ignored in the torrent of analysis and debate. This is the issue of *locus*: where PAS ought or ought not to occur. In this essay, I propose that if PAS is legalized, it would be best that it not be introduced into the practice of hospital medicine; assistance in suicide ought not to be provided to patients while they are hospitalized. Important ethical and social objectives which have already been recognized by both advocates and opponents of PAS will be best served by the exclusion of PAS from hospital practice.

The arguments I will present in support of a policy of excluding PAS from hospitals are constructed in a way that mirrors the debate about PAS. Putting aside absolutist views about the moral impermissibility of suicide or of a physician's participation in a suicide, arguments against the legalization of PAS have often taken the form of predicting that ethically and socially undesirable consequences will flow from the legal and medical acceptance of PAS. Advocates have responded by agreeing on the undesirability of these outcomes; they then go on to argue that either these negative outcomes probably will not occur or that the frequency of their occurrence can be reduced to an acceptable minimum through improvement in the clinical care of ill and dying patients and through social regulation and monitoring of the practice.

Let me lay out an example of this kind of argument. Opponents of PAS point out that current medical practice is seriously deficient in helping patients with pain and that legalization of PAS will lead to requests for assistance by patients who are suffering from inadequately treated pain. In such a circumstance, the decision to end life results not from autonomous deliberation and decision-making concerning the value of the remainder of life but from desperation and helplessness produced by chronic or severe pain. Advocates of PAS agree on the ethical and social undesirability of assisting the suicides of patients who would not choose to kill themselves if their pain were relieved. They go on to argue that improving the treatment of pain and mandating the evaluation of pain and pain management as a prerequisite for suicide assistance will go a long way toward preventing this undesirable consequence of PAS.[2]

My arguments for excluding PAS from hospitals consist of two steps which parallel this kind of exchange. In the first step, I delineate a potential consequence of legalizing PAS which both advocates and opponents regard as socially or ethically undesirable. In the second step, I try to show that incorporating PAS into hospital practice would increase the likelihood of that undesirable outcome and that excluding PAS from the hospital would serve to reduce its likelihood. Basing these arguments on points of agreement about the undesirable potentialities of PAS bridges the divide between advocates and opponents of PAS. These arguments provide reasons for excluding legalized PAS from the hospital that are valid and, I hope, compelling for both.

A clarification about a limitation of these arguments will be useful at this point. Their objective is to show that in-hospital PAS will tend to produce certain undesirable outcomes and that excluding PAS from hospital practice will reduce the frequency of these outcomes. However, this does not entail that excluding PAS from the hospital will lower the risk of these negative outcomes occurring outside of the hospital. The fact that there are ethical and social reasons to keep PAS out of the hospital does not entail that PAS will be ethically unproblemmatic elsewhere.

Four Preliminary Observations
The Locus of PAS as an Ignored Issue

To my knowledge, the question of locus has not been explicitly addressed in the debate about PAS. It is useful to speculate about why. There are, I think, two explanations for this. The first is normative and philosophical. The second is empirical and clinical.

First, PAS is conceptualized as the voluntary suicide of autonomous individuals. It is implicitly assumed that the place in which a person ends his or her life is a matter of individual choice and that the locus of a suicide does not have intrinsic significance in so far as the moral status and social regulation of suicide is concerned. It follows that from an ethical point of view the hospital is, *ceteris paribus*, as suitable a location for PAS as any other place, such as the person's home. Autonomous individuals with terminal illnesses who decide to end their lives with the assistance of their physicians should be able to do so wherever they are. Like many undertakings in the hospital, PAS would require a regulatory protocol to insure compliance with state law and administrative regulations. But the fact that a person makes a request for suicide assistance while in the hospital would not disqualify the request.

This moral view of place as ethically neutral is buttressed by an empirical, social explanation of why locus has been ignored in the debate about PAS. Paralleling what Willie Sutton said of money and banks, hospitals are where very ill patients are. Most people now die in hospitals. It is reasonable to expect that patients with progressive diseases sometimes will request assistance in dying during a hospitalization. If we decide to allow physicians to assist their patients' suicides when they are ill, it would seem heartless and paradoxical to adopt a policy of forbidding physicians to provide assistance when their patients are so ill as to be admitted to the hospital.

These two considerations explain why the hospital as a locus of PAS has not been viewed as problematic. Later, as I argue against in-hospital PAS, I shall have to explain why the hospital is not an ethically neutral place with respect to PAS and why the social and clinical ramifications of a policy of disallowing suicide assistance to hospitalized patients are neither paradoxical nor heartless.

The Locus of Assisted Suicide as an Iconographic Element in the Debate About PAS
The locus of suicide has already had a role in the public discussion of PAS. Locus has operated as a subtly persuasive factor in representations of the assisted suicides that have been reported in the media. Images of place have operated emotionally and aesthetically to buttress analysis and argument.

In narratives of "good deaths" achieved through voluntary suicide, the person is sometimes represented at home surrounded by the people and things that have comprised his or her life. Family, friends, the accumulations of a lifetime, and sometimes a pet are in attendance. The poignancy and sometimes even the beauty of dying in a place with personal history and meaning create a powerful pull toward accepting the legalization of PAS. In addition, in an ironic twist under current law, families and friends must absent themselves in the final moments in order to protect themselves from prosecution, which heightens the poignancy of the image of dying at home: The person dies at home, but alone because of a readily reversible legal sanction.[3]

In a contrary vein, in the accounts of suicides arranged by Dr. Jack Kevorkian, motel rooms far from home and rear compartments of vans have served as the settings for an exit from life in which the person is cut off from the rest of her or his life. These images heighten the grisliness of Kevorkian's *modus operandi*. Indeed, the ugliness of these scenes is sometimes explicitly recruited into the debate. Defenders of Kevorkian point to them as evidence of what current prohibitions on PAS compel people to do to get relief from their suffering; opponents view them as an indication of the debasing and horrifying practices we will have to tolerate if PAS is legalized. Either way, the locus of the suicide has meaning which is recruited into the normative argument.

Locus as an Explicit Factor in the Evaluation of Other Aspects of Medical Care
The idea that locus is a relevant factor in the social regulation of medical care is not novel. The importance of locus is well understood in current attempts to reduce the costs of medical services. A major component of this effort is to reduce the utilization of the hospital as a locus of care. This is manifested in the trend toward shortening the length of hospitalizations by shifting care to home or other facilities, and in the transfer of diagnostic and therapeutic procedures to outpatient settings. It is reasonable to move a medical service out of the hospital when the change results in lower costs without an increase in clinical morbidity.

Recognition of the importance of locus is also reflected in critiques of the discharge policies of insurance and managed care corporations which speed up discharges for the sake of profit. In these critiques, the hospital is recognized as a place in which patients receive benefits in addition to medical services. For the patient, the hospital is a locus of rest and recuperation; for the patient's family, the continuation of inpatient care provides temporary relief from often burdensome home care.

If the planning of healthcare services routinely involves the question of whether a particular service or procedure ought to be performed in the hospital or elsewhere, then it seems worth asking whether a similar question ought to be formulated with respect to PAS: If it is legalized, should it be incorporated into hospital medical practice of caring for patients with terminal illnesses? Just as the transfer of procedures and services out of the hospital reduces economic costs, it might turn out that excluding PAS from hospital practice would reduce the ethical and social costs of legalizing PAS.

The Moral Permissibility of Excluding PAS from Medical Practice in the Hospital
It may seem paradoxical to propose a policy of excluding PAS from the principal institution in which the ill and dying are found. Such a policy makes suicide assistance unavailable at a time when seriously ill and dying people can be expected to request it; when their illness has worsened and necessitated admission to the hospital, or when they are dying. The sense of paradox is reduced a bit if one reflects on the fact that the moral permissibility of excluding assisted

suicide from a hospital's practice has already been implicitly accepted without challenge in the course of the debate.

A person's right to end life with the assistance of a physician has been advanced as a claim against governmental prohibition of the physician's assisting suicide. It has not been advanced as an indefeasible claim on physicians for assistance. It seems to be universally agreed that if PAS were legalized, the decision to provide assistance should be regarded as a matter of a physician's individual choice. Physicians would be free to choose not to help patients to end their lives as a matter of personal moral conviction. So far, no model legislative code or electoral referendum for the legalization of PAS has envisaged an arrangement in which physicians have a moral or legal obligation to provide suicide assistance. The choice may be based on a physician's view of medical ethics, or on the religious beliefs or moral principles to which the physician is committed. If a physician were to elect not to help a patient to end his or her life for reasons of principle or conscience, the patient would have to seek assistance from a different doctor or could remain in the care of the physician without receiving suicide assistance.

For physicians whose clinical work regularly involves them in the care of the people with serious and terminal diseases, this moral freedom is a critical matter. Without it, some would find themselves obligated to act against their understanding of their professional ethic, or against their own moral or religious beliefs. Even the most ardent advocates of PAS do not propose that the legalization of PAS would entail a correlative obligation of physicians to assist suicides. In order for society to curtail this moral freedom of physicians by establishing a professional obligation to assist patients when they want to die, there would need to be far broader and deeper public acceptance of the legitimacy and urgency of autonomous suicide by the terminally ill.

Thus, PAS is unlike any other ministration to an ill or dying patient that a physician can offer. All the rest—such as symptom relief or pain control—is owed the patient: The physician is remiss in not providing the requisite care or finding specialists to do so. In this respect, PAS occupies a place in our moral outlook which is similar to the place of abortion in medical ethics and public policy. Physicians are free to choose not to perform abortions. This choice is important, of course, only to physicians who actually are requested by patients to terminate a pregnancy and who are trained to perform the surgery. They are free to choose not to do so even though they are able to.

The moral freedom not to perform abortions has also been extended to healthcare institutions. Hospitals owned or operated by, or closely affiliated with, religious organizations which regard abortion as morally forbidden are not obligated to provide elective abortions to patients. As a matter of law and public policy, hospitals operated by the Roman Catholic Church are permitted not to provide abortions, tubal ligations, or reproductive counselling to their patients.

It takes only a moment's reflection to realize that if PAS is legalized, it will also be permissible for hospitals with religious affiliations not to provide suicide assistance to hospitalized patients even if their suicide requests fulfill the requirements of the legal regulations. Opinion about both abortion and assisted suicide is too sharply divided and the conflict with traditional morality is too stark to sustain a public policy of requiring all hospitals to provide these services. Clearly, we are not about to reorder basic relationships between government and religion in order to insure that suicide assistance is available to ill or dying patients when they have been admitted to a Catholic hospital.

Given the stringency of Roman Catholic law and theology concerning the immorality of suicide and euthanasia, the governing boards of Catholic hospitals will not need to look beyond church canon for a rationale for prohibiting intramural PAS. The traditional Christian norm prohibiting suicide provides a sufficient foundation for this decision. A handful of hospitals affiliated with fundamentalist Protestant groups will probably also decide against PAS on similar grounds. To my knowledge, there are no orthodox Jewish organizations that have a proprietary relationship to a hospital; but if there were, it is probable that PAS would not be permitted in such hospitals.

Four Arguments for a Policy of Exclusion

Religiously affiliated hospitals have their reasons for not permitting in-hospital PAS. The question at this point is whether there are also ethical or policy considerations, which are not grounded in religious morality, for excluding legalized PAS from private secular hospitals or public sector hospitals. These would be reasons relevant to the governing boards of hospitals and the professional medical organizations be responsible for integrating PAS into medical practice if and when it is legalized.

The Nexus of Autonomy, Depression, and Hospitalization

People who are ill with chronic, progressive, fatal diseases have high rates of clinically significant depression. Depression is one of those neuropsychiatric conditions which (along with dementia and delirium) can interfere with or impair the process of deliberation which results in autonomous decision-making. Medically ill, depressed patients frequently express a desire to end their lives and relinquish that desire when their depression remits. Unfortunately, clinical recognition of depression is haphazard. For a variety of longstanding and unfortunate reasons, depression is underdiagnosed both in the general population and in the medically ill.[4]

Opponents of PAS regard this nexus of illness, depression, and suicidal ideation as one of the pitfalls of legalized PAS. Physicians will facilitate the suicides of clinically depressed patients who would not choose to end their lives if they were relieved of their depressive disorder. In response, supporters have proposed model codes of medical-legal regulation which require a physician whose assistance has been requested to evaluate the mental functioning of the patient and, in some codes, to arrange for an evaluation by a second physician.

This nexus of illness, depression and suicidality has been well described in the medical literature. It has to be addressed in clinical practice whether or not PAS is legalized. But if PAS is legalized, this nexus becomes significantly more problematic. The availability of suicide assistance will make it essential to differentiate between two phenomenologically similar states of a patient. In one state, the patient expresses a decision to die which results from a process of reflection and deliberation about (among other things) the meaning of one's remaining life and of the suffering one expects to endure. In the other state, the expression of a wish to die arises from a condition of clinical depression in which feelings of hopelessness and helplessness color the future as grim in outlook and full of suffering without redeeming meaning.

Even for psychiatrists and internists who regularly care for severely ill and dying patients, distinguishing between these two states of mind is sometimes quite difficult. One reason for this stems from the problem of diagnosing depression in the medically ill. Diagnostic criteria for clinical depression (or Major Depression in current psychiatric nosology) overlap with physical symptoms that are prevalent in the medically ill: low energy, loss of appetite or weight loss, sleep disturbance, impaired concentration and short term memory. A second impediment to the diagnosis of Major Depression is an understandable tendency to view a state of clinical depression in a seriously ill person as an appropriate emotional response to a terrible ordeal. The suicidal ideation which issues from the patient's depression is then regarded as reasonable and warranting assistance even though psychotherapeutic and/or psychopharmacological intervention might relieve the depression and extinguish the patient's interest in suicide.[5]

Thus, there is real potential for the legalization of PAS to lead to doctors helping clinically depressed, suicidal patients to kill themselves. The question at this point is how the question of locus affects the probability of this occurring. My contention here is that permitting PAS in the hospital makes this aspect of PAS more troublesome.

There are several interconnected reasons for this. The first has to do with the role of hospitalization in the care of patients with the kinds of diseases which, in their later stages, might elicit a desire to end one's life: prolonged, progressive, and usually fatal diseases, such as cancer, neurodegenerative disorders (e.g., multiple sclerosis and amyotrophic lateral sclerosis), congestive heart failure, and AIDS. These diseases unfold over extended periods of time, only a small part which is spent in the hospital. Generally, patients are admitted to the hospital when they become more symptomatic from progression of the disease (e.g., pain resulting from metastases to bone of lung cancer that had been in remission) or from some complication of the treatment (e.g., renal failure caused by a medication which is used to treat the viral retinitis that occurs in AIDS patients). Patients are admitted when their diseases make them so ill that they need the medical services of the hospital. Their stay may be short, or it can stretch on for months if complications of the disease or of the treatment accumulate, or anything in between. Because these patients are often quite ill when they are hospitalized, the clinical task of differentiating between an autonomous desire for suicide and suicidal depression is much more difficult than it would be when their medical conditions are more stable. Hospitalization may be the worst of times to address this question.

The second reason has to do with the psychological impact of admission to a hospital. Admission to the hospital is necessitated by deterioration after a period of some degree of medical stability. This is a time of setback and patients, understandably, become demoralized. They feel helpless; their hope and confidence in their capacity to endure are deflated. People in this state are depressed, but medical improvement enables them to reorganize their psychological resources—to pull themselves together and prepare for returning to life outside of the hospital. In contrast, a patient with a serious clinical depression responds weakly to feeling better, or not at all. If the hospitalization is prolonged because new clinical problems arise, the state of demoralization may also be prolonged and may deepen over time.

Thus, admission to the hospital is a time of both medical deterioration and psychological demoralization. These are circumstances in which it is likely that some patients will request suicide assistance. It also a time when it is most difficult to distinguish between the suicidal ideation of clinical depression, temporary demoralization, and a well thought out desire to bring life to an end. A hospital policy of permitting PAS makes it available when there is the greatest potential for PAS to lead to the suicide of patients who are temporarily overwhelmed and demoralized by illness. Its unavailability to patients when they are hospitalized protects against this kind of possibility.

As a coda to this discussion, it merits acknowledgement that some model legal codes of PAS try to address this problem.[6] They specify a waiting period in order to prevent acquiescence to transient or impulsive requests for assistance and to establish the stability of a patient's desire to bring life an end. However, illness and demoralization do not always clear up in seven or fourteen days, or whatever period the code stipulates. In addition, there will be patients who have requested assistance from their physician long before their hospitalization. When they are admitted to the hospital, they may ask for the assistance because they are demoralized by their current but possibly temporary deterioration. For these patients, the waiting period has already passed. There may also be patients whose conditions are stabilized after many weeks in the hospital; they then approach a discharge into an unknown, discouraging and possibly terrifying future. For example, patients with new onset end stage renal disease must incorporate renal dialysis into their lives, and weakened, cachectic patients may be compelled to move to a skilled nursing facility instead of going home. Patients in these predicaments may request suicide assistance to avoid futures which they are understandably afraid of trying but might be fruitful if they were tried. They may sustain their suicidal intention in the hospital long enough to satisfy the requirement of a waiting period.

In-Hospital PAS and the Legitimation of Euthanasia

A principal moral concern of opponents of PAS has been the possibility of a transition along a slippery slope from the assistance of voluntary suicide by physicians to voluntary euthanasia and then to involuntary euthanasia. In order to understand how the issue of in-hospital PAS intersects with this slippery slope, we need to keep in mind both the conceptual distinction between PAS and euthanasia and the practical difference in how each is effectuated. In essence, the conceptual distinction has to do with the identity of the agent who administers a lethal agent.[7] In the case of PAS, the physician provides the patient with the technical means of ending life which the patient later utilizes without the further participation of the physician. In the case of euthanasia, the physician (or some other person) is directly involved in causing death through the administration of the lethal agent. Whether the euthanasia is voluntary or involuntary depends upon factors other than the technical means of suicide and the identity of the agent who administers them.

There is also a concrete, practical difference between PAS and euthanasia. As PAS is now understood by advocates and practiced by physicians, the physician writes a prescription for barbiturate capsules; the patient takes a sizeable number of these pills at a time and place of her or his choice. In the case of euthanasia, the physician administers an intravenous infusion of a central nervous system depressant; high dose intravenous morphine acts rapidly and reliably to induce sleep, coma, and then suppress respiration. For the most part, the conceptual and the practical distinction between PAS and euthanasia match up in practical terms. As commonly envisaged and currently practiced out-of-hospital, in PAS the physician prescribes and the patient administers the medication, possibly with the help of others; in the case of euthanasia, the physician directly administers a lethal intravenous agent.[8]

Advocates of PAS are divided about the undesirability of moving down the slope even to this point. Some are ambivalent about or opposed to voluntary euthanasia. They may have moral reservations about doctors' intentionally and directly killing their patients. Or, along with opponents of PAS, they may worry that voluntary euthanasia carries a significant risk of leading to involuntary euthanasia; patients might be killed without their knowledge or consent.

Other advocates of PAS have no moral qualms about voluntary euthanasia. They regard prescribing a barbiturate and administering a lethal intravenous drug as having the same moral status: Neither is morally blameworthy if a terminally ill person makes an autonomous decision to die. Because euthanasia has had a bad history and the legalization of PAS is a politically more realizable goal, they may not actually advocate euthanasia. But in principle, voluntary euthanasia is not morally different from assisted suicide.

For all these differences, there is agreement that involuntary euthanasia is murder. Descent down a slippery slope to involuntary euthanasia is one of the agreed upon potential undesirable consequences of the legalization of PAS. It is morally abhorrent and fraught with social dangers of all sorts. In order to question what effect introducing PAS into hospital practice will have on the possibility of descending this slope, we need to think concretely about the technical means of ending life which are used in PAS and euthanasia. Oral barbiturates do not lend themselves to the killing of unknowing and unwilling people. For barbiturates to reliably kill a person, many pills have to be taken in a short time. This takes a knowing, intending person who is determined to die. Intravenous medications, on the other hand, are more reliable and do not require knowledge, will, intention, or even cooperation from the recipient. Thus, intravenous administration of lethal medications is the technological gateway to the slippery slope leading to involuntary euthanasia.

It is my contention here that the introduction of PAS into hospital practice can be expected to give rise to clinical situations in which powerful, collectively experienced pressures of compassion and common sense will compel hospital staff to substitute lethal intravenous infusion in place of self-administered oral medication. Three features of hospital acute care units make this a worrisome likelihood.

First, intravenous access is ubiquitous and routine, which means that euthanasia does not require a step beyond the simplest everyday technology of hospital medicine. Almost all seriously ill patients in the hospital have established intravenous access. If, contrary to fact, euthanasia required access to expensive, advanced technology, the bureaucratic process of obtaining approval and arranging access would undoubtedly serve as a brake on the practice of euthanasia. The routine technology of intravenous catheters and pumps to dispense medication is no hurdle at all. Second, there will be seriously ill and dying patients in the hospital who cannot swallow, retain, or absorb enough oral medication to end their lives. It is hard to imagine that euthanasia will not be provided in hospitals legally permitting PAS when a request for assistance in dying comes from a patient for whom oral barbiturates are useless but who, in all other respects, qualifies for assistance in dying. We should expect that compassion for a patient in this predicament will at times generate an emotional intensity among medical, nursing, and support staff which will be relieved only by euthanizing the patient. Over time, it will be morally and psychologically unsustainable for the staff to assist in-hospital suicides of some patients with oral medication while withholding intravenous medication from patients who cannot utilize oral medication to die.

Third, death is achieved more quickly and more reliably with intravenous medication. Patients do not have to worry about retaining medication in the stomach. They do not have to potentiate the barbiturate with alcohol. They do not have to endure anxiety about the effectiveness of the medication before and after they ingest it. Even for patients whose gastrointestinal function permits the use of an oral barbiturate, euthanasia with an intravenous agent is a superior method of suicide.

This analysis should be troubling to advocates of PAS who are ambivalent about voluntary euthanasia as well as confirmatory to outright opponents of PAS. The confluence of these reasons imply that concern about PAS leading to euthanasia is not misplaced if PAS enters hospital medical practice. Conversely, the exclusion of PAS from the hospital serves to prevent the substitution of voluntary euthanasia for PAS.

It might be objected that keeping PAS out of the hospital does not prevent euthanasia for patients at home. This is true. Euthanasia at home may occur because seriously ill patients sometimes have indwelling catheters for infusion of medications or for parenteral nutrition. Undoubtedly this access will be used because intravenous agents are techically preferable to oral agents. Moreover, even if a patient who has decided to die does not have an indwelling catheter, inserting one is a simple, basic procedure.

Granting that euthanasia may occur outside of the hospital, this is not the whole story. What matters is whether excluding PAS from the hospital will *increase* the risk of euthanasia outside of the hospital. I do not think this is the case. Physicians and patients in the community may consider opting for euthanasia, but there are greater psychological and moral hurdles for them to overcome. More importantly, in the locus of the home, the substitution of intravenous for oral medication will not be fostered by the force of collective emotional and moral validation which would be generated in the locus of the hospital.

PAS and the Destabilization of the Ethos of Medicine

My concern in this argument is with the impact of PAS on the medical units in which ill and dying patients are cared for. The undesirability of introducing PAS into the hospital stems from its impact on the milieu of the medical unit, on the psychological and interpersonal dynamics of hospital staff and on the quality of care that will be provided to the ill and dying. This approach to the issue of in-hospital PAS is similar to a broad range of issues which opponents of PAS have raised about its impact on the ethical conduct of conduct of physicians and on the quality of care for ill and dying patients. For instance, adherents of the Hippocratic tradition in medical ethics have seen PAS as a threat to the moral integrity of the medical profession and to its identity as a healing profession. From a socioeconomic point of view, critics contend that an environment ill suited for the legalization of PAS is being created by the absorption of healthcare institutions into profit-maximizing corporate structures, the entry of physicians into the salaried work force of profit-seeking organizations, and the curtailment of the professional independence of doctors through reimbursement and review policies of insurers. For instance, some critics of PAS argue that in a capitation system of managed care, instead of counselling and supporting patients in their efforts to live as fruitfully as possible with their afflictions, physicians will be inclined to agree to, or even to subtly encourage, a request for suicide assistance in order to avoid the increasing cost of care which accompanies disease progression. Fortunately, because I have the limited objective of arguing for a policy of not assisting in-hospital suicides, I can bypass these broader ethical and socioeconomic issues.

The assisted suicides which have been described in published reports and media accounts have, of course, all occurred out of the hospital. These suicides differ from one another in innumerable respects. Patients who elect to end their lives differ in age, disease, and severity of illness, personal history, current station, future prospects in life, and in their reasons for ending life. They may arrive at their decision by themselves or through deliberation in concert with others who are important to them. They may inform others of their plan or keep it to themselves. They may have a long-standing relationship with a physician who fully supports their action; or their physician may disagree with the decision to die but agree to write a prescription out of respect for their freedom of choice; or they may request assistance from a physician they barely know.

These myriad differences will also be characteristic of legalized in-hospital suicides. However, intramural suicides will differ from extramural suicides in one fundamental respect. In-hospital suicide will take place in a public space and will necessarily involve many individuals who do not belong to the personal world of the patient. If assisted suicide becomes an organized and regulated activity of hospital practice, it will have to be intercalated into the hospital's usual way of doing business. The care of patients in the hospital is carried out through the systematic organization of the activity of physicians, nurses, and other staff on a twenty-four-hour basis. The retinue of physicians is comprised of the primary physician of record, house officers, and specialist consultants. Nursing care involves two or three shifts of nurses; in the course of a prolonged hospitalization, this may amount to a dozen or more nurses. If a patient in the hospital deliberates about suicide, the patient and family members will speak with many of these staff members about prognosis, about treatment and palliative options, about the circumstances under which the patient might want to die, and about the arrangements for suicide. They might seek the counsel of the nurses with whom they feel most open and trusting.

Information among this cadre is transmitted orally and written in the chart, which is reviewed by other hospital staff, such as utilization reviewers, infection control officers, and discharge planners who have no direct contact with the patient. They will routinely, and appropriately, read the chart and thereby know of the patient's deliberations and plans. In the rule-governed, risk-aversive, bureaucratic structure of the hospital, it is a near certainty that hospital administrators will establish a protocol for institutional review and authorization of a suicide, which will necessitate the involvement of yet another cadre of hospital personnel. One can readily imagine that hospital ethics committee and psychiatric consultants will be mandated to play some kind of regulatory role. Inevitably, many individuals will be engaged in the patient's suicide, not because the patient chooses to involve them, but because of the magnitude and complexity of the organization and its legal-bureaucratic necessities.

The occurrence of PAS outside of the hospital in the patient's home (or the home of family or friend), places it in a private space in which the patient can control the extent to which others participate and the dispersal of information about his or her plans. Even then, the suicide would have an open, public dimension. For instance, governmental regulation may mandate consultation and review by a second physician, but this is a highly circumscribed breach in the patient's privacy. The health professionals who come to the home may be privy to the patient's thinking about and planning to bring life to an end. But in contrast to the hospital, contact in the home with professionals like a visiting nurse, a physical therapist, or a psychotherapist is episodic; the patient retains control over whether these individuals will be aware of or participate in his/her deliberations about suicide.

For those who believe that a person's suicide ought to be a private, quiet matter protected from the scrutiny of strangers, the patient's loss of control over who knows of and becomes involved in the suicide will be an undesirable aspect of in-hospital PAS. However, the experience of the patient is not my concern in this argument. If the loss of privacy and intimacy in ending life in the hospital is too distressing for a patient, the alternative is discharge to a more suitable environment.

The public character of suicide in the hospital is disturbing from a broader clinical and ethical point of view. For an individual patient, an assisted suicide is a singular experience; for the staff, it is repetitive. The staff who care for seriously ill and dying patients will be repeatedly drawn into this kind of emotionally charged process. Emotional intensity and distress are, of course, not unknown in the care of the seriously ill. Clinical training, a grounding in morality and professional ethics, and accumulated clinical experience prepare physicians and nurses to handle the intrapsychic and interpersonal stresses that abound in hospital work. Training, ethics, and experience serve to keep staff pulling in the same direction and to maintain interpersonal equilibrium in medical units even when there are sharply divergent beliefs and feelings about what is appropriate care for a particular patient.

The clinical and psychological demands on physicians and nurses who care for the very ill are complex and considerable. They must find a balance in themselves between their realism about the patient's prognosis, the potentialities and limitations of existing therapies, and their drive to achieve a stabilization or reversal of the patient's disease to make a return to life outside of the hospital possible. They also must help the patient achieve a livable synthesis of realism and hope and to respond as best they can to the increasing encroachment of the disease on his or her life and to an approaching death.

It is very difficult to do this well. At present, many physicians are not adept at achieving this kind of balance for themselves. They do not know how to prepare their patients for progression of their diseases without undermining their hope. They are unable to engage their patients in the kind of collaborative planning for care at the end of life which would help bolster the patient's sense of control over a terrifying process and which would provide reassurance of the physician's continuing presence and commitment to caring for the patient until the end of life. The need to develop these abilities and to learn how to transmit them to physicians in training is now being recognized and seriously addressed in training programs.

The possibility of assisted suicide in the hospital will make it harder for physicians and nurses to deal with these questions. When a decision to end life does not arise from clinical depression or transient demoralization, it stems from the patient's existential judgment that nothing further of value can outweigh the burden of living with the adversities of the illness and its treatments. Individual physicians will have to learn to respond to this kind of judgment and to the premature resignation or despair that may sometimes lead to it. The physicians, nurses, and other staff who become aware of or directly involved in a patient's moving toward suicide will be compelled to address core existential issues about what gives life and suffering meaning as well as moral issues about aiding another person's suicide.

As hard as it is, and ought to be, for individual physicians to achieve a settled view of these questions, it will be all the more difficult because of the public character of PAS in the hospital. Many minds with tremendous disparities in their existential, moral, and religious outlooks will become engaged in these questions in the hospital. So there will be many different judgments about the wisdom of each patient's decision and the appropriateness of acceding to each patient's wishes. Training, professional ethics, and clinical experience do not pull health professionals in medical units together on these kinds of issues.

In units where patients die frequently, this can work badly for clinical practice. The engagement of staff with requests for suicide assistance would become a regularly recurring phenomenon. Reflecting on the appropriate conditions for suicide, in general and with respect to particular patients, would become part of staff discourse. When talk of the appropriateness of a suicide becomes routine, patients who request assistance and their families will inevitably hear some of it. If the comments are unsolicited, they will be inappropriate; if sharply disparate views are offered, the patient's burden could be made heavier. Moreover, when talk of the appropriateness of suicide becomes routine, patients who do not request assistance may have the subject raised for them by members of the staff. This would begin a transformation of assisted suicide as an existential choice of the patient into suicide assistance as a modality of care—as a "procedure" the medical system can offer patients in the later stages of their disease.

The involvement of staff with questions of suicide in this kind of ethical hothouse might also be deleterious to the care of patients whose death is imminent. At present, terminal sedation—the intravenous infusion of morphine to ease the suffering of a patient with diffuse pain, respiratory insufficiency, or agitation—is underutilized as a palliative modality. It is not initiated when it should be, or it may be done inadequately because a physician mistakenly believes it is wrong to use a medication that has the potential of hastening a patient's death. These deficiencies in medical practice are correctable through improved clinical and ethical training. However, if PAS were to be introduced into hospital practice, these inadequacies might, paradoxically, become more entrenched. Currently, it is physicians' fears that terminal sedation will hasten death that keeps them from initiating or using terminal sedation effectively. If suicide (and possibly volun-

[handwritten marginal notes:] can't this happen w/ any # of choices the patient is given? That's the why it's the patients choice for medical treatment of any kind. Why is PAS different? Should we go back to the time when the patient didn't have the right to his/her choice of medical treatment? No.

tary euthanasia by means of lethal intravenous infusion) begins to occur in hospital, a physician considering terminal sedation will have to wrestle with the added fear that starting terminal sedation as a palliative modality may provoke suspicions of unrequested euthanasia.

[handwritten: No. That's why it's the patient's choice!]

The Hospital in Society

The hospital as a social institution has never been an unalloyed object of social affection or reverence. Whatever luster it enjoys now is of recent origin, having been garnered from the extraordinary scientific and technological advances in medicine since the Second World War. But admiration for the hospital as a locus of basic medical competence, technological marvels, and occasional clinical miracles is tempered by its status as a locus of disease, illness, and suffering. No one looks forward to needing the best stuff the hospital has to offer.

Ambivalence about hospitals has been heightened in recent years by the tension patients (and families) feel when they need both to rely on their doctors for care and at the same time to protect themselves from what they regard as excessive therapeutic efforts. This ambivalence is now being further intensified by the economic transformation of the healthcare system, which adds a new tension running in the opposite direction. Patients (and families) increasingly feel they have to battle to extract what they need from hospitals and doctors dominated by profit-seeking insurance companies and managed care corporations. Thus, the perception of the hospital as an institution in which it might be necessary to battle to get enough care is being intertwined with the already existing perception of it as a locus in which it is necessary to fend off too much care.

The question arises, then, of what impact the legalization of PAS will have on the hospital as an object of public consciousness—i.e., in the mind of patients in the future. In this final argument, I want to sketch two undesirable states of affairs which can be avoided by a policy of excluding PAS from hospital practice. The first is, I think, probable; the second is at best conjectural.

If PAS is introduced into hospital practice, the hospital as a locus of care would acquire another identity which would generate ambivalence and even foreboding. Over and above all the other things it is perceived to be, the hospital would become a place in which human lives are, *in fact*, intentionally brought to an end. If PAS is legalized, this would take the morally acceptable form of patients' ending their own lives. However, in sectors of society in which the distrust of social institutions is an important feature of the group's social outlook, it is a small step from the actuality of the hospital as a locus in which some people kill themselves for their own good to the perception of the hospital as a locus in which some people are killed by others for someone else's benefit. The readiness of people to come to hospitals when they are ill, to accept medical advice when they are hospitalized, and to remain in them for treatment is undermined by this kind of mistrust.

Obviously, an estimate of how much distrust of this sort might be generated by the in-hospital practice of PAS is an act of imagination. There are two reasons

misconduct

slippery slope

to believe that some degree of mistrust will actually arise. First, because there is already public knowledge of intentional institutional medical malfeasance in the recent past, the fear of involuntary euthanasia will have a tangential relation to fact. Second, the substantial distrust of the government and other important social institutions can readily generate increased distrust of the hospital when it becomes perceived as a place in which intentional killings occur under official auspices.

Although this picture of distrust of doctors and hospitals might seem like an unreal, far fetched vision of paranoia, something like this state of mistrust already obtains in American society. The fear of being killed for the convenience of others is evidenced in low rates of organ donation among minorities. For many African-Americans, mistrust of hospitals and doctors has a basis in the exploitation of African-Americans in the Tuskegee experiment. Moreover, while there is no basis in fact for the belief that the United States government developed and used the Human ImmunodeficiencyVirus to kill off poor black people, this belief was, for a time, entrenched enough in the minds of inner city African-Americans to impede efforts at case identification for treatment and education as a public health measure. It is counterproductive to the mission of hospitals, particularly for hospitals serving African-American communities, to introduce a practice which will nurture the perception of the hospital as a place where an ill, defenseless person might be killed without requesting it.

The second reason for excluding PAS from hospitals is a matter of political conjecture. In the political and legal process which may result in the legalization of PAS, one unknown is whether traditional, religious moralists will become engaged with the same passion and persistence they have manifested in their campaigns against abortion. For religious moralists, suicide is the destruction of life and is on a par with abortion. It is not inconceivable that they will turn their sights on institutions which abet suicide. Since *Roe* v. *Wade*, we have had ample and painful evidence of what their passion can lead to when it is harnessed by a political will. Although abortion is a medical procedure, hospitals have largely been spared the traumas inflicted on clinics in which abortions are available to women. If politically organized religious traditionalists should mobilize against PAS after losing battles against its legalization, then in-hospital PAS might lead to hospitals bearing the brunt of an unpleasant and possibly poisonous *Kulturkampf*.

Like the previous argument, this one may seem to have a trace (or more) of paranoia. It is admittedly conjectural. But dismissing it without some concern about the potential for this turn of events is an option only for those who believe they know to a near certainty that politics in America will not take another turn to the right in the next ten years.

This is no reason not to have PAS available, just a reason to illegalize abortion

Clinical Implications

I want to return to an issue raised in the preliminary observations of this essay. This is the apparent incongruity of making PAS available to patients when they are not in the hospital but not making it available to them when their illness has necessitated hospitalization. This would seem to withhold PAS just when patients are most likely to request or need it. The way to unravel the incongruity is to attend to the differing clinical circumstances of hospitalized patients with progressive and terminal diseases. Consider the following clinical situations.

For patients whose deterioration can be reversed so that a return to life outside of the hospital is possible, consideration of suicide can be deferred until after the reconstitution of extramural life. Suicide delayed is not like justice delayed; it is not autonomy denied. Deferral until after leaving the hospital may lead, autonomously, to a different outlook on the future.

Patients who can return home only with intensive interventions to control symptoms and maintain an acceptable level of comfort need to have comprehensive, sophisticated hospice services in the home. In time, when the need for more and better end-of-life, out-of-hospital palliative care is met, it will become unacceptable not to offer palliative home services to severely ill patients. In this case too, consideration of the request for suicide assistance can be deferred until living at home is reestablished.

The final two situations are more vexing. First, for hospital patients whose survival depends on the continuation of intensive medical support, life sustaining interventions can be discontinued. When cardiovascular or respiratory support is withdrawn, death is imminent; the patient can be kept comfortable until it occurs. But if death is not a predictably imminent consequence of the discontinuation of support, the patient may request suicide assistance. For instance, a hospitalized patient decides to discontinue renal dialysis and requests assistance in ending life to eliminate the delay in dying. For patients whose clinical condition permits leaving the hospital, the decision to end life can be reviewed and, if sustained, can be enacted at home. Second, patients in their final days who have begun to die may request suicide assistance. They may be too fragile to leave the hospital, and there are no life sustaining therapies whose discontinuation will promptly end the patients' lives.

When a dying patient cannot leave the hospital, the request for suicide assistance is most psychologically and morally pressing. Death is already on its way. In this circumstance, a policy of not acceding to the request of a dying patient for suicide assistance does seem pointless or cruel. But in a hospital which has labored to achieve excellence in the care of dying patients, it is neither pointless nor cruel. It isn't pointless because the policy of excluding PAS is intended to prevent an ethical and clinical deterioration in the care of seriously ill and dying patients. And it isn't cruel because the alternative to intentionally ending a patient's life is the compassionate, skillful easing of the way to death.

When this kind of end-of-life care is possible, the principal difference between excellence in end-of-life care and intentionally ending life in these two in-hospital situations is the rapidity with which the patient dies. As I have tried to show, the costs of achieving this acceleration of dying in the hospital will be substantial and unwarranted.

Concluding Personal Remarks

This essay has been addressed to both advocates and opponents of the legalization of PAS. It is not about *whether* PAS ought to be legalized but *how* it ought not be introduced into hospital practice if society decides to legalize it. The elaboration of the argument has not required a statement of my own views about the issue of legalization. In this concluding section, I want to state them.

The fact that this argument straddles two opposing viewpoints mirrors my own deep personal ambivalence. Like many opponents of PAS, I am concerned about its potential for a seriously deleterious impact on medical practice in the United States. I believe that this potential is substantial. So I do not want to see PAS legalized quickly or widely in the country. I have argued for excluding legalized PAS from the hospital because I believe that, along with other reasonable professional and legal regulations, this policy of exclusion will reduce the potential for harm to patients, the medical and nursing professions, and the institution of the hospital.

On the other hand, I do not believe that suicide violates a law commanded by God or that it is intrinsically wrong from the moral point of view. Hence, it is hard to resist the powerful moral force of the idea that a reflective adult capable of deliberation about what is the best course of action in life ought to have the freedom to choose not to endure the deterioration and suffering inflicted by a progressive, terminal disease and also ought to have humane effective assistance to end life.

The moral validation of suicide as a response to disease and death derives from the Kantian/postmodern conception of autonomy as the foundation of moral choice, value, and judgment.[9] Hence, I regard a person's decision to end life in response to illness and declining health as a personal, existential moral choice. The physician has several important and proper services to render for a person who decides to end life. The physician can ascertain that the decision does not arise from the hopelessness and helplessness of clinical depression, from a confusional state stemming from dementia, delirium, or medication effects, or from despair over the future which is based on limited clinical information or misunderstanding. The physician can counsel the patient about future prospects and address the sources of the patient's pessimism or despair.

And finally, when the circumstances are appropriate, the physician can provide the patient with medication to end life and with instructions about how to use it effectively. But with this last service to the patient, I believe that the physician steps beyond the boundary of the therapeutic domain. Assisting a person's suicide is not medical care of the *patient's* disease or illness. It is support of the *person's* decision about how to respond to disease and illness out of respect for the individual's moral freedom.

Because I view a person's decision to end life as a personal, existential choice, I think it is fitting for a private space of the person's choice to serve as the locus of the suicide. Patients who want to kill themselves should do so in their homes or other suitable spaces but not in the public space of the hospital, in which the harmful effects of assisted suicide are more likely to ramify and propagate. Assisted suicide ought to be done at home (or in some other chosen place) because it is a personal phenomenon, and not in the hospital because it is not a medical phenomenon.

I am not distressed by the idea of making the option of suicide unavailable to the very ill and dying whose diseases compel them to remain in the hospital. From my medical and psychiatric training in several hospitals in New York City, I know how haphazard, insensitive, and deficient the care of patients can be. But from my clinical experience as a psychiatrist caring for people with AIDS, I also know that it is possible (if difficult) to achieve excellence in care of dying patients. Patients who are dying in the hospital can receive skillful, compassionate care that addresses fully the pain, physical discomfort, and anguish that are often present in the last days of a person's life. When we do these things well, we have met our human and professional responsibilities to dying patients. We do not fail them in their final days by not assisting their suicides while they are in the house of medicine.

Notes

The author wishes to acknowledge the patient and thorough assistance of Dr. Bert Hansen.

1. Daniel Callahan and Margot White, "Legalization of Physician-Assisted Suicide: Creating a Regulatory Potemkin Village," *University of Richmond Law Review* 30 (1) (1996): 1–83. Ronald Dworkin, "Assisted Suicide: What the Court Really Said," *New York Review of Books* 44 (14) (1997): 40–44.

2. F. G. Miller, T. E. Quill, H. Brody, J. C. Fletcher, L. O. Gostin, and D. E. Meier, "Regulating Physician-Assisted Death." *New England Journal Medicine* 331 (2) (1994): 119–23. Franklin G. Miller, Howard Brody, and Timothy E. Quill, "Can Physician-Assisted Suicide Be Regulated Effectively?" *Journal of Law, Medicine and Ethics* 24 (3) (1996): 225–232.

3. Timothy E. Quill, *A Midwife Through the Dying Process: Stories of Healing and Hard Choices at the End of Life* (Baltimore, MD: Johns Hopkins University Press, 1996). Andrew Solomon, "A Death of One's Own," *New Yorker*, May 22, 1995, pp. 54–69.

4. W. Breitbart, E. Bruera, H. Chochinov, and M. Lynch, "Neuropsychiatric Syndromes and Psychological Symptoms in Patients with Advanced Cancer," *Journal of Pain Symptom Management* 10 (2) (1995a): 131–41. F. Gil, P. Arranz, P. Lianes, and W. Breitbart, "Physical Symptoms and Psychological Distress Among Patients With HIV Infection," *Aids Patient Care* 9 (1) (1995): 28–31. H. M. Chochinov, K. G. Wilson, M. Enns, N. Mowchun, S. Lander, M. Levitt, and J. J. Clinch, "Desire for Death in the Terminally Ill," *American Journal of Psychiatry* 152 (8) (1995): 1185–91. William Breitbart, "Suicide Risk and Pain in Cancer and AIDS Patients," in *Current and Emerging Issues in Cancer Pain: Research and Practice*, C. R. Chapman and K. M. Foley, eds. (New York: Raven Press, 1993), pp. 49–65.

5. H. M. Chochinov, K. G. Wilson, M. Enns, and S. Lander, "Prevalence of Depression in the Terminally Ill: Effects of Diagnostic Criteria and Symptom Threshold Judgments," *American Journal of Psychiatry* 151 (4) (1994): 537–40.

6. Callahan and White, "Legislation."

7. A detailed exegesis of the conceptual distinction would be tangential to the objective of this essay. For a thorough discussion, see Brock, Dan, "Voluntary Active Euthanasia." *Hastings Center Report* 22 (March–April 1992): 10–22.

8. The principal exception to this mapping of the conceptual and practical distinction on to one another is the case in which the patient administers a lethal intravenous agent

without the physician's direct participation. Dr. Kevorkian has attempted to structure the suicides of his clients in this fashion. By connecting the patient to an infusion contraption which the patient controls, he intends to combine the technical advantages of euthanasia with the ethically desirable distancing of the physician from the act of killing. This distancing is fatuous to the point that it actually adds to the opprobrious quality of what he does.

9. H. Tristram Engelhardt, Jr., "Death by Free Choice: Modern Variations on an Antique Theme," in *Suicide and Euthanasia: Historical and Contemporary Themes*, ed. Baruch A. Brody (Dordrecht: Kluwer Academic Publishers, 1989), pp. 251–80.

Part Four

Considering the Impact
of Legalization

CONTRIBUTORS TO THE PREVIOUS TWO SECTIONS considered how the position of putatively vulnerable groups of citizens, and how the practice of medicine, might be affected if the circumstances under which physicians may legally assist their patients to die were broadened. The essays in this section explore another dimension of the debate. They directly address the outcomes of public policy changes that would reduce the opportunity for intervention by the criminal justice system.

The initial response to this possibility is simple but may be deceptively so. For a policy which narrows the conditions under which physicians face prosecution for providing life-ending services is, it might seem, a policy which reduces the protection the criminal justice system can give patients to prevent their being killed by their physicians. But second thought warns against imagining this to be the clear policy implication of legalizing physician-assisted suicide.

How effective are laws against assisting in suicides and what is their impact on medical personnel? Although American physicians theoretically face prosecution for assisting in the suicides of their patients, studies have shown that some nevertheless pursue the practice. And only in the very rare instance, usually where there clearly is intent to create a test case, have physicians who do so been pursued by the criminal justice system. Indeed, at least in the last twenty years, physicians who are the subject of litigation over their right to assist their patients to commit suicide are more likely to have themselves initiated an open challenge to the law than to have been discovered breaking it by law enforcement officials.

The essays in this section weigh the prospective benefits of changing the criminal status of physician-assisted suicide against the putative harms of doing so. Lance Stell distinguishes between legalizing and decriminalizing the practice. The latter is more nuanced and more felicitous, he argues, warning that the former approach has the potential to disrupt the delicate balance of public policy. Helga Kuhse concludes, on the other hand, that it is safer to legalize physician-assisted suicide than to allow hollow threats of prosecution to continue to obscure what physicians actually do to their patients. To substantiate her point, she invokes a comparison of the outcomes of the different policies pursued in the Netherlands and in Australia.

In contrast, John Arras believes that the changes implicit in modifying public policy to legalize physician-assisted suicide invite too many dangers. Consequently, despite the public's toleration of underground practice through which physicians provide the means, and sometimes even do the deed, legalizing physician-assisted suicide would have dire policy consequences, he warns. In a similar vein, Don Marquis holds that those who argue for policy change have not provided a reasonable level of proof as to the harmlessness of such an alteration. The cases made for legalizing physician-assisted suicide are too weak, he says. But David Orentlicher believes, instead, that the greater weakness lies with the case for continuing the current policy. We now permit procedures that are direct forms of killing patients, he worries, but we dangerously disguise them as something else.

Finally, Merrill Matthews, Jr., investigates the economic dimensions of changing the legal status of physicians' service in aid of patients' suicide. It sometimes is charged that, absent the legal sanctions against physician-assisted suicide, greed will place patients in mortal danger. In an increasingly competitive business environment, would this change of policy invite healthcare providers to kill rather than try to cure their patients? Matthews considers what the competitive advantage of such a strategy might be and concludes that its economic benefits are so negligible as to be no incentive for harming rather than helping individuals. Assuming that healthcare providers are accurate and rational in weighing the economic impact of their practices, he declares, economic considerations do not weigh in as reasons for maintaining, rather than modifying, our present public policy stance on the criminality of physicians who assist their patients' suicide.

14

Physician–Assisted Suicide

To Decriminalize or to Legalize, That Is the Question

LANCE K. STELL

Two conceptual lines have played important roles in the development of the right to die: that between natural and unnatural death and that between informed refusals of life-sustaining treatment and suicide. Both lines have become decrepit. A natural death is now virtually impossible for hospitalized patients. And the idea that a physician's abating life-sustaining treatment at patient request is *inherently different* from physician-assisted suicide is philosophically untenable. *One way* for physicians to assist suicide is for them to write orders that withhold or withdraw life-sustaining treatment at patient request. I argue that analysis and experience have washed these lines away. Only memory and force of habit preserve them. Further, I argue that physician-assisted suicide (already *effectively* decriminalized) should be fully and formally decriminalized. It should not be "legalized-but-strictly-regulated" unless such a regime would extend to medically managed, physician-facilitated deaths generally.

*   *   *

Introduction

OVER THE LAST FORTY YEARS OR SO, the concept "natural death," (where disease or aging processes rather than misfortune or human choice determine when and how life ends), has become decrepit. Our persistence in applying the concept to medically managed deaths makes its decrepitude all the more remarkable. According to the amicus curiae brief filed by the American Hospital Association in *Cruzan*,[1] 70 percent of the 1.3 million people who die in U.S. hospitals annually, die subsequent to someone's decision to withhold or withdraw life-sustaining medical interventions.[2] Since the decision to stop treatment is made in full awareness of it's life-shortening effect, since it may be made for that very reason, and since it is carried out by physician's order, "letting nature take its course" is a euphemism. For a patient under the supervision of physicians and nurses in a modern hospital, a "natural death" is virtually impossible.[3]

More recently, the conceptual line between a physician's abating life-sustaining treatment at the request of a decisionally capable patient and physician-assisted suicide, until recently regularly discerned in right-to-die case law[4] and proclaimed in living will statutes,[5] has become decrepit too. The line could hold as long as deaths occurring subsequent to removal of treatment were taken *not* to implicate the state's interest in preventing suicide at all.[6] For example, this position would follow from the proposition that refusing of life-sustaining treatment does not express specific, self-destructive intent, or by virtue of a causal theory that abating such treatment does not *make the patient die*, but merely enables or allows underlying disease processes to cause death.[7] However, once it is acknowledged that abating treatment can *cause* death, a patient's choice to abate treatment when death will (foreseeably) result will tend to implicate the state's interest in preventing suicide, because prima facie, he displays an intent to die. If so, it is difficult to resist the further inference that *cooperating* with refusals of life-sustaining treatment implicates the state's interest in preventing *assisted* suicide. And if it is *permissible* for a patient intentionally to cause his own death with the knowing cooperation of his physician, how can the determination whether the physician's cooperation counts as assisting suicide hinge solely on which medical privilege he uses, whether to order life-sustaining treatment stopped or to prescribe a lethal dose of medicine?

We now face important questions regarding the lines that separate natural death from unnatural death and suicide from refusals of life-sustaining treatment. If these old chestnuts, so well-roasted in the fires lit to illuminate the right to die, are now charred and crumbling, must we undertake a conceptual preservation project to avoid the ethically slippery slope many commentators warn of? Or would it be better to retire them from use and seek better tools to protect the underlying values at stake?

I will argue that we have roasted these old chestnuts long enough. The ideas that "letting nature take its course" is *inherently different* from causing death and that a physician's abating life-sustaining treatment at patient request is *inherently different* from physician-assisted suicide are philosophically untenable. *One way* to cause death is to "let" nature take its course. *One way* for physicians to assist suicide, while remaining within their professional capacities, is for them to write orders that withhold or withdraw life-sustaining treatment at patient request. The latter claim implies only that it is *possible* for physicians to assist suicide by acting within their well-recognized authority to abate life-sustaining treatment at patient request. It does *not* imply that their abating life-sustaining treatment at patient request amounts to, constitutes, is equivalent to assisted suicide. To refute my modest claim, one would have to prove that it is *not possible* for physicians to assist suicide in this way. Further, I will argue that physician-assisted suicide (already *effectively* decriminalized) should be fully and formally decriminalized.[8] It should not be "legalized-but-strictly-regulated" unless such a regime would extend to medically managed, physician-facilitated deaths generally.

Is the Refusal-of-Life-Sustaining-Treatment/Suicide Line Breached and Crumbling?

I think so.[9] In writing for the majority in *Cruzan*, Chief Justice Rehnquist pointed out that "All agree that such a removal [of artificial nutrition and hydration] would cause her [Nancy Cruzan's] death."[10] He allowed, *arguendo*, that "the United States Constitution would grant a competent person a constitutionally protected right to refuse lifesaving hydration and nutrition." But, he continued, "this does not end the inquiry" because, whether the individual's "constitutional rights have been violated must be determined by balancing his liberty interests against relevant state interests." And what state interests are those? The "interest in the protection and preservation of human life . . ." as evidenced by its treating homicide as a serious crime. And (the Chief Justice continued) "the majority of States in this country have laws imposing criminal penalties on one who assists another to commit suicide. We do not think a state is required to remain neutral in the face of an informed and voluntary decision by a physically able adult to starve to death." This reasoning forces the question: How could the interest in preventing suicide be a "relevant" countervailing state interest if the decision to cause death by stopping treatment failed to implicate it?

Associate Supreme Court Justice Antonin Scalia breached the line completely. In his concurring opinion, he denied perceiving any inherent difference between a patient's refusing life-sustaining treatment and suicide.[11] Thus he wrote that "there is nothing distinctive about accepting death through the refusal of food or through the failure to shut off the engine and get out of the car after parking in one's garage after work." Scalia argued that if the state's interest in preventing suicide is strong enough to interfere with the latter, it is strong enough to interfere with the former. Indeed, Justice Scalia reacted strongly to Justice Brennan's dissent in *Cruzan*, where his colleague had proclaimed that "The State has no legitimate general interest in someone's life completely abstracted from the interest of the person living that life, that could outweigh the person's choice to avoid medical treatment. . . ." Scalia retorted that "One who accepts it [Brennan's proposition] must also accept, I think, that the State has no such interest that could outweigh the person's choice to put an end to her life . . . that it is none of the state's business if a person wants to commit suicide."

The logical implications have been under-appreciated, even by Rehnquist and Scalia! If refusing life-sustaining treatment challenges the state's interest in preventing suicide, then it becomes a question *when* a decisionally capable patient's liberty interest might become strong enough to outweigh the competing state interest.[12] This naturally and minimally invites the inference that the liberty interest of *decisionally capable, terminally ill patients* trump the state's interests ("naturally and minimally" because it is not reasonable to suppose that a bona fide constitutionally protected liberty interest could *never* become strong enough to trump).[13] If so, we get the additional conclusion that the state's interest in preventing assisted suicide *by physicians* must *eventually* fall before the liberty interests of the terminally ill too. Otherwise how do we explain the physician's duty to write orders abating the unwanted treatment when the patient intends to end his life thereby?[14]

Scalia's reasoning kicked the ladder from under those who had grown accustomed to standing on the claim that committing suicide requires an "affirmative act."[15] One can commit suicide by omissions (e.g., omitting to get out of the car whose engine continues to run in a closed garage). But this implies that it is possible to *assist* suicide by omissions. Once this is granted, no logical barrier remains to block the inference that it is *possible* for a physician to assist suicide by "letting" a patient die. Only habits of mind prevent inferring it.

What Rehnquist and Scalia did not additionally infer, but should have, is that there is no constitutionally permissible, practical way for the State to protect it's interest in preventing suicide (and assisted suicide) in a medical context once it is tacitly acknowledged that terminally ill patients may indeed commit suicide, and secure medical assistance in doing so, by exercising a constitutionally protected liberty interest to refuse life-sustaining treatment. Indeed, as Richard Epstein observes, a physician's cooperation in these circumstances "is no more suspect than a routine joint decision to suspend treatment or terminate life-support."[16] Such logic moved the Federal Court of Appeals for the Second Circuit to strike down New York's prohibition of assisted suicide on equal-protection grounds. The statute could not stand because New York allows "those in the final stages of terminal illness who are on life-support systems ... to hasten their deaths by directing the removal of such systems; but those who are similarly situated, except for the previous attachment of life-sustaining equipment, are not allowed to hasten death by self-administering prescribed drugs."[17]

Remarkably, in reversing the Second Circuit in *Vacco et al.* v. *Quill*, the Chief Justice proclaimed that the line still holds firm. To prove it, he cited the fact that "the overwhelming majority of state legislatures have drawn a clear line between assisting suicide and withdrawing or permitting the refusal of unwanted lifesaving medical treatment by prohibiting the former and permitting the latter." Since he had noted this when he wrote for the Court in *Cruzan*, Rehnquist concluded that "Cruzan ... provides *no support* for the notion that refusing life-sustaining medical treatment is 'nothing more or less than suicide'" [emphasis added].

Does this undermine my associating Rehnquist's *Cruzan* opinion with the "crumbling line" theory? No, it doesn't. Explicitly recognizing that stopping treatment can cause death, and tacitly acknowledging that a refusal of life-sustaining treatment *may* convey self-destructive intent (and so implicate a specific, contrary state interest) does not entail that refusing life-sustaining treatment *necessarily* conveys such intent.[18] It may or may not. Similarly, for Rehnquist to reject that a death resulting from a knowing refusal of life-sustaining treatment is "nothing more or less than suicide" does not rule out that *some* such deaths are or may be suicides. Indeed, it would be illogical for Rehnquist to argue that a (hypothetically recognized) constitutionally protected liberty interest in refusing unwanted life-sustaining treatment would not be absolute on the ground that it *competes with* and must be *weighed against* two competing state interests (preserving life and preventing suicide) and then assert that there is a "clear line" between refusals of treatment *per se* and suicide. If the latter claim were true, then the right to refuse life-sustaining treatment cannot challenge, cannot be limited by, and cannot be weighed against the state's interest in preventing suicide.

More interesting, however, is the question of how far the law can plausibly go with disclaimers regarding suicide and assisted suicide. Such disclaimers impress

Rehnquist, but not consistently. In reversing the Ninth Circuit in *Glucksberg*, Rehnquist noted that voters in California and in Washington had rejected legalizing assisted suicide. "On the other hand," he continued, "in 1994, voters in Oregon enacted, also through ballot initiative, that state's 'Death with Dignity Act,' *which legalized physician-assisted suicide* for competent, terminally ill adults" [emphasis added]. This claim is false according to Rehnquist's own theory of statutory construction, namely, that statutes containing explicit "construction" provisions must be so interpreted.

The official explanatory statement for Oregon's law says it "allows an informed and capable adult resident of Oregon, who is terminally ill and within six months of death, to voluntarily request a prescription for medication to take his or her life. The measure allows a physician to prescribe a lethal dose of medication when conditions of the measure are met. The physician and others may be present if the medication is taken." But at Sec. 3.14, under *"Construction of Act,"* the law says, *"Actions taken in accordance with this Act shall not, for any purpose, constitute suicide, assisted suicide, mercy killing or homicide, under the law"* [Emphasis added].

If the line between deaths resulting from refusals of treatment and suicide holds because statutory construction says so, then mutatis mutandis, the line between a physician prescribing a lethal dose of medication for the purpose of a patient's taking his life and physician-assisted suicide should hold also. On the other hand, if the law's power of linguistic legerdemain fails in the latter case (as it has, at least for Rehnquist), whence its power in the former case?

Acknowledging that it is possible for physicians to assist suicide by ordering treatment stopped implies (for those who oppose any and all forms of assisted suicide) that the line must be redrawn, namely, *within* the category of stopping life-sustaining treatment at patient request. If some instances of *ordering* life-sustaining treatment stopped are (or might be) instances of physician-assisted suicide, and if these are unethical and illegal (as opponents of assisted suicide contend), then each instance of withholding and withdrawing life-sustaining treatment must be scrutinized (by whom?) to determine on which side of the line it falls. Failing to do so effectively decriminalizes physician-assisted suicide—those instances of it where the physician's assistance takes the form of ordering treatment stopped. The only way to resist these inferences is to block them at the start. Stomp one's foot! Dogmatically assert that it is *not possible* to commit suicide by refusing treatment, hence *not possible* for a physician to assist suicide by using his authority to order treatment stopped. Such dogmatism is indefensible.

Unless it is per se worse for a physician to use his privileges to write prescriptions for a lethal dose of medicine (which his patient may or may not take) than to use his authority in other ways which almost certainly will make a hospitalized patient's death occur sooner (e.g., writing a DNR order or ordering antibiotics stopped despite sepsis), his doing so should cause no more concern (and probably less) than his writing orders to stop treatment on which the patient's life totally depends (e.g., discontinuing mechanical ventilation or stopping enteral and/or parenteral nutrition and hydration).

Definitions and Clarifications

Suicide implicates tragic, stigmatizing paradigms—a young person's destroying herself because of an overwhelmingly negative, but inaccurate evaluation of her future; a despairing, sick and lonely, uncared for elderly person's inflicting death on himself while an indifferent society goes about business as usual. Where intentional self-destruction fails to mar the memory of the suicide, it tends to indict the callousness of survivors. Often it does both.

The power of paradigms makes it hard to call by the same name instances of reasonable, intentional self-destruction. Nevertheless, clear thinking about suicide requires avoiding distraction by paradigms. Giving them dominion tempts us to suppose that cases of reasonable, intentional self-destruction aren't "real" suicides. This is as bad as thinking that illnesses which fail to make a pathognomonic presentation aren't "real" diseases. A painstaking analysis of the relevant concepts will help us better to appreciate how common physician-assisted suicide *probably* is as well as our current arbitrariness in thinking about it.

What Makes a Death a Suicide?

At common law, suicide was "self-murder," wrongful self-killing. More precisely, a person "of years of discretion, and in his senses," was guilty of the crime of suicide if he "deliberately puts an end to his own existence." Blackstone reasoned that the suicide committed a double offense—one against God "for rushing into the presence of the Almighty uncalled for," the other against the King, "who has an interest in the preservation of all his subjects."[19] Neither one's motive nor the means by which one intentionally brought about one's death could decriminalize it.

Unlike homicide, which could (and still can) be justified in certain circumstances (e.g. killing in self-defense by a non-provocateur, killing of condemned murderers by the state's executioner), the common law made suicide wrong by definition. Since the offense contained no "without justification or excuse" clause, one who deliberately put an end to his life was guilty of wrongful self-killing. It could not be legally permissible, all things considered.

Decisional capacity was an element of the common law's definition of suicide. If one lacked sufficient capacity to act "deliberately," (one was a minor or out of one's senses), then there was no *mens rea*, hence, no suicide. Since being out of one's senses negated an element of the crime, there has always been an incentive to avoid adding felonious stigma to private tragedy when determining cause of death. Thus, self-destructive behavior tends to be taken not as evidence of derangement, but inherently deranged. Perhaps the remarkable psychology of many individuals who intentionally take their own lives when we think they shouldn't makes such question-begging seem reasonable.

Except for making suicide inherently wrong ("self-murder"), Blackstone's definition, "deliberately putting an end to one's own existence," captures suicide's conceptual core, provided that "deliberately" is understood to imply sufficient decisional capacity for intentional self-destruction, but not necessarily implying that the self-destruction results from deliberation. Thus, *a suicide is a death one brings on oneself, by doing or omitting something with the specific intent that one will die as a result, and where it is reasonable for one to believe that what one does or omits is substantially certain to produce that result.*[20]

For one's death to be a suicide, one must have (a significant degree of) *control* over performing an act that will make one die or omitting to perform a death-delaying/preventing act; one must have *sufficient capacity* to intend that one's death result from how one exercises that control; one's *death must in fact result* from the act or omission over which one has control and one must have good reasons to believe that acts or omissions of that sort reliably produce death.

Whether self-destructive intent is made effective by an act or omission doesn't matter.[21] Nor do motives matter. Motives to suicide may be self-regarding (ranging from selfish to prudent) or other-regarding (ranging from vindictive to altruistic). The reasons may be admirable, despicable, foolish, stupid, ill-informed, or some mixture.

Nor does temporal proximity of the act or omission to the resulting death matter conceptually. For example, suppose Alzheimer's runs in one's family. To avoid such a death, one has implanted in one's brain a device which somehow measures telltale plaque build-up. It is calibrated to trigger a lethal, comparatively painless cerebral event, when, but only when, it detects a pre-determined amount. Twenty-five years after the implant, the device triggers as planned, causing one's death. Despite the twenty-five-year interval, one's death is a suicide. (Would it still count as suicide if one forgot about the implant? What if one forgot because of memory loss associated with the disease and concomitantly developed an obsessive fear of suicide? Suppose one changed one's mind about the implant, wanted it removed, but it couldn't be done for some reason. Would this be like jumping off Golden Gate Bridge and thinking on the way down that this really wasn't such a good idea?)[22]

It is a mistake to define suicide as self-*inflicted* death.[23] Death is not always a harm to the one who dies.[24] To describe a death as "inflicted" implies its badness or harmfulness (one does not "inflict" benefits on oneself). Common sense supports thinking that dying too late can be a harm just as dying too soon can be. If so, death can benefit the one who dies. When death is the least-bad thing that can happen to a person, and nothing better can happen to him, it benefits him.[25]

Reflexivity in the making die or letting die is a logical feature of suicide.[26] Thus one can commit suicide by doing at least one of the following.

- *Making oneself die.* To avoid capture, torture and humiliation by the Philistines, King Saul falls on his sword intending to die as a result.[27] A quadriplegic, ventilator-dependent, competent patient has an engineer-friend build a device which enables him to turn off his ventilator by means of a timer. He asks his physician to give him a sedative to alleviate anticipated air-hunger. He triggers the device, intending to die as a result.[28] The patient's request for a sedative is an essential part of the self-destructive plan. The sedative insures against the power of air-hunger overwhelming his self-destructive resolve.

- *Letting oneself die or allowing oneself to be killed.* A woman in her late 50s becomes despondent over the death of her husband and the loss of her job. She takes a massive overdose of her blood pressure medicine (verapamil). She is discovered unresponsive by her son who rushes her to the hospital. The efforts of the doctors temporarily stabilize her and she regains consciousness—ventilator-dependent, in an ICU. She indicates a desire to communicate with those attending her. She is provided with a chalk board. On it she writes, "Let me die! Stop the vent, remove the breathing tube, discontinue all treatment. Do not start any treatment!" Not only does the precarious nature of her medical condition make it "suicidal" for her to refuse treatment, but also, her demand, "Let me die" makes it clear that she intends to die as a result.[29] If her doctors comply, it is a white lie to say they "let nature take its course."
- *Getting oneself killed.* One commits a capital crime, writes a detailed letter of confession, mails it to authorities, and surrenders to police, intending to be convicted and executed as a result. One takes out a "contract" on one's own life with an end-of-life service. The contract specifies that, in the event one is hospitalized with a terminal illness in a right-to-life hospital, an agent of the service will surreptitiously "pull one's plug" in the middle of the night.

Someone might object that counting some instances of getting oneself killed as suicides has the absurd consequence that some people will die two ways at once (both a suicide and a homicide). Intuitions about this can vary. I see no logical reason for insisting that a death cannot count as both a suicide and a homicide. Real life can provide stories stranger than philosophers can dream up. Consider the strange case of the suicidal forgery.

On 17 July 1786, Samuel Burt signed two documents—a counterfeit bank draft and a letter confessing his deed. The first act apparently amounted to a capital offense. Burt's lawyer argued an insanity defense on his troubled client's behalf (and against his client's will!). The judge wasn't buying. During jury instructions, he attributed to the defendant "a criminal purpose of destroying his own life" (thus finding sufficient evidence of *mens rea)* but allowed that the jury might reach a different conclusion. The jury returned a guilty verdict with a sentence of death but recommended that the judge show mercy to Burt because it suspected that he "laboured under some degree of mental disorder." Sensing that the jury's benevolence threatened his plan, Burt implored the jury, "[I]t is death that I wish for, it is death that I seek; for nothing but death can extricate me out of the troubles which my follies have brought upon me." Burt's outburst provoked the judge. Echoing Blackstone, he chided, "To come uncalled for into the presence of your Creator is highly criminal in itself; he who made you best knows when you shall have fulfilled those purposes for which you were created [and] it is therefore the highest degree of presumption in you, to take the secret judgment to yourself . . . [as for the punishment which your crimes have merited] it is your duty to submit to, but not to desire."[30]

Doing something or letting something happen intending to die as a result entails nothing about what one might do in case of failure. A failure might result in changing one's mind about self-destruction for some reason. It might result in a rerun or substituting other acts or omissions. Indeed, one might find self-destruction to be acceptable only if it can be accomplished by a particular kind of act or omission but not otherwise—taking an overdose of pills or refusing life-sustaining treatment, okay. Shooting oneself between the eyes with a nail-gun, not okay. Such preferences might reflect a desire to render one's self-destructive intent ambiguous to others and perhaps to oneself.[31]

Someone might object that my analysis results in counter-intuitively inflating the number of suicides. I answer: There is a distinction between what makes a death a suicide and when we can be appropriately certain in affixing that label to it. Our epistemology of suicide reflects the judgment that it is worse falsely to pronounce it than falsely to fail to do so. Since diagnosing a death as a "suicide" stigmatizes, there's an incentive to withhold this diagnosis when an alternative cause of death seems plausible. Despite the fact that suicide is the eighth leading cause of death in the United States (approximately 31,000 annually), suicide is almost certainly underdiagnosed and underreported. Probably many more occur where we fail to have sufficient evidence.[32]

Intending that one's death result from what one does or lets happen distinguishes risky behavior performed voluntarily and bad habits from suicide. It follows from one's intending to die as a result of what one does or lets happen that one expects to die. However, it does not follow from expecting one's death to result from what one does or lets happen that one intends to die. This implies that it is possible to perform "suicidal" acts intentionally, expect to die as a result, but not intend to die.[33] When this happens, one's death, if it occurs, is not a suicide. How so? Consider: A traumatically injured Jehovah's Witness (JW) whose hemoglobin has fallen to 2 (normal adult male values = 14–17 gm/dl) is informed that it would be "suicidal" for him to continue refusing transfusion. Perhaps no one with similar injuries whose hemoglobin had fallen below 2 had ever survived. The JW refuses nevertheless. Suppose, on the basis of the information he has been given, the JW expects to die as a result. If he dies, must we in honesty count his death as a suicide (leave aside well-meaning deception in reporting)? Not necessarily. Despite that he expected to die as a result of his refusal, the Witness may have hoped and prayed that he wouldn't die. (He wanted to be a reportable case. His refusal was up to him, whether his death resulted was up to God, and so on). Since hoping and praying that he wouldn't die rules out his intending to die, his death isn't a suicide. Consider another case: A soldier intentionally enters a field he knows to be heavily mined. He believes that crossing it is the only way to warn his comrades of impending danger. It is consistent with common usage to label his rash act "suicidal," but incorrect to label his death a suicide even if he'd made a rational calculation of the odds and expected to die as a result of entering the field. He hoped to beat the odds and miraculously to cross the field without getting himself blown up. Another case: A ventilator-dependent patient judges continued ventilatory support worse than death. His pulmonologist warns him that, in light of his respiratory status, it would be suicidal to demand removal from the vent in the circumstances. He gives the patient strong inductive evidence for his medical opinion. Suppose the patient persists in his demand. He may also hope and pray that he will not die, despite the fact that he does not disbelieve his pulmonologist's description of the risk. If so, his death is not a suicide.

Since it is possible to expect something to result from what one does or lets happen but also possible to hope that it won't, and since hoping that something won't happen rules out intending that it does, we cannot deduce intent from what a person expected to happen. But for very good reasons, our epistemological principles permit an inductive inference of intent from a person's (reasonable) expectations. Evidence about what a person expected to result from what he does or lets happen is often the best evidence for inferring what he intended. Our common-sense principles help us better to track the truth in situations where a person is strongly motivated to deny his intending to die, (because he couldn't count on the cooperation of others, say, were he candid about his intent, or perhaps he wants to spare their feelings) but is willing to admit that he is risking death and even expects it.

Assisting Versus Facilitating Suicide

Intending to die as a result of what one does or omits is necessary for a death's being a suicide. Similar reasoning applies to assisting it. One can assist in another's suicide by doing something or omitting to do something (just stand by, where doing so counts as "letting" or "allowing" or providing an opportunity). Control and intent are key. If one intends that another's suicide result from how one exercises one's control over whether it occurs, one assists it.

One can unintentionally facilitate suicide, but one cannot unintentionally assist it. One can also intentionally do what facilitates suicide (e.g. extubate a ventilator-dependent patient at his request knowing that he intends to die as a result), expect the patient's death to result, but not assist suicide because one did not intend the patient's suicide to result from respecting his request. Perhaps one hopes the patient will survive despite expecting that he won't. Thus one might avoid sedating the patient in hope that his expectable air-hunger will lead him to request reintubation.

Suppose a suicidal ICU patient has attempted self-extubation several times, only to be reintubated and finally physically restrained. A unit nurse sympathizes with his plight. They agree that somehow his restraints will be removed and that he will time his next self-extubation for the nurse's next scheduled break. The nurse also agrees to delay, somehow, anyone who might intervene. The plan succeeds. The patient commits suicide. The nurse assisted. He intended his cooperation to result in the patient's suicide. Not only did the nurse assist, he assisted *in his capacity as a nurse*. He coordinated his occupational activities, used his authority, privileges, knowledge of institutional procedure, his knowledge of what coworkers would be doing, etc., in a manner he intended to result in the patient's suicide.

Again, it would not be sufficient to attribute assistance to him were he only to have "expected" his acts/omissions to result in the patient's suicide. It would have been consistent with his expecting the patient to commit suicide for him to hope that the patient wouldn't do it. Maybe he thought the patient's killing himself was not what he would have chosen for himself but he recognized that the patient's was not an ill-considered plan, but on the contrary, one he had a right to complete.

Physician-Facilitated Suicide, Physician-Assisted Suicide, and Assisting Suicide in One's Capacity as a Patient's Doctor

"Physician-assisted suicide" is ambiguous. Sometimes it means nothing more than that someone who happens to be a physician knowingly provides the means for a suicide. Here's an example. Suppose someone with a medical degree assists his neighbor to commit suicide. This medical school graduate has no license to practice medicine, cannot authorize prescriptions, cannot issue medical orders to anyone. He's a retired pathologist. He never took care of patients. Nor is the neighbor his patient. The nonlicensed, retired pathologist provides a section of hose retrieved from his basement which the neighbor uses to asphyxiate himself with carbon monoxide. Suppose, in a backyard conversation on the previous day when responding to the neighbor's questions concerning various ways of dying, the pathologist had said, "carbon monoxide poisoning isn't a bad way to die."

In this case, the fact that suicide assistance came from a someone with a medical degree is purely accidental. Since there was no physician/patient relationship with all its special obligations to care for, attend to, and act as a fiduciary of the patient, no use of medical authority or privilege, no use of legally restricted medical means, it is not a case where someone *acting in his capacity as the patient's doctor* assists in suicide. In short, hardly a paradigm case of physician-assisted suicide!

A death should not count as a physician-assisted suicide *in the proper sense* unless the assistance comes from a physician licensed to practice medicine, and in his capacity as a care-giving fiduciary for the one who commits suicide, counsels the patient regarding life-ending medical options, and/or uses his medical authority (to write orders to discontinue life-support or to withhold life-saving medical measures such as CPR or to regard the patient's foreseeable medical instability as not counting as a medical emergency, or merely to create "an opportunity space" for the patient to do himself in) or uses his prescribing privileges (to prescribe a lethal dose of legally restricted medicine) with the intent that these various acts or omissions contribute to the patient's suicide.

A physician may prefer to restrict his cooperation to writing orders to withdraw or withhold life-sustaining treatment at his patients' request. This restriction can make the physician's intent ambiguous to others and to himself. Thus he may use his medical authority to write the appropriate orders out of respect for the patient's right to refuse treatment, expect the patient to die as a result, but as psychological insurance against intending death, somehow hope the patient won't die, which, if he manages it, would rule out his intending to play a contributory role in any suicidal plan the patient may or may not have.

If he writes the orders, fully resigned to (with no residual hope or prayer to avoid) the patient's dying as a result, and in fact secretly hopes that death will result quickly, it gets harder to describe the psychology which avoids his intending the patient to die as a result of his orders being obeyed. If the physician would be disappointed (as opposed to relieved) that the patient's death failed to occur as quickly as he expected, then it becomes all but impossible to withhold ascribing to him the intent that the patient's death result from his orders being obeyed. Needless to say, it is not uncommon for physicians and nurses to intend that the patient die as result of medical orders being obeyed and to acknowledge this privately off the record or in anonymous surveys.[34]

Implications

First Implication

Commentators who categorically deny that a physicians's stopping life-sustaining treatment at a patient's request do not intend the patient's death are self-deceived. As my analysis shows, it is certainly *possible* for a physician to intend a patient's death to result from stopping treatment. When the psychological facts are such as to support a diagnosis of intent in any particular case depends on what our standards of proof are. I haven't said anything about that. It is also *possible* for a physician to stop treatment, expect his patient to die as a result, but hope he won't, in which case she did not intend the patient to die. This proves that physicians *do not necessarily intend* patient death to result from stopping life-sustaining treatment. It can't prove that they necessarily do not intend the patient's death.

Second Implication

Often, commentators opposed to physician-assisted suicide don't bother to analyze suicide, neglect to distinguish facilitating from assisting it, or fail to lay out what makes physician-assisted suicide distinctive. Instead they give a cursory definition of physician-assisted suicide, often accompanied by an example which implicitly suggests that all *bona fide* instances must somehow be like it. For example, physician Ezekiel Emanuel, writing in the March 1997 issue of *Atlantic Monthly*, says, "In physician-assisted suicide a doctor supplies a death causing means, such as barbiturates, but the patient performs the act that brings about death" (p. 73). Emanuel goes on to declare that "a patient's refusal of life-support technology, such as a respirator or artificial nutrition, or a patient's request that it be withdrawn" despite that a physician must "supply" the orders implementing the request, do not count as suicide and the physician who honors the patient's refusal does not assist suicide." And why is that? Because, says Emanuel, "patient's refusal or requests have had ethical and constitutional sanction for years." Emanuel's reasoning suggests that a patient who refuses life-sustaining treatment or requests that the doctor order it withdrawn *may expect, but never intends, that he will die as a result,* or that when he does intend to die, it doesn't count as a "real" suicide and the physician's supplying the orders needed to make the request effective never "assist" because patients' refusals or requests have had ethical and constitutional sanction for years.

That a patient does not necessarily commit suicide if he intentionally "pulls his own plug" and dies as a result, does not entail that a patient who does this and dies as a result necessarily does not commit suicide. Similarly, that a doctor does not necessarily assist suicide when he pulls the plug at the patient's request, does not entail that a physician who does this with a lethal result necessarily does not assist suicide. What each intends makes the difference.

Too, Emanuel fails to recognize that the "means" physicians furnish to patients who intend to die as a result of their choices are often "opportunities" to die, created by medical authority. Such opportunities can be hard to come by for hospitalized patients. A "No-CPR" order can forestall resuscitation once a cardiopulmonary arrest has occurred. But this order does not preclude efforts to prevent the arrest. A patient who becomes hemodynamically unstable and decompensates is at risk for arrest. Ordinarily, this is a medical emergency. Measures *not requiring informed consent* will be employed to treat it. However, when hemodynamic instability is an expectable result of stopping ventilatory and pressor support at the patient's request where the patient intends to die as a result, the patient's decompensation must be covered, by a tacit physician-endorsed judgment that not every instance of patient decompensation should be regarded as a medical emergency. Were this understanding not put in place, mechanical ventilation and pressor support (and probably much else) would be rapidly restarted, to the frustration of the patient's will.

A patient who disagrees with his doctor about whether he can "fly" off the vent may demand extubation and cessation of ventilatory support, but also instruct that, in case he's mistaken, these measures should be reintroduced promptly. Obviously different understandings apply for patients who elect a "terminal wean."

Third Implication

Intent and control play central roles in my analysis. I have not analyzed them. I won't either. But it's clear that I cannot import the criminal law's theory of intent. According to its construction, a person is presumed to intend the natural and foreseeable consequences of what he does or omits. This rule economizes on arguments which implausibly deny intent in order to escape liability. For example, a defendant denying an intent to cause his victim's death despite admitting that he expected his victim's death to result from shooting him. He will offer expert psychological testimony tending to show that people do not always intend what's foreseeable, and that at the time he pulled the trigger, it will be the expert's opinion that he sincerely hoped his victim wouldn't die! Nor can defendant argue justification on the ground that he had a signed, notarized affidavit from victim conditionally consenting to the shooting. (Defendant was the survivor of a voluntarily fought duel where the parties exchanged such affidavits). When applied to medically managed deaths, the criminal law's rules of construction effectively transform all instances of withholding or withdrawing life-sustaining treatment into assisted suicides (in jurisdictions where this is a crime) when done at patient request; or into premeditated homicide or at least manslaughter otherwise.

Obviously, this theory of intent won't do. Yet, explaining why physicians who cause their patients' death (by making them die or letting them die) ordinarily do not and should not come within the ambit of the criminal law is harder than it looks. For an example of an unconvincing attempt, see the reasoning in *Barber* v. *Superior Court* (California, 1983).[35] This is not an idle, "philosophical" problem. If physician-facilitated/assisted deaths were to come within the ambit of the criminal law's construction of intent, proving physicians' *mens rea* would be "duck soup," benevolent motivation notwithstanding.

A dissenting judge in the Ninth Circuit Court of Appeals' opinion in *CID* v. *Washington*, Andrew Kleinfeld, seems to appreciate the problem of importing the criminal law's construction of intent into doctor's decisions to stop life-sustaining treatment. But in the process he shows how one can combine logical insight (physicians *do not necessarily intend* patient death to result from stopping life-sustaining treatment) with wishful thinking (physicians *don't intend* patient death). Thus he attempted a reductio ad absurdum on the majority by pointing out that when General Eisenhower ordered troops onto the beaches at Normandy, he knew (reasonably expected) many would die as a result. But Eisenhower's purpose was to liberate Europe. From this Judge Kleinfeld inferred, "The majority's theory of ethics would imply that this purpose was legally and ethically indistinguishable from a purpose of killing American soldiers."[36]

Kleinfeld's reductio fails! He confuses "purpose" with "intent." One's broader purposes cannot negate the strict construction of intent imposed by the criminal law. Suppose a nihilistic physician has a twenty-five-year-old female patient who suffers from refractory depression. Nothing he prescribes works. She remains suicidal. She mentions various ways of committing suicide at every office visit. She asks him if he would help her "get dead." He replies that the only way he could "help" her would be for her to become dependent on life-sustaining treatment and for her to request that he discontinue it. He documents their understanding in the chart. In a suicide attempt, she drives her car into a bridge abutment, suffering severe but not fatal injuries. When she regains consciousness, ventilator-dependent in the ICU, she writes on a note pad "Let me die!! You promised." He stops the vent and extubates her. She expires. What, besides access to the facts, would prevent prosecution for "assisting suicide"?

Fourth Implication

Rights to self-determination in medical care require that physicians use their medical authority in myriad ways that will cause death—not infrequently while aiming (more or less tentatively) at that outcome. Whether a physician's causal role is not only that of intentionally facilitating patient death but is also an instance of his assisting the patient's suicide depends on what both the physician and patient intend. *Without objectionable sacrifice of protected privacy interests, there is no practical way to discern "true intent" for either party.*

Unless some uses of medical authority and privilege should never facilitate suicide, per se, (e.g., prescription writing) it is arbitrary to "draw lines" in the sand. As my examples should suggest, the waves of clinical reality will wash them away. Better to acknowledge that all the physician's authority and privileges operate under the rules of informed consent/refusal, where all medical offers are regulated by the idea of patient benefit, as the doctor and his patient can best discern it in the circumstances. These principles may permit physician-assisted suicide when death has become *the least bad thing* that can happen to a patient and nothing better can happen to him. When this point is reached, the physician should not enjoy conscientious "opt-out." He should not be too quick to decide for death when he harbors sincere doubts that death isn't what's best for his patient *at that particular time.* But if the idea of a covenant between a doctor/healer and his patient means anything, it means a shared commitment to see things through to the least-bad end. *Anything less harms the patient.* Sometimes this covenant may require writing a lethal prescription. When it does, the physician's hand may (and should) tremble, but it had better write that prescription (or document that arbitrariness prevented acting in the patient's best interests). The physician's hand should similarly tremble when it writes DNR orders and other orders which may (and often likely do) aim at letting the patient die.

Fifth Implication

Susan M. Wolf has argued that Constitutional jurisprudence relevant to charting the limits of patient control over medical decisions making does not implicate any bona fide right to physician-assisted suicide.[37] It implicates only a right to accept or to refuse treatment, the core idea of which is bodily integrity—veto power over what goes into one's body and power to get "unwanted stuff" out of one's body. That these rights are not compromised by a patient's suicidal intent does not imply a right to physician-assisted suicide. The physician's duty to respect one's refusal of treatment is not contingent on the motive one may have for refusing, nor on what one intends to bring about by refusing. Physicians have a duty to respect decisionally capable refusals of treatment although that the patient may intend to commit suicide by means of refusing treatment. Thus a physician should remove an unwanted pacemaker, even though that doing so will facilitate a patient's suicidal plan.

Suppose a heart transplant recipient requests its removal. (Every beat of the transplanted heart can be regarded as a "mini-treatment.") The patient refuses to authorize any measure that would prevent his dying as a result of the removal. He makes it plain that bringing about his death is what he intends. To comply requires the doctor to do more than merely remove an unwanted mode of treatment—the pump that circulates his blood. Honoring the patient's refusal of treatment will make the patient dead. Where's the fine-but-still-perceptible line between removing the patient's transplant and making him dead?

Wolf's argument shows that a patient's right to bodily integrity, when exercised with suicidal intent, imposes a duty on physicians *to facilitate* but *not necessarily to assist* suicide. This is a legitimate philosophical distinction, one which gives logical if not psychological force to the "fine line" in this example. But the law cannot accommodate her distinction without abandoning its own strict construction of intent.

Preserving a "Natural Death":
Shoring Up the Line Between Causing Death and Letting it Happen

In 1975, James Rachels proved that killing is not per se morally worse than letting die by constructing a now-famous pair of cases.

> In the first, Smith stands to gain a large inheritance if anything should happen to his six year old cousin. One evening while the child is taking his bath, Smith sneaks into the bathroom and drowns the child, and then arranges things so that it will look like an accident.... [The second situation, involving Jones, is the same.] [H]owever, just as he enters the bathroom, Jones sees the child slip and hit his head, and fall face down in the water. Jones is delighted; he stands by, ready to push the child's head back under if it is necessary, but it is not necessary...."

Rachels argued that if it were true that killing is per se worse than letting die, we should be able to explain how Smith's conduct is worse than Jones's. We can't, because they are equally bad. Since we have one pair of cases, alike in all ethically relevant respects, where the difference between killing and letting die makes no ethical difference, it can't be true that killing is worse per se than letting die.

Rachel's argument also suggests that only some of the things that failed to prevent the child's drowning can be candidates for having caused it in a sense relevant for culpability. Obviously and trivially, both Smith and Jones failed to prevent the child's drowning. Indeed, everyone in the world failed to prevent it. The bath water's not suddenly and unexpectedly draining from the tub also failed to prevent it, and so on. But none of these nonoccurrences, *despite being necessary conditions* of the child's drowning, are serious candidates for being causes of it.[38]

In Smith's case, there is only one candidate for "the one who killed the child." No one in the Smith case let the child die. In Jones's case, there is only one candidate for "the one who let the child die." Only Jones had *sufficient control over the situation to have prevented it*, a necessary condition for "letting" something happen. He also intended the child's death to result from how he used the control he had.

Lettings-happen are among the necessary conditions of some events which are causes of them (or causal factors in their occurring). A physician who claims not to have caused her patient's death because she "didn't do anything" is liable to the retort, "Yes, you did do something—you let your patient die." If the physician intentionally or negligently let the patient die, (because she missed an obvious diagnosis, say) she is culpable for the death as well as being the cause of it.[39]

Conceptual conservationists who claim to oppose physician-assisted suicide but approve of physicians' honoring informed refusals of life-sustaining treatment, attempt to preserve the idea of a natural death by rediscovering differences (ethical and/or causal) between killing and letting die. Having discovered some, they suppose that letting die secures a space where nature can still take its course, despite the presence of medical supervision. Thus, Daniel Callahan argues that "killing and letting die are causally different.... There must be an underlying fatal pathology if allowing to die is even possible. Killing by contrast, provides it's own fatal pathology."[40]

The truth of Callahan's claim notwithstanding, it does not follow that lettings die don't cause death.[41] It is tempting to suppose otherwise only if we ignore the difference between *failing to prevent* and *letting or allowing to happen*. Trivially, one must fail to prevent the unpreventable. However, one cannot *let happen* something one was powerless to prevent. Letting or allowing to happen implies (some degree of) control over what happens or how or when. When death results from how one uses one's control, (e.g., by intentionally withholding efforts which could have postponed it) one causes or one at least is a causal factor in determining the moment and manner of death. That letting die is "causally different" than making die doesn't diminish that letting die is one way to cause death, sometimes intentionally so. When one *decides* to let die, one *takes advantage of* an "underlying fatal pathology."

David Orentlicher makes the point forcefully. "If I were to enter an intensive care unit and shut off every patient's ventilator, I would be charged with murder for every patient who died. And, it would be no defense that the patients' deaths were caused by their underlying illnesses [as determined at autopsy]."[42] This would be clearly true of all patients who died of respiratory failure. It might not be so clearly true of a patient who was successfully resuscitated, survived for several years in a persistent vegetative state, later to die from overwhelming sepsis because antibiotics were discontinued at family request.

Another conceptual conservationist, Yale Kamisar, confesses "a deep need ... to draw a boundary somehow between the withholding or withdrawal of life-sustaining medical treatment and ... 'ordinary' suicide."[43]

Kamisar's deep need cannot be satisfied. No one can deny that pulling one's own plug is one way to commit suicide. Another way to commit suicide is to get one's plug pulled. One way to assist the suicide is to help him to pull his plug. Another way is to write orders that his plug be pulled.

I do not claim that every instance of pulling one's own plug is suicide. Nor do I claim that writing orders to pull someone's plug is equivalent to assisted suicide.

Intent makes the difference. Nevertheless, when patients and their physicians think it is time for death to occur, there are myriad ways they can let it happen or make it happen.

Baruch Brody is another prominent commentator who argues for retaining the killing/letting die distinction in medical ethics on ethical and on metaphysical grounds. On ethical grounds, he claims that the obligation to refrain from killing can be present when the obligation to save life or to refrain from letting die is absent and that even when both are present, the former is more stringent than the latter. "The obligation not to take life is clearly of a higher priority than the obligation to save lives and is present in a great many cases where the latter is not. I am normally under an obligation to another not to take her life even when my own life or my well-being is at stake. I certainly am not normally under an obligation to another person to save his life. . . ."[44] Brody further claims that even if one is under a credible threat of death which can be removed only by killing a third (innocent) person, he is not permitted to do it. However, if one were under a credible threat of being killed unless one lets a third innocent person to die, one would (or at least might) be permitted to remove the threat by letting another to die.

If Brody's gambit is successful, he staves off the conceptual decrepitude of a natural death and provides support for the belief common among physicians that they don't necessarily cause death by stopping life-sustaining treatment.

Brody avoids the categorical, counter-intuitive declaration that physicians don't intend their patients to die from withholding or withdrawing treatment. He thinks this is unfaithful to the clinical facts. Nor does Brody deny that it is possible to cause death by letting die. What Brody denies is that all physicians' lettings die of their patients are causes of patient death. He thinks this because some lettings die are (merely) necessary conditions for the patient's dying when and in the manner that he does, but since not all necessary conditions are causes, there is space for physician's to let nature be the cause of death. In sketching a metaphysical basis for his view, Brody points out that not all necessary conditions for death are causes of death. And some causes of death are not necessary (over-determined deaths).

Brody is correct to claim that "normally" the stringency of the duty to avoid killing is greater than that to avoid letting die. But this reflects nothing deeper than the fact that most people, most of the time, are *more vulnerable* to killing than they are to letting die or to failures to save. For most of us, survival from day to day depends more on others refraining from killing us than from their refraining from letting us die. We fear the comparatively common danger more too. Thus the more stringent duty tracks the more common vulnerability.

Does Brody's suggestion help? No it doesn't. To preserve the idea of a natural death (where disease processes determine the moment and manner of death rather than the patient's and/or physician's decision to let it happen), Brody encourages playing charades with responsibility. Namely, the thought that since some lettings die aren't causes of death, some medically supervised lettings die import no (or at least lesser) physician responsibility. This is not an obvious net-gain ethically. His proposal is dubious on causal grounds too.

All killings cause death. Yet, not all killers are blamed for the deaths they cause (justifiable killings, excusable killings). Not all failures to prevent death are lettings die. Not all failures to prevent death are coupled with the control which could have enabled its prevention or marginal delay. All lettings die cause death (or are causal factors in death). Yet, not all those who let others die are blamed for the deaths they cause (e.g., some bad Samaritans, some of those that let themselves or others die unintentionally, but not negligently). Obviously, both killings and lettings die can be unintentional. (Namely, where it is true to say, "I didn't mean to kill her. I didn't mean to let her die," etc.)

It is also dubious for Brody to imply that, just like the rest of us, physicians' duty to avoid making their patients die is more stringent than the duty not to let them die. Consider two cases. In the first, a murderer threatens to kill the physician unless he makes his patient die by bolusing him with a massive overdose of barbiturates. In the second, a murderer threatens to kill the physician unless he lets his patient die by abstaining from calling a code to treat the witnessed arrest of his patient who has just suffered an iatrogenic anaphylactic reaction. Others' intuitions may differ from mine, but it isn't obvious to me that the physician's ethical bind is looser in the second case than the first.

Brody might respond by saying that "normally" (i.e. for non-medical contexts) his point holds. But doesn't the whole discussion (Brody's included) aim to illuminate how *physicians* may or may not use their medical authority and privileges to end their patients' lives, whether by killing or by letting die? Physicians have duties to take care of their patients, to attend to them, to refrain from harming them, to benefit them. Against these background duties of care, it matters comparatively little whether a physician wrongs his patient by killing him or wrongs him by letting him die. A sloppy surgeon who kills his patient through careless cutting is not obviously worse than the slack surgeon who leaves the OR for a smoke, failing to notice that his patient has started to bleed, letting his patient exsanguinate while he adjusts his nicotine level.

Too, people's moral intuitions divide sharply over the limits of what one may do under the general doctrine of necessity. *Regina* v. *Dudley and Stephens,* is a case that involved shipwrecked, starving sailors, cast adrift in a life boat, far from shipping lanes.[45] To preserve as many lives as possible, the first mate killed the cabin boy, who had been drinking sea water and who seemed near death (at least nearer than the others). The survivors ate the boy. At the time, public opinion was divided whether the desperate seamen did anything wrong at all. Yet, in a highly publicized trial, Dudley and Stephens were convicted of murder in the House of Lords only to receive Queen's pardons within six months. If Brody's claims were obviously right, there should have been a clear, stable consensus condemning the survivors on the ground that it would have been preferable for the castaways to let the cabin boy die by omitting to postpone his expectable death than to do what they did—kill him by cutting his throat in order to eat him.

But, on the contrary, the case has become a "classic" in the law of necessity because there wasn't then and isn't now a consensus about it.

Letting Go Old Chestnuts

Concepts are mental tools. When used with apparent success for a long time, they become more than tools, they become media of ethical exchange—they denominate the world and enable good-faith intellectual interaction with others. We tend to form attachments to such concepts, to have affectionate regard for them, to defend them. We imagine that they have never let us down, that we can't get on without them. We tend to forget why we have them—to solve problems. This point has been well-made by David Orentlicher.[46]

In the boundary between life and death, we have a problem to solve—to distinguish deaths improperly caused from those properly caused, to distinguish deaths which should not have occurred when and how they did from those which should have occurred when and how they did, to distinguish those we should refer to the criminal justice system from those we shouldn't. This is a hard problem. We need good concepts to help us address it rationally. We need good theories (ethical, metaphysical, and epistemological) to regulate their use. This is the context in which our old concept "natural death " has worked for so long.

Many kinds of death are preventable. Yet, everyone dies from something. So death, per se, is not preventable. We have used natural deaths as a surrogate for deaths that are not preventable. In theory, natural death occurs when a person's "time has come." But we also know that the quality of such deaths ranges from benign to horrible.

Unnatural deaths tend to be untimely. In homicides and suicides, human agency is key. In accidents, usually not (although negligence plays a role in some of them too). The moment and manner of death tends to be preventable with unnatural deaths. Often (*but not always*) we should have negative attitudes toward them. Even so, some homicides are justifiable (e.g., of aggressors in self-defense, of combatants in just war, of murderers by the state). Some suicides are at least excusable or even admirable (e.g., those that are prudent, heroic, or altruistic, martyring oneself for a worthwhile cause). Some accidental deaths are unavoidable. This sketch of our traditional conceptual scheme for distinguishing properly caused from improperly caused deaths should remind us that it has never enabled us to construct leak-free categories.

Another piece of the puzzle is the widely shared belief that decisionally capable adults have a near-absolute right to make death-causing (and not merely death-risking) medical decisions. They can refuse artificial nutrition and hydration. They can have feeding tubes removed. They can refuse CPR, and so on. By and large, these decisions (and the counseling/facilitating/executing role physicians play in them) may be made without much regulation, without court permission or even stringent medical review. Indeed, so much has been already conceded and accepted in this regard, that it is a puzzle how physicians' writing lethal prescriptions (which may or may not be taken) for their terminally ill patients has become such a hot controversy.

However, many commentators retain nagging worries about the sweep of the liberty. They want to hedge their support for it depending on whether the patient's project is suicide (impermissible) or letting nature take its course (permissible), on whether the physician's use of medical authority actively assists in producing death (impermissible) or merely serves to remove obstacles to the patient's dying (permissible), on whether medical authority is used to withhold/withdraw life-sustaining treatment (permissible) or to write a lethal prescription (impermissible). These conceptual mediators cannot help us distinguish permissible deaths from impermissible deaths.

The implications of my argument are that either all uses of medical authority which produce death with reasonable foreseeability ought to be prohibited (untenable) or, since physician-assisted suicide is already effectively, but informally, decriminalized, that physician-assisted suicided ought to be either formally decriminalized or legalized.

Physicians routinely do what would be criminal for non-physicians to do. Neither homicide laws, nor the criminal law's construction of intent generally, contain exceptive clauses for physicians. Yet, no physician, acting within his capacity as a licensed, medical fiduciary for his patient, has ever been convicted of homicide or for assisted suicide. When a New York State prosecutor invited a grand jury to indict Dr. Timothy Quill for assisting his patient Diane's suicide, the jury declined, despite that Quill had "confessed" to all the elements of the crime in the *New England Journal of Medicine*![47]

Physicians already have the tacitly recognized liberty to provide suicide assistance by ordering life-sustaining medical treatment stopped. We make no systematic effort to discern the "intent" that makes the crucial difference between facilitating death and assisting it, nor do we rationally distinguish causal pathways which produce death. Currently, turning off a respirator counts as letting die when a patient's physician does it, but as making die when his enemy does it. On reflection, formally recognizing their having the incremental liberty to prescribe lethal medications for the purpose of patients' ending their lives is substantially less imposing than the wide-ranging, non-judicially supervised power physicians already have.

To Decriminalize or to Legalize?

Mine is an argument for full, formal decriminalization of *physician*-assisted suicide. It is compatible with but does not make the argument for decriminalization of *assisted* suicide, per se.[48] Similarly, it is compatible with but does not make the argument for legalization. The distinction is this. Laws that criminalize conduct (whether at common law or by statute) define acts that are wrongful, specify elements of the offense, and (in the case of statutory prohibitions) prescribe punishment(s) which may be imposed for committing the offense.[49]

Decriminalization of conduct may occur by legislative removal from the criminal law of statements which define the conduct as wrongful and punishable. For example, Section 14–17.1 in Article 6 of North Carolina's law concerning homicide says, "The common-law crime of suicide is hereby abolished as an offense." (1973, c.1205). North Carolina's criminal code does not include "promoting suicide" or "aiding suicide" or "assisting suicide," as offenses. Nor does its homicide law specify any of these as a way of committing manslaughter. Obviously, when an offense is abolished, one can no longer be indicted for it. (After Jack Kevorkian's first highly publicized assisted suicide, it was discovered that, apparently, "assisted suicide" was not defined as a specific offense in Michigan. So he was indicted for homicide instead, and acquitted).

Conduct can also be decriminalized by courts' striking down statutes (in whole in or in part, on constitutional grounds) which define offenses and provide punishments for them. With uncertain and arbitrary effect, conduct can be decriminalized by police discretion, prosecutorial discretion and jury nullification—conveying more or less clearly that physicians' using their medical privileges to assist patient suicide in certain circumstances will not be punished.

Decriminalization confers no special privileges or immunities—not on physicians, nor on anyone else. Decriminalization provides no course to a "safe harbor" securing qualified persons from criminal or civil penalties.

Legalization of conduct defines acts that are *authorized* by specifying what, how, when and by whom they may be performed. Legalization may also confer criminal and civil immunity upon eligible persons who follow the law's provisions in good faith. For example, Oregon's Proposition 16, despite explicitly denying that it does so, legalizes physician-assisted suicide. Its procedures,

> allow an informed and capable adult resident of Oregon, who is terminally ill and within six months of death, to voluntarily request a prescription for medication to take his or her life. The measure allows a physician to prescribe a lethal dose of medication when conditions of the measure are met.

The distinction between decriminalization and legalization matters because stringent regulation of lethal-prescription writing enabling terminally ill patients to take their lives with the law's blessing, by implication, ignores the myriad other unregulated uses of medical authority which can be deployed to the same end. Thus, not only is it dishonest for Oregon to proclaim that it doesn't authorize physician-assisted suicide, it is arbitrary for it to single out one use of medical privilege by which physicians may assist, (the prescribing privilege), and offer a shield of immunity to physicians who follow the procedures outlined for that use of privilege. If this is a wedge, opening the way to stringent regulation of all medically managed deaths, patient self-determination will have been effectively extinguished. The wedge interpretation threatens to turn lose the dogs of the criminal law on physicians, potentially destroying the control patients have won over life-sustaining treatment. If legalization/regulation of lethal prescription writing isn't a wedge, it perpetuates dishonesty and strategic behavior.

Coda

Opposition to my argument favoring decriminalization over legalization/regulation may reflect pragmatic concerns rather than philosophical ones. For example, the amicus brief filed by law professors supporting the Ninth and Second Circuits argued that current law is both conceptually untenable (because it is based on a bogus distinction between suicide and letting nature take its course by stopping treatment) and is more dangerous to the interests of vulnerable populations than legalization of physician-assisted suicide, which involves regulatory oversight. By insisting on a broad distinction between "merely letting patients die" and physician-assisted suicide, the states take (and encourage others to take) decisions to engage in the former much less seriously than decisions to engage in the latter. This works to the detriment of vulnerable populations, because the patient who asks to be allowed to die by removal from a ventilator is at least as likely as a patient who requests a prescription for lethal drugs to be making the request because of undue influence, financial pressure, clinical depression, or inadequately treated pain.

By implication, the Law Professors' Brief would oppose my position favoring simple decriminalization of physician-assisted suicide. Although they would seem to agree that placing on a par prescribing lethal doses of medication and ordering life-sustaining treatment stopped is philosophically consistent and ethically necessary, they would seem to disagree with decriminalization. The brief urges that both uses of medical authority should be subjected to the *heightened regulatory oversight* commonly envisioned for prescribing lethal medication (perhaps along the lines of those outlined in Proposition 16).

Is legalization superior to decriminalization? I don't think so. Ratcheting up the scrutiny of all decisions to withhold or withdraw life-sustaining treatment to the level outlined in Oregon's lethal prescription law is manifestly unworkable. Heightening regulatory oversight for decisions to withdraw life-sustaining treatment is possible, but not for decisions to withhold life-sustaining treatment. How could a regulatory system require prospective evaluation of decisions not to start life-sustaining treatments without permitting infliction of treatment while the decision to refuse/not institute treatment was reviewed (and appealed if it went against the patient)?

On the other hand, if it is infeasible and undesirable to demand prospective evaluation of decisions not to institute life-sustaining treatment, it should be objectionable ethically to demand extensive review of decisions to stop treatment. The decisions are symmetrical as far as patient self-determination is concerned (requiring informed consent to treat presupposes a right to informed refusal). Too, if review of decisions not to institute treatment escape the level of scrutiny imposed on decisions to stop, there would be a tendency to push more decisions into the "don't start" category—to the potential harm of patients. Therefore, either simple decriminalization beats legalization/regulation, or legalization/regulation should be offered as an "optional and nonexclusive" means for securing "good faith" immunity—as current living will statutes commonly provide.

Notes

I am grateful to the following people for comments that improved this essay: Rosamond Rhodes, Al Mele, Haavi Morreim, Norman Cantor, Dan Dugan, B. James Kellenberger, Irwin Goldstein, Ann-Dudley Goldblatt and Tom Hill.

1. *Cruzan v. Director, Missouri Department of Health*, 497 U.S. 261.
2. Cited in the National Center for State Courts, *Guidelines for State Court Decision Making in Authorizing or Withholding Life-Sustaining Medical Treatment* (St. Paul, MN: West Publishing Company, 1991), p. 13.
3. For example, Norman Cantor has argued, "The physician has unavoidably become a manager of the dying process . . . the approaches already available to the physician (in response to a stricken patient's request) include the removal of life-support, administration of risky analgesics, and deferral to a patient's determination to resist feeding." See "Two Opinions in Search of a Justice: The Constitution and Physician-Assisted Suicide," *Rutgers Law Journal*, 28, pp. 435, 440.
4. Norman Cantor, "The Permanently Unconscious Patient, Non-Feeding and Euthanasia," *American Journal of Law and Medicine* 15 (1989): 381–437, at 433.
5. Statutes recognizing the validity of advance directives typically provide that a patient's death resulting from the withholding or withdrawing of treatment pursuant to his or her living will does not constitute suicide. For example, North Carolina's law specifies, "The withholding or discontinuance of such extraordinary means or artificial nutrition or hydration shall not be considered the cause of death for any civil or criminal purpose." (Sec 90–322 ART. 23 at 461). Washington's law states, "that acts in accordance with a directive are not deemed suicide . . ." (1989 URTIA sec. 11(a), 9B U.L.A. 96, 113 (Supp. 1992).
6. The elements of suicide are two: (1) self-initiated action performed with (2) the specific intent to end one's life thereby. Courts avoided interpreting refusals of life-sustaining treatment as challenges to the State interest in preventing suicide by failing to find one or both elements. Thus refusals of treatment merely *allowed* an underlying disease to *cause* death and besides, the patient did *not necessarily* have the specific intent to die as a result of refusing treatment. This gambit is besides the point. The prior question concerns what the legal presumption is or should be. For example, the law ordinarily assumes that a person intends the natural and foreseeable consequences of what he does (intentionally). This assumption is rebuttable, but ordinarily it must be rebutted. For example, to say, as the court did in *Conroy* (486 A. 2d at 1224) "People who refuse life-sustaining medical treatment *may not* harbor a specific intent to die . . ." invites the response, "Yes, but they *may!*" What are "the priors"? What sort of argument does it take to overcome them?
7. See *Superintendent of Belchertown State School* v. *Saikewicz* holding that a competent adult's refusal of treatment does not constitute suicide because "(1) in refusing treatment the patient may not have the specific intent to die, and (2) even if he did, to the extent that the cause of death was from natural causes the patient did not set in the death producing agent in motion with the intent of causing his own death." 373 Mass. 728, 370 N.E. 2d 417 (1977) at 426.
8. For example, in the state of Washington, physician-assisted suicide seems to be as common as it is in the Netherlands. See, Anthony L. Back, et al., "Physician-Assisted Suicide and Euthanasia in Washington State: Patient Requests and Physician Responses," *Journal of the American Medical Association* 275 (1996): 919. Other studies suggest that Washington state is not unique. See, for example, D. J. Doukas, et al, "Attitudes and Behaviors on Physician-Assisted Death: A Study of Michigan Oncologists," *Journal of Clinical Oncology* 13 (1995): 1055; R. S. Shapiro, et al., "Willingness to Perform Euthanasia: A Survey of Physician Attitudes," *Archives of Internal Medicine* 154 (1994): 575; S. H. Miles, "Physicians and their Patient's Suicides," *Journal of the American Medical Association* 271 (1994): 1786.
9. The "line" seems to have been drawn in the *Quinlan* case. (See, *In re* Quinlan, 355 A.

2d at 670). However, only five years earlier, the New Jersey Supreme Court held that a patient's refusal of a blood transfusion and life-saving surgery would implicate the State's interest in suicide. (See, *John F. Kennedy Memorial Hospital* v. *Heston*, 58 N.J. 576, 279 A. 2d 670 (1971). The line has been hammered by philosophers for years. For a recent, influential example, see Dan W. Brock, "Voluntary Active Euthanasia," *Hastings Center Report* 22 (2): 10–22 (1992).

10. *Cruzan v. Director, Missouri Department of Health*, Supreme Court of the United States, 1990. 497 U.S. 261, 110 S. Ct. 2841, 111 L. Ed. 2d 224.

11. *Cruzan v. Director, Missouri Department of Health*, 497 U.S. 261, 280 (1990).

12. See Alan Meisel, *The Right to Die*, 2d ed., vol. I (New York: John Wiley and Sons, 1995), p. 516.

13. To hold that an individual's liberty interest could *never* trump suggests that the State interest which it challenges is absolute. Strictly, nothing weighs against an interest which is absolute.

14. One should not underestimate the ability of judges to resist logical inferences. Even when a patient has said "he was suffering so much, he wanted to die," a New York court found that stopping treatment persuant to the patient's wishes did not constitute suicide. See, *In re* Lydia E. Hall Hosp., 455 N.Y. 2d at 709.

15. In *Bouvia v. Superior Court* (Glenchur), the court recongized that "a desire to terminate one's life is probably the ultimate exercise of one's right to privacy,. . ." but it flatly denied that physicians who cooperate with that desire assist suicide, because assisted suicide involves, "affirmative assertive, proximate, direct conduct suchy as furnishing a gun, poison, knife. . . . Such situations are far different than the mere presence of a doctor during the exercise of his patient's constitutional rights." (179 Cal. App. 3d 1227, 225 Cal. Rptr. 297). As I explain below, it's not the presence or absence of "affirmative conduct" that transforms physician-facilitated death into physician-assisted suicide, it's intent.

The "affirmative act" theory has been well refuted by Richard Epstein. "Disconnecting a respirator or removing a feeding tube is as much as 'act' as hooking up that same respirator or inserting a feeding tube. No one would regard disconnecting respirators or removing feeding tubes as the cessation of treatment, to be treated as a mere omission, if that act (what other word can we use) were performed by a stranger."

16. Richard A. Epstein, *Mortal Peril: Our Inalienable Right to Health Care?* (New York: Addison Wesley, 1997), p. 305.

17. Timothy E. Quill, M.D.; Samuel C. Klagsbrun, M.D.; and Howard A. Grossman, M.D. v. Dennis C. Vacco. *Quill* v. *Vacco*, 80f. 3rd. 716 (2nd Cir 1996).

18. The 2d Circuit claimed, "The ending of life by these means [withdrawal of life-support] is nothing more nor less than assisted sucide." This is a mistake, as I shall argue below. However, if one adopts the standard legal fiction that a person intends the reasonably foreseeable consequences of what he does or omits, then inferring the intent necessary for "assisting" is valid.

19. 4 Blackstone 189.

20. Richard Brandt has defined suicide "as doing something which results in one's death, either from the intention of ending one's life or the intention to bring about some other state of affairs (such as relief from pain) which one thinks it certain or highly probable can be achieved only by means of death or will produce death." "The Rationality of Suicide," in *Suicide: The Philosophical Issues*, M. Battin and D. Mayo eds., (1980) 117–18. I don't use Brandt's definition because it cannot accommodate a situation where one fully expects to die as a result of one's pain-relief plan, but hopes one won't. I think this is psychologically possible. This matters because hoping that an expected result won't occur, rules out intending to die as part of one's plan.

Too, Brandt's definition seems vulnerable to wayward-causation counter-examples. Suppose one were to think it certain or highly probable that uttering an special incantation will produce one's death. One utters the incantation with the intent of ending one's life. One's attendant emotional state causes a strong catacholamine reaction leading one's coronary arteries to spasm, which triggers an arythmia causing a fatal myocardial infarction. It seems counter-intuitive to label this death a suicide on these facts.

21. Justice Lynch, dissenting in *Brophy*, argued "Suicide is primarily an crime of commission, but can, and indeed must, also be conceived as an act of omission at times. If nutrition and hydration are terminated, it is not the illness which causes the death but the decision (and acts in accordance therewith) that the illness makes life not worth living. There is no rational distinction between suicide by deprivation of hydration or nutrition in or out of a medical setting—both are suicide." *Brophy v. New England Sinai Hospital, Inc.*, 398 Mass. 417, 497 N.E. 2d 626 (1986) at 446–47, 642–43.

22. I am indebted to Professor John Fisher for the "Golden Gate" example.

23. For example, Dan Brock argues, "The refusal of life-sustaining treatment is their means of ending life; they intend to end their life [sic] because of its [sic] grim prospects. Their death [sic] now when they otherwise would not have died *is* self-inflicted, whether they take a lethal poison or disconnect a respirator." "Death and Dying," in *Medical Ethics*, ed. Robert M. Veatch (Boston: Jones and Barlett Publishers, 1989), p. 345.

24. In a *Health* magazine survey, death was cited by only 28 percent of respondents to the question what they feared most about growing old. Most feared was "nursing home or long term illness." 56 percent feared "Alzheimer's," 47 percent feared "becoming a financial burden on children," 36 percent feared "loneliness," while 34 percent feared "losing their looks." Cited in *Contemporary Long Term Care*, January 1997, p. 16. Also see J. Kellenberger, *Relationship Morality* (University Park, PA: Penn State Press, 1995), pp. 144–45).

25. See Margaret Pabst Battin, "The Least Worst Death," *Hastings Center Report* 13(2): 13–16 (April 1983), also in her *The Least Worst Death* (Oxford: Oxford University Press, 1994).

26. George Smith, "All's Well That Ends Well: Toward a Policy of Assisted Rational Suicide or Merely Enlightened Self-Determination?" *University of California Davis Law Review* 22 (1989): 275–419, 279.

27. I Samuel 31:4.

28. The facts in *State v. McAfee*, 385 S.E. 2d 651 (Ga. 1989). Georgia's Supreme Court found no State interest strong enough to justify interfering with the patient's plan.

29. Professor Gregory Pence of the University of Alabama at Birmingham posted the facts of this case on the Bioethics Discussion Forum run by the Medical College of Wisconsin at Milwaukee on 4 February 1997.

30. Joel Peter Eigen, *Witnessing Insanity: Madness and Mad-Doctors in the English Court* (New Haven: Yale University Press, 1995), pp 47–48.

31. See N. Ann Davis, "The Right to Refuse Treatment" in T. L. Beauchamp, ed., *Intending Death: The Ethics of Assisted Suicide and Euthanasia* (Upper Saddle River, NJ: Prentice Hall, 1995), p. 118.

32. M. J. McGinnis and W. H. Foege, Actual Causes of Death in the United States, *Journal of the American Medical Association*, 270 (1993): 2207–12.

33. Alfred R. Mele, Paul K. Moser, "Intentional Action," *NOUS* 28 (1) (1994): 39–68.

34. "Poll shows that 1 in 5 internists has helped a patient die," in *American Medical News*, March 16, 1992, p. 9. David A. Asch, "The Role of Critical Care Nurses in Euthanasia and Assisted Suicide." *New England Journal of Medicine* (1996) 334: 1374–79.

35. 147 Cal. App. 3d 1032, 195 Cal. Rprt 484.

36. 79 F. 3d at 858 (Kleinfeld, J., dissenting).

37. Susan M. Wolf, "Physician-Assisted Suicide in the Context of Managed Care," *Duqesne Law Review* 35 (1996): 455.

38. See Joel Feinberg, *Harm to Others: The Moral Limits of the Criminal Law* (New York: Oxford University Press, 1984), 118–25.

39. Howard Brody, "Causing, Intending, and Assisting Death," *The Journal of Clinical Ethics* 4 (2) (Summer 1993): 112–17, 112.

40. Daniel Callahan, *The Troubled Dream of Life: Living with Mortality* (New York: Simon and Schuster, 1993), chapter 2.

41. Allen Buchanan, "Intending Death: The Structure of the Problem and Proposed Solutions." T. Beauchamp, ed., *Intending Death: The Ethics of Assisted Suicide and Euthanasia* (Upper Saddle River, NJ: Prentice Hall, 1995), pp. 23–41.

42. David Orentlicher, "The Legalization of Physician Assisted Suicide: A Very Modest Revolution," *Boston College Law Review* 28 (3) (May 1997): 444–75, 447–48.

43. Yale Kamisar, "Are Laws Against Assisted Suicide Unconstitutional?" *Hastings Center Report* 23 (3) (1993): 32–41, 34.

44. Baruch Brody, "Withdrawal of Treatment versus Killing of Patients." T. Beauchamp, ed., *Intending Death: The Ethics of Assisted Suicide and Euthanasia* (Upper Saddle River, NJ: Prentice Hall, 1995), pp. 90–108, 92.

45. *Queen's Bench Division*, 14 Q.B.D. 273 (1884).

46. See note 22, *supra*.

47. Timothy Quill, "Death and Dignity: A Case of Individualized Decision Making," *New England Journal of Medicine* 324 (1991): 691.

48. Contrary to uninformed reports, assisted-suicide remains a criminal offense in the Netherlands whose criminal code provides, "... a person who on the clearly expressed and serious request of another person takes that other person's life will be sentenced to a maximum of twelve years imprisonment ..."; and "... a person who deliberately incites another person to suicide or who helps or provides him/her with the means to do so, will, if suicide follows, be sentenced to a maximum of three years imprisonment ..." P. J. Van der Maas, et. al. "Euthanasia and Other Medical Decisions Concerning the End of Life." *Lancet* 338 (1991): 669–74.

49. For example, Washington criminal law provides, "A person is guilty of promoting a suicide when he knowingly causes or aids another person to attempt suicide. [A violation of the statute] constitutes a felony punishable by imprisonment for a maximum of five years and a fine of up to $10,000." RCW 9A.36.060 and RCW 9A.36.060(2) and 9A.20.oso (1) (c).

15

From Intention to Consent

Learning from Experience with Euthanasia

HELGA KUHSE

It is often assumed that a morally relevant and practically workable distinction can be drawn between cases of the intentional termination of life, on the one hand, and the provision of potentially life-shortening palliative care and the withdrawal and withholding of life-sustaining treatment, on the other. It is also often assumed that a restrictive public policy approach which prohibits voluntary euthanasia and medically assisted suicide, but allows other medical end-of-life decision, can be justified on the grounds that it is more protective of the rights or interests of patients than a liberal approach. In this article, I challenge some of these assumptions. While the issue of moral significance may ultimately be irresolvable, there appear to be good public policy reasons to support the decriminalization of voluntary euthanasia. Not only are restrictive public policies arbitrary and unjust; they are also unable to prevent doctors from intentionally terminating the lives of some of their patients. Comparative data from the Netherlands and Australia suggest that a liberal public policy approach which focuses on the patient's consent, rather than on the doctor's intention, is more protective of the rights and interests of patients than a restrictive approach.

*   *   *

O N 25 MAY 1995, the Legislative Assembly of the Northern Territory of Australia passed the *Northern Territory Rights of the Terminally Ill Bill 1995.*[1] With this, the Assembly became the first parliament in the world to legalize voluntary euthanasia and medically assisted suicide.[2] The legislation became operative in July 1996, and in the following nine months four terminally ill patients died under the provisions of the Act with the help of their doctor. The Act was annulled in March 1997, when federal parliamentarians passed the *Commonwealth Euthanasia Laws Bill 1996*. That Act effectively prohibits Australian territories from enacting legislation that permits "the form of intentional killing of another called euthanasia ... or the assisting of a person to terminate his or her life," but allows the making of laws regarding the withdrawal or withholding of life-sustaining treatment and the provision of palliative care to the dying, provided these do not sanction the intentional killing of the patient.

In this article, I shall not specifically focus on the *Northern Territory Rights of the Terminally Ill Act*, nor on the *Euthanasia Laws Act*. Rather, I want to challenge two widely held assumptions that underpin not only the *Euthanasia Laws Act*, but much of Anglo-American law as well. The first assumption is that a morally relevant and practically workable distinction can be drawn between cases of the intentional termination of life, on the one hand, and the provision of palliative care and the withdrawal and withholding of life-sustaining treatment, on the other. The second is that a restrictive public policy approach which prohibits voluntary euthanasia and medically assisted suicide can be justified on the grounds that it is more protective of patients than a liberal approach. This second assumption was a chief plank in an Australian Senate Committee's support for the *Euthanasia Laws Bill*. As the committee warns, in its majority report: "Laws relating to euthanasia are unwise and dangerous public policy. Such laws pose profound risks to many individuals who are ill and vulnerable."[3] Nor does the Australian Senate Committee stand alone in counselling against the legalization of voluntary euthanasia and medically assisted suicide on these grounds. Similar reasons have been put forward by many others as well—for example, by members of the House of Lords Select Committee on Medical Ethics,[4] and the New York State Task Force on Life and the Law.[5] As the House of Lords Committee put it in its report:

> Th[e] prohibition [of intentional killing] is the cornerstone of law and of social relationships. It protects each of us impartially, embodying the belief that all are equal. We do not wish that protection to be diminished. . . .[6]

In line with contemporary debates, much of my article will focus on competent and terminally ill patients, although I will, for the sake of brevity, generally write "patients" only. Some of my discussion may, of course, have implications for other groups of patients as well, but this is not my present concern. Again, for the sake of brevity, I shall, unless otherwise indicated, use the term "voluntary euthanasia" to refer to both medically assisted suicide and voluntary euthanasia. While some writers take the view that the two practices are morally distinct,[7] I do not share that view. Voluntary euthanasia and medically assisted suicide can be distinguished in terms of the *causal* roles performed by the doctor and the patient. In voluntary euthanasia, the doctor deliberately or intentionally ends the patient's life, at the patient's request; in assisted suicide, the patient deliberately or intentionally ends her life, with the purposeful assistance of her doctor. But no such distinction can be drawn in terms of the two agents' *moral* responsibility.[8] I also believe that it would be bad public policy to limit legislation to medically assisted suicide. Not all patients are capable of ending their own lives, and attempts at suicide may fail.[9] Within the above parameters, I shall argue that the present public policy approach—which permits the foregoing of treatment and the administration of potentially life-shortening palliative care,[10] whilst prohibiting voluntary euthanasia—ought to be rejected on the following grounds:

- Focus on the doctor's intention does not prevent doctors from intentionally terminating the lives of patients.
- A restrictive public policy approach does not protect all patients equally, but is inherently arbitrary and unjust.
- A restrictive public policy approach based on intention may be less protective of the rights and interests of patients than a liberal approach which—instead of focusing on the doctors' intention—focuses on the patient's consent.

Medical End-of-Life Decisions

For many patients, death is no longer the natural event it once was. Rather, it is very often the result of a deliberate medical end-of-life decision. According to a 1995 Dutch survey, 43 percent of all deaths in that country were preceded by a medical end-of-life decision, that is, by an action or omission undertaken by the doctor in the knowledge or belief that the patient would die earlier as a consequence of that decision than she would if that decision were not taken.[11] A 1996 Australian study found that 65 percent of all deaths were preceded by such decisions.[12] In some particular healthcare settings the incidence may be even higher. A 1994 United States study, focusing on patients nearing the end of their lives, for example, found that 84 percent of these patients had died after a decision had been taken to forego at least one type of life-sustaining treatment.[13]

Doctors who engage in medical end-of-life decisions are not necessarily acting contrary to the law. Rather, in many countries it is lawful for doctors to implement decisions that will have the effect of shortening the patient's life. With the patient's consent, doctors may withhold or withdraw life-sustaining treatment and a legal consensus is developing according to which doctors may administer life-shortening doses of pain and symptom control, in full knowledge of their "double effect."

In most countries doctors are, however, not permitted intentionally to terminate a patient's life. This means that the contemporary debate is not about doctors being/not being permitted to at least sometimes collaborate with their patients in actions or omissions that will foreseeably lead to death, but rather about the drawing of plausible distinctions between permissible and impermissible end-of-life decisions.[14]

This distinction between permissible and impermissible medical end-of-life decisions is often expressed in terms of the distinction between deliberately or intentionally ending a patient's life and merely allowing the patient to die. Medical decisions implemented with the intention of causing the patient's death are often described as "killings" or "euthanasia", and are deemed impermissible; cases of withholding or withdrawing treatment and of administering life-shortening palliative care are often described as cases of "allowing" to die, and are—at least sometimes—thought to be permissible.

But when does a doctor deliberately or intentionally end a patient's life, and when does she merely allow a patient to die? Consider the following four hypothetical examples:

- *Dr. Adams's* patient—Mr. Angels—is dying from a progressively debilitating disease. He is almost totally paralysed and needs a respirator to keep him alive. He is suffering considerable distress and wants to die. He asks his doctor to disconnect the respirator. Dr. Adams complies, and Mr. Angels dies three hours later, from respiratory failure.
- *Dr. Bernard's* patient—Mr. Brown—is dying from the same disease as Mr. Angels, needs a respirator to keep him alive and wants to die. He asks Dr.

Bernard to give him a lethal injection and Dr. Bernard complies by administering potassium chloride. Mr. Brown dies a few minutes later.

- *Dr. Clemens's* patient—Mr. Charles—is suffering from cancer of the throat, which threatens to choke him. In great pain and distress, he asks Dr. Clemens to end his life. She explains that this is not possible, but that she will steadily increase the amount of pain and symptom control. In a day or two, she says, the doses will be such that Mr. Charles will die as a consequence of her efforts to relieve his distress. Dr. Clemens starts the infusion and eighteen hours later Mr. Charles dies.
- *Dr. Daisy's* patient—Mr. David—is in virtually the same situation as Mr. Charles. When asked to end his life, Dr. Daisy complies by injecting a lethal dose of potassium chloride, and Mr. David dies within minutes.

It is commonly assumed that Drs. Adams and Clemens acted lawfully, but that Drs. Bernard and Daisy performed unlawful acts. But is it possible to draw morally relevant distinctions between these actions?

Dr. Adams, it might be said, "allowed" her patient to die. Her patient died from an underlying disease, respiratory failure, and not from the effects of a lethal injection in the way Dr. Bernard's patient did. In this sense, it might be said that the two cases are distinguishable—that Mr. Angel's disease, not Dr. Adams, caused the patient's death, but that, in Mr. Brown's case, Dr. Bernard's action was the cause of death. But even if one accepts this not uncontroversial view of causation, this does not settle the question of moral responsibility. To the extent that Dr. Adams foresaw that her patient would die as a consequence of what she did—turn off the respirator—it would be odd to say that she is somewhat less morally responsible for the consequences of her action (the patient's death) than is Dr. Bernard.[15]

Matters become even more complex when we turn to the next pair of cases. Dr. Clemens clearly seems to have caused her patient's death in a way seemingly similar to the way Dr. Daisy caused her patient's death. Both doctors administered drugs that they thought would hasten their patient's death. It is true, Dr. Daisy used potassium chloride, whereas Dr. Clemens administered drugs commonly used in pain and symptom control, but this difference in the type of drugs used can hardly allow us to distinguish, in causal or in moral terms, between the two cases. Nor can it make a moral difference that one drug acted quickly, and the other more slowly. (To see why this must be so consider the case of a would-be inheritor who uses large doses of a slow-acting therapeutic drug to end her rich uncle's life. It would be odd to say that she is, either causally or morally, less responsible for her uncle's death than she would be were she to use a fast-acting non-therapeutic drug.)

The issue of drawing a valid distinction between currently permissible and impermissible end-of-life decisions was raised in the United States Ninth Circuit Court of Appeals decision *Compassion in Dying* v. *State of Washington*.[16] For the state to justifiably uphold the prohibition of medically assisted suicide, it would be necessary, Judge Reinhardt wrote in the 8:3 majority opinion, to point to a relevant difference between voluntary euthanasia and "conduct ... the state has explicitly recognized."

Here it would not do, he argued, to point to the distinction between actions and omissions. In many cases of foregoing treatment, doctors unquestioningly perform actions that lead to the foreseen deaths of their patients. Nor would it help to bring in the notion of causation. A doctor who ceases treatment causes death—often with the same certainty as she would were she to administer a lethal injection. While some would say that it is the disease that causes death, this is not, he continued, the case when the doctor administers life-shortening palliative care. In that case the doctor, not the disease, causes death.

In all these cases, Reinhardt concluded, "there can be no doubt that ... the doctor intends that, as the result of his action, the patient will die...." Justice Reinhardt's conclusion that the distinctions between actions and omissions, and between causing and not causing death, cannot be used to distinguish between medical end-of-life decisions widely held to be permissible and those that are not is convincing and fairly uncontroversial. More sophisticated defenders of the so-called "sanctity of life" view have long recognized that these distinctions are not central.[17] Rather, on this view, it is the agent's intention that makes an action permissible or impermissible—not the mere fact that a given event, such as death, is the outcome of the agent performing/not performing a bodily movement that in some objective sense causes death. As the Roman Catholic Church's *Declaration on Euthanasia* puts it, euthanasia, or mercy killing, is "an act or an omission which of itself or by intention causes death."[18] Provided an agent does not intend death, she may, other things being equal, administer life-shortening palliative care and withhold or withdraw burdensome treatment, knowing or expecting that the patient will die as a consequence of what she does.[19]

While the sanctity-of-life view has its source in the Judaeo-Christian tradition, it is now enshrined in professional codes of conduct, in public policies and the law. This means that Justice Reinhardt's conclusions that there "can be no doubt" that the withholding of treatment and the administration of life-shortening palliative care are cases of the intentional termination of life is highly controversial. On his view, not only Drs. Bernard and Daisy, but also Drs. Adams and Clemens would intentionally have shortened their patients' lives. This conclusion is at odds with traditional morality and with contemporary mainstream interpretations of the law. On these views only Drs. Bernard and Daisy would be presumed to have terminated their patients' lives intentionally; Drs. Adams and Clemens, on the other hand, would be presumed to have practiced good and lawful medicine. In asserting that doctors who discontinue life-sustaining treatment and/or administer potentially life-shortening palliative care are intending the patient's death, Judge Reinhardt has thus challenged a whole body of traditional ethical thinking and the very coherence of existing laws.[20]

Should we accept Reinhardt's rejection of the intention/foresight distinction, and of the Principle of Double Effect? The Principle of Double Effect has been much debated in the philosophical literature. Some see the distinction between intention and foresight as having profound moral significance, while others regarding it as a hypocritical device that allows particularly those who subscribe to absolute rules to avoid some of the starkly counter-intuitive consequences of a strict adherence to those rules. After seemingly endless debates, no consensus is in sight and none seems likely. The reason is that questions relating to moral significance cannot be answered other than from within particular moral perspectives. Different moral perspectives, or value systems, will give rise to different answers—and these answers cannot be shown to be true or false, in the ordinary sense of those terms.[21]

While the question of the intrinsic moral significance of the intention/foresight distinction may thus ultimately be unanswerable, this does not mean that public policy questions are equally intractable. Rather, there appear to be good extrinsic reasons why the distinction should be rejected in public policies and laws that regulate medical end-of-life decisions.

Discrimination

One reason is that—contrary to what the House of Lords Select Committee on Medical Ethics alleged—the continued prohibition of the intentional termination of life in the practice of medicine does not seem to "protect[-] each of us impartially," and does not "embody the belief that all are equal." The legal presumption that a doctor who, following her patient's request, withholds or withdraws life-sustaining treatment does not intentionally terminate the patient's life, whereas a doctor who, at the patient's request, administers a lethal drug does intentionally end life, leads to unequal and discriminatory treatment of terminally ill patients. Existing laws allow one group of dying patients—those who are fortunate enough to require life-support—to bring about their own deaths, with the help of their doctors. Another group of patients—those who are in the unfortunate position of not requiring life-support—are denied that opportunity. Thus, rather than protect "each of us impartially," existing laws show partiality towards one group of dying patients, while disregarding the equal interests or rights of another.

This issue was raised in the case of *Timothy E. Quill et al. v. State of New York*, when one of the plaintiffs, Timothy Quill, argued:

> The removal of a life-support system that ... results in the patient's death requires the direct involvement by the doctor. ... When such patients are mentally competent, they are consciously choosing death as preferable to life under the circumstances that they are forced to live. ... Unfortunately, some dying patients who are in agony that can no longer be relieved, yet are not dependent on life-sustaining treatment, have no such options under current legal restrictions. It seems unfair, discriminatory and arbitrary, and inhumane to deprive some dying patients of such vital choices because of arbitrary elements of their condition which determines whether they are on life sustaining treatment that can be stopped.[22]

While the Appeals Court concurred and struck down the prohibition on medically assisted suicide, this ruling was not subsequently upheld by the United States Supreme Court.[23] In rejecting a constitutional right to medically assisted suicide, the court seemed to uphold the distinction between the withdrawal of life-sustaining treatment, on the one hand, and voluntary euthanasia or the intentional termination of life, on the other. Could this distinction and the discrimination to which it gives rise be justified on the grounds that the legalization of voluntary euthanasia would, as the Australian Senate Committee held, "pose profound risks to individuals who are ill and vulnerable"?

Before addressing that question, it is necessary to look at an argument that seeks to by-pass the issue of voluntary euthanasia. At the heart of the argument is the claim that there is no need for voluntary euthanasia because contemporary palliative care can give all patients a dignified and painfree death.

Terminal Sedation

There is little doubt that modern palliative care can help many patients, but it can, unfortunately, not help all of them. At the end-of-life, some 15–50 percent of patients referred for palliative care may experience intolerable pain, delirium, shortness of breath, nausea, and persistent vomiting that is refractory to the usual therapies.[24]

Seemingly, even refractory pain and other intolerable symptoms can be relieved, but there can be little doubt that the method—terminal sedation—involves doctors in the intentional termination of life, or in what has been termed "slow euthanasia."[25] As one Australian palliative care specialist describes terminal sedation:

> The patient enters a kind of "pharmacological oblivion," and appears at peace—it is usually assumed that in that state there is freedom from pain and distress. The patient cannot eat and drink, has a dampened cough reflex, develops retained airway secretions which "rattle" and become infected, all of which hasten death.[26]

In most cases, the patient's life will be shortened by only a few hours or days, but in some cases it may be shortened by several weeks.[27] Even if one were to accept the truth of the Principle of Double Effect, it would be difficult to deny that terminal sedation involves the intentional termination of life. As David Orentlicher puts it:

> In many cases, terminal sedation amounts to euthanasia because the sedated patient often dies from the combination of two intentional acts by the physician—the induction of stupor or unconsciousness and the withholding of food and water.... It is the physician-created state of diminished consciousness that renders the patient unable to eat, not the patient's underlying disease.[28]

When the Northern Territory *Rights of the Terminally Ill Act* was invalidated by the passage of the *Euthanasia Laws Act,* one patient, Esther Wild, had fulfilled all the requirements under the Act, but her doctor, Philip Nitschke, was no longer able to end her life by way of a quick-acting lethal drug. Instead, he administered terminal sedation, and after four days of drug-induced unconsciousness, Esther Wild died.

At the time of writing, Philip Nitschke is under coronial investigation. The question is: Did he, or did he not, intend Ester Wild's death? According to Nitschke himself, he did nothing wrong. His main intent, he says, was to ease his patient's terrible pain and suffering. He merely did what many other palliative care specialists do routinely: ease the passing of a suffering dying patient.[29]

What made the case of Esther Wild special is that Nitschke is an outspoken advocate of the legalization of voluntary euthanasia. It was perhaps because of this that many people assumed that Nitschke had intentionally shortened his patient's life. Most Australian palliative care specialists, on the other hand, are adamantly opposed to voluntary euthanasia and it is perhaps because of this that their practice fails to attract the attention of the criminal law. The assumption is that in distinction from Philip Nitschke they practise lawful medicine.

Intentions

But how can we be sure what Dr. Nitschke's intentions were, or what other doctors intend when they implement palliative care or non-treatment decisions, knowing or foreseeing that their patients will die as a consequence of what they do? The answer is frequently far from clear. Under the Principle of Double Effect, an outwardly identical action or omission, such as administering life-shortening palliative care, can be a case of either euthanasia, or of pain-relief depending on what it is that the agent intends to bring about as a consequence of her action or omission. Since intentions are internal mental states, this means that ultimately only the agent herself will be able to say what she intended to do when she did what she did.

The legal presumption is that doctors administering palliative care to dying patients, and those who withhold or withdraw life-sustaining treatment from the terminally ill, are not intentionally terminating these patients' lives. But what do doctors actually intend to do when they engage in medical end-of-life decisions? Do they merely intend to relieve pain and suffering, and to withhold or withdraw burdensome treatment, or are they acting with the direct intention of shortening the patient's life?

A recent nationwide Australian study—conducted in 1996 before the *Northern Territory Rights of the Terminally Ill Act* became operative—will give some answers.[30] The survey used an English translation of the questionnaire used in the 1995 Dutch study into voluntary euthanasia and other medical end-of-life decisions.[31] The questionnaire was sent to a random sample of 3,000 medical practitioners (working in disciplines where there was an opportunity to make medical end-of-life decisions) from all Australian States and Territories. The response rate to the anonymous questionnaire was 64 percent.

To determine the incidence and proportion of different end-of-life decisions, respondents were asked the following questions with regard to the most recent non-acute death attended by them:

3. Concerning this death, did you or a colleague take one or more of the following actions or omissions (or ensure that one was taken), taking into account the probability or certainty that this action or omission would hasten the end of the patient's life?
   a. withholding a treatment?
   b. withdrawing a treatment
   c. intensifying the alleviation of pain and/or symptoms using morphine or a comparable drug?
4. Was hastening the end-of-life partly the intention of the action indicated in 3 c.?
5. Was death caused by one or more of the following actions or omissions which you or a colleague decided to take *with the explicit intention* of not prolonging life or hastening the end-of-life?
   a. withholding a treatment?
   b. withdrawing a treatment?
6. Was death caused by the use of a drug prescribed, supplied or administered by you or a colleague with the explicit intention of hastening the end-of-life (or of enabling the patient to end his or her own life? This may mean one or more drugs. Morphine is also sometimes used for this purpose.)

The following are the results:

End-of-life decision		*Percent of Australian deaths*
The administration or prescription of a drug, administered or prescribed with the explicit intention of hastening the end-of-life:		5.3%
Withholding or withdrawing treatment, taking into account the probability or certainty that this action or omission would hasten the end of the patient's life:		28.6%
No intention to hasten death:	3.9%	
Explicit intention to hasten death:	24.7%	
Alleviation of pain and symptoms in doses large enough that there would be a probability or certainty that this would hasten the patient's death:		30.9%
No intention to hasten death:	24.4%	
Decision partly intended to hasten death:	6.5%	
		Total:
		64.8%

This means that 30 percent of all Australian deaths were preceded by a decision explicitly intended to hasten death or not to prolong life. Doctors prescribed, supplied, or administered drugs (which may have included morphine) with the explicit intention of ending life in 5.3 percent of all deaths, and withdrew or withheld life-prolonging treatment with the explicit intention of not prolonging life or of hastening death in 24.7 percent of all deaths. In addition to that, 6.5 percent of all deaths were preceded by a palliative care decision that was partly intended to hasten death. The study also shows that many more deaths (24.7 percent) were intentionally brought about by non-treatment decisions than by the administration or prescription of drugs (5.3 percent). If we understand "euthanasia" as "an action or an omission which of itself or by intention causes death," 30 percent of all Australian deaths (or 37,000 cases) would be cases of euthanasia.[32]

The results indicate that existing laws which prohibit the intentional termination of life are not being observed by Australian doctors. While such laws may prevent some doctors from using fast-acting, non-therapeutic drugs to end the life of a dying patient, they do not, and cannot, prevent doctors from intentionally ending their patients' lives by some other means. The reason lies in the mainstream legal assumption that doctors do not intend all the foreseen "natural" consequences of their actions or omissions. Rather, like the Principle of Double Effect, existing laws rely, at least in part, on a subjective notion of intention. If the notion of intention were understood in a wide "objective" sense, then the death resulting from each and every deliberate medical end-of-life decision, to the extent that the death is not accidental or unintended, would be taken to be the intended consequence. Since this is not the mainstream view, it entails that current regulatory frameworks and laws are at least to some extent based on a subjective notion of intention.

This makes for the extreme malleability and "constructability" of medical end-of-life decisions and with this, for the unworkability of existing laws.[33] Such laws can neither prevent doctors from intending what it is impermissible to intend—their patient's death—nor effectively prevent them from implementing those intentions. A doctor who does not, for whatever reason, wish to practise euthanasia in the way Drs. Bernard and Daisy did, will often have the opportunity to intentionally end her patient's life in the way Drs. Adams and Clemens did.

In addition to treating dying people arbitrarily and unfairly, the existing legal focus on the doctor's intention, and the assumption that a doctor who administers a fast-acting, non-therapeutic drug practises "euthanasia," whereas a doctor who withholds or withdraws life-sustaining treatment and administers life-shortening palliative care does not, thus offers neither transparency nor regulatory protection. It does not encourage honesty and openness in the doctor/patient relationship nor does it, as will be shown below, encourage consent.[34]

Consent

A central reason for the Senate Committee's support for the *Euthanasia Laws Bill* was that, in the Committee's view, the legalization of voluntary euthanasia "poses profound risks to many individuals who are ill and vulnerable." This danger is often perceived in terms of a so-called "slippery slope" that leads from voluntary euthanasia to non-voluntary euthanasia. In arguing against the acceptance of voluntary euthanasia in Australia, the Cambridge academic J. Keown thus pointed to evidence from the Netherlands which, he asserted, demonstrates that that country is on a slippery slope: "... since [voluntary] euthanasia became widely tolerated in the Netherlands, thousands of patients have had their lives intentionally shortened without an explicit request."[35]

Since the early 1980s Dutch doctors have been able to openly practice voluntary euthanasia. While voluntary euthanasia remains subject to criminal law, doctors will not be prosecuted if they comply with certain guidelines developed by the Courts and, more recently, by Parliament.[36]

Has the open practice of voluntary euthanasia in the Netherlands led to abuse? A central aim of the Australian survey into medical end-of-life decisions was to estimate the incidence of various end-of-life decisions in Australia and to compare these data with those derived from the 1995 Dutch study. A comparison of these sets of data—one from a country where voluntary euthanasia cannot be practiced openly (Australia) and the other from a country where it can (the Netherlands)—should provide some answers. Australia and the Netherlands have similar population sizes (18 million and 15.3 million, respectively) and comparable annual death rates (7.1 and 8.7 per thousand, respectively). In the Netherlands in 1995 there were 135,546 deaths, while in Australia there were 125,771 deaths from July 1994 to June 1995.

As already noted, one of the main findings of the Australian study was that 30 percent of all Australian deaths were preceded by a medical decision explicitly intended to hasten the patient's death. The Australian study also showed that Australia had a significantly higher rate of intentional ending of life without the patient's consent than the Netherlands, both through the administration of drugs and by withholding or withdrawing treatment. While the difference in the rates of the administration or the prescription of drugs with the explicit intention of hastening the end-of-life *with the patient's consent* was not significant (1.8 percent of all deaths in Australia; 2.6 percent in the Netherlands), the rates of intentionally ending life by the administration of drugs *without an explicit request from the patient* were significantly higher in Australia (3.5 percent) than the Netherlands (0.7 percent). In addition to that, in 22.5 percent of all Australian deaths doctors withheld or withdrew treatment from patients without the patient's explicit request with the explicit intention of ending life. No comparable 1995 Dutch figure is available, but a comparable earlier Dutch survey found the figure to be 5.3 percent,[37] and the 1995 figure for *all* decisions to forego treatment with the explicit intention of hastening death or not prolonging life in the Netherlands was 13.3 percent.

Cultural differences between Australia and the Netherlands and possible differences in the sampling methods could have accounted for some of the differing responses to the Australian and Dutch questionnaires. Nonetheless, the Australian study undermines suggestions that the rate at which doctors intentionally end patients' lives without an explicit request is higher in a country where voluntary euthanasia is practised openly (the Netherlands) than in a comparable country which prohibits the practice (Australia).

Conclusion

Although Australian law recognises a right to refuse treatment, and condones the administration of life-shortening palliative care, it prohibits the intentional termination of life by an action or an omission.[38] The Australian study demonstrates that large numbers of Australian doctors are intentionally ending the lives of patients: 30 percent of all Australian deaths were preceded by an action or an omission explicitly intended to end the patient's life. It also demonstrates that doctors are frequently doing so without the patient's consent. In only 4 percent of all deaths was the decision taken in response to an explicit request from the patient, and far more Australian doctors intentionally hastened death by foregoing treatment than by prescribing, supplying, or administering drugs with the explicit intention of ending life. Finally, considerably more Australian than Dutch doctors are intentionally ending their patients' lives without the patients' consent.

These findings raise the question of why more Australian than Dutch doctors chose intentionally to end the lives of some of their patients without the patient's consent, especially in situations where the patient was competent and could be consulted. While this issue must remain the subject of further empirical research, it may well be that since existing laws prohibit the intentional termination of life, doctors are reluctant to discuss medical end-of-life decisions with their patients lest these be construed as collaboration in the intentional termination of life. The point is this: If a patient indicates to the doctor that she wishes to die and the doctor subsequently implements an end-of-life decision, it might be argued that the doctor, regardless of the means used, has intentionally ended the patient's life. If the subject is not raised, if consent is not sought, it will be much easier to describe a medical end-of-life decision as merely constituting "good medical practice."

To sum up, then: There seems to be good evidence to suggest that laws prohibiting the intentional termination of life, but permitting the withholding or withdrawing of treatment and the administration of life-shortening palliative care, do not prevent doctors from intentionally ending the lives of some of their patients. There are also good reasons to believe that such laws are discriminatory and unjust, that they encourage hypocrisy and unconsented-to termination of patients' lives.

For the purposes of public policies and laws governing end-of-life decisions for competent patients, we should stop asking whether a doctor "intends" death or merely "allows" it to occur, whether death comes about as the result of an action or an omission, or as the result of doctors administering a slow-acting therapeutic or a quick-acting non-therapeutic drug. While some of these distinctions may have moral relevance in the context of some religious or moral views, they are not a proper basis for public policies regulating medical end-of-life decisions. What is needed is a single regulatory framework for all medical end-of-life decisions for competent patients, a framework that does not rely on the largely unworkable notion of intention, but on the substantive notion of respect for the patient's autonomy, which finds expression in the procedural requirement of consent. Under such a framework, patients and doctors would be free to jointly decide on a mode of dying that best meets the needs of the patient. For many patients this would involve foregoing life-sustaining treatment, and accepting palliative care. But for some patients this would also involve voluntary euthanasia or medically assisted suicide through the administration or prescription of a non-therapeutic drug.

The Australian Senate Committee was wrong to support the invalidation of the Northern Territory *Rights of the Terminally Ill Act*. In their so doing they lent support to replacing a workable public policy instrument based on the patient's consent with unworkable laws based on the doctor's intentions.

Notes

1. This paper draws on chapter 8 of Helga Kuhse, *Caring Nurses, Women and Ethics* (Oxford and Boston: Blackwell, 1997); on Helga Kuhse, Peter Baume, Malcolm Clark, and Maurice Rickard: "End-of-Life Decisions in Australian Medical Practice," *Medical Journal of Australia* 166 (17 February 1997): 191–96; and on Helga Kuhse: 'No' To the Intention/Foresight Distinction in Medical End-Of-Life Decisions," *Medicine and Law* 16 (1997): 199–200.
2. While doctors in the Netherlands have, for a number of years, been able to practice voluntary euthanasia and medically assisted suicide under guidelines laid down by the courts and written into the Burial Act by parliament in 1993, direct help in dying remains a crime under Dutch statute law. Legislation permitting medically-assisted suicide had been passed in the U.S. State of Oregon by way of a citizen initiated referendum in 1994, but its implementation was held in abeyance due to challenges to its contitutionality. In June 1997, the Oregon Senate decided to put the matter once again before the voters. On November 4, 1997, the proposal was passed with an increased majority but, at the time of writing, is still awaiting implementation.
3. Senate Legal and Constitutional Legislation Committee: *Consideraton of Legislation Referred to the Committee—Euthanasia Laws Bill 1996* (Canberra: The Parliament of the Commonwealth of Australia, March 1997) p. 123.
4. House of Lords, *Report of the Select Committee on Medical Ethics*, vol. 1, *Report* (London: HMSO, 1994).
5. New York State Task Force on Life and the Law: *When Death is Sought: Assisted Suicide and Euthanasia in the Medical Context* (New York, 1994).
6. House of Lords, *Report of the Select Committee on Medical Ethics*, op. cit., p. 48.
7. See, for example, Sidney H. Wanzer et al., "The Physician's Responsibility Toward Hopelessly Ill Patients," *New England Journal of Medicine*, 310 (1991): 1304–1307.
8. See chapter 2 of Helga Kuhse, *The Sanctity-of-Life Doctrine in Medicine—A Critique* (Oxford: Clarendon Press, 1986).
9. See, for example, Gerrit K. Kimsma, "Euthanasia and Euthanizing Drugs in the Netherlands," in M. P. Battin and A. G. Lipman, eds., *Drug Use in Assisted Suicide and Euthanasia* (New York: Pharmaceutical Products Press. 1996), especially pp. 200 and 207.

10. Not all palliative care will shorten the patient's life. In some cases good palliative care may even prolong life. There is however, no doubt, that the administration of some forms of palliative care, such as terminal sedation (see Section IV), will often hasten the patient's death. In addition to that, many doctors will intensify pain and symptom control through the use of opioids to a level where, in the doctor's opinion, there is a probability or certainty of a hastened death (see Section V).

11. P. J. van der Maas, G. van der Wal, I. Haverkate, et al., "Euthanasia, Physician-Assisted Suicide, and Other Medical Practices Involving the End of Life in the Netherlands, 1990–1995," *New England Journal of Medicine* 335 (1996): 1699–1705 (in the following "the 1995 Dutch survey").

12. Helga Kuhse, Peter Singer, Peter Baume, et al., "End-of-life Decisions in Australian Medical Practice," *Medical Journal of Australia* 166 (17 February 1997): 191–96 (in the following "the Australian survey").

13. K. Faber-Langendoen, "Humane Care of the Dying Patient Project," *Newsletter—The Center for Biomedical Ethics*, University of Minnesota, Spring 1994, p. 1.

14. See, for example, Margaret Otlowski, *Voluntary Euthanasia and the Common Law* (Oxford: Clarendon Press, 1997).

15. Helga Kuhse, *The Sanctity-of-Life Doctrine in Medicine*, op. cit., chapter 2.

16. *Compassion in Dying versus State of Washington*, No. 94–3534, United States Court of Appeals, Ninth Circuit, March 6, 1996. WL94848 (9th Circ. [Wash]).

17. See chapter 3, Helga Kuhse, *The Sanctity-of-Life Doctrine in Medicine*, op. cit.

18. Sacred Congregation for the Doctrine of the Faith, *Declaration on Euthanasia* (Vatican City, 1980), p. 6.

19. Ibid., pp. 8–11.

20. See however, also the ruling in the British case of Tony Bland, *Airedale N.H.S. Trust v. Bland* (C.A.), 19 February 1993, 2 Weekly Law Reports, p. 350. The case is discussed by Peter Singer in chapter 4 of *Rethinking Life and Death* (Melbourne: Text Publishing, 1994).

21. See, for example, Alasdaire MacIntyre, "Why is the Search for the Foundation of Ethics so Frustrating?" *Hastings Center Report* 9 (1979): 16; H. T. Engelhardt, *The Foundations of Bioethics* (New York: Oxford University Press, 1986).

22. *Vacco v. Quill*, 80f. 3rd 716 (2nd Cir. 1996).

23. *Vacco v. Quill*, 117 S. Ct. 2293 (1997).

24. Roger Hunt, "Palliative Care—The Rhetoric-Reality Gap," in Helga Kuhse, ed., *Willing to Listen—Wanting to Die* (Melbourne and Auckland: Penguin Books Melbourne, 1994), pp. 115–37; N. I. Cherny, R. K. Portenoy, "Sedation in the Management of Refractory Symptoms: Guidelines for Evaluation and Treatment," *Journal of Palliative Care* 10 (2) (1994): 31–38; R. E. Enck, *The Medical Care of Terminally Ill Patients* (Baltimore: Johns Hopkins University Press, 1994), pp. 166–72. David Orentlicher, "The Supreme Court and Physician-Assisted Suicide—Rejecting Assisted Suicide but Embracing Euthanasia," *New England Journal of Medicine* 337 (17) (October 23, 1997).

25. See Roger Hunt, "Palliative Care," Ibid., p. 125; J. A. Billings, S. D. Block, "Slow Euthanasia," *Journal of Palliative Care* 12 (4) (1996) 21–30.

26. Roger Hunt, "Palliative care," ibid., p. 123.

27. David Orentlicher, "The Supreme Court and Physician-Assisted Suicide," op. cit.

28. Ibid.

29. Roy Eccleston, "Last Rights," *The Australian*, May 16, 1997.

30. Helga Kuhse, Peter Singer, Peter Baume, et al., "End-of-Life Decisions in Australian Medical Practice," op. cit.

31. P. J. van der Maas, G. van der Wal, I. Haverkate, et al.: "Euthanasia, Physician-Assisted Suicide, and Other Medical Practices Involving the End of Life in the Netherlands, 1990–1995," op. cit.

32. Sacred Congregation for the Doctrine of the Faith, *Declaration on Euthanasia*, op. cit., p. 6.

33. John Griffiths, "The Regulation of Euthanasia and Related Medical Procedures That Shorten Life in the Netherlands," *Medical Law International* 1 (1994): 137–58.
34. See Roger Hunt, "Palliative Care—The Rhetoric-Reality Gap," op. cit.
35. Senate Legal and Constitutional Legislation Committee, *Euthanasia Laws Bill 1996*, op. cit., p. 103.
36. G. van derWal, R.J.M. Dillmann: "Euthanasia in the Netherlands," *British Medical Journal*, 308 (1995): 1346–49.
37. P. J. van der Maas, J.J.M. van Delden, L. Pijnenborg, "Euthanasia and Other Decisions Concerning the End of Life," *Lancet* 338 (1991): 669–74.
38. *Crimes Act* 1900 (NSW) s. 19 (1)(a).

16

The Weakness of the Case for Legalizing Physician–Assisted Suicide

DON MARQUIS

The purpose of this essay is to consider with some care the argument from mercy and the argument from self-determination for legalizing physician-assisted suicide. Various versions of the argument from mercy are distinguished. Each version suffers from some weakness. Acceptance of the argument from self-determination opens the door to far more life-terminating behavior than often realized. Offering the choice of life-ending behavior to those in need of care is incompatible with treating them as having intrinsic worth.

*   *   *

THE CASE FOR LEGALIZING physician-assisted suicide (hereafter PAS) rests on two well-known arguments. The argument from mercy is based on the claim that the pain and suffering produced by terminal or debilitating illnesses are often so severe that life is a burden. Therefore, helping a patient with such suffering kill herself is an act of mercy. Acts of mercy should not be against the law.

The argument from self-determination rests on the generally accepted claim that, in a free society, individuals should be permitted as much freedom as possible, as long as they do not harm others. Therefore, patients should be free to seek assistance in ending their own lives, since such acts primarily affect themselves. Both the argument from mercy and the argument from self-determination seem compelling when considered alone. Therefore, the case for the legalization of physician-assisted suicide seems overwhelming.

In addition, many standard arguments against legalization seem quite weak. One argument is based on the claim that the wrongness of killing the innocent is a moral absolute. However, because the absolute form of this rule seems to have only a religious basis, we lack good reasons for accepting it. Another argument is based on the claim that killing is worse than letting die. However, because the wrongness of killing rests on the nature of the misfortune of premature death, and because both killing and letting die result in death, this supposed moral asymmetry seems quite implausible. Still another argument is based on the claim that there is a conflict between assisting a suicide and the professional ethic of physicians. However, professional codes are subject to change. In cases where medical assistance is requested for a merciful act, the claim that there *ought* to be a conflict between assisting a suicide and the professional ethic of physicians seems hard to defend. Still another argument is based on the claim that legalization of physician-assisted suicide will result in abuses. This claim is hard to establish. There are disagreements about what should count as an abuse. There are disagreements about how widespread abuse must be in order to count against legalization. There are real problems about gathering accurate data concerning this practice. This argument requires empirical research, not philosophical analysis, so I shall not consider it.

Therefore, appraisal of the issue of legalizing PAS involves taking the arguments for legalization head on. The purpose of this essay is to show that those arguments are far less compelling than they initially appear to be and that analysis of one of them yields at least one reason for not legalizing PAS.

The Argument from Mercy

The Intolerable Pain Version

There are many versions of the argument from mercy. The standard version of the argument is the intolerable pain version.[1] According to this version of the argument, legalization of physician-assisted suicide is necessary to spare terminally ill patients the painful agony of dying. This argument has been frequently attacked with the statement that the use of up to date techniques of pain management can alleviate severe pain in all but very rare cases.[2] Even Dan Brock, a well-known proponent of legalization, does not dispute this.[3]

Another difficulty with the intolerable pain version of the argument from mercy is that no one seems to hold the view that it is wrong to give patients whatever amount of morphine is necessary to relieve their pain even if death occurs sooner as a result.[4] Therefore, physician-assisted suicide is never necessary for the relief of intolerable pain.[5] Thus, if the case for physician-assisted suicide is to rest on the argument from mercy, a version of the argument different from the intolerable pain version must be adopted.

The Intolerable Physical Suffering Version

A proponent of the argument from mercy might substitute an intolerable physical suffering version. Thus, it has been argued that a significant number of dying patients experience untreatable severe physical suffering of kinds other than pain, such as severe nausea, severe air hunger, morphine-induced unpleasant hallucinations, and severe constipation. However, many specialists in palliative care will argue that these other very unpleasant complications of extensive disease also can be adequately treated in all but rare cases.[6]

[handwritten annotation: sometimes quite difficult to control]

The Realistic Version

The defender of physician-assisted suicide might respond by offering what could be called a realistic version of the argument from mercy. Pain, indeed, physical suffering, is often not treated well by physicians in this country. No doubt, a suffering dying patient is not comforted by the realization that her physical suffering *might* have been treated well by her physician when, in fact, it *is not* being treated well. In such cases the realist would argue that assisting in a suicide is an act of mercy.

Difficulties with this realistic version of the argument from mercy emerge when one asks how this version of the argument justifies a change in the law. The legalization of PAS and the use of better pain management techniques by physicians are both practices, albeit of different sorts. So a necessary condition of legalizing PAS would require showing that adopting the practice of physician-assisted suicide is better than adopting the practice of better pain management. One huge advantage of the latter practice over the former is that it leads to more life that can be a positive experience for the patient. Another is that it is not subject to the possibility of abuse. Therefore, the realistic version of the argument from mercy does not seem to support the legalization of PAS.

There is a practical difficulty with the realistic version of the argument from mercy. If the (generic) argument from mercy were used by a legislature to justify physician-assisted suicide, then it would not be unreasonable to require a palliative care specialist to certify that a patient's physical suffering cannot be relieved as a condition of any legal physician-assisted suicide. This would plainly vitiate the realistic version of the argument from mercy.

The Psychological Version

A psychological version of the argument from mercy deserves extensive, special consideration. It more accurately reflects the real reasons physician-assisted suicide is practiced.[7] Furthermore, it is not subject to the difficulties of the previous versions of the argument from mercy.

The psychological suffering of a seriously ill or debilitated patient can cause life to be a burden to her until she dies. This burden to a patient may continue even if her physical suffering can be relieved by medical means. The proponent of physician-assisted suicide might argue as follows: What makes a condition a misfortune for a patient when she is a candidate for physician-assisted suicide is that the condition involves suffering. The cause or the nature of the suffering is, strictly speaking, morally irrelevant. Accordingly, suffering that has psychological causes can be as great a misfortune as suffering that has physical causes. Therefore, it is no less merciful to relieve psychological suffering than to relieve suffering which is directly physical in origin.[8]

Opponents of physician-assisted suicide apparently disagree with this last point. Dan Callahan, Ezekiel Emanuel, and Herbert Hendin have all argued that if physician-assisted suicide is legalized, patients who experience hopelessness, or anxiety, or who are fearful of the loss of dignity, or who are depressed will ask for and obtain the assistance of their physicians in committing suicide.[9] They regard this claim as showing that PAS should not be legalized. Surely none of these writers are opposed to being merciful. Nevertheless, the kinds of patients alluded to above all are suffering psychologically. What could there be about these cases that might prevent the argument from mercy from succeeding?

Consider some differences between physical suffering that is so great that one wishes for death and psychological suffering that is so great that one wishes for death. On the one hand, we can all imagine physical pain that would cause us to suffer no matter what our attitude toward it. We can imagine pain so horrible that anyone would wish to be rid of it, even if death were necessary to do so. On the other hand, severe psychological suffering requires a judgment by the patient that death would be preferable to a life of the psychological quality the patient experiences. Indeed, the attitude that life of a given psychological quality is a life of suffering also requires a judgment by the patient. These are not judgments everyone would make. Thus, the causes of severe psychological suffering do not *inevitably* produce psychological suffering. By contrast, the causes of severe physical suffering do inevitably produce their result.

This difference in inevitability is important. On the one hand, one can *imagine* physical suffering so great that physician-assisted suicide would be necessary to relieve it. This yields an easy argument from mercy for the legalization of PAS. On the other hand, psychological suffering is such that physician-assisted suicide is not *necessary* to relieve it, A patient can avoid psychological suffering by rejecting the judgment necessary to produce it.

Another difference between psychological suffering and physical suffering is that psychological suffering often, and perhaps, always, has a social component. Consider some person who is disabled by illness. Her views of those life situations that are undignified or hopeless or an unreasonable burden to place on others are socially conditioned. Such views are socially influenced in two ways. In the first place, our views concerning those conditions of life to which death would be preferable are a result of our education in ways that are complex and poorly understood. In the second place, our judgments about those conditions of life are affected by our judgments concerning how others perceive us. Physical suffering does not have the same social component. Severe pain will cause any human being—or any mammal, for that matter—to suffer, whatever her socialization or the attitudes of others. Both of these social factors count against the inevitability of suffering, and therefore, undercut the argument that legalization of PAS is *necessary* in order to reduce suffering. Thus, the burden of defending the psychological version of the argument from mercy is thrown back on the defender of the legalization of PAS, for, apparently, she has to show that alternatives to the reduction of suffering through PAS are not feasible.

Presumably the defender of PAS would, at this point in the analysis, defend her view in something like the following way. Plainly, there are kinds of psychological suffering that can be relieved short of PAS. Suppose that a patient suffers from clinical depression that can be alleviated by drugs or psychotherapy. Suppose that a patient suffers from depression resulting from an error of factual judgment. For example, suppose he is more pessimistic about the consequences of treatment or what dying will involve than he should be for any of a number of reasons. These kinds of psychological suffering are treatable. There are alternatives available that are better than death from the patient's point of view. Therefore, PAS is not the most merciful course of action for that patient. Hence, in these cases, the argument from mercy fails.

However, not all psychological suffering is of this sort. Suppose that the life that the patient has to look forward to is a burden when viewed from the perspective of that patient's fundamental values. Suppose that this patient is not suffering from depression that can be treated by drugs or psychotherapy and has not made an error of factual judgment. Let us call this kind of psychological suffering, fundamental psychological suffering. The proponent of the legalization of PAS might ask: Why should our failure to legalize PAS condemn such a patient to suffer?

The opponent of legalizing PAS might respond that our failure to legalize PAS would not necessarily condemn patients with fundamental psychological suffering to a life of misery. In the first place, many such patients could commit suicide without assistance. In the second place, such patients are not condemned to suffer. It is possible for them to change their fundamental values.

Proponents of the legalization have a basis for objecting to this hard line. The essence of a free society is to respect the fundamental values of the individuals in it. Therefore, when a patient's psychological suffering is fundamental, considerations of both mercy and respect support legalization of PAS. This seems to be the only version of the argument from mercy that is not, so far, open to serious objection.

The Argument from Self-Determination

The Nature of the Argument from Self-Determination

Although a defensible version of the argument from mercy appears to involve essential appeal to the value of self-determination, the argument from self-determination can be set out independently of considerations of mercy. In an essay in the *New York Review of Books* that appeared before the June 1997 Supreme Court decisions, six well-known American philosophers, Ronald Dworkin, Thomas Nagel, Robert Nozick, John Rawls, Thomas Scanlon, and Judith Jarvis Thomson argue that there is a constitutional right to physician-assisted suicide on the grounds of "a very general moral and constitutional principle—that every competent person has the right to make momentous personal decisions which invoke fundamental religious or philosophical convictions about life's value for himself."[10] That is the *sole* ground on which their case was made. This should not be surprising. Any case for the Constitutional right of physician-assisted suicide must rest on Fourteenth Amendment liberty interests.

The Constitution is not required to make this case. In his book *Life's Dominion: An Argument about Abortion, Euthanasia and Individual Freedom*, Ronald Dworkin has defended the right to physician-assisted suicide solely on the basis of the right of self-determination.[11] Dan Brock, in his defense of PAS, regards the argument from self-determination as an independent argument for PAS. [12]

What would it be like to choose physician-assisted suicide under circumstances in which the suicide did not prevent one's suffering? Here are some cases: One might believe that a life in which one would be pleasantly senile is a life not worth living, even though that senility is not accompanied by suffering.[13] One might believe that a life in which one is severely physically disabled is a life not worth living. If one did, one might prefer to die rather than live that life even if that life involved neither physical or psychological suffering.[14]

The Wide Scope of Physician-Assisted Suicide

Discussions and news accounts of PAS give the impression that the right to PAS would be a right exercised by the dying. However, there are reasons for thinking that if PAS were legalized on the basis of the right of self-determination, its scope would be very broad. This can be seen by noting how the scope of the right to refuse life saving medical care has been extended in the medical ethics literature in the past twenty-five years.

Some people originally conceived of this right as the right of a competent patient, when dying, to refuse extraordinary medical care that might minimally prolong life. However, since the basis of this right is a right to reject any bodily intrusion, it cannot be limited to dying patients or to care that only minimally prolongs life or to care that is extraordinary. Furthermore, this right was correctly extended to the right to refuse medical care in advance of a situation in which a patient might no longer be competent to refuse care. Thus, advance directives are justified. The right was extended to the right of a patient to appoint someone else to refuse medical care on the patient's behalf when the patient was no longer competent to refuse. Thus, durable powers of attorney for healthcare are justified. The right was extended to the right of a family to make a decision to refuse medical care on a patient's behalf on the grounds that the family would best know a patient's fundamental values. Thus, surrogate decision-making was justified. There is now an extensive literature on the right to refuse medical care, and the arguments for all of these extensions are generally accepted.[15]

If the right to refuse extraordinary medical care offered to dying patients can be extended in this way, then, by parallel argument, surely the legal right of physician-assisted suicide could be extended in the same way. If the right of self-determination justifies the right to physician-assisted suicide, then it does not justify this right only for dying patients and it does not justify this right only for patients with a minimal time to live. It justifies PAS for any patient. Suppose that a competent person decides that she does not want to live once she becomes incompetent. If the right of self-determination justifies the right to refuse treatment by advance directive, then surely it also justifies the right to physician-assisted suicide by advance directive. (One imagines the deadly drug, prescribed by her personal physician, mixed in her applesauce at the nursing home). Because the right of self-determination justifies the appointment of someone with a durable power of attorney to refuse medical care, it could also justify the appointment of someone with a durable power of attorney to decide, on the basis of one's fundamental values, that one should take a deadly drug after one lacks decision-making capacity. Indeed, perhaps families, because they best know a patient's fundamental values, could decide when the suicide of their (now incompetent) loved one would take place.

We can look at this matter in a slightly different way, not in terms of the ways in which the right of self-determination would naturally be extended in the case of assisted suicide, but in terms of some of the cases that these extensions would cover. The right of self-determination includes the right of a competent adult to arrange in advance for PAS if he believes that spending his last years in a debilitated or dependent state in a nursing home would warp the contours of his life. The right of self-determination includes the right of a patient who discovers that he is experiencing the early onset of Alzheimer's disease to arrange for his physician-assisted suicide when his dementia has reached a point at which he *now* chooses not to live. It includes the right of families to arrange for the physician-assisted suicide of their loved ones who now lack decision making capacity and who, they believe, would not have wanted to live in the condition in which they are now living. To legalize physician-assisted suicide solely on the grounds of self-determination may be to legalize a different mode of exit from this life for a great many people.

Consider some objections to this argument that the scope of physician-assisted suicide would be far greater than usually supposed if it is legalized in a principled way. One might argue that just as extensions of the right to refuse medical care have not resulted in refusals that have greatly changed the contours of our lives, so the right to physician-assisted suicide would not greatly change those contours either. This argument is mistaken. The right to refuse medical care is the right to reject a medical treatment. The refusal does not kick in until the treatment is offered. The act of physician-assisted suicide based upon the right of self-determination kicks in whenever a future arrives that a competent adult decided he did not want for himself. Thus, legalization of physician-assisted suicide on the ground of self-determination alone involves far greater changes in life-ending behavior than the right to refuse medical care.

Proponents of physician-assisted suicide might also argue that the apparently overly broad extensions of this right of self-determination could be forestalled by legislation restricting the conditions under which physician-assisted suicide is legal. But what can justify such restrictions? Proponents of self-determination, let us recall, have spent almost two decades arguing that restricting the right to refuse medical care only to medical care not refused in advance, or only to extraordinary medical care, or only to medical care not yet provided, or only to medical care that was not also the provision of nutrition and hydration was a restriction on one's right of self-determination. These arguments are (a) sound and (b) generally accepted. They apply just as easily to the right to choose PAS as they did to the right to refuse unwanted medical care.

Finally, proponents of physician-assisted suicide might argue that no advance directive requesting physician-assisted suicide could be regarded as having force if, when the time came for one's physician to offer her patient the lethal dose, the patient says that he would rather go on living. I think that, *ceteris paribus,* this is correct, for contemporaneous decisions about the conditions of one's life rightly trump past decisions. Nevertheless, the *ceteris paribus* clause will frequently not apply. For example, it will not apply when my later self is demented. Surely decisions made by a competent adult trump decisions made by an incompetent one.

Accordingly, the legalization of physician-assisted suicide on the basis of the right of self-determination applies to a class of life-ending decisions far more extensive than the scenarios prominent in the public debate. This argument does not require the assumption that individuals are making choices that should be respected when they are clinically depressed or when they are misinformed. The choices the proponent of PAS is committed to respecting are rational choices made in accordance with an individual's fundamental values. Whether we wish to open the door to such radical changes in the courses of our lives is something that should be the subject of wide public debate.

Why the Right to PAS Is Harmful

There is an argument for the view that the legalization of physician-assisted suicide would be harmful.[16] If physician-assisted suicide were legalized, then people with disabilities, elderly people, and people with illnesses that typically result in death would have a legally provided-for choice of whether to stay alive or die. Many of the people in the classes I am considering are people in need of some kind of care. Would legalization be a good thing for people needing care?

In order to answer this question, we need to consider what the future holds for individuals who need care. On the one hand, such persons are often major consumers of social resources. They often require a great deal of medical care for which they do not pay. They frequently require custodial care. Their last six months of life will often require very expensive medical care. They often require more attention from their relatives than ordinary healthy individuals. They often require more economic resources from them also. On the other hand, often such persons are too sick or too disabled to hold a job. They cannot make as great a contribution to the lives of their communities as they would have if they were younger or healthier or more able-bodied. Often they make no tangible economic contribution to the community at all. Furthermore, when they are old or have a death-producing illness, their contribution will not increase. When they are disabled, often their contribution will not increase.

Finally, such people typically have diminished life prospects, either relative to other nondisabled individuals or relative to their prospects earlier in their lives. They often cannot get as much out of life. Would it be a good thing for people in this class, that is, individuals who need care, to have the legally sanctioned right to decide whether to live or die?

For individuals who do not need care, and who are not children, there is a lot to be said for classical liberalism, that is, for a society that provides people with as wide a range of freedoms as possible. It does not follow that so much freedom is a good thing for people who need care. If the consequences of having the choice of PAS are worse than the consequences of not having that choice from the point of view of individuals who need care, then having the choice of PAS is not a good thing for them. If that is so, then we have a good reason for not legalizing PAS.

There appears to be an obvious argument that the choice of PAS would be good for the people who have the choice. Presumably, one would choose PAS just in case the burdens of one's continued life outweigh the benefits. One would not choose PAS just in case the benefits of one's continued life outweigh the burdens. It seems to follow that having the choice of PAS could not make one worse off.

It does not follow. It follows only if the burdens and benefits being considered are the burdens and benefits to the person making the choice. It follows, that is, only if the choice a person considering PAS would make is entirely self-regarding. Why should persons who need care make a self-regarding choice? Morality involves taking into account the interests of others. Therefore, it simply does not follow that the decision that persons needing care ought to make is to continue to live if the benefits of their lives to them outweigh the burdens of their lives to them.

Consider the following argument: Persons in need of care are often net drains on the resources of their families and societies. Therefore, if they take into account the burdens and benefits to everyone, including themselves, affected by a PAS decision, then many of them ought to end their lives either now or in the near future.[17] On this line of reasoning, however, many individuals in need of care will be worse off with the choice of PAS than without it.

Someone might object that this conclusion was arrived at through a crude utilitarian ethical analysis. And, as John Rawls once remarked, the trouble with utilitarianism is that it does not take seriously the distinction between persons.[18]

But what are the alternatives? If the individual in need of care has the choice of life or death and if she is supposed to make neither a selfish decision nor a decision on utilitarian grounds, then how does she decide what to choose? The virtue ethicist will tell her to choose what is virtuous, but that is of as little help here as in other areas of virtue ethics. Appeals to religion seem, as they do in other cases, either ambiguous or arbitrary.

Perhaps the person with the choice of PAS can appeal to Kantian ethical theory. But how is this supposed to go? We have some idea of how respect for the rational agency or for the dignity of *others* determines the morality of a choice. But what are the implications of respect for one's own rational agency or one's own dignity? Kant's account of the duty not to commit suicide is notoriously unsuccessful, given his own fundamental moral tenets. Telling a person contemplating physician-assisted suicide to respect his rational will is unhelpful. We lack an independent criterion for discerning the rule that a rational will would prescribe in this case.

Consider the matter less abstractly. I can tell a loved one that her worth, to use a Kantian phrase, is beyond all price.[19] When she tells herself the same thing, she appears, to herself, to be selfish. She may also appear to us to be selfish. In this case who is doing the deciding makes all the difference.

Consider the argument that since the utilitarian appeal leads to an obviously absurd answer in the case of PAS and there seems to be no other adequate ethical framework, PAS decisions ought not take into account the interests of others. There are three problems with this proposal. The first is that not to take into account the interests of others flagrantly violates our moral common sense. The second is that this proposal is unrealistic. Joanne Lynn reports that many of her dying patients are concerned with not being a burden.[20] The third is that persons needing care who wish to be remembered well after they die will not want to be remembered as the persons who were selfish until the very end. These three problems with this proposal are enough to do it in.

Thus, for people needing care, there are major costs associated with having the choice of PAS. There are costs associated with the selfish alternative and costs associated with the other-regarding alternative. Therefore, people needing care are better off if they do not have the choice of PAS.

If people needing care are better off if PAS is not legalized, then we have a good reason for not legalizing PAS. I assume that the attitude of the moral persons toward people who need care is that we should help them live in ways that are best for them. If this is so, then we must not evaluate their worth on the basis of balancing their social contributions and the value of their lives to themselves with the costs of providing for their needs, for that is not best for them. If they have the choice of PAS, then *they* will evaluate their worth by balancing their social contributions and the value of their lives to themselves with the costs of our providing for their needs, for there is no other way for *them* to do it. To give them the choice of PAS is, in effect, to put them in the position of doing to themselves what we believe it is wrong to have done to them.

Legalization of physician-assisted suicide will make many of those in need of care worse off. Making those in need of care worse off is incompatible with the attitude of care, concern, and support toward them that are the dictates of moral common sense.[21] Therefore, there is a good reason for not legalizing physician-assisted suicide.

There are precedents for having laws that deny people the right of self-determination when having that choice would result in a fundamental loss of well-being. People do not have the right to sell themselves into slavery, to engage in a duel, or (in many cases) not to take part in the Social Security system. It is clear that if any of these practices were legalized, many people who would engage in them would be *much* worse off. Physician-assisted suicide is the same kind of practice.[22]

Notes

1. James Rachels has set out this version of the argument on a number of occasions. See especially his *The End of Life: Euthanasia and Morality* (New York: Oxford University Press, 1986).
2. For example, see The New York State Task Force on Life and the Law, *When Death Is Sought: Assisted Suicide and Euthanasia in the Medical Context*, May 1994; Kathleen M.

Foley, "Doctoring the Doctor," *Hastings Center Report* 24 (3) (May–June, 1994): 45–46; and Shannon Brownlee and Joannie M. Schrof, "Effective Pain Treatments Already Exist. Why Aren't Doctors Using Them?" *U. S. News and World Report*, March 17, 1997, pp. 54–67.

3. Dan Brock, "Voluntary Active Euthanasia," *Hastings Center Report* 22 (2) (March-April, 1992): 16.

4. See Sacred Congregation for the Propagation of the Faith, *Declaration on Euthanasia* (Vatican City, 1980), Thomas Cavanaugh, "The Ethics of Death-Hastening or Death-Causing Palliative Analgesic Administration to the Terminally Ill," *Journal of Pain and Symptom Management* 12 (4) (October, 1996): 248–54; and Norman L. Cantor and George C. Thomas III, "Pain Relief, Acceleration of Death, and Criminal Law," *Kennedy Institute of Ethics Journal* 6 (2) (1996): 107–27. The Michigan law prohibiting physician-assisted suicide contained an exception allowing for necessary pain relief. There is an interesting discussion of this matter in Gina Kolata, "When Morphine Fails to Kill," *New York Times*, July 23, 1997, p. B10. The point of Kolata's article is that some prominent palliative care physicians report giving very high doses of morphine to patients who required such dosages for pain relief and finding no evidence that the patients died sooner as a result.

5. Proponents of PAS may want to insist that giving high doses of morphine under such conditions is euthanasia. However, even if it is, it is not PAS. Furthermore, the point is merely terminological, and therefore, not interesting. Yet, there are some very interesting, nontrivial, deep issues here concerned with the adequacy of the doctrine of double effect. Those issues are far beyond the scope of this essay.

6. This was the view of the palliative care specialists I consulted. I hasten to add that one of them remarked that these symptoms were sometimes quite difficult to control adequately.

7. A careful reading of Timothy Quill's famous case of Diane reveals that it was primarily her psychological suffering with which Quill was concerned. See "Death and Dignity, A Case of Individualized Decision Making," *New England Journal of Medicine* 324 (10) (March 7, 1991): 691–94. Jack Kevorkian's cases seem to concern psychological suffering.

8. Brock, "Active Euthanasia," p. 16 *appears* to endorse this argument. Presumably Timothy Quill would also (see previous note).

9. Dan Callahan "When Self-Determination Runs Amok," *Hastings Center Report* 22, #2 (March–April 1992), 52–55. Ezekiel Emanuel, "The Painful Truth About Euthanasia," *Wall Street Journal*, Tuesday, January 7, 1997 A22; and Herbert Hendin, *Suicide in America* (New York: W. W. Norton, 1995) chapter 11.

10. Ronald Dworkin's introduction to the Philosophers' Brief: "Assisted Suicide: What the Court Really Said" *New York Review of Books*, March 27, 1996, p. 41.

11. Ronald Dworkin, *Life's Dominion* (New York: Knopf, 1993).

12. Dan Brock, op. cit.

13. Ronald Dworkin discusses a case like this. *Op., cit.* chapter 8.

14. The main character in the movie *Whose Life is it Anyway?* does not seem to suffer.

15. For a standard account, see Allen Buchanan and Dan W. Brock, *Deciding for Others; The Ethics of Surrogate Decision Making* (Cambridge: Cambridge University Press, 1989).

16. My account of this difficulty is indebted to the wonderful paper by J. David Velleman, "Against the Right to Die," *The Journal of Medicine and Philosophy* 17 (6) (December, 1992): 664–81.

17. John Hardwig does not endorse this conclusion, but this is where, I think, his argument leads. See his "Is There a Duty to Die?" *The Hastings Center Report* 27 (2) (March–April, 1997): 34–42.

18. John Rawls, *A Theory of Justice* (Cambridge, MA: Harvard University Press, 1971), p. 27.

19. Immanuel Kant, *Grounding for the Metaphysics of Morals*, tr. James W. Ellington, 3rd ed. (Indianapolis: Hackett Publishing Co., 1993), AK 434.

20. Joanne Lynn, "Why I Don't Have a Living Will," reprinted in John Arras and Bonnie Steinbock, *Ethical Issues in Modern Medicine*, (Mountain View, CA: Mayfield, 1995), p. 219.

21. Christians will find support for this in the last verse of the Gospel according to St. Matthew.

22. An earlier version of this essay was read and discussed at the 1997 Pacific Division meeting of the American Philosophical Association, at Central Missouri State University, and at the Ethics Journal Club at the Univesity of Kansas Medical Center. I wish to thank all those who made helpful comments concerning this essay. Ron Stephens, Ann Allegre, Joe Fitschen, and Rosamond Rhodes were especially helpful.

17

Physician–Assisted Suicide

A Tragic View

JOHN D. ARRAS

This essay approaches PAS not as a problem of individual morality but rather as a social policy challenge. Two distinct slippery slope arguments are deployed to demonstrate that the legalization of PAS would pose serious and eminently predictable social harms. The prospect of such harms undermines the adequacy of a case-driven, "backward-looking," rights-oriented casuistry of PAS such as we find in the two federal circuit court decisions. I thus argue for a more "forward-looking" policy approach, one more favorable to genuine democratic deliberation, an approach whose natural habitat is the legislature rather than the courts. I conclude by noting that PAS poses a "tragic choice" for society in the sense that whichever policy we embrace, there are bound to be victims. The best policy, then, is one that attempts to limit social harms by maintaining legal barriers to PAS while vigorously addressing the medical and social deficiencies that give rise, quite unnecessarily, to most requests for an early death.

*   *   *

FOR MANY DECADES NOW, the calls for PAS and euthanasia have been perennial lost causes in American society. Each generation has thrown up an assortment of earnest reformers and cranks who, after attracting their fifteen minutes of fame, inevitably have been defeated by the combined weight of traditional law and morality. Incredibly, two recent federal appellate court decisions suddenly changed the legal landscape in this area, making the various states within their respective jurisdictions the first governments in world history, excepting perhaps the Nazi regime in Germany, to officially sanction PAS. Within the space of a month, both an eight-to-three majority of the United States Court of Appeals for the Ninth Circuit[1] on the West Coast, and a three-judge panel in the United States Court of Appeals for the Second Circuit,[2] in the Northeast, struck down long-standing state laws forbidding physicians to aid or abet their patients in acts of suicide. Within a virtual blink of an eye, the unthinkable had come to pass: PAS and euthanasia had emerged from their exile beyond the pale of law to occupy center stage in a dramatic public debate that eventually culminated in the United States Supreme Court's unanimous reversal of both lower court decisions in June 1997.[3]

Judge Reinhardt, writing for a majority of an *en banc* decision of the Ninth Circuit,[4] held that competent, terminally ill patients have a powerful "liberty interest," what used to be called a Constitutional right, to enlist the aid of their physicians in hastening death via prescriptions for lethal drugs.[5] He argued that, just as the right to privacy guarantees women the right to choose an abortion, this liberty interest protects a right to choose the time and manner of one's death.[6]

In response to warnings against the expansion of this right to broader categories of patients (e.g., to the mentally incapacitated) and against the great likelihood of mistake and abuse, Judge Reinhardt permitted the regulation of PAS in order to avoid such evils; however, he pointedly ruled out any and all blanket prohibitions.[7] In response to the traditional objections that allowing PAS would subvert the state's interests in preventing suicide and maintaining the integrity of the medical profession, Judge Reinhardt contended that our society already has effectively erased the distinction between merely allowing patients to die and killing them.[8] Reinhardt claimed that by allowing patients or their surrogates to forgo life-sustaining medical treatments, including artificially administered nutrition and hydration, and by sanctioning the administration of pain-killing drugs that might also hasten death, our society already permits a variety of "death inducing" practices. Thus, the social risks of allowing PAS are only different in degree, not in kind, from risks that we already countenance.

Writing for the Second Circuit in striking down a similar New York statute, Judge Miner explicitly rejected the claim of the Second Circuit majority that a "substantive due process" right of PAS exists in the Constitution. While presciently conceding that the Supreme Court was unlikely to extend the boundaries of the so-called right to privacy, Judge Miner found nevertheless that the statute violated the equal protection clause of the Constitution.[9] Echoing Judge Reinhardt's assertion that only a difference of degree separates PAS from the foregoing of life-sustaining treatments—claiming in effect that the administration of potentially death hastening analgesics constitutes a kind of suicide—Judge Miner observed that New York's law allowed some people relief from the ravages of terminal illness (i.e., those connected to some form of removable life-support) while denying relief to those not so connected, for whom PAS was the only remaining exit.[10] Concurring with Judge Reinhardt that the social risks of PAS are identical to those of our more socially approved "death inducing" practices, Judge Miner concluded that this kind of differential treatment serves no legitimate state purpose. Thus, he held that the law was unconstitutional even in the absence of a new fundamental right to PAS.[11]

What to think of these startling decisions? Were they harbingers of a new world brave enough to overcome centuries of religious censure and fear-mongering, a world that will no longer permit human beings to suffer unwillingly the torments of terminal illness? Or were they dangerous aberrations, decisions that simultaneously affirmed the autonomy of some, while endangering the lives of society's most vulnerable citizens?

The Supreme Court has finally left little doubt about where it stands on these questions. In a set of majority and concurring opinions remarkable for their ideological restraint, compassion, and thoughtfulness, the various Justices have concluded that extant state laws barring PAS and euthanasia violate neither the

Fourteenth Amendment protection of liberty nor the Fifth Amendment's due process provision.[12] While thus issuing a painful rebuke to the partisans of liberalization, each of the Justices tempered his or her final judgment with the recognition that their collective decision would by no means end public debate, but would rather displace it onto the agendas of the fifty state legislatures.

As a firm believer in patient autonomy, I find myself to be deeply sympathetic to the central values motivating the case for PAS and euthanasia; I have concluded, however, that these practices pose too great a threat to the rights and welfare of too many people to be legalized in this country at the present time. Central to my argument in this essay will be the claim that the recently overturned decisions of the circuit courts employ a form of case-based reasoning that is ill-suited to the development of sound social policy in this area. I shall argue that in order to do justice to the very real threats posed by the widespread social practices of PAS and euthanasia, we need to adopt precisely the kind of policy perspective that the circuit courts rejected on principle. Thus, this essay presents the case for a forward-looking, legislative approach to PAS and euthanasia, as opposed to an essentially backward-looking, judicial or constitutional approach.[13] Although I suggest below that the soundest legislative policy at the present time would be to extend the legal prohibition of PAS into the near future, I remain open to the possibility that a given legislature, presented with sufficient evidence of the reliability of various safeguards, might come to a different conclusion.

Arguments and Motivations in Favor of PAS/Euthanasia

Let us begin, then, with the philosophical case for PAS and euthanasia, which consists of two distinct prongs, both of which speak simply, directly, and powerfully to our commonsensical intuitions. First, there is the claim of autonomy, that all of us possess a right to self-determination in matters profoundly touching on such religious themes as life, death, and the meaning of suffering. Just as we should each be free to make important choices bearing on how we shall live our own lives, so we should be equally free in choosing the time and manner of our deaths. For some, more life will always be welcome as a gift or perhaps even as a test of faith, but for others, continued life signifies only disfiguring suffering and the unrelenting loss of everything that invested their lives with meaning and dignity. As philosopher Ronald Dworkin has eloquently argued, it is a form of *tyranny* to force someone to endure terrible suffering at the end-of-life merely for the sake of someone else's values.[14] Each of us should be free to live or die as we see fit according to our own conceptions of the meaning of life and death.

Second, PAS and/or euthanasia are merciful acts that deliver terminally ill patients from a painful and protracted death. According to the utilitarian, acts are morally right insofar as they promote happiness and alleviate unhappiness, and wrong insofar as they cause or allow others to suffer needlessly. Even according to the traditional ethic of the medical profession, physicians have a solemn duty not merely to extend life whenever possible (and desirable), but also to alle-

viate pain and suffering whenever possible. For patients suffering from the final
ravages of end-stage AIDS or cancer, a doctor's lethal prescription or injection
can be, and often is, welcomed as a blessed relief. Accordingly, we should treat
human beings at least as well as we treat grievously ill or injured animals by
putting them, at their own request, out of their misery.

These philosophical reflections can be supplemented with a more clinical
perspective addressed to the motivational factors lying behind many requests to
die. Many people advocate legalization because they fear a loss of control at the
end-of-life. They fear falling victim to the technological imperative; they fear
dying in chronic and uncontrolled pain; they fear the psychological suffering
attendant upon the relentless disintegration of the self; they fear, in short, a bad
death. All of these fears, it so happens, are eminently justified. Physicians routinely ignore the documented wishes of patients and all too often allow patients
to die with uncontrolled pain.[15] Studies of cancer patients have shown that over
50 percent suffer from unrelieved pain,[16] and many researchers have found that
uncontrolled pain, particularly when accompanied by feelings of hopelessness
and untreated depression, is a significant contributing factor for suicide and
suicidal ideation.[17]

Clinical depression is another major factor influencing patients' choice of suicide.[18] Depression, accompanied by feelings of hopelessness, is the strongest pre-
dictor of suicide for both individuals who are terminally ill and those who are
not.[19] Yet most doctors are not trained to notice depression, especially in complex cases such as the elderly suffering from terminal illnesses. Even when doctors succeed in diagnosing depression, they often do not successfully treat it with
sufficient amounts of readily available medications.[20]

Significantly, the New York State Task Force on Life and Law found that the
vast majority of patients who request PAS or euthanasia can be treated successfully both for their depression and their pain, and that when they receive
adequate psychiatric and palliative care, their requests to die usually are withdrawn.[21] In other words, patients given the requisite control over their lives and
relief from depression and pain usually lose interest in PAS and euthanasia.[22]

With all due respect for the power of modern methods of pain control, it
must be acknowledged that a small percentage of patients suffer from conditions,
both physical and psychological, that currently lie beyond the reach of the best
medical and humane care. Some pain cannot be alleviated short of inducing a
permanent state of unconsciousness in the patient, and some depression is
unconquerable. For such unfortunate patients, the present law on PAS/euthana-
sia can represent an insuperable barrier to a dignified and decent death.[23]

Objections to PAS/Euthanasia

Opponents of PAS and euthanasia can be grouped into three main factions. One
strongly condemns both practices as inherently immoral, as violations of the
moral rule against killing the innocent. Most members of this group tend to harbor distinctly religious objections to suicide and euthanasia, viewing them as

violations of God's dominion over human life.[24] They argue that killing is simply wrong in itself, whether or not it is done out of respect for the patient's autonomy or out of concern for her suffering. Whether or not this position ultimately is justifiable from a theological point of view, its imposition on believers and nonbelievers alike is incompatible with the basic premises of a secular, pluralistic political order.[25]

A second faction primarily objects to the fact that physicians are being called upon to do the killing. While conceding that killing the terminally ill or assisting in their suicides might not always be morally wrong for others to do, this group maintains that the participation of physicians in such practices undermines their role as healers and fatally compromises the physician-patient relationship.[26]

Finally, a third faction[27] readily grants that neither PAS nor active euthanasia, practiced by ordinary citizens or by physicians, are always morally wrong. On the contrary, this faction believes that in certain rare instances early release from a painful or intolerably degrading existence might constitute both a positive good and an important exercise of personal autonomy for the individual. Indeed, many members of this faction concede that should such a terrible fate befall them, they would hope to find a thoughtful, compassionate, and courageous physician to release them from their misery. But in spite of these important concessions, the members of this faction shrink from endorsing or regulating PAS and active euthanasia due to fears bearing on the social consequences of liberalization. This view is based on two distinct kinds of so-called "slippery slope" arguments. One bears on the inability to cabin PAS/euthanasia within the confines envisioned by its proponents; the other focuses on the likelihood of abuse, neglect, and mistake.

An Option Without Limits

The first version of the slippery slope argument contends that a socially sanctioned practice of PAS would in all likelihood prove difficult, if not impossible, to cabin within its originally anticipated boundaries. Proponents of legalization usually begin with a wholesomely modest policy agenda, limiting their suggested reforms to a narrow and highly specified range of potential candidates and practices.[28] "Give us PAS," they ask, "not the more controversial practice of active euthanasia, for presently competent patients who are terminally ill and suffering unbearable pain." But the logic of the case for PAS, based as it is upon the twin pillars of patient autonomy and mercy, makes it highly unlikely that society could stop with this modest proposal once it had ventured out on the slope. As numerous other critics have pointed out, if autonomy is the prime consideration, then additional constraints based upon terminal illness or unbearable pain, or both, would appear hard to justify.[29] Indeed, if autonomy is crucial, the requirement of unbearable suffering would appear to be entirely subjective. Who is to say, other than the patient herself, how much suffering is too much? Likewise, the requirement of terminal illness seems an arbitrary standard against which to judge patients' own subjective evaluation of their quality of life. If my life is no longer worth living, why should a terminally ill cancer patient be granted PAS but not me, merely because my suffering is due to my "nonterminal" arterio-lateral sclerosis ("ALS") or intractable psychiatric disorder?[30]

Alternatively, if pain and suffering are deemed crucial to the justification of legalization, it is hard to see how the proposed barrier of contemporaneous consent of competent patients could withstand serious erosion. If the logic of PAS is at all similar to that of forgoing life-sustaining treatments, and we have every reason to think it so, then it would seem almost inevitable that a case soon would be made to permit PAS for incompetent patients who had left advance directives. That would then be followed by a "substituted judgment" test for patients who "would have wanted" PAS, and finally an "objective" test would be developed for patients (including newborns) whose best interests would be served by PAS or active euthanasia even in the absence of any subjective intent.[31]

In the same way, the joint justifications of autonomy and mercy combine to undermine the plausibility of a line drawn between PAS and active euthanasia. As the authors of one highly publicized proposal have come to see, the logic of justification for active euthanasia is identical to that of PAS.[32] Legalizing PAS, while continuing to ban active euthanasia, would serve only to discriminate unfairly against patients who are suffering and wish to end their lives, but cannot do so because of some physical impairment. Surely these patients, it will be said, are "the worst off group," and therefore they are the most in need of the assistance of others who will do for them what they can no longer accomplish on their own.

None of these initial slippery slope considerations amount to knock-down objections to further liberalization of our laws and practices. After all, it is not obvious that each of these highly predictable shifts (e.g., from terminal to "merely" incurable, from contemporaneous consent to best interests, and from PAS to active euthanasia), are patently immoral and unjustifiable. Still, in pointing out this likely slippage, the consequentialist opponents of PAS/euthanasia are calling on society to think about the likely consequences of taking the first tentative step onto the slope. If all of the extended practices predicted above pose substantially greater risks for vulnerable patients than the more highly circumscribed initial liberalization proposals, then we need to factor in these additional risks even as we ponder the more modest proposals.[33]

The Likelihood of Abuse

The second prong of the slippery slope argument argues that whatever criteria for justifiable PAS and active euthanasia ultimately are chosen, abuse of the system is highly likely to follow. In other words, patients who fall outside the ambit of our justifiable criteria will soon be candidates for death. This prong resembles what I have elsewhere called an "empirical slope"argument, as it is based not on the close logical resemblance of concepts or justifications, but rather on an empirical prediction of what is likely to happen when we insert a particular social practice into our existing social system.[34]

In order to reassure skeptics, the proponents of PAS/euthanasia concur that any potentially justifiable social policy in this area must meet at least the following three requirements.[35] The policy would have to insist: first, that all requests for death be truly voluntary; second, that all reasonable alternatives to PAS and active euthanasia must be explored before acceding to a patient's wishes; and, third, that a reliable system of reporting all cases must be established in order to effectively monitor these practices and respond to abuses. As a social pessimist on these matters, I believe, given social reality as we know it, that all three assumptions are problematic.

With regard to the voluntariness requirement, we pessimists contend that many requests would not be sufficiently voluntary. In addition to the subtly coercive influences of physicians and family members, perhaps the most slippery aspect of this slope is the highly predictable failure of most physicians to diagnose reliably and treat reversible clinical depression, particularly in the elderly population. As one geriatric psychiatrist testified before the New York Task Force, we now live in the "golden age" of treating depression, but the "lead age" of diagnosing it.[36] We have the tools, but physicians are not adequately trained and motivated to use them. Unless dramatic changes are effected in the practice of medicine, we can predict with confidence that many instances of PAS and active euthanasia will fail the test of voluntariness.

Second, there is the lingering fear that any legislative proposal or judicial mandate would have to be implemented within the present social system, one marked by deep and pervasive discrimination against the poor and members of minority groups.[37] We have every reason to expect that a policy that worked tolerably well in an affluent community like Scarsdale or Beverly Hills might not work so well in a community like Bedford-Stuyvesant or Watts, where your average citizen has little or no access to basic primary care, let alone sophisticated care for chronic pain at home or in the hospital. There is also reason to worry about any policy of PAS initiated within our growing system of managed care, capitation, and physician incentives for delivering less care.[38] Expert palliative care no doubt is an expensive and time-consuming proposition, requiring more, rather than less, time spent just talking with patients and providing them with humane comfort. It is highly doubtful that the context of physician-patient conversation within this new dispensation of "turnstile medicine" will be at all conducive to humane decisions untainted by subtle economic coercion.

In addition, given the abysmal and shameful track record of physicians in responding adequately to pain and suffering, we also can confidently predict that in many cases all reasonable alternatives will *not* have been exhausted.[39] Instead of vigorously addressing the pharmacological and psychosocial needs of such patients, physicians no doubt will continue to ignore, undertreat, or treat many of their patients in an impersonal manner. The result is likely to be more depression, desperation, and requests for physician-assisted death from patients who could have been successfully treated.[40] The root causes of this predictable failure are manifold, but high on the list is the inaccessibility of decent primary care to over thirty-seven million Americans. Other notable causes include an appalling lack of training in palliative care among primary care physicians and cancer specialists alike;[41] discrimination in the delivery of pain control and other medical treatments on the basis of race and economic status; various myths shared by both physicians and patients about the supposed ill effects of pain medications; and restrictive state laws on access to opioids.[42]

Finally, with regard to the third requirement, pessimists doubt that any reporting system would adequately monitor these practices. A great deal depends here on the extent to which patients and practitioners will regard these practices as essentially *private* matters to be discussed and acted upon within the privacy of the doctor-patient relationship. As the Dutch experience has conclusively demonstrated, physicians will be extremely loath to report instances of PAS and active euthanasia to public authorities, largely for fear of bringing the harsh glare of publicity upon the patients' families at a time when privacy is most needed.[43] The likely result of this predictable lack of oversight will be society's inability to respond appropriately to disturbing incidents and long-term trends. In other words, the practice most likely will not be as amenable to regulation as the proponents contend.

The moral of this story is that deeply seated inadequacies in physicians' training, combined with structural flaws in our healthcare system, can be reliably predicted to secure the premature deaths of many people who would in theory be excluded by the criteria of most leading proposals to legalize PAS. If this characterization of the status quo is at all accurate, then the problem will not be solved by well-meaning assurances that abuses will not be tolerated, or that patients will, of course, be offered the full range of palliative care options before any decision for PAS is ratified.[44] While such regulatory solutions are possible in theory, and may well justly prevail in the future, we should be wary of legally sanctioning any negative right to be let alone by the state when the just and humane exercise of that right will depend upon the provision of currently nonexistent services. The operative analogy here, I fear, is our failed and shameful policy of "deinstutionalization," which left thousands of vulnerable and defenseless former residents of state psychiatric hospitals to fend for themselves on the streets, literally "rotting with their rights on."[45] It is now generally agreed that the crucial flaw in this well-intended but catastrophic policy was our society's willingness to honor such patients' negative right to be free of institutional fetters without having first made available reliable local alternatives to institutionalization. The operative lesson for us here is that judges and courts are much better at enunciating negative rights than they are at providing the services required for their successful implementation.

Two Approaches to Social Policy

We come now to the difficult task of assessing the capacity of various social policy approaches to address adequately all of the conflicting values implicated in this debate. This section shall contrast a forward-looking, policy-oriented legislative approach to the backward-looking, case-oriented judicial approach taken in the *Compassion in Dying* and *Vacco* cases. Before coming to that comparison, however, a crucial preliminary point must be noted. Central to any serious evaluation of competing policy approaches to PAS and euthanasia is the distinction between the morality of individual acts and the wisdom of social policy. Much of the debate in the popular media is driven by the depiction of especially dramatic and poignant instances of suffering humanity, desperate for release from the painful thrall of terminal illness.[46] Understandably, many of us are prompted to respond: "Should such a terrible fate ever befall me, I certainly would not want to suffer interminably; I would want the option of an early exit and the help of my trusted physician in securing it." The problem, however, lies in getting from such compelling individual cases to social policy. The issue is not simply, "What would I want?" but rather, what is the best social policy, all things considered. Social pessimists warn that we cannot make this jump from individual case to policy without endangering the autonomy and the very lives of others, many of whom are numbered among our most vulnerable citizens.

A Judge-Made Policy Based on Constitutional Law

Appellate judges in the Ninth and Second Circuits authored powerful opinions giving constitutional protection to PAS for competent patients facing terminal illness. While these opinions fully vindicated patients' important stake in having a freely chosen and pain-free death, they seriously and fatally discounted the states' important interests in preventing the kinds of slippage and abuse catalogued above.

DISMISSAL OF SOCIAL CONSEQUENCES

The opinion of the Ninth Circuit, *Compassion in Dying*, authored by Judge Reinhardt, is particularly troubling with regard to the dismissal of social consequences.[47] In response to the objection that legalizing PAS inevitably will prove "infinitely expansive," the court acknowledged the difficulty that it may be hard to distinguish the moral logic of PAS from that animating the call for direct physician-administered euthanasia. He further conceded that in some cases, patients will need the help of a physician in carrying out their choice of an autonomous and painless death.[48] Instead of carefully weighing this sobering possibility in the balance, or asking whether this likelihood of slippage should make us hesitate in taking the first step onto the slope, the court immediately dismissed it as a problem for future cases, not this one, noting that, "here we decide only the issue before us."[49] For those who worry that direct euthanasia carried out by physicians might impose too great a risk in the current social climate,[50] the dictum will prove less than comforting, especially in view of the judge's confession that "it [is] less important who administers the medication than who determines whether the terminally ill person's life shall end."[51]

Thus, although we have argued that this kind of forward-looking, policy-oriented perspective is crucial for adequately assessing the individual benefits and social risks involved in the proposal to legalize PAS, the judicial approach to the problem operates fully equipped with social blinders, and willfully dismisses the very real dangers lurking further down the slope, all in the name of individual rights. Indeed, at one point Judge Reinhardt implied that a refusal to contemplate such dangers is demanded by the judicial role itself.[52] To put it mildly and most charitably, this rights-orientated mind-set does not put us in a learning mode. When life and death are at stake, we need to base our social policy on a more comprehensive picture of the likely benefits and risks.

Judge Reinhardt's grasp of the clinical realities of depression and the ubiquitous absence of adequate pain control was no more impressive than the scope of his social vision. In response to the objection that the legalization of PAS eventually would lead physicians to treat requests to die in a routine and impersonal manner, Judge Reinhardt reassured us, in the face of massive evidence to the contrary, that "doctors would not assist a terminally ill patient to hasten his death as long as there were any reasonable chance of alleviating the patient's suffering or enabling him to live under tolerable conditions."[53] Judge Reinhardt's faith in professional and governmental regulations to ensure that all requests truly are voluntary (i.e., not due to depression), and free from the taint of untreated pain and suffering, is perhaps refreshing in the age of governmental regulation-bashing, but it is a naive and dangerous faith all the same.

EQUAL PROTECTION AND THE FATE OF RESPONSIBLE REGULATION

The ability of a constitutional right to assisted suicide to provide adequately for safeguards against abuse, neglect, and mistake is especially problematic within the context of the Second Circuit's equal protection analysis in *Vacco*. That court's assertion of the moral and legal equivalence of withholding life-sustaining treatments, the provision of potentially death-hastening analgesics, and assisted suicide raised extremely troubling questions about the constitutionality of a wide variety of possibly effective regulations.[54] The basic question is: If we have a constitutionally protected liberty interest in determining the time and manner of our deaths, then to what extent will various regulatory schemes cut too deeply into our personal choices?

We actually have seen this script played out before in the context of abortion law. Prior to *Roe v. Wade*, many states already had begun liberalizing their statutes to allow women to opt for abortion under specified conditions.[55] One regulatory constraint that had been placed on women's choice in some jurisdictions was mandatory review by a hospital-based committee.[56] Now, whether or not we think that such committee review was a good idea in the context of abortion—I do not think it was—it is still interesting to note that this regulatory mechanism, along with a host of others, was discarded unceremoniously by the Supreme Court in *Doe v. Bolton*,[57] the companion case to *Roe v. Wade*.[58] In sum, the Court held that such mechanisms only serve to encumber the woman's choice, which really belongs to her (and perhaps also her doctor) alone.[59]

Now, if the Second Circuit's equal protection analysis had prevailed, and had the Supreme Court come to see no cognizable legal or moral differences between "allowing to die" and assisted suicide, then presumably the regulatory mechanisms surrounding the two sets of practices would have been subjected to identical standards of moral analysis and judicial review.[60] This kind of legally mandated parity would have had two likely consequences. First, all the paraphernalia of surrogate decision-making that currently surrounds decisions to forgo treatment would have been extended to PAS.[61] Just as most states presently allow family or close friends to make life-and-death decisions for loved ones on the basis of so-called "substituted judgment" ("What would the patient have wanted?") or best-interests or reasonable-person determinations, so we would have to allow family members the same role in those cases in which suicide "would have been chosen" by the patient or "would have been" in his best interest.[62] Obviously, this implication of the equal protection approach would have required proponents of PAS to bite a very large bullet indeed regarding the charge of indefinite expansion.

The second implication of the equal protection analysis is that a broad range of possibly helpful regulatory mechanisms, including waiting periods, committee review, second opinions, mandatory reporting, and perhaps even the requirement of terminal illness, might well have been swept aside in the name of individual liberty.[63] Currently, we do not require these kinds of substantive and procedural constraints for most decisions to forgo life-sustaining treatments by competent, terminally ill patients.[64] If, however, there is really no moral or legal difference between "allowing to die" and "assisting suicide"—if, as Judge Miner opines, adding PAS to our repertoire of choices would not add one iota of additional risk to individuals or society over and above those we already countenance—then encumbering the choice for PAS with all sorts of extra protective devices would seemingly lack constitutional validity.[65] In sum, then, the equal protection analysis championed in the Second Circuit threatened precisely those braking mechanisms that arguably might make the slippery slope a far safer place on which to practice physician-assisted death.

THE CONFLATION OF KILLING AND ALLOWING TO DIE

Proceeding directly to the fulcrum of Judge Miner's analysis, we now consider the denial of a significant moral or legal difference between allowing a patient to die by means of forgoing life-sustaining treatments and assisting a patient in committing suicide. According to both circuit court opinions, there is no significant difference between withdrawing a ventilator, discontinuing a feeding tube, administering pain-killing but (potentially) life-shortening opioids, and prescribing a lethal dose of barbiturates.[66] In all these cases, the judges alleged, the intention is the same (i.e., to hasten death), the cause of death is the same (an *act* attributable to human agency), and the social risks of mistake and abuse are the same (e.g., misdiagnosis, undue pressure, etc.). Consequently, Judge Reinhardt concluded that PAS poses no greater threat to the state's interests in preventing suicide and in safeguarding the integrity of the medical profession than the already accepted practice of forgoing life-sustaining treatment.[67] For identical reasons Judge Miner saw no point in a more restrictive public policy towards PAS and based his entire Constitutional argument upon the purported identity of the intentions and effects of these two social practices.[68]

Along with a majority of the Supreme Court, I wish to uphold, for purposes of social policy analysis, the distinction between forgoing treatment and assisting suicide. Although the boundaries between these two practices at times are admittedly quite fuzzy, overlooking relevant differences between them leads proponents of legalization to ignore the very real social risks inherent in the judicial approach to policy.[69]

Whatever the outcome of our long-standing conceptual skirmishes bearing on the "intrinsic" distinctions between PAS, direct euthanasia, and forgoing life-sustaining treatments, the crucial question remains whether any of the purported distinctions between these activities constitute important differences for purposes of social policy.[70] As a slippery slope opponent of PAS and euthanasia, I have already conceded that individual acts involving either PAS or active euthanasia can be morally justified under certain circumstances. Having thus conceded that certain individual actions can be morally appropriate even when the intent is simply and unambiguously to end the patient's life, and even when "the cause" of death is simply and unambiguously attributable to the action of the physician, the crucial question is whether there are any remaining distinctions between allowing to die and actively killing (or assisting in a suicide) that might illuminate the negative policy implications of PAS and euthanasia.

Two points can be made in this connection. First, as the New York Task Force pointed out, the social consequences of not honoring requests to forgo treatment are very different from the consequences of failing to honor requests for PAS and euthanasia.[71] When society fails to honor requests to prescribe or deliver a lethal dose, the results can admittedly be very onerous for individual patients. The patient may face a prolonged period of deterioration before death, with increased pain and decreased dignity, contrary to what they otherwise would have wished. It is important to note, however, that in many such cases there are alternatives to prolonged and painful deaths. Under the present legal regime it is still permissible for a patient to seek out effective and compassionate hospice care, to refuse further administration of life-sustaining treatments, to request "terminal sedation" (inducing a loss of consciousness until death), and even to starve to death with the aid of a physician.[72] It is also legal for an individual truly to take matters into his own hands and to kill himself, perhaps with the guidance of a popular "self-help" book.[73] Finally, it is possible for many patients with good and trusting relationships with compassionate physicians to achieve their objectives within the bounds of private and discreet relationships, but without the cover and consolations of law.[74]

By contrast, were society, systematically and as a matter of policy, to refuse to honor requests to forgo life-sustaining treatments in order to curb possible abuses, then everyone would have to submit to the imposition of unwanted and often invasive measures. Whereas the refusal to honor a request for PAS or direct euthanasia amounts to a refusal of a positive benefit or assistance, the imposition of medical treatment against one's will represents a violation of personal autonomy and physical integrity totally incompatible with the deepest meaning of our traditional respect for liberty. Such a refusal would entail the virtual imprisonment of the entire population of terminally ill and dying patients. While the failure to offer a deadly drug to a dying patient represents a failure of mercy requiring moral justification, the forced imposition of medical treatment against a patient's will arguably constitutes a trespass, or technically a legal battery, so profound that it simply cannot be justified, especially at the level of broad-gauged social policy.[75]

Without trying to sound especially hyperbolical, we can say that the practice of forgoing treatment is by now so deeply embedded in our social and medical practices that a reversal of policy on this point would throw most of our major medical institutions into a state approaching chaos. The same cannot be said of a refusal to honor requests for PAS and euthanasia. Thus, while there may well be many overlapping similarities between withholding treatment and participating in PAS or euthanasia, their respective denial at the level of social policy would entail vastly different individual and social consequences. If our goal is to reduce the level of social risk surrounding all practices involving the treatment of incurable and/or dying patients, a blanket prohibition of PAS can arguably advance this goal without totally unacceptable moral, legal, and social consequences. The same cannot be said of a blanket prohibition of forgoing life-sustaining treatments.

The second point in this connection is that the practice of PAS and/or active euthanasia would be bound to implicate many more persons than the practice of forgoing treatment.[76] While we should definitely worry about the possibility of error, neglect, and abuse in the context of allowing patients to die, it is at least somewhat comforting to realize that just about every patient in this category must be very badly off indeed. By the time that physicians discuss forgoing treatment with a patient or family, the patient is usually well into in the process of dying.

With regard to PAS and euthanasia, however, we can expect that many candidates will be perfectly ambulatory and far from the dreaded scene of painful terminal illness depicted by advocates. Depending on how great the social slippage, this category may well come to encompass those with an incurable condition but who are not presently "terminal," such as persons in the early stagges of HIV infection or Alzheimer's disease.[77] It also may come to encompass patients suffering from prolonged and intractable depression who exhibit no other symptoms of physical illness. Although one important legislative proposal specifically excludes patients whose only symptoms are psychiatric in nature, this reluctance was likely motivated in no small measure by political considerations.[78] Once PAS or active euthanasia, or both, are firmly in place, however, it will be extremely difficult to withhold them from persons whose suffering is every bit as real but whose source is entirely psychological rather than physical. That, Judge Miner and many others would surely object, would constitute an invidious distinction and thus a form of unconstitutional discrimination against the mentally ill.

If the States Are the Laboratory, What's the Experiment?

Although the Ninth Circuit was prepared to grant that states have a legitimate interest in avoiding the possibly adverse social consequences of PAS, the court insisted that regulation, rather than prohibition, is the only constitutionally permissible means of so doing.[79] Toward that end, it would have assigned the challenging task of crafting appropriate regulations to the "laboratory of the states." In view of the very real possibility that the social and individual harms attendant upon the legalization of PAS eventually would prove disproportionate to their benefits, this division of labor between the judiciary and the state legislatures is highly problematic. Had the Supreme Court affirmed the Ninth Circuit's reasoning in granting constitutional protection to the liberty interest in choosing death, states would have been deprived of their ability to put a stop to the widespread practice of PAS even if credible studies were to demonstrate that abuses were rampant and highly resistant to procedural safeguards. Short of a Constitutional amendment, there would have been no turning back had the right to PAS been guaranteed by either the due process or equal protection clauses.

Instead of putting ourselves into this precarious position, we should assign a different and more fundamental task to the laboratory of the states. Given the very real possibilities for extension and abuse of this liberty interest, state legislatures should be entrusted with the basic questions of whether, when, and under what circumstances such a risky social experiment should be attempted in the first place. State legislatures are in a better position than federal judges to study the social and clinical facts and come to a reasonable conclusion on the likely balance of individual benefit and social risks.[80] Given the social and medical realities of this country, I would hope that most states would follow the lead of the New York Task Force in refusing to countenance the legalization and routinization of PAS at this time. However, even if some states do decide to run these risks as a social experiment, i.e., to determine for themselves on the basis of empirical evidence and moral judgment whether more good than harm will come from legalizing PAS, they would have the flexibility, absent rigidly defined constitutional mandates, both to impose very strict regulations and, if necessary, to stop the experiment cold in the face of disconcerting evidence of serious moral slippage. Such an approach is, I believe, much better suited to asking the relevant policy questions and taking appropriate and prudent action.[81]

In addition to being safer, the legislative approach is also, at least potentially, much more democratic than the judicial, rights-based orientation. The legislature is the traditional site in this country for the resolution of most difficult and divisive questions of social policy, especially those marked by deep moral questions and highly troubling empirical uncertainties involving the lives and welfare of many citizens. A court-mandated solution to the question of PAS would, I believe, have secured a decisive and irrevocable victory for one side of this controversy before a thorough and robust public debate had taken place. One significant merit of a legislative approach is that, while it would not guarantee such a debate, it would at least be compatible with large-scale efforts at the state and local levels to foster a more democratically deliberative public dialogue on this matter. Such efforts could give citizens a chance to weigh the nature and value of the liberties at stake against the extent and probability of the social dangers posed by PAS. They could thus serve as a valuable *via media* between the judicial approach, which can often short circuit public debate, and decision-making by public referendum, which is more democratic in theory but often lacks an explicitly deliberative dimension that would allow citizens a deeper understanding of the issues involved before their legislatures took action.[82]

Toward a Policy of Prudent (Legal) Restraint and Aggressive (Medical) Intervention
In contrast to the judicial approach, which totally vindicates the value of patient autonomy at the expense of protecting the vulnerable, my own preferred approach to a social policy of PAS and euthanasia conceives of this debate as posing essentially a "tragic choice."[83] It frankly acknowledges that whatever choice we make, whether we opt for a reaffirmation of the current legal restraints or for a policy of legitimation and regulation, there are bound to be victims. The victims of the current policy are easy to identify: They are on the news, the talk shows, the documentaries, and often on Dr. Kevorkian's roster of so-called "patients." The victims of legalization, by contrast, will be largely hidden from view; they will include the clinically depressed eighty-year-old man who could have lived for another year of good quality if only he had been adequately treated, and the fifty-year-old woman who asks for death because doctors in her financially stretched HMO cannot, or will not, effectively treat her unrelenting, but mysterious, pelvic pain. Perhaps eventually, if we slide far enough down the slope, the uncommunicative stroke victim, whose distant children deem an earlier death to be a better death, will fall victim. There will be others besides these, many coming from the ranks of the uninsured and the poor. To the extent that minorities and the poor already suffer from the effects of discrimination in our healthcare system, it is reasonable to expect that any system of PAS and euthanasia will exhibit similar effects, such as failure to access adequate primary care, pain management, and psychiatric diagnosis and treatment. Unlike Dr. Kevorkian's "patients," these victims will not get their pictures in the papers, but they all will have faces and they will all be cheated of good months or perhaps even years.

This "tragic choice" approach to social policy on PAS/euthanasia takes the form of the following argument formulated at the legislative level. First, the number of "genuine cases" justifying PAS, active euthanasia, or both, will be relatively small. Patients who receive good personal care, good pain relief, treatment for depression, and adequate psychosocial supports tend not to persist in their desire to die.

Second, the social risks of legalization are serious and highly predictable. They include the expansion of these practices to nonvoluntary cases, the advent of active euthanasia, and the widespread failure to pursue readily available alternatives to suicide motivated by pain, depression, hopelessness, and lack of access to good primary medical care.

Third, rather than propose a momentous and dangerous policy shift for a relatively small number of "genuine cases"—a shift that would surely involve a great deal of persistent social division and strife analogous to that involved in the abortion controversy—we should instead attempt to redirect the public debate toward a goal on which we can and should all agree, namely the manifest and urgent need to reform the way we die in America. Instead of pursuing a highly divisive and dangerous campaign for PAS, we should attack the problem at its root with an ambitious program of reform in the areas of access to primary care and the education of physicians in palliative care. At least as far as the "slippery slope" opponents of PAS are concerned, we should thus first see to it that the vast majority of people in this country have access to adequate, affordable, and nondiscriminatory primary and palliative care. At the end of this long and arduous process, when we finally have an equitable, effective, and compassionate healthcare system in place, one that might be compared favorably with that in the Netherlands, then we might well want to reopen the discussion of PAS and active euthanasia.

Finally, there are those few unfortunate patients who truly are beyond the pale of good palliative, hospice, and psychiatric care. The opponents of legalization must face up to this suffering remnant and attempt to offer creative and humane solutions. One possibility is for such patients to be rendered permanently unconscious by drugs until such time, presumably not a long time, as death finally claims them. Although some will find such an option to be aesthetically unappealing, many would find it a welcome relief.[84] Other patients beyond the reach of the best palliative and hospice care could take their own lives, either by well-known traditional means, or with the help of a physician who could sedate them while they refused further food and (life-extending) fluids. Those who find the latter option to be unacceptable might still be able to find a compassionate physician who, like Dr. Timothy Quill, will ultimately be willing, albeit in fear and trembling, to "take small risks for people [they] really know and care about."[85] Such actions will continue to take place within the privacy of the patient-physician relationship, however, and thus will not threaten vulnerable patients and the social fabric to the same extent as would result from full legalization and regulation.[86] As the partisans of legalized PAS correctly point out, the covert practice of PAS will not be subject to regulatory oversight, and is thus capable of generating its own abuses and slippery slope. Still, I believe that the ever-present threat of possible criminal sanctions and revocation of licensure will continue to serve, for the vast majority of physicians, as powerful disincentives to abuse the system. Moreover, as suggested earlier, it is highly unlikely that the proposals for legalization would result in truly effective oversight.

Conclusion

Instead of conceiving this momentous debate as a choice between, on the one hand, legalization and regulation with all of their attendant risks, and on the other hand, the callous abandonment of patients to their pain and suffering,[87] enlightened opponents must recommend a positive program of clinical and social reforms. On the clinical level, physicians must learn how to really listen to their patients, to unflinchingly engage them in sensitive discussions of their needs and the meaning of their requests for assisted death, to deliver appropriate palliative care, to distinguish fact from fiction in the ethics and law of pain relief, to diagnose and treat clinical depression, and finally, to ascertain and respect their patients' wishes for control regarding the forgoing of life-sustaining treatments. On the social level, opponents of PAS must aggressively promote major initiatives in medical and public education regarding pain control, in the sensitization of insurance companies and licensing agencies to issues of the quality of dying, and in the reform of state laws that currently hinder access to pain relieving medications.[88]

In the absence of an ambitious effort in the direction of aggressive medical and social reform, I fear that the medical and nursing professions will have lost whatever moral warrant and credibility they might still have in continuing to oppose physician-assisted suicide and active euthanasia. As soon as these reforms are in place, however, we might then wish to proceed slowly and cautiously with experiments in various states to test the overall benefits of a policy of legalization. Until that time, however, we are not well served as a society by court decisions allowing for legalization of PAS. The Supreme Court has thus reached a sound decision in ruling out a constitutional right to PAS. As the Justices acknowledged, however, this momentous decision will not end the moral debate over PAS and euthanasia. Indeed, it should and hopefully will intensify it.

Notes

The author would like to thank Carl Coleman, David DeGrazia, Yale Kamisar, Tom Murray, David Orentlicher, and Bonnie Steinbock for helpful discussions and exchanges on the issues dealt with in this paper. Longer versions of this article, published before the Supreme Court's decisions, appeared in *Biolaw* (July/August 1996), Special Section: 171–88 and *The Journal of Contemporary Health Law and Policy* 13 (1997): 361–89.
1. *Compassion in Dying* v. *Washington*, 79 F. 3d 790, 838 (9th Cir. 1996).
2. *Quill* v. *Vacco*, 80 F. 3d 716, 731 (2nd Cir. 1996).
3. *Vacco, Attorney General of New York, et al.* v. *Quill et al.*, certiorari to the United States Court of Appeals for the second circuit, No. 95–1858. Argued January 8, 1997—Decided June 26, 1997. *Washington et al.* v. *Glucksberg et al.*, certiorari to the United States Court of Appeals for the ninth circuit, No. 96–110. Argued January 8, 1997—Decided June 26, 1997.
4. See *Compassion in Dying*, 79 F. 3d at 790.
5. Ibid., 816.
6. Ibid., 813–14.
7. Ibid., 816–32, 836–37 (reviewing state interests and illustrating the application of the balancing test and holding).
8. Ibid., 822–23.
9. *Vacco* v. *Quill*, 80 F. 3d 716, 724–25 (2nd Cir. 1996).

10. Ibid., 727–29.

11. Ibid., 727.

12. *Washington* v. *Glucksberg,* 117 Sup. Ct. 2258 (1997). *Vacco* v. *Quill,* 117 Sup. Ct. 2293 (1997).

13. My stance on these issues has been profoundly influenced by my recent work with the New York State Task Force on Life and the Law (hereinafter "the Task Force") to come to grips with this issue. Following a thorough review of the moral, legal, and social arguments, this highly pluralistic advisory committee unanimously concluded against the legalization of either PAS or direct killing by physicians. A reading of the Supreme Court opinions in these cases suggests that the Task Force's analysis of the social policy of PAS was accepted by most, if not all, of the Justices. See Task Force, *When Death Is Sought: Assisted Suicide and Euthanasia in the Medical Context* (May 1994).

14. Ronald Dworkin, *Life's Dominion: An Argument About Abortion, Euthanasia, and Individual Freedom* (New York: Knopf, 1993), 217. While I agree with Professor Dworkin on the inadmissability of religious rationales for the legal prohibition of PAS, we disagree on the availability of convincing secular justifications.

15. "A Controlled Trial to Improve Care for Seriously Ill Hospitalized Patients; The Study to Understand Prognoses and Preferences for Outcomes and Risks of Treatments (SUP-PORT)," *Journal of the American Medical Association* 274 (Nov. 22, 1995): 1591–92.

16. Task Force, *When Death is Sought*, x–xi.

17. Ibid., xiv.

18. Ezekiel J. Emanuel et al., "Euthanasia and Physician-Assisted Suicide: Attitudes and Experiences of Oncology Patients, Oncologists, and the Public," *Lancet* 347 (1996): 1805. See also D. Saltzburg et al., "The Relationship of Pain and Depression to Suicidal Ideation in Cancer Patients," *Proc. ASCO* 8 (1989): 312 (abstract).

19. W. Breitbart, "Cancer Pain and Suicide," in K. M. Foley, ed., *Advances in Pain Research and Therapy* 16 (1990): 399–412 (showing that studies indicate that depression "is present in 50 percent of all suicides, and those suffering from depression are at 25 times greater risk for suicide than the general population").

20. New York State Task Force, *When Death Is Sought*, 127–28 (documenting the claim that doctors fail to diagnose and treat depression). See also Y. Conwell and E. D. Caine, "Rational Suicide and the Right to Die," *New England Journal of Medicine* 325 (1991): 1101.

21. New York State Task Force, *When Death Is Sought*, xiv.

22. As we shall see later, this fact is of enormous importance for our evaluation of PAS and euthanasia as social policies, for if the root causes or motivations for assisted death can be addressed successfully for most patients through the delivery of technically competent and compassionate medicine, the case for changing the law loses much of its urgency.

23. The above section thus signals two important points of agreement with the so-called Philosophers' Brief submitted to the Supreme Court in *Compassion in Dying* and *Vacco* by Ronald Dworkin, Thomas Nagel, Robert Nozick, John Rawls, Thomas Scanlon, and Judith Jarvis Thomson. I agree that individuals in the throes of a painful or degrading terminal illness may well have a very strong moral and even legal interest in securing PAS. I also agree that the pain and suffering of a small percentage of dying patients cannot be adequately controlled by currently available medical interventions. (*New York Review of Books* 44 (5) [March 27, 1997]: 41–47. See also appendix B of this volume.) As we shall see, however, I disagree with the philosophers' conclusion that this interest is sufficiently strong in the face of current medical and social inadequacies as to justify a legal right that would void the reasonably cautious prohibitions of PAS and euthanasia in effect in every State.

24. For religious objections to suicide and euthanasia, see St. Thomas Aquinas, "Whether It Is Lawful to Kill Oneself," in Tom L. Beauchamp and Robert Veatch, eds., *Ethical Issues in Death and Dying*, 2nd. ed. (1996), pp. 119–21. See also Dworkin, *Life's Dominion*,

193. See also Richard John Neuhaus, "The Return of Eugenics," *Commentary* 22 (1988) (arguing that life is a good of the person, not simply for the person).

25. Here too I agree with the Philosophers' Brief.

26. Willard Gaylin et al., "Doctors Must Not Kill," *Journal of the American Medical Association* 259 (1988): 2139–40 See also David Orentlicher, "Physician Participation in Assisted Suicide," *Journal of the American Medical Association* 262 (1989): 1844–45.

27. The author was a part of this faction during his tenure with the New York State Task Force.

28. See Christine Cassel et al., "Care of the Hopelessly Ill: Proposed Clinical Criteria for Physician-Assisted Suicide," *New England Journal of Medicine* 327 (1992): 1380–84 (approving of PAS but not of active euthanasia because it poses excessive social risks).

29. See Daniel Callahan, *The Troubled Dream of Life: Living With Mortality* (New York: Simon and Schuster, 1993). See also Yale Kamisar, "Against Assisted Suicide-Even a Very Limited Form," *University of Detroit-Mercy Law Review* 72 (1995): 735.

30. ALS also is known as Lou Gehrig's disease.

31. *In re Conroy*, 486 A. 2d 1209 (1985) (summarizing the logic of foregoing life-sustaining treatments).

32. Cassel et al., "Care of the Hopelessly Ill," 1380–84. See also Franklin G. Miller et al., "Regulating Physician-Assisted Death," *New England Journal of Medicine* 331 (1994): 199–23 (conceding the untenability of the previous distinction).

33. Professors Dworkin, et al. consistently fail to mention the possibility, let alone the high likelihood, of this first sort of slippage; I take this to be a serious omission both in their joint brief and in Professor Dworkin's individually authored articles on this subject. These authors simply assume (with the plaintiffs and circuit court majority opinions) that this right will be restricted by means of procedural safeguards to presently competent, incurably ill individuals manifesting great pain and suffering due to physical illness. (For evidence of Professor Dworkin's continuing failure to acknowledge this problem, see his assessment of the Supreme Court opinions in "Assisted Suicide: What the Court Really Said," *New York Review of Books* 44 (14) (Sept. 25, 1997): 40–44.) Failure to notice this sort of dynamic might be due either to the philosophers' lack of familiarity with the recent history of bioethics or to their belief that the social risks of PAS are equivalent to the risks inherent in the widely accepted practice of forgoing life-sustaining treatments, and thus that such slippage would not present any additional risk. The latter assumption is, of course, vigorously contested by the opponents of PAS and euthanasia.

34. John Arras, "The Right to Die on the Slippery Slope," *Social Theory and Practice* 8 (1982): 285 (describing the "slippery slope" argument in favor of PAS).

35. See, e.g., Cassel et al., "Care of the Hopelessly Ill"; Miller et al., "Regulating Physician-Assisted Death"; Charles H. Baron et al., "Statute: A Model State Act to Authorize and Regulate Physician-Assisted Suicide," *Harvard Journal of Legislation* 33 (1996): 1.

36. Dr. Gary Kennedy, Division of Geriatrics, Montefiore Medical Center, Albert Einstein College of Medicine, Testimony before the New York Task Force on Life and the Law.

37. Task Force, *When Death Is Sought*, 143 (illustrating discrimination against minority groups). See also C. S. Cleeland et al., "Pain and Its Treatment in Outpatients with Metastic Cancer," *New England Journal of Medicine* 320 (1994): 592–96 (illustrating a study that found that patients treated for cancer at centers that care predominantly for minority individuals were three times more likely to receive inadequate therapy to relieve pain).

38. Susan M. Wolf, "Physician-Assisted Suicide in the Context of Managed Care," *Duquesne Law Review* 35 (1996): 455.

39. Task Force, *When Death Is Sought*, 43–47. "Despite dramatic advances in pain management, the delivery of pain relief is grossly inadequate in clinical practice. . . . Studies have shown that only 2 to 60 percent of cancer pain, is treated adequately." Ibid., 43.

40. Wolf, "Physician-Assisted Suicide in the Context of Managed Care."

41. Task Force, *When Death Is Sought*, 44: "In general, researchers report that many doctors and nurses are poorly informed about, and have limited experience with, pain and symptom management. Health care professionals appear to have a limited understanding of the physiology of pain and the pharmacology of narcotic analgesics. Accordingly, many lack the understanding, skills, and confidence necessary for effective pain and symptom management." See also K. M. Foley, "The Relationship of Pain and Symptom Management to Patient Requests for Physician-Assisted Suicide," *Journal of Pain and Symptom Management* 6 (1991): 290.

42. Task Force, *When Death Is Sought*, 17.

43. One source estimates that in the early 1990s, no more than 30 percent of cases of PAS were reported. During 1994, the rate of reporting increased to roughly 50 percent of cases. See John Keown, "Further Reflections on Euthanasia in the Netherlands in the Light of the Remmelink Report and the Van Der Maas Survey," in Luke Gormally, ed., *Euthanasia: Clinical Practice and the Law* (1994) 219. See also Daniel Callahan and Margot White, "The Legalization of Physician-Assisted Suicide: Creating a Regulatory Potemkin Village," *University of Richmond Law Review* 30 (1996): 17.

44. See, e.g., Ronald Dworkin, "Introduction to the Philosophers' Brief," *New York Review of Books*, 41–42; and Dworkin, "Assisted Suicide: What the Court Really Said," 44.

45. Nancy Rhoden, "The Limits of Liberty: Deinstitutionalization, Homelessness, and Libertarian Theory," *Emory Law Journal* 32 (2) (Spring 1982): 375–440.

46. Tom Kuntz, "Helping a Man Kill Himself, As Shown on Dutch TV," *New York Times* (Nov. 13, 1994), at E-7 (describing the first national broadcast of an actual mercy killing in the Netherlands).

47. *Compassion in Dying* v. *Washington*, 79 F. 3d 790, 830–32 (9th Cir. 1996).

48. Ibid., 831.

49. Ibid., 832.

50. This group once included such distinguished physicians and advocates of PAS as Dr. Timothy Quill, Christine Cassel, and Diane Meier. See Cassel et al., "Care of the Hopelessly Ill."

51. *Compassion in Dying*, 79 F. 3d at 832.

52. Ibid., 831 ("In fact, the Court has never refused to recognize a substantive due process liberty right or interest merely because there were difficulties in determining when and how to limit its exercise or because others might someday attempt to use it improperly.").

53. Ibid., 827. Judge Reinhardt's optimism is contradicted by evidence amassed in the SUPPORT study. See note 15 above.

54. *Quill* v. *Vacco*, 80 F. 3d 716, 729 (2nd Cir. 1996).

55. 410 U.S. 113 (1973).

56. *Doe* v. *Bolton*, 410 U.S. 179, 184 (1973).

57. 410 U.S. 179 (1973).

58. Ibid., 198.

59. Ibid.

60. See Frank G. Miller, "Legalizing Physician-Assisted Suicide by Judicial Decision: A Critical Appraisal," *Biolaw* (Jul.-Aug. 1996).

61. Ibid., S-143.

62. For a comprehensive account of practices and laws governing the forgoing of life-sustaining treatment and surrogate decision making, see Alan Meisel, *The Right to Die*, 2d ed. (New York: Wiley Law Publications, 1995).

63. Miller, "Legalizing Physician-Assisted Suicide by Judicial Decision."

64. Meisel, *The Right to Die*.

65. Miller, "Legalizing Physician-Assisted Suicide by Judicial Decision."

66. *Quill* v. *Vacco*, 80 F. 3d 716, 729 (2nd Cir. 1996); see also *Compassion in Dying* v. *Washington*, 79 F. 3d 790, 822–24 (9th Cir. 1996).

67. Miller, "Legalizing Physician-Assisted Suicide by Judicial Decision," S-139.

68. *Quill v. Vacco*, 80 F. 3d 716, 729 (2nd Cir. 1996).

69. Dan Brock, "Voluntary Active Euthanasia," *Hastings Center Report* 22 (1992): 10. See also Brock, "Borderline Cases of Morally Justified Taking Life in Medicine," in Tom Beauchamp, ed., *Intending Death: The Ethics of Assisted Suicide and Euthanasia* (Upper Saddle River, NJ: Prentice Hall, 1996): 131–49.

70. For a helpful review of the arguments surrounding the distinction between "letting die" and PAS/euthanasia, see Kamisar, "Against Assisted Suicide—Even a Very Limited Form," 753–60. For those wishing to go deeper into these troubled waters, see B. Steinbock & Alastair Norcross, eds., *Killing and Letting Die* (New York: Fordham University Press, 1995). See also Beauchamp, ed., *Intending Death: The Ethics of Assisted Suicide and Euthanasia*.

71. Task Force, *When Death Is Sought*, 146–47.

72. David M. Eddy, "A Conversation with My Mother," *Journal of the American Medical Association* 272 (1994): 179 (illustrating the possibility of death by starvation).

73. Derek Humphrey, *Final Exit: The Practicalities of Self-deliverance and Assisted Suicide for the Dying*, 2nd ed., (New York: Bantam Doubleday, 1997).

74. Dick Lehr, "Death and the Doctor's Hand: Increasingly, Secretly, Doctors Are Helping the Incurably Ill to Die," *Boston Globe* (Apr. 25, 1993), p. 1 (featuring the experience of physicians who have helped patients to commit suicide).

75. *Restatement (second) of Torts*, sec. 13 (1965) (defining battery).

76. See also Seth Kreimer, "Does Pro-Choice Mean Pro-Kevorkian?: An Essay on Roe, Casey, and the Right to Die,"*American University Law Review* 44 (1995): 803, 841.

77. The prospects for slippage here are excellent. The step from a requirement of terminal illness, viewed by these courts as canonical, to one of merely "untreatable" or "incurable" illness, already has been recommended by a panel of distinguished proponents of PAS. See Miller et al., "Regulating Physician-Assisted Death." It is interesting to note in this connection that one of Jack Kevorkian's earliest "patients," Janet Atkins, reportedly was playing tennis a week or two before her assisted suicide.

78. Baron et al., "A Model State Act to Authorize and Regulate Physician-Assisted Suicide," 11. At an American Philosophical Association symposium on PAS in December, 1995, Professor Brock conceded that political-strategic considerations played a significant role in his group's decision not to sanction PAS for the chronically mentally ill.

79. *Compassion in Dying v. Washington*, 79 F. 3d 790, 832–33, 836–37 (9th Cir. 1996).

80. Carl E. Schneider, "Making Sausage: The Ninth Circuit's Opinion," *Hastings Center Report* 27 (1997): 27–28 (reviewing the shortcomings of judges in coming to terms with the complexities of highly contextualized social problems such as PAS).

81. For similar reasons, I am highly skeptical of state ballot initiatives, such as the 1994 initiative in Oregon, which do not make use of the legislatures' superior fact-finding capabilities or, for that matter, of the citizens' capacity for more deliberative approaches to democratic problem solving.

82. It does not speak well for the level of pubic understanding of this issue, as gauged by polls and referenda, that I, a middling public speaker at best, am unfailingly able to convert (or at least shake the confidence of) largely pro-PAS audiences by the end of a half-hour exploration of the social risks and available alternatives. For an excellent discussion of the promise of a more deliberative mode of democracy, see Amy Gutmann and Dennis Thompson, *Democracy and Disagreement* (Cambridge: Harvard University Press, 1996).

83. For an explication of the notion of a "tragic choice" in the sense that I employ here, see Guido Calabresi & Philip Bobbit, *Tragic Choices* (New York: W.W. Norton, 1978).

84. For a good example of how such "terminal sedation" can fit into an overall plan of palliative care, bringing relief to patients and families alike, see Ira Byock's compassionate and instructive account in *Dying Well: The Prospect for Growth at the End of Life* (New York: Riverhead Books, 1997), ch. 10.

85. Timothy Quill, "Death and Dignity: A Case of Individualized Decision Making," *New England Journal of Medicine* 324 (1991): 694.

86. Allowing for the occasional covert practice of PAS would, it is true, favor well-educated, middle-class individuals with access to willing physicians and would thus perpetuate an undesirable double standard that excludes the poor and unconnected from the benefit of a better death. (For a powerful formulation of this criticism, see Dworkin, "Introduction: The Philosophers' Brief," 41.) I take this double standard to be a definite liability of my approach, but one required by the moral necessity of avoiding other harms to other people. Describing my approach as informed by a "tragic" vision acknowledges the unhappy fact that no solution to the problem of dying in our society will be acceptable, fair, or humane to all. The most we can hope for here is "the least worst" policy.

87. In framing the question in just this way, Ronald Dworkin is guilty of posing a false dilemma in his otherwise admirable book. See Dworkin, *Life's Dominion*, p. 198.

88. This brief sketch of suggested reforms merely summarizes the careful work of the New York State Task Force. See *When Death Is Sought*, pp. 153–184.

18

The Supreme Court and Terminal Sedation

An Ethically Inferior Alternative to Physician-Assisted Suicide

DAVID ORENTLICHER

In reaffirming the distinction between the withdrawal of life-sustaining treatment and physician-assisted suicide, the U.S. Supreme Court breached the distinction between treatment withdrawal and euthanasia. For the unrelieved suffering of some dying patients, the Court pointed to the availability of "terminal sedation," a practice in which patients are deeply sedated to eliminate their awareness of their pain or other discomfort. Once sedated, the patient's food and water is typically withheld, and the patient dies, either from the underlying disease or the withholding of food and water. Often, then, terminal sedation is effectively euthanasia—the patient dies because the physician has artificially induced an inability to eat or drink and withheld nutrition and hydration. In addition, terminal sedation is a method of death that is ethically inferior to assisted suicide. Terminal sedation requires patients to linger for a few more days before they die. More importantly, it poses greater risks to patient welfare than assisted suicide. Since the death-causing act of assisted suicide is much more under the control of the patient than are the death-causing acts of terminal sedation, incompetent persons are less likely to die without their consent by assisted suicide than by terminal sedation.

*   *   *

IN DISCUSSING the United States Supreme Court's physician-assisted suicide decisions, many commentators will attack the Court for its affirmation of the distinction between withdrawal of life-sustaining treatment and assisted suicide. Others will disagree with the Court's understanding of the United States Constitution. I will make my critique from a third perspective. I will argue that, even if we accept the premises and logic of the Court, we have decisions that undermine the very distinction that the Court was trying to preserve.[1]

On the surface, the Court maintained the distinction between "passive" cases of patient death—those brought on by withdrawal of treatment—from "active" cases of patient death—those brought on by assisted suicide or euthanasia. According to the Court's decisions, states may prohibit assisted suicide (and by implication euthanasia) even while they must permit withdrawal of treatment. However, a deeper analysis demonstrates that the Court maintained the withdrawal-suicide distinction only by breaching the distinction between treatment withdrawal and euthanasia. In response to concerns about the unrelieved suffering of some dying patients, the Court indicated that these patients can turn to "terminal sedation," a practice that seems consistent with traditional medical care but often is a form of euthanasia. The Court's embrace of terminal sedation not only undermines its effort to preserve the active-passive distinction, it also results in a constitutional scheme that is ethically inferior to one in which assisted suicide is recognized as an individual right. Terminal sedation serves fewer of the purposes of right-to-die law while posing greater risks of abuse than assisted suicide.

The Supreme Court's Assisted-Suicide Decisions

In preserving the distinction between treatment withdrawal and assisted suicide, the Supreme Court justified the distinction by appealing to considerations of causation and intent. According to the Court, when life-sustaining treatment is withdrawn, the patient dies from an underlying disease. In contrast, with assisted suicide, the patient dies because of a physician's active intervention in supplying a lethal medication. Similarly, while a physician may withdraw treatment with the intent of respecting the patient's wishes to be free of unwanted medical intervention, the physician assisting suicide must necessarily do so with the intent that the patient will die.[2]

In earlier articles, I have argued that claims about causation and intent really do not justify a moral distinction between treatment withdrawal and assisted suicide.[3] Physicians do cause their patients' deaths when treatment is withdrawn. Turning off a ventilator, for example, directly results in the patient's death. As for intent, physicians prescribing a lethal dose of medication may intend only that possession of the prescription will relieve the patient's anxiety about losing control, thereby making it feasible for the patient to endure the remaining days of life. Moreover, in withdrawal cases, patients frequently harbor an intent to die, and physicians often intend the patient's death.[4]

Here, I want to show that, even if we accept the Court's claims about causation and intent, the Court's decisions end up undermining the distinction between active and passive cases of patient death. To see how this is so, we need to turn to the Court's discussion of the argument that assisted suicide is necessary to ensure adequate relief of patient suffering. According to the plaintiffs in the assisted suicide cases, there are some dying patients who experience suffering that is intolerable and that cannot be relieved by traditional medical care. For these patients, the plaintiffs said, a right to assisted suicide must be available.

The Court's response to this argument can primarily be found in the concurring opinions of Justices O'Connor and Breyer. In her concurrence, Justice O'Connor rejected any generalized right to assisted suicide.[5] However, she noted, there might be a narrow right to assisted suicide for terminally ill persons who are suffering greatly. Rather than deciding whether this narrower right exists, Justice O'Connor observed that, even if such a right did exist, a prohibition on assisted suicide would not violate the right. Dying patients who are experiencing great pain can obtain medication to relieve their suffering, even if relief can be achieved only by rendering the patient unconscious and hastening the patient's death. Justice O'Connor's opinion was joined by Justices Ginsburg and Breyer.

In his separate concurrence, Justice Breyer echoed Justice O'Connor's argument. He wrote that, while there might be a right to avoid "unnecessary and severe physical suffering," that right would not justify assisted suicide.[6] According to Justice Breyer, patients suffering greatly could always turn to pain control medications or "sedation which can end in a coma."[7]

For purposes of my argument, the key point made by Justices O'Connor and Breyer, and joined by Justice Ginsburg, is their rejection of a right to assisted suicide on the ground that treatment is available to relieve the suffering of any dying patient, with the most severe suffering avoided by sedating the patient into unconsciousness or coma. By relying on the availability of such heavy sedation, the Justices rejected assisted suicide only by embracing euthanasia.[8]

Terminal Sedation

When Justice O'Connor wrote about palliative care causing unconsciousness, and Justice Breyer wrote about physicians sedating patients into a coma, they were referring to the same practice, a practice commonly characterized as "terminal sedation."

At the end of life, dying patients may develop intolerable symptoms of pain, shortness of breath, agitated delirium, or persistent vomiting that are refractory to the usual therapies.[9] Intolerable pain may be caused by a number of conditions, including cancer metastatic to the spine with collapse of the vertebral bodies, intestinal obstruction, or headache due to massive intra-cerebral edema (i.e., massive build-up of fluid in the brain).[10] Intolerable shortness of breath also may be caused by a number of conditions, including emphysema, lung and other cancers, and congestive heart failure.[11] In cases of intolerable and refractory suffering, adequate relief can be obtained only by sedating the patients, often into unconsciousness, so that they no longer are able to feel their pain or other suffering. With terminal sedation, narcotics (e.g., morphine), benzodiazepine sedative drugs (e.g., Valium), barbiturates (e.g., amobarbital) and/or major tranquilizing drugs (e.g., Haldol or Thorazine) are used to sedate the patient.[12]

The sedation is maintained until the patient dies, from either the underlying terminal illness or from a second step that is often part of terminal sedation—the withholding of nutrition and hydration. Since the sedation leaves the patient with a depressed level of consciousness and stopping the sedation would only result in the patient reexperiencing the suffering, the patient frequently agrees to have food and water withheld rather than having life prolonged for a short time. In cases in which terminal sedation shortens the patient's life it usually does so by hours to days. For some patients, life is shortened by as much as several weeks.

At first glance, terminal sedation seems consistent with well accepted practices. It is appropriate for physicians to treat the pain and other suffering of patients aggressively, even if doing so increases the likelihood that the patient will die. It also is appropriate for patients to refuse life-sustaining treatment, including food and water. Upon closer examination, however, terminal sedation is at times essentially euthanasia, or a kind of "slow euthanasia."[13]

Terminal Sedation as a Form of Euthanasia

In many cases, terminal sedation amounts to euthanasia because the sedated patient often dies from the combination of two intentional acts by the physician—first the induction of stupor or unconsciousness and second the withholding of food and water.[14] Without these two acts, the patient would live longer before eventually succumbing to illness. In other words, if the sedation step and the withholding of nutrition and hydration step are viewed as a total package, then we have a situation in which a patient's life is ended by the active intervention of a physician.

It might be argued that these deaths by terminal sedation are not deaths by euthanasia because they result from the withholding of nutrition and hydration. Although in form terminal sedation deaths from dehydration or starvation appear to be a type of treatment withdrawal, they are in principle more like a type of euthanasia. As discussed above, the Supreme Court distinguished the withdrawal of life-sustaining treatment from assisted suicide (and euthanasia) because, with treatment withdrawal, the patient dies from the underlying disease, not from the active intervention of the physician. Patients with severe emphysema die after the removal of their ventilators because their lung disease is responsible for their inability to breathe. Similarly, a patient in a persistent vegetative state dies after the removal of a feeding tube because the patient's brain damage is responsible for the patient's inability to eat food or drink fluids. But this is not what happens in terminal sedation accompanied by the withholding of nutrition and hydration. In such a case, the patient dies from the intentionally induced stupor or coma. It is the physician-created state of diminished consciousness that renders the patient unable to eat, not the natural progression of the patient's underlying disease.

In terms of the Supreme Court's other main justification for the withdrawal-suicide distinction—the physician's intent—terminal sedation also cannot be distinguised from euthanasia. As previously mentioned, the Court observed that a physician who withdraws life-sustaining treatment may only intend to free the patient of an undesired treatment, while a physician assisting a patient's suicide must necessarily intend the patient's death. This point about intent places terminal sedation in the category of euthanasia rather than withdrawal of treatment. As the Court suggested, there are two components to the issue of intent. First, there is the subjective motivation or purpose of the actor.[15] Second, there are objective considerations like the knowledge of the actor and the consequences of the action. The law often holds people responsible for the foreseeable consequences of their acts, even if they had no desire to cause those consequences.[16] In terms of the subjective component of intent, we cannot distinguish between terminal sedation and euthanasia, or, for that matter, among withdrawal of treatment, terminal sedation, assisted suicide and euthanasia. With all four, the physician acts with a morally acceptable—indeed morally praiseworthy—purpose, to relieve the patient's suffering and/or to free the patient of an unwanted treatment.

Although treatment withdrawal is typically distinguished from euthanasia in terms of the objective component of intent, we cannot differentiate between terminal sedation and euthanasia on that basis. Treatment withdrawal is distinguished from euthanasia because, with the former, the physician can genuinely believe that the patient might survive the discontinuation of treatment. The physician may have misjudged either the patient's dependence on the treatment or the chances that the patient's condition would improve.[17] Since it is possible for treatment to be withdrawn and for the patient to survive, we can say that the physician only intends to free the patient from an unwanted treatment. We cannot make a parallel argument for euthanasia. Since euthanasia will relieve the patient's suffering only by killing the patient, the physician cannot reasonably intend that the patient not die.

In terms of this distinction between treatment withdrawal and euthanasia, terminal sedation falls on the euthanasia side of the line. Just as a physician performing euthanasia must necessarily intend the patient's death because the patient will certainly die, so must a physician providing terminal sedation intend the patient's death when the sedation is accompanied by the withholding of nutrition and hydration. In such cases, the patient will surely die. Withholding food and water will inevitably cause the patient's death, since no one can survive very long without sustenance. In other words, there is no possibility that the physician will have misjudged the patient's dependence on the treatment. Moreover, the sedation will preclude the possibility of patient survival from a mistaken prognosis. Even if there is an improvement in the patient's underlying condition, the sedation will prevent the patient from starting to eat or drink. In short, if the physician's intent is the key, then terminal sedation is still more like euthanasia than withdrawal of treatment.

Although the Supreme Court's two primary justifications for the withdrawal-suicide distinction fail to support terminal sedation, proponents of terminal sedation might defend the practice by citing the principle of double effect. Under that principle, physicians may take steps that might hasten a patient's death as long as the steps are a reasonable effort to treat the patient's suffering, and the patient's death is not intended.[18] For example, it is permissible to give analgesics or sedatives to alleviate a patient's pain even if the drugs might halt the patient's breathing. However, the principle of double effect only justifies the sedation part of terminal sedation. We cannot justify the withdrawal of food and water part of terminal sedation, for that step does nothing to relieve the patient's suffering but only serves to bring on the patient's death. If it is argued that withdrawal of food and water is a permissible act, then we are back to the previous response that it is permissible only because the patient's inability to eat or drink results from an underlying disease.

Finally, it might be asserted that, with terminal sedation, the patient's death really is the result of the underlying disease rather than the physician's action. According to this argument, it is the patient's illness that creates the need for the sedation. The underlying disease is responsible for the patient's suffering and for the patient's request for palliative care. But this logic would also justify euthanasia (and assisted suicide). With euthanasia or assisted suicide, it is the patient's underlying disease that causes the patient to ask for a life-ending drug.

Terminal Sedation Versus Assisted Suicide

Terminal sedation is not only a type of euthanasia; it is also more problematic ethically than either assisted suicide or euthanasia. With respect to euthanasia, it poses the same risks of abuse while serving fewer of the purposes of right-to-die law. With respect to assisted suicide, terminal sedation both poses greater risks of abuse and serves fewer of the purposes of right-to-die law.

How does terminal sedation serve fewer of the purposes of right-to-die law than either assisted suicide or euthanasia? We recognize a patient's right to refuse life-sustaining treatment in large part because of the pain and suffering caused by the patient's illness. With respect to this concern, terminal sedation provides the same relief as assisted suicide or euthanasia. However, the right to refuse life-sustaining treatment responds to other concerns of dying patients, concerns that are met by assisted suicide and euthanasia but not by terminal sedation. These other concerns are not met because patients who undergo terminal sedation are required to accept a dying process that is prolonged relative to the dying process with assisted suicide or euthanasia. Terminal sedation thereby forces patients to linger in a state that they may feel is profoundly compromising of their dignity, that further distorts the memory they leave behind and that involves a drawn out and debilitating process for family members.[19] Terminal sedation also prevents patients from retaining a sense of control over the timing and circumstances of their death, a sense that may be critical to the psychological well-being of dying patients. Dying patients have little control over their lives. Critical matters will be determined almost entirely by their disease: How much longer they will live, where they will spend the remaining days or months of their lives, how many of their routine activities they will be able to manage by themselves and how much discomfort they will have. In addition, if they are in a hospital or other institution, their schedules will be determined in large part by the needs of their health-care providers. The option of assisted suicide gives patients more control because they ultimately decide when they will die.[20] In sum, terminal sedation is as beneficial to patients as assisted suicide or euthanasia in terms of relief of physical pain and distress but it is less beneficial in terms of the other concerns that patients have about their deaths.

At the same time, terminal sedation raises the same risks of abuse as assisted suicide or euthanasia. Patients who are not terminally—or even seriously—ill can end their lives by terminal sedation. Similarly, patients who mistakenly believe that they are terminally ill can choose terminal sedation. Patients might also choose to end their lives by terminal sedation because their mental competence is compromised by their disease or by a depression that would respond to psychiatric therapy. Terminally sedated patients might have been pushed to end their lives by their families or their physicians because of concerns about the costs of their care or the emotional burdens of caring for them. Terminally sedated patients might have chosen to end their lives because they did not receive appropriate palliative care for their suffering.

If we look at the other concerns with legalizing assisted suicide or euthanasia, we see that they apply in the same way to terminal sedation. If physician-assisted suicide (or euthanasia) would "undermine the trust that is essential to the doctor-patient relationship" because physicians would be killers as well as healers,[21] then the practice of terminal sedation would also undermine patient trust. With terminal sedation, the physician is hastening death rather than healing disease. Commentators observe that physician-assisted suicide is dangerous also because physicians undervalue the lives of patients who are terminally ill, elderly, or disabled and therefore are less likely to question suicidal impulses when their patients are terminally ill, elderly, or disabled rather than young and healthy.[22] But terminal sedation is similarly dangerous. When deciding whether to provide terminal sedation to a terminally ill, elderly, or disabled person, the physician's undervaluation of the patient's life will make the physician more likely to provide the sedation than if the patient is a young and healthy person. Critics of assisted suicide argue that it is more dangerous than withdrawal of treatment because treatment withdrawals typically occur in institutional settings where abuses are difficult to hide. However, like assisted suicide, terminal sedation can take place in the patient's home or other noninstitutional settings. Finally, if a right to *slippery slope* assisted suicide for the terminally ill must inevitably lead society down the slippery slope to assisted suicide for patients who are not terminally ill, then terminal sedation for the terminally ill will also inevitably lead to terminal sedation for patients who are not terminally ill.[23] All of the risks of abuse that exist for assisted suicide or euthanasia are also risks of abuse for terminal sedation.

Moreover, terminal sedation shares a serious risk with euthanasia that goes beyond the risks associated with assisted suicide. While it is not possible to coerce an unconscious or severely demented person to commit suicide,[24] it is a simple matter to terminally sedate, or perform euthanasia on, any incompetent person without that person's consent or even the person's knowledge. The death-causing act of assisted suicide is much more under the control of the patient than are the death-causing acts of terminal sedation and euthanasia.

In sum, when it comes to the issues that really count in determining the morality of a death-causing act by physicians—whether the act serves the purposes of right-to-die law and whether the act threatens patient welfare—terminal sedation turns out to be a worse alternative than euthanasia or assisted suicide.

The Court's preference for terminal sedation over assisted suicide seems puzzling. Not only is terminal sedation akin to euthanasia—a practice generally considered less acceptable than assisted suicide—it also leaves patients with an option that is ethically more problematic than the rejected practice of assisted suicide. Accordingly, the Court has preserved the distinction between treatment withdrawal and assisted suicide only by creating a constitutional scheme that is inferior compared to a regime in which there is a constitutional right to physician-assisted suicide.

Note the irony here. The Supreme Court rejected a right to assisted suicide in large part because of the risks that it poses.[25] While there might be some morally acceptable cases of assisted suicide, the Court was concerned that it would not be possible to limit assisted suicide to only those cases. Once we permit assisted suicide for some persons, we will have no principle for denying it to other persons who claim great suffering. Yet, by sanctioning terminal sedation—a practice with greater risks—the Court implicitly took the view that the risks of legalizing physician-assisted suicide can be sufficiently minimized. In other words, the Court must have concluded that physicians can be trusted to offer terminal sedation in appropriate situations without offering it in all situations. More specifically, the Court must have concluded that physicians will reserve terminal sedation accompanied by the withholding of nutrition and hydration for patients who meet certain criteria, such as that they are terminally ill and suffering intolerably. If physicians can limit terminal sedation to appropriate cases, then they can limit assisted suicide in the same way. By whatever criteria physicians employ to decide when terminal sedation is appropriate therapy, they can also decide when assisted suicide is appropriate therapy.

Explaining the Court's Reasoning

If terminal sedation essentially amounts to euthanasia in many cases, and if terminal sedation is more problematic ethically than assisted suicide, then why did three Supreme Court Justices explicitly endorse the practice while rejecting assisted suicide, and why did the other Justices signal their approval of terminal sedation?

In explaining the Court's decisions, there are two issues to be addressed: (1) Why would the Court endorse a practice that is essentially euthanasia? (2) Why would the Court reject the ethically superior alternative of assisted suicide?

As to why the Court would endorse a form of euthanasia, I believe there are two parts to answering this question. First, the Court's decision suggests that it cares more about why a patient wishes to die than how the patient dies. In endorsing terminal sedation despite its amounting to euthanasia at times, the Court is essentially saying that the right to die primarily reflects a moral sentiment that people who are dying and suffering intolerably should be allowed to die even if they cannot do so simply by refusing life-sustaining treatment.[26] The second part of the explanation for the Court's acceptance of terminal sedation is that the Court saw a right to terminal sedation as necessary to preserve a patient's right to refuse life-sustaining treatment. A dying patient might decide against further medical interventions, including a feeding tube, and then require heavy sedation for relief of pain. If the prohibition of euthanasia implied a prohibition of terminal sedation accompanied by the withdrawal of nutrition and hydration, the patient could not refuse the feeding tube once the sedation was employed. The patient would be forced to choose between obtaining relief from suffering and retaining the right to refuse life-sustaining treatment. This is a choice that people should not have to make.

The Court's decision to reject assisted suicide despite its acceptance of terminal sedation can be explained by comparing the typical case of terminal sedation with the typical case of suicide. While it is true that terminal sedation *can* effectively constitute euthanasia, and it is true that terminal sedation *can* be abused more than assisted suicide, terminal sedation in practice appears to be limited to appropriate cases. No one is suggesting that physicians are administering terminal sedation to people who are not seriously ill or who really should be treated with psychological counseling and antidepressive drugs.[27] In contrast, there is real concern that Dr. Jack Kevorkian is assisting the suicides of persons who are not seriously ill or who have serious psychological problems.[28] In addition, there are many suicides in this country that are committed by people who are psychologically depressed but who have no serious physical illness. The Court may have been concerned about the message to these people if it permitted assisted suicide for terminally ill persons.[29]

Nevertheless, the Court's preference for terminal sedation comes at a substantial cost. The Court rejected assisted suicide only by embracing euthanasia; it thereby undermined its efforts to preserve the active-passive distinction in patient deaths. Moreover, the benefits of terminal sedation come at a significant cost to patients. As discussed, patients who are denied assisted suicide and who therefore must choose terminal sedation are forced into a less desirable alternative. In addition, the permissibility of terminal sedation poses greater risks than assisted suicide for incompetent patients who would not want to die.

Notes

1. This paper builds on ideas that I am presenting in 24(4) *Hastings Constitutional Law Quarterly* (in press) and parts of that article are included here with permission of the *Hastings Constitutional Law Quarterly*. I gratefully acknowledge the contributions of Judy Failer, Ph.D.
2. *Vacco* v. *Quill*, 117 S. Ct. 2293 (1997).
3. David Orentlicher, "The Legalization of Physician-Assisted Suicide," *New England Journal of Medicine* 335 (9) (1996): 663–67. David Orentlicher, "The Legalization of Physician Assisted Suicide: A Very Modest Revolution," *Boston College Law Review* 38 (3) (1997): 443–75.
4. John Arras, "News from the Circuit Courts: How *Not* to Think About Physician-Assisted Suicide," *BioLaw* July-Aug. 1996: S171–S188.
5. *Washington* v. *Glucksberg*, 117 S. Ct. 2258, 2303 (1997) (O'Connor, J., concurring).
6. *Washington* v. *Glucksberg*, 117 S. Ct. 2258, 2311 (1997) (Breyer, J., concurring).
7. Ibid. at 2311–12.
8. While Justices Stevens and Souter did not discuss whether there is a constitutional right to obtain relief from severe suffering, their opinions suggest that they would be sympathetic to that view. Ibid. at 2291 n. 16 (Souter, J., concurring) (observing that there are important reasons for distinguishing assisted suicide from both aggressive pain control and the withdrawal of life-sustaining treatment); ibid. at 2308 (Stevens, J., concurring)

(stating that "[e]ncouraging the development and ensuring the availability of adequate pain treatment is of utmost importance"). Similarly, although the majority opinion in *Glucksberg* did not explicitly address the argument that the right at stake is the right to avoid suffering, the Court did signal its approval of sedation even into coma in *Quill*. There, the majority rejected the claim that such heavy sedation "is covert physician-assisted suicide." *Quill*, 117 S. Ct. at 2301 n.11.

9. Nathan I. Cherny and Russell K. Portenoy, "Sedation in the Management of Refractory Symptoms: Guidelines for Evaluation and Treatment," *Journal of Palliative Care* 10 (2) (1994): 31–38. Timothy E. Quill, Bernard Lo and Dan W. Brock, "Palliative Options of Last Resort: A Compariosn of Voluntary Stopping Eating and Drinking, Terminal Sedation, Physician-Assisted Suicide, and Voluntary Active Euthanasia," *Journal of the American Medical Association* 278 (1997): 2099–2104. Timothy E. Quill and Robert V. Brody, "'You Promised Me I Wouldn't Die Like This!': A Bad Death as a Medical Emergency," *Archives of Internal Medicine* 155 (1995): 1250–54. William R. Greene and William H. Davis, "Titrated Intravenous Barbiturates in the Control of Symptoms in Patients with Terminal Cancer," *Southern Medical Journal* 84 (1991): 332–37. Subha Ramani and Anand B. Karnad, "Long-Term Subcutaneous Infusion of Midazolam for Refractory Delirium in Terminal Breast Cancer," *Southern Medical Journal* 89 (1996): 1101–03.

10. Cherny and Portenoy, *supra* note 9, at 32.

11. David B. Reuben and Vincent Mor, "Dyspnea in Terminally Ill Cancer Patients," *Chest* 89 (1986): 234–36.

12. Cherny and Portenoy, *supra* note 9, at 35; Robert D. Truog, Charles B. Berde, Christine Mitchell, and Holcombe E. Grier, "Barbiturates in the Care of the Terminally Ill," *New England Journal of Medicine* 327 (1992): 1678–82.

13. It is "slow" euthanasia because the patient dies after a few hours or days rather than almost immediately. The term slow euthanasia has previously been used to describe other forms of euthanasia. See, e.g., J. Andrew Billings and Susan D. Block, "Slow Euthanasia," *Journal of Palliative Care* 12 (4) (1996): 21–30 (using slow euthanasia to refer to the practice of increasing the dose of palliative medications "not for the purpose of easing identifiable discomfort but with the expectation of hastening death gradually").

14. It is true that the withholding of food and water is an "omission" and therefore a different kind of action than an injection of a drug, and it is also true that the law often distinguishes "acts" from "omissions." Nevertheless, as Justice Antonin Scalia has observed, the line between appropriate and inappropriate patient deaths is not defined simply by the distinction between action and inaction. *Cruzan* v. *Director, Dept. of Health*, 497 U.S. 261 (1990) (Scalia, J., concurring) (observing that, if "one may not kill oneself by walking into the sea," then one may also not "sit on the beach until submerged by the incoming tide"). Moreover, ethicists have long argued that withholdings are worse than withdrawals since treatment withdrawals at least come after a trial of the therapy while withholdings deny the chance for an unexpected recovery.

15. Wayne R. LaFave and Austin W. Scott, Jr., *Substantive Criminal Law*, vol. 1 (St. Paul: West Publishing, 1986), pp. 302–309.

16. Ibid. at 305–309.

17. For example, the patient thought to be dependent on a ventilator for breathing may turn out to be able to breathe without a ventilator; the patient who is unable to eat or drink without a feeding tube may recover enough to start eating and drinking again.

18. Tom L. Beauchamp and James F. Childress, *Principles of Biomedical Ethics*, 4th ed. (New York: Oxford University Press, 1994), pp. 206–11.

19. *Cruzan*, 497 U.S. at 310–12 (Brennan, J., dissenting). ("For many, the thought of an ignoble end, steeped in decay, is abhorrent.... A long, drawn-out death can have a debilitating effect on family members.... For some, the idea of being remembered in their persistent vegetative state rather than as they were before their illness or accident may be very disturbing."). James Rachels, "Active and Passive Euthanasia," *New England Journal of Medicine* 292 (1975): 78–80.

20. Robert F. Weir, "The Morality of Physician-Assisted Suicide," *Law, Medicine and Health Care* 20 (1–2) (1992): 1116–26.

21. *Glucksberg*, 117 S. Ct. at 2273.

22. Ibid., 117 S. Ct. at 2273–2274.

23. Ibid., at 2274.

24. These persons are unable to take pills themselves. Marcia Angell, "The Supreme Court and Physician-Assisted Suicide—The Ultimate Right," *New England Journal of Medicine* 336 (January 2, 1997): 50–53.

25. *Glucksberg*, 117 S. Ct. at 2272–75.

26. Orentlicher, *supra*, note 3.

27. To be sure, this might reflect the fact that terminal sedation is not used very widely. As physicians begin to use it more, the chances of abuse will grow.

28. "Clash in Detroit Over How Ill a Kevorkian Client Really Was," *New York Times,* August 20, 1996, p. A-13.

29. *Glucksberg*, 117 S. Ct. at 2272 (discussing the seriousness of suicide as a public health problem).

19

Would Physician–Assisted Suicide Save the Healthcare System Money?

(Or, Is Jack Kevorkian Doing All of Us a Favor?)

MERRILL MATTHEWS, JR.

Physician-assisted suicide is often considered only in the context of the ethical problems it creates for patients, healthcare providers, and society. However, there is also an economic aspect to physician-assisted suicide that people discussing the topic often try to avoid. In this chapter I examine some of the economic questions surrounding the debate. How much does it cost to die? Does treating one person mean we have to sacrifice the care of others? How many people would actually request a physician's assistance in committing suicide? And, would the availability of physician-assisted suicide save the healthcare system money? By looking at how much money people spend on healthcare at the end of life (the last six months for our purposes) and estimating how many people would request physician-assisted suicide, we can estimate the total amount, or upper limit, of money saved. That allows us to evaluate whether the amount of money is large enough that it must be considered in the public policy debate over physician-assisted suicide.

*　　*　　*

P HYSICIAN-ASSISTED SUICIDE is often considered only in the context of the ethical problems it creates for patients, healthcare providers, and society. However, there is also an economic aspect to physician-assisted suicide that people discussing the topic often try to avoid, in part because it is thought that questions touching on life and death ought not to be sullied by the insertion of economic considerations.[1] Even the debate over Dr. Jack Kevorkian and his indelicate attempts to make society face the dilemma of a terminal patient needing the assistance of a "healer" in order to die has completely avoided any comment about whether these untimely deaths will save the rest of us some money.

Unfortunately, however, ignoring the economic aspects of medical decisions is a fading luxury. For better or worse, medical ethics and medical economics are increasingly becoming two sides of the same coin—a coin being pinched by employers, insurers, and the federal government. Decisions to treat or not to treat a patient may have implications that affect other patients' health—or lives. This problem is most evident in the allocation of human organs, where donor scarcity keeps thousands of people waiting and hoping, while physicians and ethicists are faced with the decision of who should receive a new organ.

While most of the chapters in this volume examine the moral questions arising from physician-assisted suicide (in which a physician provides a patient with the means to end his life),[2] this essay examines some of the economic questions surrounding the debate.

1. How much does it cost to die?
2. Does treating one person mean we have to sacrifice the care of others?
3. What guidelines should be used in order to protect the patients and the physicians?
4. How many people would actually request a physician's assistance in committing suicide?
5. If there were generally agreed-upon guidelines for granting patient requests for physician assistance in committing suicide, and the assistance were legal and accepted, would the availability of physician-assisted suicide save the healthcare system money?
6. And, will we someday look back and thank Jack Kevorkian for doing us all a favor?

These questions are economic, but they lead to some that are more normative. For example, if it could be shown that physician-assisted suicide saved the healthcare system money, should that factor play a role in deciding whether to adopt physician-assisted suicide as a society? And if physician-assisted suicide made economic sense, wouldn't it only be a matter of time before proponents converted the economic arguments into moral arguments?

Whether the economic aspect of the issue or the moral aspect is more important is still open to question. What seems clear is that patients and their friends and loved ones will be increasingly confronted not with simply the high cost of living, but the high cost of dying. By looking at how much money people spend on healthcare at the end of life (the last six months for our purposes) and estimating how many people would request physician-assisted suicide, we should be able to estimate the total amount, or upper limit, of money saved. Finally, we will evaluate whether this amount of money is large enough that it must be considered in the public policy debate over physician-assisted suicide.

How Much Does It Cost to Die?

As most people who have recently lost a loved one know, dying can cost a lot of money. Physician and hospital bills can add up quickly, devastating family budgets and savings—especially for those who have limited or no health insurance. Add funeral bills on top of medical expenses—since people tend to blur all the costs together—and dying can become as traumatic financially as it is socially.

However, even though personal experience and anecdotal evidence implies that it costs a lot to die, it is hard to say just how much. Estimating healthcare utilization costs for those at the end of life is difficult because there is no consistent tracking system that encompasses all expenses. Furthermore, some studies imply that many of our common assumptions about the high costs of dying are wrong. For example, it is often argued that the higher expenses at the end of life are a result of overutilization of more expensive hospitals rather than less expensive home or hospice care. But according to a study by the National Center for Health Statistics, more than half of all seniors die in nursing homes or in their own residences (1994).[3]

While several studies over the past fifteen years have tried to quantify the financial burden those in the last stages of life impose, the conclusions have varied significantly based on the assumptions and the medical conditions involved. The most accurate source of healthcare costs at the end of life comes from the Health Care Financing Administration (HCFA), which regularly tracks healthcare costs for Medicare recipients in their last year of life. According to HCFA:[4]

- 6.4 percent (1.9 million) of Medicare beneficiaries died in 1994, with an average annual cost of $15,761 per beneficiary, or 20.6 percent ($30.2 billion) of all Medicare spending for the year.
- That is about 3.8 times higher than the average annual cost imposed by beneficiaries who survived the year ($4,131).[4]

While HCFA's figures are helpful, they are limited. For example, seniors spend money out of pocket on healthcare for services such as nursing home care that Medicare does not reimburse and HCFA does not track.

By one estimate, HCFA's figures are only 45 percent of seniors' total healthcare costs at the end of life. If we add in the other 55 percent, as Ezekiel J. and Linda L. Emanuel have done in a *New England Journal of Medicine* article estimating the cost of care in the last year of life, we arrive at a total cost of $35,020 (adjusted to 1994 figures).[5]

But what about those under age sixty-five?

- Based on a study by Anne Scitovsky of under-age-sixty-five deaths in California, the Emanuels argue that they are justified in assuming that end-of-life costs for those under age sixty-five are approximately equivalent to those of seniors who are in the sixty-five to seventy-nine year old range—which run about 15 percent higher than the average for all seniors ($15,761), or about $18,125 for 1994.[6]
- Then they assume that, like Medicare, this figure only covers about 45 percent of the total healthcare costs incurred, and so they increase the number by the other 55 percent. Using this methodology would make last-year costs for those under sixty-five about $39,875 for 1994.

Are these figures accurate? It's impossible to know for sure. It seems likely, however, that the Emanuels' attempt to use the same methodology (i.e., assuming the recorded costs are only 45 percent of total healthcare costs) for both those under sixty-five and over sixty-five probably overstates under-sixty-five patients' expenses. The Emanuels' primary justification for raising seniors' estimated healthcare costs from Medicare's estimate of $15,761 per year to $35,020 is the nursing home factor, which can lead to high out-of-pocket expenditures. But nursing homes play a far smaller role for those under sixty-five.

However, even if the Emanuels' methodology overstates the healthcare costs of those under sixty-five, and perhaps those over sixty-five as well, their approach is still useful in trying to establish an upper limit on healthcare spending for those at the end of life. Healthcare costs can vary significantly, depending on the medical condition that is afflicting the patient. A person who is dying of old age will likely have much lower costs, on average, than cancer and AIDS patients. Since those seeking assistance in dying are more likely to have a costly medical condition—e.g., requiring a ventilator, constant nursing home or intensive care—high-end cost estimates are probably justified.[7] Moreover, even if the Emanuels' methodology overestimates the costs somewhat, other surveys seem to indicate that they are not unreasonable.[8] Therefore, we shall use the estimates presented by Medicare and Scitovsky as our low-end costs, and the Emanuels' methodology to establish our high-end costs.

There are other points that must also be considered. As the end nears, healthcare spending rises. For many seniors, costs in the last month of life will be significantly higher than those who are twelve months away from death. That means that any cost estimates over periods of less than a year must be weighted toward the final months. In an analysis of Medicare patients with cancer during their last six months, from July 1 to December 31, 1992, Lewin-VHI (now the Lewin Group) found that:

- The healthcare costs of patients who did not go into a hospice were $1,436 during the sixth month before death, while those in their last month of life spent $8,723.[9]
- For the total twelve-month period preceding death, costs were $26,206, which means that about three-fourths of the total spending for the last year came in the last six months and that one-third of the last year's costs came in the final month.[10]
- If we now take three-fourths of our upper-end estimates of the cost of care for the last year of life—$35,020 for seniors and $39,875 for those under sixty-five—we arrive at an outside estimate of the cost of care for the last six months of $26,265 for seniors and $29,906 for those under sixty-five. (Low-end costs would be $11,820 and $13,593, respectively.)

Does Treating One Person Mean We Have to Sacrifice the Care of Others?

One of the most difficult encounters healthcare professionals face is saying no to a patient:

- No, we don't know what's causing your illness.
- No, we know what's wrong, but we do not have what we need to cure your condition.
- No, we don't have a suitable organ available at this time.
- No, with such a poor prognosis, we cannot justify spending the money necessary to cure your condition while others who would benefit so much more are denied care.

Of the four "nos" listed above, surely the last is the one that causes the most anguish, largely because we do not think that people's healthcare needs should be captive to their checkbooks. Rejections due to a lack of knowledge, a lack of skill, or a scarcity of organs just seem less objectionable than a rejection due to a lack of money. Nevertheless, the economic "no" is increasingly heard around the world—probably less in the United States than in most other countries because we do not have a "zero-sum system." But even that is changing.

A "zero-sum system" in economic parlance means a society in which total economic resources are capped so that a dollar spent on Smith means one less dollar available to Jones.[11] Most countries with socialized medicine operate under such a system. Through the political process, the government determines how much money will be spent on healthcare services, as well as other services such as welfare, education, and defense. Because it is a political process, compromises are made, and no one program gets all the money its defenders think it needs. As a result, there is never enough healthcare money—or education or welfare money, for that matter—to go around.

That situation can create some extremely difficult decisions for providers in a national health system. If there is not enough money to provide everyone with everything they need—and there never is—some will lose out as healthcare is rationed. But how should a country make those determinations? On a first-come-first-served basis? On a greatest need basis? On a sliding scale based on income? By determining who contributes the most value to society? Fortunately, most United States healthcare providers and their patients have been able to avoid the rationing decisions that come as a result of a zero-sum system. Most, but not all. The limited funds available in Medicaid, the federal-state health insurance program for the poor, have forced some providers and even state legislatures to look for arguments to justify rationing.

Case Study: Oregon

In 1987 the Oregon legislature decided to cancel Medicaid funding for about thirty organ transplant recipients so that the state could expand services to poor women and children and still balance the Medicaid budget. Since then, the state has been openly advocating healthcare rationing.

In 1991 Oregon decided to rank medical treatments in terms of priority, taking into consideration such factors as costs, benefit to the patient, the extent to which treatment would affect the patient's quality of life, and community values.[12] The original list of 709 procedures was established by a first-of-its-kind public process that included hearings, community meetings, and telephone surveys. The legislature was not permitted to change the order on the list. It could only determine at what procedure to cease funding, based on the available money for that year. Those whose medical condition fell above the line would receive treatment; those with conditions that fell below the line would be out of luck. When Oregon asked the federal government for a waiver from normal Medicaid regulations in order to implement its new plan, the Bush administration denied the request on the grounds that it would allow treatment to be denied patients with advanced stages of AIDS since, at the time, there was no hope of a cure (and, thus, no "benefit").[13] Once Oregon had made a few changes, President Clinton approved the waiver request.[14]

Other states have not followed Oregon's lead. Rather, they are moving their poor populations into managed care, primarily health maintenance organizations (HMOs). From a state legislator's standpoint, this is a good political move. The HMOs that receive the contract charge less per patient than the state was spending under traditional Medicaid, saving the state some money. That's a "win" for the legislators because it frees up money for other needs. The politicians also pass most of the responsibility for ensuring the quality of care to the HMO. Thus, if a Medicaid patient is found scamming or abusing the system, the HMO, not the legislators, is deemed responsible. That's also a "win" for the politicians. Finally, the HMO, not the Medicaid system, rations the care, deciding which physician the poor patient can or cannot see and what treatment he can or cannot have. Of course, when middle- and upper-income patients get squeezed by the HMOs, we often hear about it in the news—albeit after the patient's death—when the families complain and file a lawsuit. The poor usually suffer their rationing in silence.

But that's Medicaid, which covers only about 14 percent of the population. Most Medicaid recipients are healthy and need little care. Most other patients encountering the U.S. healthcare system will find it to be an open-ended system rather than a zero-sum system. That is, an extra dollar spent on Smith does not necessarily take anything away from Jones. If Smith spends a dollar on healthcare, we just add that dollar to total healthcare spending. Even if seniors spend more Medicare money than the U.S. government has budgeted, bills do not go unpaid and doctors and hospitals do not shut down. The federal government pays whatever bills come in from Medicare, and the government shows that it underprojected the program's growth for that year.

However, the open-ended nature of most of the United States healthcare system doesn't mean it provides a blank check—at least not anymore. Increasingly, employers are clamping down on employee healthcare utilization, primarily by turning to managed care plans that impose a type of internal rationing by not allowing patients a full range of choices in physicians, medical procedures, pharmaceuticals, length of hospital stays, and so on. And Medicare keeps ratcheting down its provider reimbursements, giving healthcare providers a financial incentive to reduce the amount and quality of care.

But even though the various elements that make up the American healthcare system are becoming more circumspect in ensuring that money is not wasted, the cap that marks a zero-sum healthcare system is largely absent in the United States. Of course, ethicists and physicians might still argue that physician-assisted suicide is justified on moral or other grounds. But, considering the way we finance healthcare in the United States, it would be hard to make a case that there is a financial imperative compelling us to adopt physician-assisted suicide in an effort to save money so that others could benefit.

What Guidelines Would Be Used for Physician-Assisted Suicide?

Several proposals have been made by physicians and other groups that would establish clinical criteria for physician-assisted suicide in the United States. When Drs. Timothy Quill et al. opened the discussion of clinical criteria with their 1992 article in the *New England Journal of Medicine,* they suggested several elements that should be included.[15] Since then, a number of others have weighed in with proposals, including several states. And Oregon's legislation ultimately placed the issue of whether patients had a right to a physician's assistance in committing suicide before the United States Supreme Court. (The Court did not find that a patient has a constitutional right to such assistance.)

One of the most recent attempts at consensus came from a group of medical ethics committees located in San Francisco, where the high incidence of AIDS has forced a disproportionately large number of physicians and hospitals to consider requests for physician-assisted suicide.[16] Like many other proposals, this new set of guidelines includes second opinions, a waiting period and psychiatric evaluation for depression.[17] For purposes of this paper, we will adopt the guideline that requires a diagnosis that the patient has less than six months to live.

Would physicians strictly follow these, or any other, guidelines if they became law? Indications from the Netherlands imply that guidelines may provide physicians with some direction in the beginning, but eventually they fade into the background—especially if the government does not hold doctors criminally liable for bypassing the guidelines.[18] The Dutch Royal Society of Medicine endorsed a set of guidelines in 1984, even though euthanasia and physician-assisted suicide were, and still are, officially against the law. But physicians began to ignore the guidelines shortly after they were passed. For example, the most recent analysis of euthanasia and physician-assisted suicide in the Netherlands found that 23 percent of the physicians interviewed had ended a patient's life without a specific request—even though the guidelines require informed consent for proceeding.[19]

Quill et al. wanted to be sensitive to the notion that not every patient would fit into a specific mold and wanted to leave physicians some discretion in making the decision about who should be assisted in dying. He considered recognizing a window in which a terminal patient might be approved for assisted suicide, but rejected the notion on the basis that a few cases might be worthy of physician assistance even if the patient was not terminal or if the physician does not know how much time was left. However, it would be very unlikely that such an open-ended approach has any possibility of being adopted in the near future. Thus, we will stick with the more palatable guideline of less than six months to live for purposes of estimating how much money physician-assisted suicide would save the healthcare system.

How Often Do Patients Request Assistance in Dying?

Much more often than they actually receive it, if the Dutch experience with physician-assisted suicide can serve as a basis for making an estimate. While euthanasia and physician-assisted suicide are illegal in the Netherlands, as mentioned earlier, both are accepted by the state and by the medical profession—with euthanasia being much more common than physician-assisted suicide. Two studies, one in 1990 and a follow-up comparative study in 1995, evaluated both the number of requests from patients and the extent to which physicians complied. According to the study, "88 percent [of the physicians responding] said they had received at least one request for euthanasia or physician-assisted suicide at a later time in the course of disease, whereas 77 percent had received at least one explicit request for a particular time."[20]

However, the compliance rate was much smaller. In 1990, 0.3 percent of the deaths examined by the investigators were due to physician-assisted suicide; and in 1995, 0.4 percent of deaths were. Euthanasia accounted for 1.9 percent and 2.3 percent, respectively.[21]

There are enough similarities between the Dutch and U.S. populations to speculate that, were physician-assisted suicide accepted in the United States, requests and compliances would be similar to those in the Netherlands. Fortunately, we do not have to speculate too hard. Back et al. have already conducted a survey of physicians in the state of Washington. They came up with almost identical responses to those in the Netherlands. According to the study:

- Washington physicians received requests for euthanasia or physician-assisted suicide (0.2 requests per year) about as often as Dutch physicians received them (0.25 to 0.8 per year).
- 24 percent of Washington physicians had complied with a request, as opposed to a little less than a third in the Netherlands.

Back et al. did not examine deaths as van der Maas et al. have done in Holland, but, based on the similarities of the patient requests and physician compliance, it is reasonable to say that we could expect—indeed, may already be experiencing—that 0.4 percent of all deaths would involve a physician's assistance. Since approximately 2.3 million Americans died in 1994, we can estimate that about 9,200 patients would be categorized as physician-assisted suicide.[22]

Would Physician-Assisted Suicide Save Money?

The answer to the question seems almost certainly no, at least not enough to justify legalizing physician-assisted suicide. The primary reason is that the number of people seeking physician-assisted suicide and being granted that assistance is extremely small. If, based on the Dutch experience, we could expect about 9,200 patients to die from physician-assisted suicide, and their medical care costs for the last six months of life would range between $11,820 and $26,265 for seniors and $13,593 and $29,906 for those under sixty-five, we can conclude that we would save $179 million at the high end for seniors, and $72 million for those under sixty-five, for a total of $251 million.[23]

While one might reasonably argue that $251 million is a lot and would indeed support the proposition that physician-assisted suicide would save the healthcare system money, two very important points should be considered. First, $251 million is a "worst case" (or "best case") scenario. That is, it assumes that those granted assistance in dying are doing so six months out, and thus saving all the money that would have been spent in the interval. In fact, most requests for physician assistance come in the last month, or even the last days of life, which would drastically reduce the actual amount of money saved. For example, in the survey of Dutch physicians, 64 percent said they had shortened a patient's life by less than twenty-four hours, and in 16 percent it was shortened less than a week.[24]

Second, as the survey of Washington physicians indicates, many U.S. physicians are already granting patients' requests for assistance in dying—in numbers almost as large as those in the Netherlands where physician assistance is overt rather than covert. While the total number of patients seeking assistance and the number of physicians complying would likely increase were physician-assisted suicide legal and open—it would probably increase even more if, heaven forbid, it were encouraged—there is little indication that it would grow significantly, if the Dutch experience is any guide. Thus, if we as a society decide to adopt physician-assisted suicide, it should be for other than economic reasons.

Is Jack Kevorkian Doing Us All a Favor?

The debate over physician-assisted suicide has revolved entirely around the ethical dilemmas it creates, and this examination of the economic side of the issue implies that ethics rather than economics should continue to be our primary concern. If countless Americans were suffering while money was being wasted on terminal patients who were receiving no therapeutic benefit, then perhaps an economic—and ultimately utilitarian—case for physician-assisted suicide could be made. As we have seen, however, only a small percentage of Americans fall under a zero-sum healthcare system. The vast majority do not and are therefore not deprived of care because there is not enough money to go around.

Moreover, it is possible that legalization of physician-assisted suicide would cost society *more* money. By helping a number of people end their lives early, Kevorkian has saved some healthcare expenditures, but he has surely offset these savings in attorneys' fees and court costs. Since American physicians generally act covertly in providing suicide assistance to dying patients, families may often remain ignorant of the physician's role. Open that system up for discussion and scrutiny in our litigious society and we will surely see the number of wrongful death cases rise significantly.

Thus, it is hard to see how, given our current healthcare system, its sources of financing, and the small number of people seeking assistance in dying, one could make an economic case for physician-assisted suicide—now, or for a long time to come. So if Jack Kevorkian is doing us a favor, it stems from the fact that he is forcing society—albeit in a somewhat crude manner—to face an ethical question, rather than an economic question, that it would prefer to ignore.

Notes

1. Discussing the cost savings that might accrue from physician-assisted suicide, Daniel Callahan of the Hastings Center notes, "This has never been the stated view of most prominent proponents of this measure, but as in the case for advanced directives, sometimes it is quietly advanced as a nice byproduct." "Controlling the Costs of Health Care for the Elderly—Fair Means and Foul," *New England Journal of Medicine* 335 (10) (September 5, 1996): 745.

2. In euthanasia, by contrast, a physician terminates a patient's life at the patient's or family's request—at least that's how it's supposed to work.

3. "Seven Deadly Myths: Uncovering the Facts About the High Cost of the Last Year of Life" (Washington, D.C.: Alliance for Aging Research, no date): p. 6.

4. Health Care Financing Review, *1996 Statistical Supplement* (Baltimore: U.S. Department of Health and Human Services, 1996): p. 32. While Medicare recipients' end-of-life costs have remained remarkably consistent over the years, costs of those who survive have increased significantly.

5. Ezekiel J. Emanuel and Linda L. Emanuel, "The Economics of Dying: The Illusion of Cost Savings at the End of Life," *New England Journal of Medicine* 330 (8) (February 24, 1994): 540–44.

6. Anne A. Scitovsky, "Medical Care in the Last Twelve Months of Life: The Relation Between Age, Functional Status, and Medical Care Expenditures," *Millbank Quarterly* 66 (4) (1988): 640–60.

7. In a survey of Washington state physicians, Anthony L. Back, et al., found that two-thirds of the patients requesting physician-assisted suicide had either cancer or AIDS or had a neurological disease. Anthony L. Back, et al., "Physician-Assisted Suicide and Euthanasia in Washington State: Patient Requests and Physician Responses," *Journal of the American Medical Association* 275 (12) (March 27, 1996): 919–25.

8. See, for example, Ezekiel J. Emanuel, "Cost Savings at the End of Life: What Do the Data Show?" *Journal of the American Medical Association* 275 (24) (June 26, 1996): 1907–14; A. Maksoud, D. W. Jalmigen and C. I. Skibinski, "Do Not Resuscitate Orders and the Cost of Death," *Archives of Internal Medicine* 153 (1993): 1249–53; Peter A. Singer and F. H. Lowy, "Rationing, Patient Preferences and Cost of Care at the End of Life," *Archives of Internal Medicine* 152 (1992): 478–80.

9. Lewin-VHI, Inc., "An Analysis of the Cost Savings of the Medicare Hospice Benefit" (Miami: National Hospice Organization, 1995). Cited in Emanuel, "Cost Savings at the End of Life."

10. While this figure is lower than the estimate by the Emanuels, it includes medical care and not nursing home care.

11. Lester C. Thurow, *The Zero Sum Society: Distribution and the Possibilities for Economic Change* (New York: Basic Books, 1980).

12. See Timothy Egan, "Oregon Shakes Up Pioneering Health Plan for the Poor," *New York Times*, February 22, 1991.

13. "Oregon's Bid to Boost Coverage Gets Federal Red Light," *Congressional Quarterly* (August 8, 1992): 2362.

14. A few years ago I had the opportunity to be on a program with the person in charge of implementing Oregon's new Medicaid system. Oregon had just recently become the first state to pass a physician-assisted suicide provision. I pointed out during the debate that, while it may be only a coincidence, I thought it very interesting that the first state to openly embrace healthcare rationing was also the first state to adopt physician-

assisted suicide. The administrator denied any connection, but still the coincidence invites conjecture.

15. Timothy E. Quill, Christine K. Cassel, and Diane E. Meier, "Care for the Hopelessly Ill: Proposed Clinical Criteria for Physician-Assisted Suicide," *New England Journal of Medicine* 327 (19) (November 5, 1992): 1380–84.

16. Lee R. Slome, et al., "Physician-Assisted Suicide and Patients with Human Immuno-deficiencyVirus Disease," *New England Journal of Medicine* 336 (6) (February 6, 1997): 417–21.

17. Gina Kolata, " 'Passive Euthanasia' Is the Norm in Today's Hospitals, Doctors Say," *New York Times*, Saturday, June 28, 1997.

18. Herbert Hendin, Chris Rutenfrans, and Zbigniew Zylicz, "Physician-Assisted Suicide and Euthanasia in the Netherlands: Lessons from the Dutch," *Journal of the American Medical Association* 277 (21) (June 4, 1997): 1721. Among the most disturbing lapses from the guidelines reported by Hendin et al. are these: "50 percent of physicians reported that they considered it appropriate to suggest euthanasia to patients"; the lack of consultation with another physician; and ending the patient's life without the patient's consent.

19. Peter van der Maas, et al., "Euthanasia, Physician-Assisted Suicide, and Other Medical Practices Involving the End of Life in the Netherlands, 1990–1995," *New England Journal of Medicine* 335 (22) (November 28, 1996): 1699–705.

20. Ibid, 1701.

21. Ibid.

22. *Statistical Abstract of the United States, 1996* (Washington, D.C.: U.S. Department of Commerce, October 1996): Table no. 131; See also Kathleen M. Foley, "Competent Care for the Dying Instead of Physician-Assisted Suicide," *New England Journal of Medicine* 336 (1) (January 2, 1997): 55.

23. Ibid. About 1.7 million seniors died in 1994. The other 600,000 were under sixty-five. Therefore, 6,800 of the assisted deaths would be seniors and 2,400 would be under sixty-five.

24. Van der Maas, et al., "Euthanasia, Physician-Assisted Suicide, and Other Medical Practices Involving the End of Life in the Netherlands, 1990–1995," p. 1702.

Part Five

Considering Religious Perspectives

EVEN IN A SOCIETY that accepts the principle of separation of church and state, religious attitudes come into play. Individual voters and their political representatives may have religious convictions, and those beliefs are sometimes reflected in the positions those individuals adopt. We cannot fail to acknowledge the religious forces at work in our society's conflict over abortion. Physician-assisted suicide is another issue where religious convictions may come to play a significant role in the public debate.

Because religions have traditionally provided comfort to the dying, rituals for dealing with the death of a loved one, accounts of death and an afterlife, interpretations of the meaning of death, and sanctions against killing, we can expect that religions will offer perspectives on assisted suicide. In this section we have asked Catholic, Protestant, and Jewish theologians to offer their positions on physician-assisted suicide based on their own religious sources. Significant controversy on assisted suicide can be found within each of these religious traditions and these papers are clearly not intended, and should not be understood, as definitive answers or as even consensus reports from these religious perspectives. The contributions in this section are offered merely as examples of the tone of religious debate within these religious communities. They are intended to reveal the kinds of considerations that will be relevant in the religious dialogue of three prominent religious traditions.

In that spirit, John Paris and Michael Moreland's essay, "Catholic Perspectives on Ending Life" considers the evidence to be taken into account in Catholic reasoning. Cynthia Cohen's chapter provides the reasoning of the Committee on Medical Ethics of the Episcopal Diocese of Washington and their account of alternative Anglican positions. Allen Verhey's essay, "A Protestant Perspective on Ending Life: Faithfulness in the Face of Death," offers an argument in the voice of a sermon. And Noam Zohar's chapter, "Jewish Deliberation on Suicide: Exceptions, Toleration, and Assistance," presents a carefully crafted talmudic argument.

20

A Catholic Perspective
on Physician–Assisted Suicide

JOHN J. PARIS AND MICHAEL P. MORELAND

This essay explains the Catholic understanding of life as a gift from God, something over which we have stewardship, not dominion. According to this view, it
is not for us to end life when it becomes overly burdensome, difficult, or
demanding. The duty to preserve life, however, is not absolute. There is no moral
obligation to utilize measures that the individual perceives to be disproportionately burdensome. In the words of the Vatican *Declaration on Euthanasia*, "One
cannot impose on anyone the obligation to have recourse to a technique which
is not the equivalent of suicide (or euthanasia); on the contrary, it should be
considered as an acceptance of the human condition, or a wish to avoid the
application of medical procedure disproportionate to the results that can be
expected."

*   *   *

To die proudly when it is no longer possible to live proudly. Death freely chose,
death at the right time, brightly and cheerfully accomplished amid children
and witnesses. . . . From love of life, one should desire a different death: free,
conscious, without accident, without ambush.

—Nietzsche, "Morality for Physicians—Twilight of the Idols"

IN ITS RULING ON PHYSICIAN-ASSISTED SUICIDE, the United States
Supreme Court rejected the argument that an individual's constitutionally
protected "liberty interest" extends to the right to assistance in suicide. In the
course of its sweeping opinions in the companion cases of *Washington* v. *Glucksberg* and *Vacco* v. *Quill* the Court noted the limited character of personal autonomy.[1] Though we are free, we are not fully free; individuals cannot do whatever
they want indifferent to the implications of their actions on themselves or on
others. This concern for the well being of the individual and that of the "common good" was among the "rationally related interests" that a state may constitutionally impose on individuals' behavior.

Such interests, the court observed, are broad based and far reaching. In the
area of physician-assisted suicide they include such societal concerns as prohibiting intentional killing and preserving human life; preventing the serious
public health problem of suicide, especially among the young, the elderly, and
those suffering from untreated pain or from deep depression; protecting the
integrity and ethics of the medical profession; maintaining the physician's role
as healer; protecting vulnerable populations from psychological and financial

pressure to end their lives; and avoiding the slide toward voluntary and involuntary euthanasia.

In the course of its opinion, the Supreme Court also rejected the Second Circuit Courts of Appeals' equation of treatment with suicide.[2] As the Court stated, "We think the distinction between assisting suicide and withdrawing life-sustaining treatment, a distinction widely recognized and endorsed by the medical profession and our legal traditions, is both important and logical." In making that argument the Supreme Court made it clear that the circuit court erred when it had held the Supreme Court ruling in *Cruzan* authorizing the withdrawal of life-sustaining medical treatments was implicit approval of suicide.[3] In the Court's words: "[W]e certainly gave no intimation [in *Cruzan*] that the right to refuse unwanted medical treatment could be somehow transmitted into a right to assistance in committing suicide."

The Court buttressed its support for the distinction between killing and letting die with reference to the fundamental legal principles of causation and intent. As Chief Justice William Rehnquist put it in his opinion for the Court: "When a patient refuses life-sustaining medical treatment, he dies from an underlying fatal disease or pathology; but if he ingests lethal medication prescribed by a physician, he is killed by that medication." Further, as the Court noted in a citation to Dr. Leon Kass, "a physician who honors a patient's wish to cease doing useless and futile or degrading things to a patient when [the patient] no longer stands to benefit from them," even though that death may be foreseen or anticipated, does not intend the patient's death. That, however, is not true of one who assists in a suicide. There, in the Court's phrasing, the physician "must necessarily and indubitably, intend primarily that the patient be made dead."

Though the Supreme Court rejected the claim of constitutional protection for physician-assisted suicide, its opinion, and more particularly the concurring opinions of Justices O'Connor and Breyer, and especially Justice John Paul Stevens, did not exclude the possibility of approval of physician participation in a dying patient's suicide. As the Court opinion put it: "Our holding permits the debate to continue, as it should in a democratic society."

As is clear from the Court's opinion and the comments of the concurring justices, constitutional argument and legal reasoning alone have not and will not settle the debate over physician-assisted suicide. In a diverse pluralistic society there are and will continue to be widely differing values and sharply clashing choices on the issue of how we should live and when and how we should die.

Even within the unanimous court, there was disagreement if not dissent on the role physicians should have in the death of a patient. As Justice Stevens's lengthy concurrence made obvious, those differences "are not necessarily resolved by the opinions announced today." The debate and the persuasion necessary for the enactment of policy choices remains an on-going process.

One voice in the debate on how we are to understand the meaning of life and of death is that of religion. Are we, as the Supreme Court put it in the rhetorical extravagance that marked its *Casey* opinion, entities who have "the right to define one's own concept of existence, of meaning, of the universe, and the mysteries of human life?"[4] Or do we have a different and more modest role than as "masters of the universe?" If, as the Ninth Circuit held in its opinion on physician-assisted suicide, the "mastery of life" argument from *Casey* is the lodestone of our analysis, there is and ought not be any limit on "self-sovereignty." Personal choice with regard to lifestyle as well as "how and when to die" are but corollaries of our autonomy.

Catholic View of Death

The Catholic tradition views life—and death—differently. Life is seen not as "self-creation" but as a gift of the Creator, a gift over which we are to exercise stewardship, not dominion.[5] That stewardship demands that we be responsible for life—its protection and enhancement. We will in turn be held accountable before God not only for how we protected and developed our individual lives, but for all life. We are in the words of scripture, "Our brother's keeper."

The implication of a stewardship approach for the issue of physician-assisted suicide is, as University of Notre Dame law professor M. Cathleen Kaveny notes, that we do not have total control over our lives. Life is not ours to dispose of when we choose. It is not property which we can trade, sell, or destroy at will. In her words, "By aiming at our own deaths we usurp God's proper providence in allotting the span of our lives."[6] In attempting to do so, we transgress what Harvard Divinity School's J. Bryan Hehir labels "the definitive limits that are entrusted to us with life—we do not own it."[7]

Life, though, is not an end in itself. It has been given to us, as Richard McCormick, S.J., phrased it in his now-landmark 1974 *JAMA* essay "To Save or Let Die," that we might achieve salvation through fidelity to the Great Commandments of love of God and love of neighbor.[8] To achieve that goal one must enter into and be active in relationships. When the potential for those relationships is either nonexistent or exhausted, one's purpose in creation is fulfilled. When that moment is reached—in advanced old age or merely moments after birth—the duty to maintain life is ended.

McCormick elaborated on the limited duty to preserve life in a recent essay on assisted suicide:

> Life is a basic good but not an absolute one. It is basic because, as the Congregation for the Doctrine of the Faith worded it, it is the "necessary source and condition of every human society and all of society." It is not absolute because there are higher goods for which life can be sacrificed [such as the] glory of God, salvation of souls, service of one's brethren.[9]

Seen in this context, death is not an unmitigated evil, nor is it the enemy. Rather, it is but a stage in the pilgrimage of life. It is a hollowing out of the earthly that we might be filled and fulfilled in God.[10] Within this understanding of life, suicide is a violation of God's dominion. It is the ultimate act of defiance—the assertion of self over divine sovereignty.

Death in the Christian context is not defeat or failure. It is rather a transformation from earthly to eternal life. As such it is a necessary and integral aspect of life, one that both marks and makes possible the completion of a process that begins and ends in God. As St. Augustine wrote in his *Confessions*, "Thou stir man to take pleasure in praising thee, because thou have made us for thyself and our heart is restless until it rests in thee."[11] Given this perspective on life and death, there is no obligation to act officiously to preserve life, when life itself is ebbing away. Such attempts which but ensnare us in technology—trapped as it were in a twilight game between life and death—serve no Christian purpose.

This theology on life and death is the basis for the four-hundred-year-old tradition in Catholic moral theology that there is no obligation to employ what has in the past been labeled "extraordinary" means of preserving life.[12] That term, now outmoded and at times even detrimental to an appropriate understanding of Catholic teaching on care of the dying, indicated that no one had an obligation to employ measures that were disproportionately burdensome to the patient.[13] Thus, if a technique were available that could extend life but was "overly costly, burdensome, or painful"—or even if it were inexpensive, readily available, and easily administered—and did not offer a realistic expectation of substantial reversal of the disability, there was no obligation to use it.[14] The patient could be allowed to die.

The liturgical expression of that moral teaching was the prayer fervently made on behalf of the gravely ill patient "for a speedy recovery or a happy death." The prayer was made with the conviction that with life places us in the face of a mystery that is larger that we are, a mystery in Fr. J. Bryan Hehir's terms, "that comes *to* us and will be taken *from* us."[15] Death in this faith-filled context is perceived, then, not as an enemy but, in the words of the dying Joseph Cardinal Bernadin, as "a friend."[16] This is a friend sent not sought. Received not summoned. The time and manner of our "being called home," as Bernadin noted it, is not of our choosing. As the twentieth century's greatest Catholic theologian, the late Jesuit Karl Rahner, described it, death is "an act in which the person either willingly accepts or definitely rebels against his own utter impotence, in which he is utterly subject to a mystery which cannot be expressed, that mystery which we call 'God.' "[17]

The theological understanding of death as a part of the Divine Plan is the basis of the distinctions made in the Catholic moral theology between "killing and letting die"; "active and passive euthanasia"; "omission and commission"; "foreseeing and intending"; "allowing and causing." The clarity of these traditional distinctions has often been obscured. In recent years, philosophers and jurists alike have with regularity dismissed the distinction between killing and letting die as at best "a mere quibble."[18] But as the Supreme Court has now ruled, though the distinction might at times be difficult to discern, "the two acts are widely and reasonably regarded as quite distinct."

Issue of Physician Participation in Suicide

Though the role and meaning of death have been the focus of the Catholic critique of physician-assisted suicide, it is not suicide itself that is the focal point of the present policy debate. What is new in our era is the desire to medicalize suicide and active euthanasia. We want physicians to provide the means to end life in an antiseptically acceptable fashion. Knives, guns, ropes, and bridges tend to be messy. We seek a more aesthetically pleasing way of terminating life, one that leaves the patient looking dead, but not disgusting. For this, as in so much else in the twentieth-century quest for happiness, we turn to the physician.

What has led to this situation, one so fundamentally at odds with the 2500-year-old Hippocratic tradition that the physician as healer was never to administer a lethal potion? In large part, today's demands are a result of medicine's successes. We have come to believe that the "miracles" of modern medicine can not only defeat disease but conquer death. With the rise of technological medicine, lives which once were beyond rescue can now be saved. Sometimes, however, that success comes at too great a price: a life suffused in suffering, pain, and despair.

Once the quest for salvation through science and immortality through medicine proves unavailing, we seek a different medical "fix" for our problem. Since we fear death and the unrelieved suffering that prolonged dying can produce, we turn to medicine for relief from both. Commenting on that issue, Daniel Callahan writes that the movement to legalize euthanasia and assisted suicide is an "historically inevitable response to that fear."[19] He traces that response to what Joseph Cardinal Bernardin has described as the "increasingly mechanistic, commercial, and soulless" process of modern medicine.[20] "Caring" which traditionally characterized the profession is now being pushed aside for profit. In such an environment it is not surprising that Jack Kevorkian is held up as the model of a "good doctor."

Kevorkian is, in George Annas's description, not simply an aberrant physician; he is "a symptom of a medical care system gone seriously wrong at the end of life."[21] It is a system that treats death not as the Church teaches, as integral a part of nature as birth and life itself, but as "an offense against nature"—something to be fought off at all cost or, if that battle is not successful, to slay.

The inability of modern medicine to reassure us that it can manage our dying with dignity and comfort, a reality documented in the recent SUPPORT study finding that half of all conscious patients who died in the hospital experienced moderate to severe pain at least half the time during their last three days of life, leads to the demand that we be allowed to take back control of our fate.[22] In the face of this powerful, almost relentless dynamic, Callahan asks how we accomplish that goal. He observes that "for many, the answer seems obvious and unavoidable, that of active euthanasia and assisted suicide."

The 1991 referendum in Washington state was the first public attempt to achieve that end. Though defeated in a close vote, that referendum set the stage for the successful ballot measure three years later in Oregon where, for the first time in our nation's history, voters sanctioned state approval of physician-assisted suicide. The outcome in Oregon was not surprising. Public opinion polls in this country consistently show 65 percent of the populace supporting such a proposition. In great part that support is a reflection of two cultural phenomena that have emerged and flourished over the last twenty-five years: an emphasis on individual autonomy and the transformation of American medicine from a caring profession into a business designed to serve demands for medical services.

One of the striking features of this shift was the triumph of the patient "rights" movement over and against the long-standing tradition of medical paternalism. The corollary of the emphasis on patient autonomy was the obligation of medicine to respond to patient desires. The legislative response to that emphasis was the Patient Self-Determination Act of 1990 in which Congress mandated that healthcare facilities must inform patients of their right to decline any unwanted medical treatment, including those that were potentially life-prolonging.

Catholic View of Suicide

In enacting the PSDA, the Congress was implicitly following four hundred years of consistent Catholic moral teaching that no one is obliged to undergo a proposed medical treatment that is disproportionately painful or burdensome. That doctrine is best summed up in the Vatican's 1980 *Declaration on Euthanasia*, where we read:

> [O]ne cannot impose on anyone the obligation to have recourse to a technique which is already in use but which carries a risk or is burdensome. Such a refusal is not the equivalent of suicide (or euthanasia); on the contrary, it should be considered as an acceptance of the human condition, or a wish to avoid the application of a medical procedure disproportionate to the results that can be expected.[23]

That *Declaration*, however, makes a sharp distinction between refusing measures that would serve "only [to sustain] a precarious and burdensome prolongation of life" and suicide or active euthanasia. The former is permitted; the latter is prohibited.

The word euthanasia ("a good death") is subject to widely differing understandings, and the distinction between active and passive euthanasia (killing and letting die) is, as we have seen in the appellate court rulings, frequently collapsed into the one term. James Rachels' now famous 1975 *New England Journal of Medicine* essay on "Active and Passive Euthanasia" was the first to deny that there is any real difference between the two.[24] For him, "if a doctor lets a patient die, for humane reasons, he is in the same moral position as if he had given the patient a lethal injection."

The supporters of unlimited patient autonomy agree. They place no constraint and no limitation on an individual's autonomous "right" to direct medical treatment. The patient alone determines not only what medical intervention will be undergone, but whether medicine should be enlisted in the ending of life itself. As the highly publicized Philosophers' Brief to the Supreme Court in the physician-assisted suicide case starkly puts it:

> If it is permissible for a doctor deliberately to withdraw medical treatment in order to allow death to result from a natural process, then it is equally permissible for him to help a patient hasten his own death more actively, if that is the patient's express wish.[25]

That brief, as does the ruling of the Second Circuit Court of Appeals in *Quill*, rejects any distinction between killing and letting die. As Ronald Dworkin, the principle author of the Philosophers' Brief , noted in a commentary on the oral argument before the Supreme Court in the physician-assisted suicide cases:

> One justice suggested that a patient who insists that life support be disconnected is not committing suicide. That's wrong: he is committing suicide if he aims at death, as most such patients do. Just as someone whose wrist is cut in an accident is committing suicide if he refuses to try to stop the bleeding.[26]

If that thesis is correct, we land in one of two seemingly untenable positions:

1. If killing is seen as morally wrong, then we cannot withdraw life-prolonging medical procedures that are overly burdensome to the patient. That was the argument made by the trial court in the *Quinlan* case when Judge Robert Muir ruled that removing the ventilator would subject the physicians to charges of homicide.[27] Such rulings, which allow "no exit" from medical technology, are characterized by Daniel Callahan as "a clear case of slavery to technology."[28] They also lead to cries for relief, including demands for active euthanasia.

2. Alternatively, if there is no distinction between killing and letting die and one holds, as do all of the courts of final jurisdiction that have addressed the issue, that it is morally and legally acceptable to withhold or withdraw unwanted medical interventions, then there is no barrier to "killing" the patient. As Rachels puts it, the physician is in the same moral position "if he [gives] the patient a lethal injection as in withdrawing a respirator." In fact, Rachels argued since the latter action spares the patient from suffering, it is "actually preferable."

To avoid confusion in this debate, it is imperative to have a clear definition of terms. Here euthanasia is defined as the deliberate action by a physician to terminate the life of a patient. The clearest example is the act of lethal injection. Singer and Siegler's 1991 *New England Journal of Medicine* essay on "Euthanasia—A Critique" provides the helpful distinction between that action and such other acts as the decision to forego life-sustaining treatment (including the use of ventilations, cardio-pulmonary resuscitation, dialysis, or tube feedings); or the administration of analgesic agents to relive pain; or "assisted suicide" in which the doctor prescribes but does not administer a lethal dose of medication; or "mercy killing" performed by a patient's family or friends.[29]

Catholic tradition, as the Vatican *Declaration* makes clear, opposes euthanasia or the direct intentional killing of innocent life, whether of "a fetus or an embryo, an infant or an adult, an old person, or one suffering from an incurable disease, or a person who is dying." Furthermore, the Church holds that "no one is permitted to ask for this act of killing for himself or herself," nor is it morally licit to consent to such an action for one entrusted to your care. The reason for these moral imperatives is found in the *Declaration's* statement: "Only the Creator of life has the right to take away the life of the innocent." To arrogate that right to ourselves, whether as patient, guardian, or caregiver would be a "violation of the divine law" and "an offense against the dignity of the human person."

Referenda, legislative enactments, or judicial approval of state-sanctioned physician assistance in death stand as a challenge to that tradition. What is being asked for in these movements is most clearly seen in the Washington state referendum where voters were asked to approve what its proponents labeled "a new medical service": authorization for physicians actively to assist a terminally ill patient to die. The ballot initiative was circulated with the title, "Shall adult patients who are in a medically terminal condition be permitted to request and receive from a physician aid-in-dying?" Beneath that innocuously worded heading was the reality that "aid-in-dying" meant "aid in the form of a medical service, provided in person by a physician, that will end the life of a conscious and mentally qualified patient in a dignified, painless, and humane manner, when requested voluntarily by the patient through a written directive . . . at the time the medical service is to be provided."

From the time of Hippocrates through the 1997 *Current Opinions* of the Council on Ethical and Judicial Affairs of the American Medical Association, Western medicine has regarded the killing of patients, even on request, as a profound violation of the deepest meaning of the medical vocation.[30] Leon Kass undertook to explain the reasons for the societal change on this question in a probing essay in *The Public Interest* entitled "Why Doctors Must Not Kill."[31] There he argued that the basis for the shift in attitude, which has already led to some 5,000 cases of active euthanasia or assisted suicide a year in the Netherlands, is an overemphasis on freedom and personal autonomy, expressed in the view that each one has a right to control his or her body and life, including the end of it. In this view, physicians are bound to acquiesce not only to demands for termination of treatment, but also to intentional killing through poison, because the right to choose—freedom—must be respected even more than life itself. The second reason advanced for killing patients is not a concern for choice but the assessment by the patient or others that the patient's life is no longer deemed worth living. It is not autonomy but the miserable or pitiable condition of the body or mind that warrants, in Kass's words, "doing the patient in."

Both of these positions, individual autonomy and a life so devoid of dignity it should be destroyed, run counter to the Catholic understanding of life as a divine gift over which we exercise stewardship not dominion. Rather than the complete control over life demanded by the Philosophers' Brief in which life is to be ended when we conclude that living on "would disfigure rather than enhance the lives we have created," the Christian finds death's meaning in the example of the suffering Savior who abandoned himself in perfect obedience to the Father's will.

The recent example of Joseph Cardinal Bernardin's very public dying, which *Newsweek* captured in a cover story as "Teaching Us How to Die," stands in sharp contrast to the view that control and domination over death should be our goal.[32] As Bernardin expressed it in his parting legacy, *The Gift of Peace*, "I now realize that when I asked my doctor for the test results [of his metastatic cancer], I had to let go of everything. God was teaching me how little control we really have." Bernardin's conclusion when he understood that he was dying was uncomplicated: "[God] is now calling me home."

Self-abandonment to the will of God, not self-determination or the triumph of the human will, is the Christian response when medicine is unable to reverse the dying process. This is because in the Christian tradition death is not the final victor; it is, rather, a "transition from earthy life to life eternal," That truth is movingly set forth in the final movement of Mahler's *Resurrection Symphony*, where amidst the soaring music we hear the words of hope in the face of death: "I am from God and to God I shall return!"

The message of the triumph of Christ's resurrection over death, which Mahler heard at a friend's funeral, lead him from despair at the friend's death to hope in the promise of the resurrection, a hope he expressed musically in the glorious finale of his second symphony. It is also the counterpoint to the belief that death is something "freely chose," when "it is no longer possible to live proudly."

Notes

1. *Washington v. Glucksberg*, 177 Sup. Ct. 2258 (1997). No. 96–110. June 26, 1997. *Vacco v. Quill*, 177 Sup. Ct. 2293 (1997). No. 95–1858. June 26, 1977.
2. *Quill v. Vacco*, 80 F. 3rd 716 (2nd Cir. 1996).
3. *Cruzan v. Director Missouri Dept. of Health*, 110 Supreme Court 2841 (1990).
4. *Planned Parenthood v. Casey*, 505 U.S. 833 (1992).
5. John Paul II, *Evangelium Vitae*. (Washington, D.C.: USCC, 1995).
6. M. Cathleen Kaveny, "Assisted Suicide, Euthanasia, and the Law," *Theological Studies* 58 (1977): 124–48.
7. J. Bryan Hehir, "Intentity and Institutions," *Health Progress*, November–December 1995, pp. 17–23.
8. Richard A. McCormick, "To Save or Let Die: The Dilemmas of Modern Medicine," *Journal of the American Medical Association*, 299 (1974): 172–76.
9. Richard A. McCormick, "Technology, the Consistent Ethic and Assisted Suicide," *Origins* 25 (1995): 459–64.
10. Teilhard de Chardin, *The Divine Milieu* (New York: Harper and Row, 1960), pp. 88–89.
11. St. Augustine, *Confessions*, trans. Henry Chadwick (Oxford: Oxford University Press, 1991), p. 3.
12. James J. Mc Cartney, "The Development of the Doctrine of Ordinary and Extraordinary Means of Preserving Life in Catholic Moral Theology Before the Karen Quinlan Case," *Linacre Quarterly* 47 (1980): 215–28.
13. Sacred Congregation for the Doctrine of Faith, *Declaration on Euthanasia* (Vatican City: Polyglot Press, 1980).
14. Gerald Kelly, "The Duty of Using Artificial Means of Preserving Life," *Theological Studies* 16 (1950): 203–20.
15. J. Bryan Hehir, "Identity and Institutions," p. 23.

16. Joseph Bernadin, *The Gift of Peace* (Chicago: Loyola Press, 1996).
17. Karl Rahner, quoted in "The Moment of Death," *Newsweek*, November 25, 1966, 65.
18. Judge J. Skelly Wright in *Application of President and Direction of Georgetown College*, 331 F. 2d 1000 (D.C. Cir. 1964).
19. Daniel Callahan, "Frustrated Mastery: The Cultural Context of Death in America," *Western Journal of Medicine* 163 (1995): 226–30.
20. Joseph Cardinal Bernadin, "AMA Address: Medicine's Moral Crisis," *Origins* 25 (1995): 454–57.
21. George Annas, "Physican Assisted Suicide—Michigan's Temporary Solution," *New England Journal of Medicine* 328 (1995): 1575–76.
22. SUPPORT, "A Controlled Trial to Improve Care for Seriously Ill Hospitalized Patients: The Study to Understand Prognosis and Preferences for Outcomes and Risks of Treatments (SUPPORT)," *Journal of the American Medical Association* 274 (1995), 1591–98.
23. Sacred Congregation for the Doctrine of Faith, "Declaration on Euthanasia," *Orgins* 10 (1980): 154–57.
24. James Rachels, "Active and Passive Euthanasia," *New England Journal of Medicine* 292 (1975): 78–80.
25. Ronald Dworkin, et al. "Assisted Suicide: The Philosophers' Brief," *New York Review of Books*, March 27, 1997, pp. 41–47.
26. Ronald Dworkin, "Introduction to the Philosophers' Brief," *New York Review of Books*, March 27, 1997, p. 42.
27. *In Re Quinlan*, 70 N.J. 10, 355 A.2D 647 (1976).
28. Daniel Callahan, *The Troubled Dream of Life* (New York: Simon and Schuster, 1993).
29. Peter A. Singer and Mark Siegler, "Euthanasia—A Critique," *New England Journal of Medicine* 322 (1991): 181–83.
30. Council on Ethical and Judicial Affairs, AMA, *Code of Medical Ethics: Current Opinions* (Chicago: American Medical Association, 1997).
31. Leon R. Kass, "Neither for Love Nor Money: Why Doctors Must Not Kill," *The Public Interest* 94 (1989): 24–45.
32. Kenneth L. Woodward and John McCormick, "The Art of Aging Well," *Newsweek*, November 25, 1996, pp. 61–63.

21

Christian Perspectives on Assisted Suicide and Euthanasia

The Anglican Tradition

CYNTHIA B. COHEN

As we develop a social consensus about assisted suicide and euthanasia, religious voices should be heard, for they share with secular voices an embedded common morality and raise significant questions concerning human finitude at the end of life. To promote and inform public debate, this article presents a brief history of Christian thought, particularly that of the Anglican tradition, concerning these practices. It also offers the major arguments for and against assisted suicide and euthansia along with an intermediate position, and presents significant areas of agreement among Christians that can be brought to public discussion.

*   *   *

WE HAVE ALWAYS HAD THE ABILITY to commit suicide or request euthanasia in times of serious illness. Yet these acts have been prohibited within the Christian tradition from early times. Some Christians, as they see some relatives and friends kept alive too long in poor condition through the use of current medical powers, however, are beginning to question that tradition. Are assisted suicide and euthanasia compassionate Christian responses to those in pain and suffering who face death? Or are they ways of isolating and abandoning them, of fleeing from Christian compassion, rather than expressing it?

The Committee on Medical Ethics of the Episcopal Diocese of Washington recently issued a report addressing the issue of assisted suicide and euthanasia.[1] This matter cries out for religious contributions and perspectives, the Committee believes. The group recognizes that religious voices should not determine public policy, but believes they should be heard as we develop a social consensus about assisted suicide and euthanasia.[2] Therefore, the Committee chair has culled from the group's extensive report a brief history of Christian thought about these practices and some of the major arguments concerning them found in Christian thought, particularly the Anglican tradition.

Christians bring a distinctive theological and moral framework to these questions. Moreover, they bring centuries of experience of seeking meaning in death and meaning in life in the shadow of death. They are grounded in the conviction that the purpose of existence is to respond to God's call to a loving relationship with the Creator, Sustainer, and Redeemer of life. Their understanding of the moral life is embedded in that relationship and looks to the transformation of character through the imitation of Christ. Christians are called by God as a community to embody relations of trust, care, and mutual dependence. In short, there are certain ends that shape the way Christians should live—and die.

Anglican moralists, although adopting many traditional Christian moral principles and distinctions, have not set up an authoritative system of teachings to apply to assisted suicide and euthanasia.[3] They appeal to scripture, tradition, and reason as complementary guides in morals, belief, and worship.[4] No one of these alone, however, is taken by the Anglican tradition as the exclusive basis for moral action. They are to be interwoven, yielding a sense of what conclusion is fitting to the moral question at hand.[5]

Views About Ending and Extending Life in the Christian Tradition

Intentionally to end our own life or deliberately to kill another is considered seriously wrong within the Christian tradition, except in self-defense, war, and often in capital punishment. At the same time, that tradition has not viewed life as an absolute good that must be extended for as long as possible.

The Christian tradition has consistently and unequivocally prohibited euthanasia. The scriptural roots of this prohibition are in the horror of shedding innocent blood attested in the story of Cain and Abel and throughout scripture, most notably in the Sixth Commandment.[6] Those who kill the sick in order to spare them from pain are to be viewed as murderers, according to the Hebrew tradition. There also is a widespread conviction among Christians that euthanasia is forbidden.[7] St. Paul, when faced with what has been taken as a physical ailment, expressed a desire to die, but he went on living, accepting his affliction as necessary for God's purposes.[8]

The commandment against murder has almost universally been interpreted to apply to taking one's own life. In the few accounts of suicide in the Bible, it is, for the most part, committed by figures whose actions have brought them to a final act of despair or who wish to avoid shame and dishonor.[9] The silence of scripture on the moral status of suicide cannot be counted as approval of or indifference to the practice. Indeed, some conclude from the fact that suicide occurs only rarely and without endorsement in scripture that it was not approved in that writing.

Like St. Paul, the early Christians did not counsel the faithful to escape pain and suffering by asking others to kill them. The Church accepted a position that honored martyrdom, but stressed the importance of doing all one could, short of betraying one's faith, to avoid being killed. There is no evidence of any Christian committing suicide for any reason in the first 250 years of the Christian era, a period when persecution and suffering were rampant.[10] A succession of theologians took a strong stand against suicide, including Augustine, who denounced it in *The City of God* as a cowardly way of escaping pain and suffering in this life.

The prohibition against killing innocent persons (those not guilty of committing a serious crime or deliberately threatening the life of others) continued into the later church. Aquinas adopted the view of the Jewish scholar Maimonides that killing an innocent person, "whether he is healthy or about to die from natural causes," is wrong. He also expressed classical objections against suicide, arguing that it was absolutely prohibited because 1) it violates our natural self-love and inclination to preserve our being, 2) it offends the human community, of which each human being is a part, and 3) it offends God, who offers life as a gift.[11]

During the sixteenth century, some Christians explicitly discussed suicide and euthanasia in the face of illness.[12] In an imaginary land named Utopia depicted by Thomas More, a Roman Catholic, suicide and euthanasia were encouraged for those suffering from incurable diseases accompanied by continuous pain. Speculation that the book offers a satire of, rather than serious argument for, suicide and euthanasia is supported by the fact that as More awaited his own execution, he wrote *A Dialogue of Comfort: Against Tribulation*, in which he argued against these acts.[13] John Donne, the poet and Anglican divine, wrote the first defense of suicide in English in *Biathanatos*. However, he did not permit suicide undertaken for self-interest, and did not defend suicide for those who were seriously ill and near death.

In the *ars moriendi*, or art-of-dying literature, the recommendation to those caring for the dying was to provide ease and comfort, rather than to bring about their death. Seventeenth-century works such as *The Rule and Exercise of Holy Dying* by Anglican Jeremy Taylor explained the importance of preparing for death and argued that we should not choose to cause our own death. More recently, however, some Anglicans, such as Hastings Rashdall, W. R. Inge, and Joseph Fletcher have maintained that euthanasia and suicide might be permissible to end extreme and incurable physical suffering.[14] In short, with few exceptions, the Christian tradition, including Anglicanism, has condemned euthanasia and assisted suicide.

The term "sanctity of life" has been used by Christians to convey the enormous value that God ascribes to our lives. Although biological life is a fundamental good, it is not an absolute one. Christians are called to risk—not take—their lives at times for the sake of God and others. Christ's own death revealed this. Although life is an extremely high value, certain other values, such as love of God and others, are even weightier.

Nothing in the central Christian tradition, however, requires its adherents to extend their lives for as long as possible. Though there is a presumption that we have a duty to nurture and preserve our lives, this may be overcome when treatment is useless or overwhelmingly burdensome.[15] Christians, although called by God to life, have reason not to fear death. The meaning that they find in death is not the nothingness of final extinction, but the complete revelation of the being and love of God.

Arguments for Assisted Suicide and Euthanasia

Those in the Christian tradition who favor assisted suicide and euthanasia tend to make two basic claims: 1) We have an obligation to respect individual human choice; and 2) We have an obligation to relieve suffering, even if this means ending human life. Other considerations, such as our loss of control over dying and the need to regulate socially approved killing, figure in their thought.

Respect for Autonomy or Self-Determination. Christians have distinctive reasons for taking the claims of autonomy with great seriousness. An essential aspect of the image of God we bear is our ability to make free choices. Therefore, some maintain, we have a right to choose to end our lives when we can no longer serve God or others by remaining alive while in great pain and suffering. A report issued by the Episcopal Diocese of Newark in 1995, for instance, states that it would be right to allow assisted death when "[t]he decision to hasten death is a truly informed and voluntary choice free from external coercion."[16] The *Newark Report* adds the related criterion that "[t]he plan for voluntary assisted death places maximum autonomy and command of the process in the hands of the dying person."

Upholding God's Purposes and Sovereignty. Joseph Fletcher argued that if Christians allow exceptions to the Sixth Commandment in wartime and for capital punishment, they should also allow an exception for killing to alleviate pain and suffering near death.[17] The Hebrew in which the Sixth Commandment is written, he observed, is not correctly translated "Thou shalt not kill," but, as in the Episcopal *Book of Common Prayer*, "Thou shalt do no murder." To murder is to kill wrongfully. To end the lives of those who are sick and suffering, Fletcher argued, is not to kill them wrongfully, and would therefore not violate the Sixth Commandment.

Further, the doctrine of creation, according to the *Newark Report*, means that some destruction of life is inevitable within creation, since "life can be sustained only at the expense of other life." The report goes on to claim that "[t]he willful taking of life ... can be morally justified only if the good desired outweighs the potential evil and only if that good cannot be achieved in a less destructive manner."[18] When killing brings about a balance of good over evil, it can be justified by its good consequences. The report concludes that we do not intrude on God's purposes and prevent the realization of God's intentions for our lives when we make intelligent, voluntary decisions to end them in light of the good results this would entail.

Responding to Pain and Suffering. Because human beings are created in the image of God, we have an inherent dignity. This is violated, those who favor assisted suicide and euthanasia maintain, when we are forced to go through an agonizing period of pain and suffering before our lives end. Dean Inge, a noted Anglican theologian, wrote in the early 1930s:

> I confess that in this instance I cannot resist the arguments for a modification of the traditional Christian law, which absolutely prohibits suicide in all circumstances. I do not think we can assume that God willed the prolongation of torture for the benefit of the soul of the sufferer.[19]

Our Christian dignity is assaulted, advocates hold, not only by physical pain, but also by the depersonalization associated with prolonged use of life-sustaining technology, loss of control over bodily functions, and the deterioration of our health. Such diminishment serves no discernible spiritual or other purpose. Indeed, they believe it can be destructive of moral and spiritual values. It can amount to "radical suffering," which has been defined by Wendy Farley as suffering which "is destructive of the human spirit and cannot be understood as something deserved."[20]

God's will for humanity is to alleviate suffering. Biblical passages where St. Paul rejoices in the virtue of suffering and the abundance of grace that flows through it do not glorify suffering for its own sake, the Newark Report maintains. Instead, these passages validate suffering *only when* it is for the sake of Christ. The *Newark Report* thus states:

> Unless an individual somehow understands suffering due to serious illness as a direct consequence of one's faithful response to the Gospel, endurance of such suffering cannot be seen as a mandate, either moral or theological, on the basis of the scriptural witness. It is not a moral failing to view such suffering as devoid of purpose, and thus without redemptive value. This, coupled with the clear precedent of Jesus' countless efforts to alleviate suffering through his healing ministry, makes clear that there is no obligation incumbent upon the Christian to endure suffering for its own sake.[21]

On this view assisted suicide provides a way of ending the non-redemptive suffering of those who do not elect to undergo it.

Curbing medical technology. Many of us fear that our deaths will involve the overzealous employment of technological "miracles" that will keep us alive too long. Some Christian thinkers argue that accepting assisted suicide and euthanasia would return a measure of control over the dying process to individuals to whom God has given this responsibility. These practices represent a final use of our God-given power to govern technology in a death-denying culture that would use all available technological means to keep people alive.

Overcoming dangers to the community. A legitimate concern arises, some proponents of assisted suicide and euthanasia recognize, that adopting these practices as a matter of public policy endangers society. A practice could develop of ending the lives of patients without their request or under different circumstances than they detailed when competent. This is a serious concern for Christians, who are called to care for and preserve fellow members of the community. Further, the institutionalization of these practices could undercut the value ascribed to life by Christians and encourage a practice pattern based on social utility rather than individual need. However, proponents argue, the failure to legitimize these practices also has its dangers. It could allow secret and uncontrolled killing according to no agreed moral criteria.

Precautions against financial coercion. Another legitimate concern recognized by proponents of assisted suicide and euthanasia is that the seriously ill might be pressured to end their lives for financial reasons. They acknowledge that the attempt to lower health costs may subtly encourage those who are dying to do so more quickly.[22] However, they maintain that Christians are called to protect the sick from such coercive influences. Consequently, some who accept assisted suicide and euthanasia hold that it is essential to enact regulations to provide stringent safeguards against financially coerced decisions to end life.

Arguments Against Assisted Suicide and Euthanasia

Opponents do not find that our new medical powers provide reason to discard the long-standing Christian prohibition against suicide and euthanasia. Their most significant arguments focus on 1) God's purposes for us and the world and 2) the meaning and role of suffering in human life. The Christian view of autonomy, concern about pressure on the critically ill to justify remaining alive, and the dangers of abuse give added force to their position.

Impeding God's purposes and violating God's sovereignty. Our lives belong to God. As Paul declares, "Do you not know that your body is a temple of the Holy Spirit within you, which you have from God? You are not your own...."[23] We hold our lives in trust and are accountable to God for how we live them—and for how we die. The ultimate sources of the inviolability of our lives are God's creative and loving purposes for us; these do not include self-annihilation opponents maintain. We intrude on those purposes and deny God's sovereignty when we intentionally cause the death of an innocent person. The authors of *On Dying Well*, a 1975 Anglican Working Group report, observed of the Christian, "[H]e can claim no inalienable right to death on the grounds that his life is his own, and that after due consideration has been given to the interests of other men and women, he may do with it exactly as he pleases."[24]

Moreover, we are created by God to live in community with one another, caring for one another and working to achieve the common good. Assisted suicide and euthanasia would diminish our bonds with others, opponents state, for the acts would cut out of human and Christian fellowship those most in need of it. Care for the sick and suffering requires that we ameliorate their suffering, not end their lives.

The *Newark Report* argues that the doctrine of creation opens the door to assisted suicide, and implies that killing is built into the very nature of things.[25] Yet opponents note that this seems to suggest that life involves a struggle in which the strong destroy the weak. This Nietzschean approach is contrary to the Christian view of the goodness of God's creation. Moreover, critics hold that it is morally unacceptable to couple a doctrine of creation with a social utilitarian doctrine that condones taking human life for the greater good. The Christian tradition does not accept a consequentialist calculus of benefits and burdens to society as the basis for determining who should live and who should die.

Alleviating pain and suffering by moral means. Because we are finite and limited beings, suffering is an inevitable consequence of our human condition. Throughout Church history, Christians have struggled to understand the meaning and mystery of suffering. The question in scriptures is not whether we should suffer, but how and why.[26]

Suffering can sanctify and transform us, opponents of assisted suicide and euthanasia declare. It can give us a clearer perspective on the meaning of our lives and on eternal life, show us our limitations, refine our faith, make us more Christ-like, and produce perseverance and character.[27] Even as we suffer, and ultimately die, God shares in our brokenness and calls us to share in his.[28] Contrary to the *Newark Report*, much suffering is redemptive, not just that which is explicitly borne for the sake of Christ.[29] This, for instance, was displayed by St. Paul, who willingly accepted the physical suffering caused by his own illness.[30]

It is immensely important to recognize, however, that Christians are not obligated to endure all suffering, opponents of assisted suicide and euthanasia observe. We have been brought into this world to prevent or end nonredemptive suffering where we can through moral means. The suffering that some who are seriously ill unnecessarily endure today should be alleviated by medical and pastoral means—not by killing. This is the time when the adequate and appropriate use of narcotics should be encouraged as a matter of compassionate Christian stewardship.

Moral constraints on autonomy. To acknowledge the importance of human freedom of choice is to recognize the great worth and dignity that God has bestowed on us. The God whom we love is the God "whose service is perfect freedom," the *Book of Common Prayer* proclaims. But this freedom is not the freedom to do whatever we wish. Our call to live out God's purposes places moral limits on what we may choose at the end of life. Opponents hold that the Christian prohibition of these practices is one such moral limit.

Moreover, they argue, the dominion God gave us in Genesis 1:28 does not mean that we are to take complete control of our own living and dying. Instead, that dominion is better understood as taking responsibility for stewardship in this world, as we live in community with one another. We are to cede some of our autonomy, according to God's plan, for the good of the community. And that good would be seriously injured were we to allow socially sanctioned killing of the innocent through assisted suicide and euthanasia.

Having to justify our existence. Although the availability of assisted suicide and euthanasia might increase the choices open to us, opponents observe, it would eliminate others. It would eliminate our God-given choice to remain alive without having to justify our continued existence. Having the option of assisted suicide and euthanasia would pressure us to end our lives or else explain our continued existence.[31] How can those who remain alive during terminal illness respond to the implicit—and unChristian—question: Why aren't you dead yet?

Dangers of abuse. Christians and others are concerned that it would be difficult—indeed impossible—to draw stable moral boundaries around assisted suicide and euthanasia were these practices legalized. After all, opponents ask, if a right to be killed is grounded in Christian self-determination, why wait until individuals are dying before they can exercise that right?[32] Without any limiting principles, an expansion of killing to the chronically ill and incurable seems inevitable. Similar problems of definition emerge for a standard that requires some degree of pain and suffering before assisted suicide and euthanasia can be provided. How are we to define the degree of physical or mental suffering that goes beyond what God would have us endure that would justify killing the sufferer? Moreover, critics claim, if the rationalization for assisted suicide and euthanasia is to relieve suffering, why should these practices be limited to those who are competent? This is acknowledged by Dan Brock, a leading proponent of voluntary euthanasia, who states, "There is reason to expect that legalization of voluntary active euthanasia might soon be followed by strong pressure to legalize some nonvoluntary euthanasia of incompetent patients unable to express their own wishes."[33]

Once we cross the vital line between allowing to die and killing, Christian thinkers caution, where do we stop? Do we hit the bottom of the slippery slope?[34] Acts of assisted suicide and euthanasia threaten to destroy the human community at the heart of the Christian faith by deliberately eliminating its members.

Succumbing to financial pressures. As we move rapidly into managed care health plans, whose *modus operandi* is to cut costs, some who are critically ill may conclude that they cannot afford to remain alive. Assisted suicide and euthanasia may seem their only alternative.[35] This can be the case for those without health insurance and therefore without access to medical treatment and palliative care. It may also hold true for the insured, for cost-saving limitations on services may lead them to doubt they will receive appropriate therapeutic and palliative care at the end of life. Given the harsh economic realities that many patients face today, critics think it would be difficult to avoid the conclusion that those who request assisted suicide and euthanasia have been coerced into doing so by financial pressures. Christian charity should not condone a practice that would wrongly push individuals to choose death because they cannot afford to live.

The impact of social isolation on the vulnerable. The institutionalization of dying creates a profoundly alienating experience for many who are seriously ill. The elderly and persons with disabilities can face structural impediments and lack of companionship in nursing homes and hospitals. Moreover, reports of abuse in nursing homes are increasing.[36] The requests of persons in such institutions for assistance in killing themselves may arise from an experience of isolation, mistreatment, and dehumanization. We are created by God in a social dimension; our lives are built on mutual dependence. Therefore, we must ask whether the relational bonds of those requesting assisted suicide and euthanasia have been disrupted and whether such requests arise from despair. Rather than providing an occasion for severing social relations, the suffering of the dying, elderly, and disabled should provide an occasion for a Christian ministry that offers compassionate bonding, care, and fidelity. We can provide those who are chronically and terminally ill a presence affirming that "none of us lives or dies to himself alone."[37]

Justifying or Excusing Assisted Suicide and Euthanasia
in Extreme Circumstances

Some Christian thinkers who accept and some who reject assisted suicide and euthanasia find common ground in those extraordinary circumstances when suffering becomes intolerable and no means, such as pain relieving drugs, alleviate it. A body of Christians within the larger group of those who accept assisted suicide and euthanasia maintain that the Christian tradition should allow exceptions to the prohibition against killing the innocent in extreme circumstances. Some who reject assisted suicide and euthanasia also hold that in rare circumstances these would be excusable. Thus, the first set of thinkers holds that assisted suicide and euthanasia in such circumstances amount to a justified exception to the Christian prohibition of killing the innocent. The second set holds that these acts are wrong, but excusable.

In what rare situations would both sets of thinkers agree that it would be morally allowable to kill or assist in committing suicide? The example often given is that of a person trapped in a fiery car wreck with no way to escape. A loving, compassionate God, "whose mercy endureth forever," would not will such an excruciatingly painful death for that person and would allow others to kill him.

It is important to recognize, however, that those who come to this conclusion apply it only to the rare and catastrophic case. Most instances of terminal illness are not analogous to the highly unusual case of burning to death, either in the degree of pain and suffering involved or the nearness of death. Those allowing this justification or exception do not believe that in most cases where patients experience pain and suffering as part of the normal course of dying it would be morally acceptable for them to commit suicide or for others to provide euthanasia.

Other Christian thinkers are concerned that justifying the compassionate killing of those who are dying in extreme circumstances may lead to killing those who are not. The class of rare cases is bound to expand until its boundaries vanish. Decisions that seem morally acceptable in individual circumstances can slide into loose general policy, which could lead to killing in cases where it would be clearly wrong.[38] Robert Wennberg explains that

> It is important to remind ourselves that there is a danger in doing ethics by relying heavily on extreme cases, and the case of the soldier who commits suicide as the only alternative to being burned alive in a tank is just such a case. By focusing on extreme cases, we can unfairly undermine confidence in the firmness of moral rules that in the context of normal human existence are in fact sound and virtually exceptionless.[39]

Consequently, the position of those who would allow exceptions for assisted suicide and euthanasia or who would excuse them has not been adopted as a general rule within the Christian tradition.

Finding a Christian Approach to the Question of Assisted Suicide and Euthanasia

Paradoxically, both those Christians who accept and reject assisted suicide and euthanasia begin with similar convictions. Both have a sense of the sovereignty of God and view life as a gift not entirely at the disposal of humanity. Both want to protect human dignity and to preserve the freedom of individuals to choose how to confront their finitude and death. They recognize that human life, especially in situations of death and dying, often confronts us with a conflict of goods where physical life clashes with other purposes. Both feel compassion toward those who suffer near death and desire to relieve this in ways they deem consonant with God's purposes. They call on healthcare providers and pastoral counselors to improve their care of those in pain and suffering, not only pharmacologically, but also psychologically and spiritually. Moreover, both recognize that Christ's charge to love our neighbor obligates us to look beyond our own immediate health needs to those of the community.

How can those in the Christian tradition respond to the poignant and divisive matters of assisted suicide and euthanasia? A recent Episcopal study group noted that

> Differences in moral judgments are not simply or narrowly matters of right and wrong. Rather, differences in judgment reflect differences in understandings that can be articulated, respected, and debated. . . . Christian ethics and moral theology provide the basis for critical reflection that informs moral judgments and promotes respect for those who may differ.[40]

When disagreement about a significant moral issue such as assisted suicide and euthanasia persists, even in light of central Christian teachings, Christian thinkers have a responsibility to explore common ground as they weigh all arguments. Further, they must realize, as Bishop Kirk observed, that moral truth can have some uncertainties attached to it due to "the limitations of the human mind, the imperfection of the human vocabulary, and the needs of different ages."[41] Only through dialogue will Christians discover what Kirk called "something outside ourselves—something the same for all—something in the eternal will of God" that points to the approach for Christians to take to assisted suicide and euthanasia.[42]

What value has this exploration within one Western religious tradition to a secular, pluralistic society? Views of various religious traditions are not irrelevant to the process of informed public debate in such a society. Although religious voices are undergirded by references to a distinctive canon and tradition, they share with secular voices an embedded common morality concerned with respect for humans and their choices, as well as the will to promote social justice and the common good. Perhaps the distinctive contribution that religious traditions can make to the public debate is to offer a way of thinking that moves beyond the boundaries set by public regulation of private choices to what Campbell terms "a context of meaning and ultimacy."[43] Religious voices raise those significant questions that surge forward when we face our finitude at the edge of life. These focus on how we might live a meaningful life and die a good death, the significance of suffering in our lives, and what it means to be human. They bring to public attention the ultimate dimensions of the question of assisted suicide and euthanasia that social policy must address. In the words of the seventeenth-century Anglican, Robert Sanderson, we are

> sociable creatures, contrived ... into policies and societies and common-wealths ... fellow members of one body and every one another's members. As, therefore, we are not born, so neither must we live, to and for ourselves alone; but our parents and friends, and acquaintances nay, every man of us hath a kind of right and interest in every other man of us, and our country and the com-monwealth in us all.[44]

Notes

1. Committee on Medical Ethics, Episcopal Diocese of Washington, *Assisted Suicide and Euthanasia: Christian Moral Perspectives* (Harrisburg, PA: Morehouse, 1997). Members of the committee who developed the full report are Cynthia B. Cohen, Ph.D., J.D., Chair, The Rev. Dr. David J. Bird, Co-Chair, Jean Galloway Ball, J.D., Priscilla Cherouny, M. Div., Frank W. Cornett, M.D., J.D., Alex Hagerty, Patricia Lusk, M.P.H., R.N.C., L.N.H., Virginia Oler, M.D., Dorothy Rainey, The Rev. George P. Timberlake, The Rev. Dr. Joseph W. Trigg.

2. D. H. Smith, *Health and Medicine in the Anglican Tradition* (New York: Crossroad, 1986), pp. 17–18; C. S. Campbell, "Religious Ethics and Active Euthanasia in a Plural-istic Society," *Kennedy Institute of Ethics Journal* 2 (1992): 253–77.

3. See K. E. Kirk, *Some Principles of Moral Theology and their Application* (London: Long-mans, 1920); Frederick Denison Maurice, *The Kingdom of Christ*, vol. II (London: SCM Press, 1958), at p. 331; Smith, *supra*, note 2; T. Sedgwick and P. Turner, eds., *The Cri-sis in Moral Teaching in the Episcopal Church* (Harrisburg, PA: Morehouse, 1992).

4. S. Sykes and J. Booty, eds., *The Study of Anglicanism* (London and Philadelphia: SPCK and Fortress, 1988), part III.

5. G. R. Dunstan, *The Artifice of Ethics* (London: SCM Press, 1974), at p. 52; "The Author-ity of a Moral Claim: Ian Ramsey and the Practice of Medicine," *Journal of Medical Ethics* 13 (1987): 189–94.

6. Exodus 20:13.

7. H. Y. Vanderpool, "Death and Dying: Euthanasia and Sustaining Life: I. Historical Aspects," *Encyclopedia of Bioethics*, revised edition, vol. 1, (New York: Macmillan, 1995), pp. 554–63.

8. 2 Corinthians 5:1–10; 12:8–9.

9. Ahitopel hanged himself after David's son failed to take his advice in his rebellion against his father (2 Samuel 17: 23). Abimelech, who was mortally wounded by a woman in battle, ordered his armor-bearer to kill him to save him from public disgrace (Judges 9: 50–66). Saul was wounded in battle and committed suicide to spare himself mockery by a victorious enemy (1 Samuel 31:1–6; 2 Samuel 15:1; 1 Chronicles 10:1–13). Zimri set a house afire and burned himself to death when he was about to be captured after having wrongfully killed the king of Israel and all his house (1 Kings 16:18–19). The warrior, Razis, killed himself rather than suffer dishonor (2 Maccabees 14:41–6). Judas hanged himself after betraying Christ (Matthew 27:5). Paul, on the other hand, prevented his jailer from committing suicide (Acts 16:27–28).

10. D. W. Amundsen, "Suicide and Early Christian Values," in B. A. Brody, ed., *Suicide and Euthanasia* (Dordrecht, Netherlands: Kluwer, 1989): 77–153.

11. T. Wood, "Homicide," in *Westminster Dictionary of Christian Ethics*, J. F. Childress and J. Macquarrie, eds. (Philadelphia: Westminster Press, 1986), pp. 270–71.

12. G. B. Ferngren, "Ethics of Suicide in Renaissance and Reformation," in B. A. Brody, ed., *Suicide and Euthanasia* (Dordrecht, Netherlands: Kluwer, 1989): 155–81.

13. We are indebted to Daniel P. Sulmasy, O.F.M., M.D., Ph.D., for bringing this our attention.

14. Hastings Rashdall, *The Theory of Good and Evil: A Treatise on Moral Philosophy*, vol. 1 (Oxford: Clarendon Press, 1997), pp. 208–12. W. R. Inge, *Christian Ethics and Moral Problems* (New York: Putnam, 1930). Joseph Fletcher, *Morals and Medicine* (Princeton, NJ: Princeton University Press, 1954): 172–210.

15. J. F. Childress, "Life, Prolongation of," in *Westminster Dictionary of Christian Ethics*, J. F. Childress and J. Macquarrie, eds. (Philadelphia: Westminster Press, 1986), pp. 349–50.

16. *Report of the Task Force on Assisted Suicide to the 122nd Convention of the Episcopal Diocese of Newark*, January 27, 1996, at p. 8. [Hereafter referred to as *Newark Report*.]

17. Fletcher, *supra* note 14, pp. 195–96.

18. *Newark Report*, *supra* note 16, at p. 4.

19. Inge, *supra* note 14, at p. 397.

20. Wendy Farley, *Tragic Vision and Divine Compassion: A Contemporary Theodicy* (Louisville, KY: Westminster/John Knox Press, 1990): at 21.

21. *Newark Report*, *supra* note 16, at p. 7.

22. D. P. Sulmasy, "Managed Care and Managed Death," *Archives of Internal Medicine* 155 (1995): 133–36; P.A. Singer, M. Siegler, "Euthanasia—A Critique," *New England Journal of Medicine* 322 (1990): 1881–83; R. I. Misbin, "Physicians' Aid in Dying," *New England Journal of Medicine* 235 (1991): 1307–11.

23. 1 Corinthians 6:19–20.

24. General Synod Board for Social Responsibility, *On Dying Well. An Anglican Contribution to the Debate on Euthanasia* (Newport: Church Information Office, 1975), at p. 16.

25. *Newark Report*, *supra* note 16, at p. 4.

26. Sondra Ely Wheeler, *Stewards of Life: Bioethics and Pastoral Care* (Nashville: Abingdon, 1996), at p. 33.

27. 1 Peter 1:5–7; Hebrews 12:1; Romans 5:3–5; Psalm 119:71.

28. Matthew 16:21; D. H. Smith, *supra* note 2, at pp. 6–8; D. H. Smith, "Suffering, Medicine, and Christian Theology," *On Moral Medicine: Theological Perspectives in Medical Ethics*, S. E. Lammers, A. Verhey, eds. (Grand Rapids, Michigan: Eerdmans, 1987), pp. 255–61; A. C. McGill, *Suffering: A Test of Theological Method* (Philadelphia: Westminster, 1982), pp. 10–11.

29. C. S. Lewis, *The Problem of Pain* (New York: Macmillan, 1943), p. 168.

30. 2 Corinthians 12:7–10.

31. A. Verhey, "Choosing Death: The Ethics of Assisted Suicide," *Christian Century*, July 17–24, 1996, pp. 716–19.

32. D. Callahan, "When Self-Determination Runs Amok," *Hastings Center Report* 22 (1992): 52–55.

33. D. Brock, "Voluntary Active Euthanasia," *Hastings Center Report* 22 (1992): 10–22, at 20.

34. H. Bouma III, D. Diekema, E. Langerak, T. Rottman, A. Verhey, *Christian Faith, Health, and Medical Practice* (Grand Rapids, MI: Eerdmans, 1989), p. 300.

35. R. J. Blendon, U. S. Szalay, R. A. Knox, "Should Physicians Aid their Patients in Dying?" *Journal of the American Medical Association* 267 (1992): 2658–62; G. J. Annas, "Death by Prescription—The Oregon Initiative," *New England Journal of Medicine* 331 (1994): 1240–43.

36. M. Tousignant, P. Davis, "Nursing Homes in Area, Nationwide Plagued by Reports of Abuse," *Washington Post*, October 13, 1996, p. B-1.

37. Romans 14:7.

38. *On Dying Well*, *supra* note 24, p. 11.

39. R. N. Wennberg, *Terminal Choices: Euthanasia, Suicide, and the Right to Die* (Grand Rapids, MI: William B. Eerdmans, 1989), pp. 86–7.

40. T. Sedgwick, "Introduction," *supra* note 3, pp. 9–10.
41. K. E. Kirk, *Conscience and Its Problems: An Introduction to Casuistry* (London: Long-mans, Green, 1927), p. 79.
42. Ibid., p. 33.
43. Campbell, *supra* note 2, p. 275.
44. R. Sanderson, Sermon IV, *Sermons ad populum Works*, vol. III: 101. Quoted in Thomas Wood, *English Casuistical Divinity during the Seventeenth Century* (London: SPCK, 1952), p. 58.

22

A Protestant Perspective
on Ending Life

Faithfulness in the Face of Death

ALLEN VERHEY

This chapter distinguishes minimal notions of justice and mercy from the richer notions available to story-formed communities, and suggests reasons to be suspicious of the minimal notions. It provides a theological defense of the distinction between killing and accepting death and theological backing for attention to the identity and integrity of medicine. Finally, it responds to arguments which urge public policy to permit physician-assisted suicide as a way to maximize freedom.

*   *   *

PETER DEVRIES died a few years ago. He grew up in a Dutch Calvinist home, much like the one I grew up in. He went to Calvin College, my alma mater. He was a wonderful satirist, the author of novels like *The Blood of the Lamb* and *Slouching Towards Kalamazoo*.[1] He was, if you will, a Calvinist comic. Unfortunately, there is no parallel set of accomplishments in my c.v. I am a theologian, and frankly, a funny Dutch Calvinist is a rarity. Many people regard "Calvinist comic" as an oxymoron. Even so, Peter DeVries provides the lines that introduce this effort to articulate a Protestant perspective on ending life.

There is first, his wonderful acknowledgement of our mortality. "Like the cleaning lady," he said, "we all come to dust."[2] There is, moreover, a little piece of conversation that reminds religious people that they are not exempt from that mortality: A character in *The Tunnel of Love* says, "I see Reverend Bonniwell . . . died," and another replies, "Yes, death is no respecter of parsons."[3] Finally, there is a line in his *The Glory of the Hummingbird* that provides something like a text for this paper: "Suicide is not a viable alternative."[4]

Suicide is not a viable alternative. Faithfulness in the face of one's own death need not do everything possible to preserve life, but it should not choose suicide. Faithfulness in the face of another's death will always care, but it will not kill or assist in suicide. "Suicide is not a viable alternative." That is the text for—and the burden of—this paper. I will develop that text in four sections, attending, first, to notions of justice and mercy; second, to notions of suffering and dying; third, to notions of healing and caring; and finally, to the notion of maximizing freedom. I hope to show in the first section that the notions of justice and mercy used to defend physician-assisted suicide are *minimal* notions and that, if their minimalism is not acknowledged, they can distort the moral life and a moral dying. In the second section I will provide a *theological* defense of the distinction between allowing to die and killing. I will admit that it is getting harder to defend that distinction without appealing to the story within which it is embedded, but I will claim that Christian communities have very good reasons of their own for preserving the traditional distinction and the Christian consensus that we need not always preserve life but ought not deliberately kill ourselves or another. The third section turns to the identity of medicine and to the issue of faithfulness to that identity. The fourth part, finally, argues that a shift in public policy which is undertaken for the sake of maximizing freedom may have the *ironic* result of eliminating an important option. I hope that at the end of the paper readers will agree with Peter DeVries and with me that "suicide is not a viable alternative."

Justice and Mercy

First then, justice and mercy: "Do justice!" "Love mercy!" Who can argue with such advice? Surely not a Protestant, not one who has been formed by scripture. The prophet Micah, after all, gave such advice in summary of what the Lord required (Micah 6:8). One may well ask, however, what such advice means. "Justice" and "mercy" are slippery terms, and they shift in meaning as the background for intelligibility shifts.

In our pluralistic culture we sometimes use these terms as though they were free-standing, independent of their embeddedness in particular stories. As a result, we sometimes have and use "minimal" notions of "justice" and "mercy."

The "minimal" notion of *justice* insists on respect for the *autonomy* of each person, demands the protection of individual rights, and attempts to guarantee a space for each one to act in ways that suit one's preference as long as such actions do not violate the autonomy of another. Such a notion of justice, of course, has its own tradition, its own story. It fits the story of enlightenment individualism.

The *strengths* of such a justice should not be denied. In a pluralistic society like ours, such a notion of justice can provide a context for conversation and a challenge to the arbitrary dominance of one perspective or one person over another.

But the *weakness* of such a notion of justice should also not be overlooked, and its fundamental weakness is precisely that it is so minimal. Its minimalism shows up in a variety of ways. First, such a notion tells us nothing about what *goods* to seek, only something about certain *constraints* to exercise in seeking them. Moreover, it is attentive finally only to one constraint prohibiting any violation of another's freedom. Second, such a notion of justice tends to reduce the significance of *covenantal* relationships (like the relationships of husband and wife, parent and child, doctor and patient) to matters of *contract*. Third, by its emphasis on the procedural question, "Who should decide?" it pushes to the margins of public discourse the substantive moral questions of conduct and character, the questions, "What should be decided?" and "What character traits should mark the one who decides?" This minimalism does not make it wrong, but if its minimalism is not acknowledged, it can distort and subvert the moral life (and the moral death).

It is true, to take an example from another area, that "nonconsensual" sex is wrong—but there is more to say about a good sexual life. And if we deny that there is more to say, then we distort and subvert a good sexual life. It is true that my wife and I sometimes resort to the language of contract, to the "rights" and "duties" that belong to our contract—but usually in the middle of an argument, and if that is the only language we have for our relationship, then we distort and subvert the covenant of marriage.

The minimal notion of justice is used to defend the moral legitimacy of suicide. Suicide, after all, is (at least sometimes) an autonomous act: chosen, preferred by a free individual. Guaranteeing to each one a space to act in ways that suit one's preferences requires, we are told, making a space for decisions to commit suicide. What matters publicly, after all, is simply that there be such a space, not how it is filled.

Such a notion of justice is also used to defend the legitimacy of assistance with suicide and voluntary euthanasia, for the single-minded attention to consent as a constraint seems to prohibit only "nonconsensual killing." It is true, of course, that "nonconsensual killing" is wrong—but there is more to say about our relationships with the suffering and dying, and if we deny that there is more to say, then we may subvert and destroy the possibility of covenantal relationships with the suffering and dying.

Our culture is prepared to acknowledge that something more than justice is required in these relationships, and to name that something more "mercy." But it has, I fear, a minimal notion of mercy, too. It is prepared to acknowledge as morally appropriate the emotive response to another's suffering that we call mercy or compassion, the emotive response that moves us to action when we see suffering, to do something to ease our neighbor's pain, to put a stop to our neighbor's suffering, to put an end to our neighbor's dying.[5] The problem with the minimal notions of mercy and compassion, however, is that, while they tell us to do *something*, they do not tell us *what thing* to do. Such a notion of "mercy" can justify almost anything. The minimal notion of mercy is used to defend the legitimacy of assisted suicide and voluntary euthanasia, which at least qualify as "doing something" to put a stop to suffering. Such acts are sometimes described (and defended) in terms of their motive as "mercy-killing."

The minimal notions of justice and mercy, then, seem to justify assisted suicide and voluntary euthanasia. Assisted suicide and voluntary euthanasia, after all, are chosen by autonomous individuals and end the suffering of one who hurts. "Do justice!" "Love mercy!" Who can argue with such advice or with the validity of the inferences which justify assisted suicide and voluntary euthanasia? Well, we can, I think. We should at least be suspicious of this advice as minimal and suspicious of these inferences as a possible distortion of our relationship with the suffering and dying. We might point out, for example, that, if we begin to regard killing as a work of *mercy*, it will be hard not to be merciful (and deadly) toward those who have lost or never achieved a capacity for autonomy. Or, we might point out that, if we begin to regard being killed as a *right*, it will be difficult to limit the space for the exercise of that right to those cases where the suffering is severe and beyond human remedy.

We should ask whether such minimal notions are finally adequate to the moral life or to care for the dying. None of us is as independent and "autonomous" as the minimal notion of justice pretends, nor should we want to be. And when compassion kills, when the desire to help becomes confused with the desire to obliterate, then "taking care" of someone suggests a sinister double meaning which should make us morally cautious.[6]

Christians, among others, might provide a different context for the intelligibility of these notions, and, so, a different way to understand these notions and their implications. "Do justice!" "Love mercy!" Yes, but when the prophet Micah gave such instruction, he connected it with a third instruction, "Walk humbly with your God!" (Micah 6:8). And he presented the whole as a requirement of God, as the response of faith and faithfulness. "Justice" and "mercy" embedded in such a story are not minimal requirements.

They are, first of all, characteristics of God. The justice of God is God's own faithfulness to covenant, God's fidelity to the intentions with which God formed the world and a people, even when it meant resistance to the resistance to God's cause. And God's mercy is God's grace, God's persistence to bless, and God's presence to suffering. God's mercy intends, in spite of the powers of sin and death, even now a little space for joy and rest and finally the triumph of *shalom*. And until "the close of the age," God's mercy shares the pain while the creation groans and the tears while any creature weeps.

Justice and mercy are also, of course, standards of excellence for those who would be faithful to God, who would walk humbly with God. They are the shape of response to God—and to all things in ways appropriate to the relations of all things to God. Such justice tells us something of the goods to seek, the goods which belong to God's cause, life and human flourishing among them. Such justice exercises some constraints besides respect for the arbitrary preferences of another, constraints that include the prohibition of the intentional destruction of an embodied image of God. Such justice will nurture covenantal relations, not reduce them to contractual or instrumental relationships. It will defend the weak and be an advocate for the powerless against the powers that resist God's cause. Such mercy will persist in blessing "the least of these" (Matthew 25:40, 45) and will be present to them in the midst of hurt and harm. It will visit the sick (Matthew 25:36, 43), not abandon or eliminate them. Indeed, it will discover in "the least of these" and in their vulnerability the very image of Christ (Matthew 25:40, 45). To "walk *humbly* with God" will acknowledge that there are limits to our powers—and so to our responsibilities. We are not God; our powers are not messianic; they provide no escape finally from human mortality or from the human vulnerability to suffering. Even while we work for God's cause, we wait and watch for it. Such justice and mercy "fit" the story of scripture, but such justice and mercy do not fit assisted suicide and consensual killing.

The rule of such a justice prohibits eliminating the sufferer in the name of eliminating suffering. The reign of such a mercy will not be satisfied with simply shouting that prohibition; it will not be satisfied with a rule, however clearly stated and argued. A rule, a prohibition, even one formed out of scripture's story, will almost certainly not be sufficient as a response to suicide or to our culture.[7] Given the sort of world it is, a world not yet God's unchallenged sovereignty, there are many who quite reasonably despair. Their bodies are broken, or their spirits are crushed; their circumstances seem hopeless, or their dignity seems lost; and the One who bears down on them no longer seems to sustain them. No law, no rule, no cogent philosophical or religious argument may be sufficient to dissuade them from suicide.[8] Indeed, the prohibition may only increase the "fascination with the forbidden"—and in some cases identify a final form of rebellion and betrayal against the One (or ones) upon whom they depend but have come to distrust.

What is required in such cases is not law but a powerful and creative word of grace. That word may be mute, of course, a voiceless presence communicating a readiness to listen and to share the suffering. Or, the word may find voice in response to the complaints of the sufferer, a voice sharing the human cry of lament, enabling courage or patience. The word of grace may be a deed , some little thing that expresses faithfulness in our relations to others, some little signal that one is permitted to live, not obliged to live, even while it gives no permission to kill, or some little token that one is also permitted to die, not obliged to die, even while it gives no permission to "live on at all costs." The word of grace will sometimes take the form of the rule itself, to say "no" to the request of assistance in suicide, for such a request is sometimes deeply confused with tests of perceptions that others would prefer that one be dead. What is required is a word of joy which is capable of acknowledging the reality of their sadness, a word of hope which is capable of recognizing the limits on their real options. What is required is gospel, the good news that the human senses of dependence, remorse, and hope meet a God who can be trusted, even in the midst of suffering and dying. I do not mean to suggest that what is required is a homily, surely not a glib assurance that all is well, or the cheap advice that one engage in a little positive thinking. I mean a faithfulness that keeps company with the suffering and dying and with God, a faithfulness that walks humbly with God and humbly in the imaginations and affections of those in despair. I mean at the very least to commend hospice care as "fitting" to the story.

Even so, given the sort of world it is, even such words and deeds may not be enough to call a person from despair and suicide, and the tragedy of their lives and deaths should keep us from judging them (or ourselves) too quickly and too harshly. And sometimes, when one has mournfully assisted another in suicide, we need mercy when we render judgment, even just judgment, on another. Justice requires a verdict of guilty, but mercy might suggest, not a different verdict, but suspending the sentence in tragic circumstances.

Suffering and Dying

Permit me to turn to notions of suffering and dying. For Christians the significance of "suffering" and "dying" is determined by the story of scripture, stories of creation and fall and redemption, stories of a cross and of an empty tomb. In those stories one discovers a certain dialectic in the dispositions toward suffering and dying.

On the one hand, life and its flourishing belong to the creative and redemptive cause of God. The signs of it are breath and a blessing, a rainbow and God's own sanction, a commandment and, finally, an empty tomb. Therefore, life and its flourishing will be recognized and celebrated as goods, as goods against which we may not turn without turning against the cause of God. Life and its flourishing are gifts of God. They are to be received with thanksgiving and used with gratitude. Acts which aim at death (and acts which aim at suffering) do not fit this story, do not cohere with devotion to the cause of God or with gratitude for the gifts of God. Death and suffering are not to be intended, nor to be chosen.

On the other hand, life and its flourishing are not the ultimate goods. They are not "second gods."[9] Jesus walked a path steadily and courageously that led to his suffering and to his death. Therefore, Christians may not live as though either survival or ease were the law of their being. Sometimes life must be risked, let go, given up. And sometimes suffering must be risked or shared for the sake of God's cause in the world. The refusal ever to let die and the attempt to eliminate suffering altogether are not signals of faithfulness but of idolatry. And if life and its flourishing are not the ultimate goods, neither are death and suffering the ultimate evils. They need not be feared finally, for death and suffering are not as strong as the promise of God. One need not use all one's resources against them. One need only act with integrity in the face of them.

This dialectic is captured in the distinctions between killing and allowing to die and between choosing suffering and patiently bearing it. Those distinctions have formed a consensus in Christian communities and—until recently—in our culture. The moral significance of those distinctions, of course, is being challenged—and may be difficult to defend when the story in which they are embedded is denied or ignored.[10]

They are hard to defend, for example, in the context of a utilitarian calculus. There the only relevant consideration is outcomes, results, consequences. If the consequences are the same, it is hard to see in a utilitarian calculus why the moral evaluation of mercifully allowing one to die and mercifully killing another ought to be different. Moreover, if the standard for assessing the consequences is the maximization of preference satisfaction, and if anyone (whether arbitrarily or reasonably) prefers death to life in their particular circumstances, then it is not hard to see the moral obligation to kill the suicidal (or to inflict pain on the masochist).

The distinctions seem more at home—at least initially—in the context of the sort of moral minimalism that focuses on rights and their correlative duties. In this context, for example, one can distinguish between negative and positive rights, between rights to noninterference and rights to assistance. One can distinguish the right to life as a negative right not to be killed from the right to life as a positive right to assistance in preserving one's life. And one can also distinguish the right to die as a negative right, not to have one's dying interfered with, from the right to die as a positive right, as a right to assisted suicide. Since rights to noninterference impose much more stringent correlative duties than rights to assistance, and since the negative right to life imposes a duty not to kill, many have argued that there can be no positive right to die and no correlative duty—or even a permission—to assist in suicide. Perhaps that is why the right to life was once regarded as "unalienable." It's a good argument, I think, but it loses something of its force in the context of the moral minimalism that is attentive only to autonomy, that regards even fundamental rights as alienable. Not only does the right to die seem, then, to extend to suicide; it would also seem to extend to assistance in suicide if a contract had been freely entered. Where choice monopolizes our moral attention, there consensual killing becomes morally indistinguishable from consensual allowing to die.

If the right to life, or any right, is simply a legitimate claim, if it is *not*, as the Declaration of Independence says, unalienable, then if I simply and autonomously refuse to make this legitimate claim, if I refuse to claim my right to die, it is hard to see why killing me would be a violation of that right.

The distinction, however, still fits the story of scripture and the notions of suffering and dying formed by it. The martyrs knew the story well, and they "bore witness" to it by choosing neither death nor suffering but by being ready to endure either for the sake of God's cause in the world and their own integrity. Their comfort was that they were not their own but belonged to God, the giver of life, from whom not even death could separate them. And their comfort was their courage.[11] In more mundane and commonplace ways, many Christian patients still display the same comfort and the same courage, still bear witness to the story by their readiness to die but not to kill, by refusing both offers of assisted suicide and offers of treatment which may prolong their days but only by rendering those days (or months or years) less apt for their tasks of reconciliation with enemies or fellowship with friends or simply fun with the family.

Because there was breath and a blessing, because there was a rainbow and a commandment, because there was an empty tomb, Christians will not choose death, will not intend death. But because the one who was raised had suffered and died, Christians will acknowledge that there may be goods more weighty than their own survival and duties which override their ease, goods and duties which determine how they should live, even while they are dying. Christian communities continue to have their reasons for preserving the traditional distinctions. There remains a theologically significant difference between intending death and foreseeing it, between choosing death and choosing how to live while one is dying, between suicide and accepting death, between killing and allowing to die, and between choosing suffering and patiently enduring or sharing it. "Suicide is not a viable alternative"—not for Christian theology at any rate.

Healing and Caring

The third section turns to notions of healing and caring and to the identity of medicine. Permit me to begin also this section theologically.

According to the Reformed tradition, medicine is a "calling," a vocation. The notion of a vocation served initially to vest the work of physicians (and others) with a new dignity, a dignity not less than the vocation to a "religious" life. It emancipated the work of physicians (and others) from the control of priestly power. At the same time, by regarding medicine as a calling, it asserted that medicine, too, could serve the cause of God, could be a form of discipleship, that medical skills and knowledge should be set within the story of scripture and its demands of faithfulness. In that story Jesus came preaching that the kingdom of God was at hand and already making its power felt in his words of blessing and his works of healing, and in that story Jesus suffered and died. He called the disciples to follow him, to preach and to heal (Matthew 10:5–15), and to take up the cross (16:24). The Christian community is called to heal just as surely as it is called to proclaim "good news," and it is called to be present to those who suffer just as surely as it is called to heal and to preach. It is, and is to be, a healing and caring community. The Christian community may not surrender this calling to medicine, but part of its calling is, and is to be, the support (and reform) of medicine. Physicians who own their work as a calling, as a form of discipleship, will not dismiss the special skills and training, the special competence, of medicine. But neither will they dismiss the story of scripture as the story they long to live in and through their vocation.

Theology aside, there is today in the debate about assisted suicide and voluntary euthanasia a struggle for the identity of the profession of medicine. It is not a novel struggle, or a new debate, for that matter, but the meaning of the profession is at stake.

In ancient Greece physicians defined their role in terms of restoring health and easing pain. They saw the good of health and their powerlessness against death. When patients were mortally ill, "overmastered by their diseases," these physicians refrained from efforts to cure them—and sometimes killed them.[12] To relieve the suffering of the dying, these physicians counted poisons and other techniques to produce a painless death among the tools of their trade.

The famous Hippocratic Oath, of course, stood against such practices: "I will neither give a deadly drug to anybody if asked for it, nor will I make a suggestion to this effect."[13] The Oath was written "against the stream." It was a minority report. But this effort to reform the practice of medicine was remarkably successful. It shaped the conduct and character of medicine for centuries. Because the goods intrinsic to medicine were to heal the sick, to protect and nurture health, to relieve pain, limits could be imposed on the use of skills within the practice. The skills were not to be used to serve alien ends, and the destruction of human life was regarded as an alien and conflicting end. They saw not only the good of health and the limit of their powers but also the respect that was due life itself. They prohibited any direct taking of life. But while they would not kill, there was not yet any sense of an obligation to prolong the lives of those "over-mastered by their disease."[14]

The physician's perspective was to shift again, however, with the development of a new vision and new powers. Francis Bacon saw a "third end" for medicine, the preservation of life, and he regarded it as the "most noble of all." He rejected the old category of those "overmastered by their disease," and complained that "the pronouncing of these diseases incurable gives a legal sanction, as it were, to neglect and inattention and exempts ignorance from discredit."[15] Bacon's recommendation was innovative for its time, but it came to shape the medical community and identity as powerfully as the innovative Oath had. Physicians were enlisted on the side of life, fighting a messy but heroic battle against death. Their courage was their refusal to call any disease incurable. There weapons were forged in study and research. Their allies were the university and its laboratories.[16]

Among the effects of this shift, of course, was the ability to cure a number of those diseases which once overmastered the sick. For that, of course, we may and must be thankful. But for some other effects, we may and must be rueful. Ironically the complaint of Bacon about the neglect and inattention and ignorance that were sanctioned by the former medicine can be turned against the medicine Bacon inspired.

Where neglect is identified with a decision no longer to attempt to cure, there medical care and the project of healing are reduced to cure. Where attention to patients is identified with the effort to cure them, attentiveness to patients is reduced to attentiveness to their pathologies. Where "knowledge is power" and where such power is regarded as power over nature and celebrated as bringing human well-being in its train, care for patients is reduced to treating their bodies as manipulable nature in an effort to cure them. The ironic result is that another kind of ignorance is sanctioned, ignorance of the identities of patients, of the particular stories they tell and of the individual aims they cherish, of their communities. And when such ignorance is sanctioned, the physician will be ill-prepared to understand and to respond to the particular ways in which patients suffer, in which they experience their condition as a threat to their embodied integrity.[17] Care motivated the search for a cure, of course, but the search for a cure pushed care to the margins.

The Baconian account of medicine had great success, but the failure of that success is told in the sad stories of a lingering dying, tragic stories of physicians treating patients like manipulable nature in an effort to cure them, and sad stories of patients suffering not only from a certain pathology but from the treatment for it. Today this Baconian account of the physician's role is under attack. The identity of the physician is being revisioned and refashioned in our age. That provides both opportunity and danger.

One of the options for medicine shares Bacon's confidence in knowledge as power over nature and the assumption that the threat to human well-being is located in nature, but it shifts attention to a still more noble end, the elimination of suffering. The project then is to eliminate suffering, even if one has to eliminate the sufferer to do it. It is no longer death but suffering which is the great enemy. The physician turns now to new technologies (except, of course, that the technology itself is as old as hemlock) in an effort to master human nature's vulnerability to suffering. Knowledge is still power over nature, including human nature, and its mastery includes not only keeping people alive but killing them.

A second option for medicine—sometimes called medicine as a marketplace—is more modest about the well-being that comes in the train of technology and agnostic about any good that belongs to medicine as a practice. In this revisioning the physician has certain skills and tools which may be made available in the marketplace, available to do the bidding of the one who pays. The identity of physician is that of a contractor or entrepreneur. Well-being still comes in the train of such knowledge, but only by reducing well-being to the satisfaction of the arbitrary preferences of medical consumers and contractors. And if the consumer prefers death, a contract can be made, and *caveat emptor!*

There is, however, another option for revisioning the identity of physician. It is the option of medicine as a vocation, a calling, a form of discipleship. Such a medicine may set the practice and its skills within the story of scripture and its demands of faithfulness. It may see medicine as a response to God, as a form of service to the cause of God. But at the very least it would work to sustain and nurture certain virtues that would constitute a faithful medicine.

A faithful medicine would sustain and nurture *truthfulness* about our finitude, about the limits imposed by our mortality and about our human vulnerability to suffering. It would sustain and nurture *humility*, the readiness to acknowledge the evil we sometimes do in resisting evil. A faithful medicine would sustain and nurture *gratitude* for the gifts of life and health and for the opportunities within its limitations—not to eliminate mortality or the human vulnerability to suffering, but—sometimes to cure, sometimes to heal, sometimes to remove someone's pain, sometimes to relieve the bitterness of someone's tears, but always at least to wipe those tears away with tenderness. A faithful medicine would nurture and sustain *care*, care even for those it cannot cure. It will acknowledge in "the least of these" the very image of the Lord who calls them to serve. It will be ready as Simon of Cyrene (Matthew 27:32) to help carry the cross another bears, a stranger called, compelled, and blessed to be present to the suffering one and so to Jesus.[18] A medicine can be present to the suffering and dying without panic, without the anxious effort to substitute for an absent God. Such a medicine can nurture and sustain a more *carefree* care.

The stories of Jesus do not fit the story sometimes told by medical practice to patients (and sometimes told by patients to medical practice) that death is the ultimate enemy and the worst evil, to be put off by any means. And if people sometimes then blame physicians for keeping them alive beyond all reason, the stories of Jesus and his cross do not fit the story told by Jack Kevorkian and the Hemlock Society that suffering is the ultimate evil and life the great enemy, and that a good doctor is a good killer.

Medicine as a vocation would be disposed to cure when possible, ready to care always, ready to let go of a patient to death and to God when care requires it, but never ready to kill. "Suicide is not a viable alternative" for a faithful medicine.

Freedom

Finally, I turn to the notion of maximizing freedom and to the question of public policy. Earlier I said that there remain theological reasons for preserving the distinction between choosing death and choosing how to live while one is dying. I have just suggested why a faithful medicine may want to preserve the distinction. These arguments, I grant, may not be sufficient for public policy deliberations. In this section I hope to present an argument against physician-assisted suicide by considering the position that defends physician-assisted suicide as a way to maximize our freedom and to increase our options.

"Maximize freedom!" Who can argue with such advice? Surely not one formed by scripture, for human freedom is a gift of God and part of God's cause. "For freedom has Christ set us free" (Galatians 5:1). But one may ask, of course, what "freedom" means. Freedom, too, is a slippery term.

The Christian tradition has consistently preferred an Augustinian account of human freedom to a Pelagian account. Pelagius had described human freedom as the capacity of a neutral agent to make choices unconstrained and uncoerced, to contemplate options without internal or external restraints. Equipoised between good and evil, undetermined even by their own previous choices, neutral selves can will what they will. The evidence for freedom on this account is inconsistency, unpredictability, arbitrariness, the ability to will one thing one moment and a contrary thing the next. Augustine—and Luther and Calvin among his heirs—saw nothing to cherish or respect in such an account of freedom. In Augustine's view there are no neutral selves, no indeterminate agents who face choices unformed by the past, and there are no choices which do not form the determinate features of the future of the self.

The Augustinian tradition, therefore, has always appreciated the significance of the determinate features of human existence. Particular human beings and their choices are formed by their natural endowments (including, we may say now, their genetic endowments), their natural communities, their cultures, their past choices, and the choices of others with respect to them. These determinate features of human existence limit human freedom, to be sure, but they also *enable* freedom. There is no human freedom which does not marshall endowments, weigh the claims of particular communities, interpret their culture, assess past choices, and respond to actions upon them. Human freedom does not exist in some disinterested point in transcendence over all that; it is rather engaged in and engaged with the determinate features of our existence. Freedom in this context is the capacity of a self to establish a self, an identity, to form a whole of the disparate and determinate features of one's life, and the evidence of freedom is not arbitrariness but consistency and predictability.

The point I want to make relies on this Augustinian reminder that our choices, including our social choices, including even the presumably innocent choice to "maximize freedom," express and form the determinate features of our life and of our common life.

The point can be illustrated with response to technology. Technology is frequently introduced as a way to increase our options, as a way to maximize freedom. But it can become part of the determinate features of existence; it can quickly become socially enforced. The car was introduced as an option to the horse, but now social pressure compels us to drive. The horse remains, I suppose, a "recreational vehicle," but don't try to ride one home on the Interstate. The technology that surrounds our dying was introduced to give doctors and patients options in the face of disease and death, but such "options" have become socially required; at least we sometimes hear, "We have no choice!" Now it is possible, of course, to claim that cars and CPR represent progress, but then the argument has shifted from the celebration of options and the maximizing of freedom to something else—to the meaning of progress. The point is simply this, that we need to ask not just whether the social legitimation of suicide, assisted suicide, and voluntary euthanasia serves freedom by increasing our options but also whether it will be moral progress if the new option becomes socially (even if not legally) enforced.

Moreover, even if a particular option does not become socially enforced, simply providing the option, simply "maximizing freedom" by giving social legitimation to certain choices, can and does effect the determinate features of our life and our common life. Our choices, even to regard certain things as choices, form selves, and our social choices, even to increase options, form our common life.

Consider, for example, the life of a night clerk at the convenience store.[19] One determinate feature of her existence is frequently identified on the front door: "The night clerk cannot open the safe." In order to maximize the freedom of the night clerk, to increase her options, one might give her the option of opening the safe. But to increase her options in this way would change the determinate features of her life, and not happily—or innocently. Not happily—because, given the vulnerability of a night clerk, it would minimize her security. And not innocently—because under cover of maximizing options we would be forming ourselves to regard the vulnerability of others as a matter of moral indifference. The sick and suffering are vulnerable, too, and maximizing their freedom may render them still more vulnerable. To the vulnerability of the sick and suffering we will return, but first note that choices to increase options sometimes eliminate options.

An acquaintance invited me to a party. It was presented as an option, of course. But by increasing my options, he had effectively eliminated an option I suddenly realized I had a moment ago, but have no longer, an option I would have preferred, namely, the option of *both* not spending three hours with him *and* not explaining to him why I would rather not (or lying). The invitation increased my options, but it also eliminated an option.[20]

When we provide social legitimation of the *option* of suicide, we may increase options, but we also effectively eliminate an option, namely, staying alive without having to justify one's existence. That happens to be a option that the Christian tradition would choose if it could, an option the Christian tradition would like to protect and preserve, for it fits with the story of life as a gift, as a given. Given the new option in the name of maximizing freedom, one may choose, of course, not to be killed, but the person who makes that choice is now responsible for it, accountable for living, and can be asked to justify that choice.

With this point we return to the issue of the vulnerability of the sick and suffering, for this burden of justification will be hard to bear for those who simply do not want to be a burden. Moreover, the very giving of the choice can create some pressure to make a particular choice.

The vulnerable will be subject not just to the pressure of malicious thugs and con-artists, not just to the pressure of relatives who may be better off financially or emotionally if the vulnerable were to die, not only to the pressure of "compassionate" friends who would like to see the suffering stop, but also to the pressure of their own sense of obligation to justify their existence. And they would respond to that pressure by drawing on resources determined in part (and undermined in part) by the social choice to provide the option of assisted suicide as a way of maximizing freedom.[21]

The point is not a subtle one. It gets lost, I think, only when we overestimate our autonomy and independence. It gets lost when we lose a sense of our dependence and interdependence. Our self-concept is always confused with our interpretation of how others think and feel about us. The suicide threat is, after all, sometimes a call for help, an inquiry about whether anyone really cares. To respond to such a threat by giving the option can all too easily be read as an answer to that inquiry, and it can affect the resources a person has for choosing still to live. And if that is true in individual cases, it is also true culturally. Maximizing freedom by providing the choice of assisted suicide to the vulnerable, to the dependent, to those who are no longer in control is recommended, doubtlessly, as a way to increase their options, to enable them to assert their independence and to take control. It expresses a culture and forms attitudes that value autonomy, independence, and control, but it also forms attitudes *toward* those who suffer their way toward death, and it may make it more difficult for the sick and suffering, the dependent, those whose lives seem out of control, to refuse the option of death, harder to justify their existence. This social innovation in the name of increasing options not only eliminates the option of receiving life as a given, it may also shape the way the choice will be made.

Giving people the option of dueling is an instructive parallel.[22] We no longer give people that option. That is moral progress, I think. Of course, people still have the option, but we do not provide social legitimation for it. The point is not simply to express disapproval of dueling. The point is, rather, to observe the relationship between a culture, the options it provides, and the pressure on choices. The social choice to provide the option of dueling expressed a culture, one obsessed with honor. Providing this option reinforced that feature of the culture. And that very feature of the culture was one of the determinate features of the context within which persons made their choices, making it more difficult not to throw down or to pick up the gauntlet. *Our* culture may be obsessed with individual autonomy. But the reason we have for giving the option of assisted suicide may well make it more difficult for people not to choose death.

If we choose to give this option, we are choosing not just a discrete piece of social policy but a pattern of our life together which asks the weak and the sick to justify their existence. To refuse freely to give that option is to choose a pattern for our life where life is received as a given even when it is not cherished as a gift, and where being dependent on others and on God is accepted as our common situation.

If such is to be the pattern for our life together, then our responsibility will not be limited to leaving our neighbors alone. Our responsibility will extend to learning to care for each other in the midst of suffering. Our responsibility will surely include respect for a neighbor's capacities for agency, but it will also include attentiveness to the neighbor when the neighbor's embodied integrity is threatened. That attentiveness will require presence, and faithfulness, and finally grace rather than either law or options.

"Suicide is not a viable alternative" for public policy either.[23]

Notes

1. Peter DeVries, *The Blood of the Lamb* (Boston: Little, Brown, and Company, 1962); Peter DeVries, *Slouching Towards Kalamazoo* (Boston: Little, Brown, and Company, 1983).
2. I am sure this is a line in a DeVries novel, but I have not been able to locate it.
3. Peter DeVries, *The Tunnel of Love* (Boston: Little, Brown, and Company, 1954), p. 65.
4. Peter DeVries, *The Glory of the Hummingbird* (Boston: Little, Brown, and Company, 1974), p. 261.
5. Oliver O'Donovan makes this point compellingly. Oliver O'Donovan, *Begotten or Made?* (Oxford: Oxford University Press, 1984), pp. 10–12. Compassion, he says, is "the virtue of being moved to action by the sight of suffering," but it "presupposes that an answer has already been found to the question 'What needs to be done?'" (p. 11). In the context of our culture's confidence in technology, compassion will simply arm itself with superior technique, relying not on wisdom but on artifice against suffering (p. 12). See also Allen Verhey, "Suffering and Compassion: Looking Heavenward," *Perspectives* (February, 1995): pp. 17–21.
6. Robert A. Burt, *Taking Care of Strangers: The Rule of Law in Doctor-Patient Relations* (New York: Free Press, 1979), pp. v–vii *et passim*.
7. Karl Barth, *Church Dogmatics*, volume III, part 4, trans. A. T. Mackay, *et al.* (Edinburgh: T and T Clark, 1961), p. 406.
8. James M. Gustafson, *Ethics from a Theocentric Perspective: Ethics and Theology* (Chicago: University of Chicago Press, 1984), pp. 201–207.
9. Barth, loc cit., p. 392.
10. Gilbert Meilaender, "The Distinction Between Killing and Allowing to Die," *Theological Studies* (September, 1976): pp. 467–70; Robert N. Wennberg, *Terminal Choices: Euthanasia, Suicide and the Right to Die* (Grand Rapids: Eerdmans, 1984), pp. 150–56.

I do not mean to rest the distinction between "allowing to die" and "killing" on the distinction between omission and commission, and I surely do not mean to suggest that the distinction provides a formula for resolving hard questions. There are clearly some cases of omission which can only be described as intending the death of the patient, the failure to treat Baby Doe's esophageal atresis, for example. And there are some cases which are hard to classify as "allowing to die" or as "killing"; Wennberg's case of the diabetic with painful and terminal cancer who withholds insulin is one example, pp. 136–42. Still, "there is a theologically significant difference between *shaping* one's dying and *creating* one's dying" (Wennberg, p. 137), between intending death and foreseeing it, between choosing death and choosing how to live while one is dying.

11. Consider besides the martyrs the first question and answer of the Heidelberg Catechism: "Q. What is your only comfort in life and death? A. That I am not my own but belong—body and soul, in life and in death, to my faithful Savior Jesus Christ. . . . Because I belong to him, Christ by His Holy Spirit, assures me of eternal life and makes me whole-heartedly willing and ready from now on to live for him."

12. As the Hippocratic treatise "The Art" would put it somewhat later; in Stanley Reiser, Arthur Dyck, and William Curran, eds., *Ethics and Medicine: Historical Perspectives and Contemporary Concerns* (Cambridge: MIT Press, 1977), p. 6.

13. Ludwig Edelstein's translation, in Charles Burns, ed., *Legacies in Ethics and Medicine* (New York: Science History Publications, 1977), p. 14.

14. On the Hippocratic Oath see further Nigel M. de S. Cameron *The New Medicine* (Wheaton, IL: Crossway Books, 1991); and Leon Kass, *Towards a More Natural Science: Biology and Human Affairs* (New York: The Free Press, 1985), pp. 224–26.

15. Francis Bacon, *De Augmentis Scientiarum, The Philosophical Works of Francis Bacon*, J. M. Robertson, ed. (New York: Books for Libraries Press, 1970), pp. 487–89.

16. See further William F. May's accounts of the "fighter" and the "technician" in William F. May, *The Physician's Covenant: Images of the Healer in Medical Ethics* (Philadelphia: Westminster Press, 1983), pp. 63–106.

17. See Eric Cassell's lament about the inattentiveness of medicine to suffering; Eric Cassell, "Recognizing Suffering," *Hastings Center Report* 21 (May-June, 1991): 24–31.

18. I owe this image to Dr. Andy von Eschenbach, who used it to describe his own sense of calling to be a physician at a physician-clergy breakfast at The Institute of Religion, Houston, Texas.

19. J. David Velleman, "Against the Right to Die," *The Journal of Medicine and Philosophy* 17 (6) (December, 1992): 671.

20. Ibid., p. 672.

21. Leon Kass, "Death with Dignity and the Sanctity of Life," *Commentary* 89 (3) (March, 1990): 41; cf. also Wennberg's powerful account of "negative fallout argument," loc cit., pp. 187–92.

22. Velleman, loc cit., p. 676.

23. This paper was presented as part of the program of "Physician-Assisted Suicide: A Multi-Disciplinary Discussion," a conference of the Ethics Institute, a joint program of Lehigh Valley Area Health Education Center and Cedar Crest College. A longer version has been published previously; Allen Verhey, "Physician-Assisted Suicide and Euthanasia: A Biblical and Reformed Perspective," in Ronald P. Hamel and Edwin R. DuBose, eds., *Must We Suffer Our Way to Death?: Cultural and Theological Perspectives on Death by Choice* (Dallas, TX: Southern Methodist University Press, 1996).

23

Jewish Deliberations on Suicide

Exceptions, Toleration, and Assistance

NOAM J. ZOHAR

Classical Jewish sources mention exceptions to the suicide prohibition, notably in a case "like King Saul." Differing religious understandings of the grounds prohibiting suicide yield opposing views on whether this exception should apply to suicide to escape terminal suffering. The Halakha (the Judaic tradition of normative discourse) contains many serious controversies, and contains also a pluralistic tradition recognizing the legitimacy of opposing positions. What, then, is the proper course of action from a physician who holds a restrictive position, if faced with a request for assistance from a patient subscribing to the more permissive view? Two alternatives are examined: A "hands-off" position, which is analyzed in terms of upholding personal integrity; versus a "cooperative" position, which is analyzed in terms of interpersonal relatedness and sharing the other's viewpoint. It is suggested that this analysis can apply to non-Halakhic and non-Judaic contexts as well, as long as each party recognizes the moral legitimacy of the other's position.

*　　*　　*

Halakha and Divergent Views

THERE IS NOT ONE, uniform "Jewish view" on how to cope with terminal suffering. There are, however, some basic premises, fairly pervasive in the Jewish tradition of normative discourse (*halakha*). These include not only views on the value of human life and the prohibition of suicide, but also traditions on dealing with disagreements. I will begin with the latter, for two reasons. First, they provide a framework for appreciating the plurality of particular halakhic positions. And second, they may offer some more general insights to guide decision-making in a pluralistic setting beyond the particularly Jewish context, where various agents are likely to hold disparate religious and moral views.

Since early medieval times, commitment to *halakha* involved canonizing the Talmud with its complex dialectic form, where hardly any debate ends with a definite conclusion. Despite the system's ultimate grounding in revelation, post-talmudic authors rarely appeal to Scripture for arguing or deciding points of halakha. Instead, they focus on the oral Torah: "God's word" as mediated by tradition, precedent, and practical reason *(sevara)*. This fits well with classical Rabbinic assertions that the Torah is "not in heaven": God's will is to be determined not by prophecy but by study and interpretation.

It is not surprising that this approach yields frequent and numerous disagreements. Anyone wishing to live by "God's word" is confronted, in this tradition, with a plurality of interpretations and rival rulings. A famous talmudic passage speaks of the dispute between the two great "houses" of the last century before the destruction of the second temple:

> Rabbi Aba, citing Shemu'el, said: For three years, the Houses of Shammai and Hillel disagreed.
> These said: the Halakha should be according to us, while those said: the Halakha should be according to us.
> [Then] a voice [from heaven] pronounced: "These and those are the living words of God; and the Halakha is according to the House of Hillel."
> (Babylonian Talmud, Eruvin 13b)

The pronouncement of the heavenly voice here is very different from a mere call for toleration, that is, a stance of civility toward others despite the utter wrongness of their views. The message seems to be rather one of pluralism: There is not just one valid rendition of "God's word." Both positions—although they are mutually exclusive—are part of the oral Torah, instances of divine teaching. God speaks richly, not univocally.

How can such a conception be translated into practice? The core document of rabbinic Judaism, the Mishna, depicts a (somewhat idealized) practice of mutual respect. The Mishna relates a series of disagreements between the two Houses regarding various halakhic issues concerning marriage and preparation of (ritually) pure foods. Given these disagreements, members of each House could have had good reason to avoid marrying individuals of the other House or relying on the purity of their utensils and foodstuffs. Each, holding their own halakhic views to be correct, should arguably have seen the alternative practice as unacceptable. Even if they did not think ill of their disputants on account of their sincerely held positions, how could they themselves, in their own actions, accommodate the perspective which they disavowed? We are told, however, that

> Even though these forbid while those permit, the House of Shammai did not avoid taking wives from the House of Hillel, nor the House of Hillel from the House of Shammai. [Despite] all the items of purity and impurity, which these declared pure while those declared impure, they did not avoid relying on each other in producing pure foods. (Mishna Yevamot 1:4)
> Instead, they acted with truth and peace between them, as is written, "Love truth and peace" (Zach. 8:19; Tosefta ibid, 1:10).[1]

Thus the pluralistic doctrine of "these and those are the living words of God" had its corollary in practice. Rabbinic Judaism conveys, then, not only a host of disagreements, but also a norm of respectful accommodation and cooperation between adherents of opposing halakhic views. Against this background, we now turn to examine some traditional views on suicide and suffering.

The Prohibition of Suicide: Reasons and Exceptions

The ideal of personal autonomy implies, according to some of its proponents, that suicide is in general morally permissible, as it involves directly none but the agent himself. Whether this is a necessary implication is a question of great interest, but I shall not address it here. Rabbinic Judaism, in any case, has consistently taught a general prohibition upon taking one's own life.[2]

Why is suicide forbidden? Traditional sources seem to suggest two religious reasons which are not, strictly speaking, mutually exclusive. But although they might be offered in conjunction, the two are quite distinct (and only one involves a direct challenge to human autonomy).

One argument against suicide is put in terms of divine sovereignty, or of God's "ownership"—of the world in general or of human beings in particular. It explicitly denies human self-ownership: A person belongs to God, and therefore has no right, through suicide, to destroy that which is not hers. It is not clear how literally the language of "ownership" is to be taken; perhaps it is just a way of stating that people are God's subjects.

Another argument points to the divine not as a locus of *authority*, but as the source of supreme *value* inhering in every human being. This approach may be captioned "Religious Humanism": the rabbis, drawing on key biblical passages (such as Genesis 1:26–28, 9:1–7), placed great significance upon the notion that each human individual is created in God's image.[3]

The first line of reasoning is expressed forcefully by a leading contemporary halakhist, Rabbi E. Waldenberg, in his extended argument against voluntary euthanasia and assisted suicide:

> No creature in the world owns a person's soul; this includes also that person himself, who has no license at all regarding his own soul nor is it his property. Thus his granting license can be of no avail concerning something which does not belong to him, but rather it is the property of God, Who alone bestows it and takes it away.[4]

The doctrine of divine ownership over humans is plausibly traced by Waldenberg to earlier rabbinic sources, including the code of Maimonides (e.g., Laws of Murder 1:4). In the Talmud itself, however, we find an extended debate on the permissibility of self-harm (BT Bava Kama 88b). Can it be surmised, then, that those who permit self-harm also allow suicide?

Well, the argument from ownership is not the only religious account for the rabbinic prohibition of suicide. The main source-text forbidding suicide points, instead, to the second religious account mentioned above. This text is found in *Genesis Rabbah*, the classical collection of rabbinic exegesis on the book of Genesis. Its context is the biblical passage already alluded to, where the value of human life—and the severity of its destruction—are proclaimed in terms of the divine image, inherent in every human individual. In that context, the rabbis announce that the terrible sin of bloodshed includes also self-destruction (Gen. Rab. 34:13).

It is important to note, however, that the same rabbinic text pronounces also two exceptions to the prohibition. As is common in midrashic literature, the rabbis' work with the text (Genesis 9:5) is not constrained by its literal sense.[5] Following a common midrashic convention, the verse's first word ("But") is construed as qualifying the absoluteness of the prohibition. Two exceptions are defined, not in substantive form, but rather by pointing to biblical examples. The two examples of legitimate suicide are those of 1) Saul (I Sam. 31: 1–6; cf. also II Sam. 1: 1–16), and 2) Hananiah, Misha'el, and Azariah (Dan. ch. 3; cf. ibid 1:7). The two exceptions are significant in themselves; as will be seen below, the first one—defined by the case of King Saul—carries special relevance for our context.

But perhaps the exceptions can also tell us something about the grounds for seeing suicide as wrong. The second exception involves martyrdom: These Jewish youngsters were prepared to be thrown into a furnace rather than worship an idol. The teaching that death should be chosen over idolatry, whether by submitting to the sword of oppressors or (on some views) even by actively killing oneself to avoid forced conversion, is pervasive in rabbinic sources, both talmudic and medieval. This exception is wholly compatible, it seems, with either of the above reasons for forbidding suicide. However grievous the destruction of the divine image, an affront to the divinity itself is (arguably) even more unbearable. And the exception is equally consistent with the assertion of God's authority over life and death. A martyr, choosing death, is surely affirming, rather than contesting, God's supreme sovereignty.

With respect to the first exception, however, there is no direct evidence for a divine interest being served by the self-inflicted death. The primary biblical account reads:

> The battle raged around Saul, and some of the archers hit him, and he was severely wounded by the archers.[6] Saul said to his arms-bearer, "Draw your sword and run me through, so that the uncircumcised may not run me through and make sport of me." But his arms-bearer, in his great awe, refused; whereupon Saul grasped the sword and fell upon it.

Saul knew that he was doomed; fearing torture (and degradation, too), he took his own life—and the Rabbis made his deed a paradigm of legitimate suicide. According to the view of divine sovereignty espoused by Waldenberg, Saul's action—and the rabbis' upholding of his deed as an example of permissible behavior—may seem difficult to explain. In the next section, we shall note some ways of trying to meet this difficulty. Arguably, however, this exception is more readily understood if the prohibition of suicide is seen as grounded in religious humanism rather than in divine authority.

Escaping Torture: Rabbi Hanina and King Saul

The issue of ending life in the face of terminal suffering should be addressed, within the Jewish tradition, against the backdrop of a basic prohibition of suicide, and hence (a fortiori) of voluntary euthanasia.[7] The question, then, is: Do the special circumstances of imminent death and of inescapable suffering offer grounds for an exception to this prohibition? In order to address this question from a *halakhic* perspective, we should analyze two central statements which seem directly relevant to the plight of a suffering, terminal patient: the talmudic account of Rabbi Hanina's martyrdom and the rabbinic endorsement of Saul's deed.

Rabbi Waldenberg, in his fierce denunciation of euthanasia and assisted suicide, cites Rabbi Hanina ben Teradion, who—being tortured to death—refused to hasten his end, stating that only God should be the one to take a person's life. The context of this event is the Roman persecutions in second-century Judea; the Talmud tells the story of Rabbi Hanina ben Teradion's martyrdom by fire. The Romans had found him acting in open defiance of their decree against the public teaching of Torah.

> They . . . wrapped him in the Torah scroll, surrounded him with bundles of vine shoots, and set them on fire. They brought tufts of wool, soaked them in water, and placed them over his heart, so that his soul should not depart quickly. . . . His disciples said to him, "Open your mouth, so that the fire will enter you quickly!" Rabbi Hanina replied: "It is better that it be taken by Him who has bestowed it— a person should not harm himself!"

But Waldenberg does not cite the continuation:

> The executioner said to him: "Master, if I increase the flames and remove the tufts of wool from over your heart, will you bring me into the life of the world-to-come?" "Yes." "Swear to me!"—Rabbi Hanina swore to him. The executioner then increased the flames and removed the tufts of wool from over his heart, and Rabbi Hanina's soul departed quickly. The executioner forthwith threw himself into the fire; a divine voice announced: "Rabbi Hanina ben Teradion and his executioner are assigned to life in the world-to-come." (Avoda Zara 18a)

The language of Rabbi Hanina's initial reaction is identical to that of one side in the Talmudic debate over self-harm alluded to above. Here (unlike in the context of that debate), a theological explanation is added: God alone, who gave life, has the prerogative of taking it. Rabbi Hanina's language does not necessarily translate into an idiom of *ownership*; but the recognition of God as one's creator, expressed in a pious readiness to suffer unto death, may indeed inspire a similar attitude in the context of terminal illness—excluding both suicide and euthanasia.[8]

But, reading on, we are forced to ask: Why does Rabbi Hanina accept the executioner's offer, rather than persevere in waiting for God to take his soul? After all, the executioners' subsequent deeds amount to both passive *and* active euthanasia. While removing the tufts of wool could conceivably be explained as allowing "natural" death to occur, is not the more compassionate *increasing of the flames* (followed by the executioner's own suicide!) equally endorsed by the Talmudic storyteller and by the heavenly voice?

It is not easy to produce any simple explanation for Rabbi Hanina's apparent inconsistency. Indeed the Talmudic tale, in its very complexity, does perhaps more justice to the anguish of this kind of human situation than any one-dimensional simplification.[9] God is proclaimed as the source of life, but what this finally implies seems far from clear. Put in Waldenberg's terms of "ownership," the question is: Must we necessarily assume that God insists on such total control of His human subjects? If, as the story suggests, the answer to this question is not entirely clear, then we may conclude that even if suicide is prohibited on grounds of divine sovereignty, seeking escape from great suffering may warrant an exception.

For a more definite statement, it seems best to return to the explicit exception defined by the midrashic text cited above—that of King Saul. Saul's death has been the focus of much discussion in the *halakhic* tradition, from the Middle Ages down to the present; three basic approaches can be discerned.[10]

One approach assimilates Saul's self-inflicted death to the model of martyrdom: Saul was afraid of being tortured not only because of the physical suffering, but also—and crucially—because he would be driven to apostasy.[11] Historically, this interpretation seems rooted more in the harsh and heroic epoch of Jewish communities under the Crusades than in the Biblical account itself. Applied to the context of illness, this might suggest a legitimation of suicide where a person feared that his or her suffering might lead to blasphemy.

A second approach reads the midrashic statement about Saul not as justifying but merely as excusing. On this view, Saul's fear was indeed of physical suffering; being thus impelled by powerful emotion, he should not be held liable for killing himself. Here too, the statement about Saul is assimilated to a well-known model. Since culpable suicide entailed in principle certain social and ritual sanctions, the issue of the deceased's emotional incapacity has long been raised as a compelling excuse.[12] Thus a person facing a tortured death is never *permitted* to take his own life; insofar as he is able to abide by the proper norm, he may not commit suicide. But once he has in fact killed himself, we are to adopt the sympathetic presumption of non-liability due to compulsion.

This view has had several adherents, and is the one adopted by Waldenberg in the essay cited above. Its hermeneutic weakness lies in the disanalogy with the other exception. After all, those who give up their lives as martyrs are not merely excused but justified—indeed, highly praised—for their deed. But it seems that the proponents of this approach, like those of the first one, view suicide as a rebellion against God's authority, and assert divine authority against any kind of human self-interest. They are therefore prepared to accept hermeneutic difficulties so that Saul's death should not read as a justified *suicide to avert a painful death*.

A third approach, however, adopts just such a reading, focusing on the explicit circumstances of Saul's death in the biblical account. Rather than introducing conditions unique to the doomed king, Nahmanides writes simply:

And likewise [inculpable is] an adult who kills himself because of a menace, like king Saul, who killed himself; indeed this was permitted to him.[13] For thus we read in Genesis Rabbah: "... Could this apply to one who is trapped like Saul?"

Nahmanides—whose position became the mainstream halakhic teaching—states plainly that any person finding himself in dire straights, like King Saul, is permitted to seek escape through suicide.[14] God's sovereignty need not be confirmed through denying His human subject such an escape. Instead, the choice of an earlier death is fully accepted in divine compassion for the individual, created in God's image.

Controversy and Assistance: A Perplexing Scenario

In light of the divergent views within the halakhic tradition, we must contemplate the following perplexing possibility. The scenario I shall describe relates to two observant Jews, but I believe it can serve as a model for the problem of assistance between individuals with other disparate convictions within a pluralistic frame of reference.

Think of an individual who subscribes to the Nahmanedian view, and sees the prohibition of suicide in terms of cherishing human life. Suppose, now, that this person is afflicted with a terminal illness and faces—in the short duration remaining—no more than unwelcome suffering. The patient seeks to escape through death, and in light of his convictions, such suicide would be perfectly legitimate. Yet, given the patient's condition and other common circumstances, success of the intended suicide requires the assistance of a physician.

He therefore turns to a physician and asks her for help. But now suppose that the physician from whom aid is requested subscribes to the other view—that represented by Waldenberg—and considers suicide, even in such circumstances, to be utterly forbidden. Her first response is outright refusal: "How can you expect me to be involved in a deed which, in my view, constitutes terrible bloodshed?"

But here things get complicated. Both individuals being observant and learned Jews, the patient reminds the doctor of the practice of the schools of Shammai and Hillel, as depicted in the mishna cited above. Each side adhered to its own views, while showing the utmost respect for those of their opponents; none could claim exclusive access to divine truth, since "These and those are the living words of God." So, says the patient, cannot the doctor go along with another's choice, without herself endorsing it?

A plausible response to this might be to point to the limits of tolerance. Surely, a member of one of those ancient schools would not himself act on the other school's teachings; it was only that he would respect the *others* when they acted on their own views. So our physician might respect the patient's choice, not speak ill of him, and—more significantly, perhaps—not attempt to frustrate his choice of suicide while in progress. But such acceptance cannot extend to the actions of the physician herself. Surely she, too, should not act against her own convictions.

But would she, in fact, be so acting—say, in subscribing or handing over a lethal dose of certain pills? After all, the act of suicide would be committed by the patient himself: We are dealing here only with the question of *assistance*. The patient is arguing that the physician should adopt a *cooperative* stance, while the physician proposes to adopt a *hands-off* stance.

The problem boils down, it seems, to a moral analysis of "assistance." The argument for cooperation runs thus: "Assisting in deed X is evil only derivatively. Where X is evil, it is wrong first of all for whoever commits it, but then also wrong for anyone to participate in the same wrong act. But if, for the patient, suicide (in these circumstances, and given his convictions) is perfectly legitimate, there is no evil in the deed, and none can extend to any participant."

Adherents of the "hands-off" position might respond to this argument in two ways. First, they could contend that (a) an act of assistance should *not* be judged merely derivatively; e.g., assisting in suicide may be wrong even if suicide itself is permitted. Second, they might contest the relativism of the "for the patient" clause of the cooperative reasoning. This line of argument would admit that the evil of "assisting in X" is derived solely from the evil of X itself; but would insist that (b) the assistor is an independent moral agent, whose *own* views about X must be the ones to figure in her judgment about whether to assist in X.

Now (a) seems to me rather hard to defend. Why should it be wrong, say, to give someone pills, unless the use of those pills is deemed wrong? It can always be argued, of course, that prescribing poison is prohibited by the doctor's professional code, independently of any judgment regarding the patient's subsequent use of the poison. But if swallowing the pills—and, derivatively, supplying them—is in itself (morally) permissible, then the prohibiting item in the professional code may lack moral force. The code would, it seems, furnish merely a formal justification of the refusal to cooperate. Or rather, it would furnish a role-specific obligation, at odds with the requirements of common morality.[15] Those upholding the professional code in this context would have to explain, in plain human terms, why it is not simply callous.

It is (b), then, that seems to offer the best defense of the "hands-off" position. Against the suggestion (by adherents of the "cooperative" position) that an act of assistance may be rendered on the terms of the principal agent, this defense consists in refusing to allow the patient's perspective to eclipse that of the doctor. In the final section of this paper, I shall offer some ideas on how to understand this debate; before that, it is perhaps worth reemphasizing the nature of the debate and its precise scope.[16]

As stipulated, parties to this debate hold firm convictions. All are fairly confident of their respective interpretations of the proper exception to the prohibition (or punishment) of suicide, epitomized in the case of King Saul. Consequently, it would be perfectly correct—within the limits of civility and sensitivity—for each to try and persuade the other. Yet each respects the validity of the other's position, which—like their own—reflects "the living words of God." This entails toleration of the other's actions; specifically, for adherents of the prohibitive stance, it means refraining from attempts to "bring back to life" one who has acted on the more permissive stance.

Both parties recognize, then, that there are (at least) two valid perspectives on the proposed act of suicide. The debate is focused narrowly on the issue of assistance. In this prospective *interaction* between two individuals, what should become of their contrasting views of the same deed?

Personal Integrity and Interpersonal Relations

The plausibility of the "hands-off" positions stems, I think, from its appeal to personal integrity. For a person to preserve his or her integrity while interacting with others, it is necessary to avoid being taken over by the others' values and motives. Individuals are commonly praised for precisely such avoidance, for sticking consistently to their own values, for protecting their minds and souls against any breach from outside—that is, for remaining "whole," keeping their integrity. In our imagined scenario, the physician may feel that acceding to the patient's request would amount to surrendering her integrity.

The "cooperative" position, in contrast, would emphasize a conception of individuals as interrelated. The "integrity" of the self, kept pure by its separation from others, is here called into question—not only empirically, but also normatively.[17] Adherents of this position might ask the doctor, "Is it really such a good thing for you to preserve the integrity of your values against incursion by those of your patient?" And hence: "In the context of your relationship with him, is it not appropriate to let down part of the wall between the two selves and bring yourself to share *his* perspective?"

An obvious difficulty with this emphasis on interrelation is that it seems to prove too much. If there is little value in personal integrity, why should any individual stand up to group pressure, or resist the pull of a racist society? Should the physician be prepared to go along with any and every kind of position her patient subscribes to, however outrageous it is in her own eyes?

In response, we should recall the narrow scope of the debate under analysis. Pluralism need not entail a stance of "anything goes." Both sides, in our scenario, recognize the validity of the other's view within a joint frame of reference. They share the conception of both positions as "the living words of God." Such recognition will not, of course, extend to all other positions they might encounter. Some views may be denounced and opposed completely. To take an extreme example, suppose our physician was invited to work with Dr. Mengele in a concentration camp. We would rightly hope that she maintain her integrity and shun the evil project.

My purpose in this jarring contrast is to underscore that the cooperative stance in our scenario rests on a recognition that, however you might disagree with one who endorses suicide to escape terminal suffering, this is very different from your denunciation of Mengele's deeds. Where exactly the limits of pluralism and toleration should lie is a question I cannot address here; in our scenario it was stipulated that these limits are not exceeded, and it can obviously serve as a model only for similar situations.[18]

Another objection will espouse the readiness of encompassing the other's view, but will seek symmetry. After all, within the dyadic relationship between doctor and patient, the proposal can be reversed: Why should the patient not yield to the physician's perspective? Why should it be the physician who gives up her principles?

Questions of symmetry (or lack thereof) in the doctor-patient relationship are of great interest to bioethicists, and have myriad implications. I wish here to avoid this broad issue, and formulate a possible explanation without reference to the specific roles of the individuals involved. Instead, let us again recall the circumscribed nature of our debate: It is not about all forms of interaction, but specifically about *assistance*. In a relational context where my act consists in rendering assistance to another person, it makes sense to adopt—for the sake of that act—the perspective of that other individual.

An instructive analogy can, perhaps, be drawn here from the kind of cases in which the schools of Shammai and Hillel showed respect and a willingness to go along with each others' divergent practices. Suppose I were from the school of Shammai, and utensils prepared or treated in particular ways in my own house would not be acceptable for my use. But, going over to borrow such items from my neighbor—of the school of Hillel—I do not reject what is offered in friendship, even though it was (from my perspective) prepared illicitly. In borrowing another's property, I reasonably yield to the owner's perspective, according to which the utensil is "pure." The context of *borrowing* justifies adopting, for this act, the perspective of the other. A similar, context-specific, explanation may work for *assistance* as well.

This explanation works, of course, only if one is prepared to adopt a relational perspective in the first place. It is not meant to convince a physician, committed staunchly to personal integrity, that it would sometimes be right to act according to the patient's perspective. Given such a commitment, the "cooperative" stance seems plainly wrong. Emphasizing the asymmetrical nature of assistance is only meant to show why, given an alternative commitment to an interpersonal, relational perspective on values and action, it can make sense here for the physician to suspend her integrity and act for the patient.

Notes

Work on this essay was supported by the Kaufman Family Center for Jewish Ethics and Public Policy at the Shalom Hartman Institute, Jerusalem. Earlier versions of this discussion were presented at a meeting of the Medical Ethics Discussion Group at the University of Utah, Salt Lake City, and at Princeton University under the auspices of the Religion Department. My thanks to several participants for their illuminating comments.

1. For a fuller discussion of these and other texts, see chapter 7, "Controversy and Dissent," M. Walzer, M. Lorberbaum, N. Zohar, and Y. Lorderbaum, eds., *The Jewish Political Tradition*, vol. 1 (New Haven: Yale University Press, forthcoming, 1998).
2. This may well not be true of the Hebrew Bible. For a detailed discussion of both biblical and Rabbinic sources, see S. Goldstein, *Suicide in Rabbinic Literature* (Hoboken, NJ: Ktar, 1989).
3. See N. Zohar, *Alternatives in Jewish Bioethics* (Albany, NY: SUNY Press, 1997), part 2, and particularly pp. 91–97.

4. E. Waldenberg, section 29 of the tractate "*Ramat Rachel*," published in vol. 8 of his responsa, *Tsits Eliezer*, Jerusalem, 1965.

5. For an analysis of midrash and its relation to scripture, see N. Zohar, "Midrash: Amendment Through the Molding of Meaning," in *Responding to Imperfection: New Approaches to the Problem of Constitutional Amendment*, S. Levinson, ed. (Princeton: Princeton University Press, 1995), pp. 307–318.

6. A significantly different translation would be: "was extremely afraid of the archers" (— but not yet hit).

7. This applies mainly to active euthanasia. For a discussion of Jewish traditions on the active/passive distinction in this context—or, more precisely, the distinction between interference and noninterference in the death-process—see Zohar (1997), 37–49.

8. An alternative reading might emphasize instead the metaphor of a gift; see D. M. Holly, "Voluntary Death, Property Rights, and the Gift of Life," *The Journal of Religious Ethics* 17 (1) (1989): 103–21.

9. Within *Halakhic* discourse, it is sometimes asserted that *Aggadic* sources—that is, non-legal sections of the Talmud or Midrash—can have no authority in determining valid rulings. That this commonly cited formal rule is also frequently disregarded, should not come as a great surprise: After all, the values and attitudes expressed in *Aggada* have much to contribute to normative discourse. Still—and quite apart from the issue of authority, which is not our concern here—there is a qualitative difference between a story, which can properly maintain an unresolved tension, and legal writing.

10. For a rather comprehensive—though not entirely unbiased—survey, see Y. Go'elman, "Soul's Death as Reflected in Halakhic Literature" (in Hebrew), in *Arakhim be-Mivhan Milhama* (Jerusalem, 1984).

11. Other variants of this approach emphasize Saul's role as king: his being captured alive would dishonor Israel and its God, or drive the Israelites to desperate suicide-missions to liberate their king, costing many more lives. What is common to all these approaches is that what legitimates Saul's taking of his life is not his personal interest in avoiding a protracted and painful death, but (as in martyrdom) some "higher," external interest.

12. See generally Goldstein (1989), p. 27 ff.

13. The connective "likewise" refers back to Nahmanides's previous point, that a minor committing suicide is never to be held culpable. An adult (in a situation like that of Saul) is also inculpable, but—by contrast—is not *merely excused*, but even justified in killing himself.

14. See Nahmanides's "*Torat ha-Adam: Sha'ar ha-Hesped*," (Hebrew, ed. Chavel 1964, p. 84); cited also in R. Asher ben Yehiel's rulings on tractate *mo'ed katan*, chapter 3, section 94. The same position is recorded by R. Joseph Caro in his "Bet Yoseph" annotations to Y. D. 345, s.v. "*ve-khen gadol*."

15. For an illuminating discussion of "role morality" as against common morality, see D. Luban, *Lawyers and Justice* (Princeton, NJ: Princeton University Press, 1988), pp. 104–47.

16. I do not mean to suggest that such a debate actually exists today amongst followers of Judaic traditions. In fact, we find only various attitudes toward suicide to escape terminal suffering, often with the more or less explicit implication that the question of assistance is to be decided derivatively. Thus the "debate" I am describing is constructed, in the context of the scenario given above, for the sake of philosophical analysis.

17. Compare the dicussion on "Feminism and Individualism" in V. Held, *Feminist Morlaity* (Chicago: University of Chicago Press, 1993), pp. 182–85.

18. For a theological defense of pluralism, extending beyond the scope of Jewish views alone, see D. Hartman, *A Living Covenant: The Innovative Spirit in Traditional Judaism* (New York: Free Press, 1985), pp. 303–304, where it is argued that "A mature recognition of the implications of human finitude may help us to understand that different and often conflicting views on what makes a human life significant are intrinsic to our human condition."

Part Six

Appendices

IN 1997, the United States Supreme Court ruled for the first time on the matter of physician-assisted suicide. At issue were two 1996 federal appellate court decisions, *Compassion in Dying v. Washington* in the Ninth Circuit (covering Washington, Oregon, California, and six other Western states) and *Quill v. Vacco* in the Second Circuit (covering New York, Connecticut, and Vermont).

Both Circuit Courts had declared that state prohibitions on physicians assisting competent terminally ill patients to commit suicide were unconstitutional. The Ninth Circuit had ruled that Washington's laws deprived dying patients of a fundamental aspect of self-determination, namely, the right to determine the time and manner of one's death. The Second Circuit had ruled that New York State violated the equal protection requirement, since its laws permitted patients dependent on mechanical life support to have the machines turned off and so die, but no similar choice was available to patients not requiring mechanical life support. Taken together, those decisions would have had dramatic impact because they directly applied to jurisdictions encompassing nearly a third of the population of the United States.

The Circuit Courts' decisions were appealed to the Supreme Court, and because they concerned similar issues, the Supreme Court treated them as companion cases and issued opinions about them on the same day. It should be noted that because the defendants, listed second in the 1996 Circuit Court appeals, were the petitioners in the Supreme Court cases, they are listed first in the the Supreme Court cases.

Appendix A and Appendix B

On June 26, 1997, the Supreme Court unanimously reversed both lower courts' decisions. In *Washington v. Glucksberg*, the Court rejected the Ninth Circuit's recognition of a fundamental right; rather than a historical tradition to support a right to die, it found a long United States history of state prohibitions against suicide and before that a history in English common law. States have legitimate interests in barring any medical practice that assists patients to hasten their deaths, Chief Justice Rehnquist observed, because states have legitimate interests in preserving citizens' lives, preventing citizens from taking their own lives, protecting especially vulnerable groups against euthanasia, and maintaining trust in the medical profession's commitment not to take patients' lives. In *Vacco v. Quill*, the Court found that New York law applied equally to everyone in that all citizens have the right to refuse mechanical life support and no citizen has the right to a physician's assistance to die. However, far from resolving decisively the legal, moral, political, and conceptual questions raised by *Washington v. Glucksberg* and *Vacco v. Quill*, the Supreme Court raised the discussion of physician-assisted suicide to an unexpected level of complexity. The legal effect of the Court's decisions was to leave the issue of physician-assisted suicide with the individual states.

There is an illusory uniformity in the unanimous reversals of the lower courts' rulings. Even the briefest study of the Justices' opinions (Chief Justice Rehnquist's opinion was joined by a majority but Justices O'Connor, Stevens, Souter, Ginsburg, and Breyer voiced their separate interpretations in concurring opinions) shows how very differently they think about the implications and impact of their unanimous decision. Certainly, the Justices do not all speak with one voice about how the legal issues surrounding physician-assisted suicide should be framed. Nor do all of the Justices agree that the final word regarding constitutional dimensions of the issue has been heard. Taken together, the Justices' opinions offer a complex account of some of the many concepts, fundamental to American society, that are challenged when we consider revising our views about who should control whose deaths. Even the understanding of our historical practices in this regard is not univocal, as a comparison of the Justices' comments will show.

We have included the full text of the opinions in both. *Washington v. Glucksberg* is Appendix A and *Vacco v. Quill* is Appendix B. We do so both for their intrinsic importance and because so many of the essays in this book cite one or another of the Justices' statements.

Appendix C

In addition to the briefs of the parties and of the United States (through the Solicitor General, who also participated in the formal arguments before the Supreme Court), the Justices were swamped by a tidal wave of amicus curiae briefs filed by individuals and organizations interested in these cases. Some thirty-nine amicus briefs urged the Supreme Court to overturn the appellate courts' decisions, arguing that physician-assisted suicide should remain prohibited or that the matter should be left to the states, while sixteen briefs offered the Court reasons for upholding them. Among the proponents on each side of the debate were physicians, attorneys, bioethicists, legislators, theologians, and a wide variety of charitable, medical affinity, and other nonprofit groups. One of these briefs, the one most often cited in the essays in this volume, has become known as "The Philosophers' Brief"; it was formulated by a group of six prominent moral philosophers in support of sustaining the Appeals Courts' decisions recognizing constitutional rights to physician-assisted suicide. Both for convenience of reference, and for its usefulness in connecting this public policy issue to larger questions of political morality, we include this document as Appendix C.

Appendix D

Appendix D contains the text of Oregon's ballot measure known as Measure 16, the Death With Dignity Act, originally passed at the polls by a 51 to 49 percent margin in November 1994. This measure was then tied up in a series of court challenges for several years. In 1997, the Oregon legislature, acting under a little-used provision of the Oregon Constitution, sent the measure back to the voters. In a mail-in ballot held the November after the United States Supreme Court's decision, the voters refused by a 60 to 40 percent margin to repeal Measure 16, and despite several further legal and political challenges, it became law. The Oregon State Health Division has instructed county agencies that handle vital records not to divulge confidential information about specific cases, but it will issue an annual report as directed by law. As of early 1998, two persons had ended their lives under the provisions of the law.

The country has watched the events in Oregon with interest, taking them to indicate what future lies in store for physician-assisted suicide. Measure 16 is likely to provide Americans with the country's first experience in implementing a plan for legal physician assistance in suicide and will, therefore, merit careful scrutiny. The full text of Oregon's Death With Dignity Act is included as Appendix D.

As of this writing, thirty-five states have statutes explicitly criminalizing assisted suicide (Alaska, Arizona, Arkansas, California, Colorado, Connecticut, Delaware, Florida, Georgia, Hawaii, Illinois, Indiana, Iowa, Kansas, Kentucky, Louisiana, Maine, Minnesota, Mississippi, Missouri, Montana, Nebraska, New Hampshire, New Jersey, New Mexico, New York, North Dakota, Oklahoma, Pennsylvania, Rhode Island, South Dakota, Tennessee, Texas, Washington, Wisconsin); nine states criminalize assisted suicide through common law (Alabama, Idaho, Maryland, Massachusetts, Michigan, Nevada, South Carolina, Vermont, West Virginia); three states have abolished the common law of crimes and do not have statutes criminalizing assisted suicide (North Carolina, Utah, Wyoming); one has neither case law nor statute criminalizing suicide, but imposes civil sanctions on persons assisting in a suicide (Virginia); one state has a state Supreme Court ruling that assisted suicide is not a crime (Ohio); and in one state (Oregon) physician-assisted suicide is now legal when performed according to the requirements of the Oregon Death with Dignity Act. New measures are pending in many state legislatures. In *Washington* v. *Glucksberg* and *Vacco* v. *Quill* the Supreme Court invited a "state-by-state laboratory" concerning physician-assisted suicide. It seems clear that this is what we will have for the foreseeable future.

Appendix A

Washington et al. v. Glucksberg et al.

Text of the Supreme Court Decision Delivered by Chief Justice Rehnquist, in which O'Connor, Scalia, Kennedy, and Thomas, JJ., joined. O'Connor, J. filed a concurring opinion in which Ginsburg and Breyer, JJ. joined in part. Stevens, J., Souter, J., Ginsburg, J., and Breyer, J., filed opinions concurring in the judgment.

Washington et al., Petitioners No. 96–100 v. Harold Glucksberg et al., 117 S.Ct. 2258 (1997)

ON WRIT OF CERTIORARI TO THE UNITED STATES COURT OF APPEALS FOR THE NINTH CIRCUIT

Argued January 8, 1997–Decided June 26, 1997

CHIEF JUSTICE REHNQUIST DELIVERED THE OPINION OF THE COURT.

The question presented in this case is whether Washington's prohibition against "caus[ing]" or "aid[ing]" a suicide offends the Fourteenth Amendment to the United States Constitution. We hold that it does not.

It has always been a crime to assist a suicide in the State of Washington. In 1854, Washington's first Territorial Legislature outlawed "assisting another in the commission of self murder."[1] Today, Washington law provides: "A person is guilty of promoting a suicide attempt when he knowingly causes or aids another person to attempt suicide." Wash. Rev. Code 9A.36.060(1) (1994). "Promoting a suicide attempt" is a felony, punishable by up to five years' imprisonment and up to a $10,000 fine. §§9A.36.060(2) and 9A.20.021(1)(c). At the same time, Washington's Natural Death Act, enacted in 1979, states that the "withholding or withdrawal of life sustaining treatment" at a patient's direction "shall not, for any purpose, constitute a suicide." Wash. Rev. Code §70.122.070(1).[2]

Petitioners in this case are the State of Washington and its Attorney General. Respondents Harold Glucksberg, M. D., Abigail Halperin, M. D., Thomas A. Preston, M. D., and Peter Shalit, M. D., are physicians who practice in Washington. These doctors occasionally treat terminally ill, suffering patients, and declare that they would assist these patients in ending their lives if not for Washington's assisted suicide ban.[3] In January 1994, respondents, along with three gravely ill, pseudonymous plaintiffs who have since died and *Compassion in Dying*, a nonprofit organization that counsels people considering physician assisted suicide, sued in the United States District Court, seeking a declaration that Wash Rev. Code 9A.36.060(1) (1994) is, on its face, unconstitutional. *Compassion in Dying* v. *Washington*, 850 F. Supp. 1454, 1459 (WD Wash. 1994).[4]

The plaintiffs asserted "the existence of a liberty interest protected by the Fourteenth Amendment which extends to a personal choice by a mentally competent, terminally ill adult to commit physician assisted suicide." *Id.*, at 1459. Relying primarily on *Planned Parenthood* v. *Casey*, 505 U.S. 833 (1992), and *Cruzan* v. *Director, Missouri Dept. of Health*, 497 U.S. 261 (1990), the District Court agreed, 850 F. Supp., at 1459–1462, and concluded that Washington's assisted suicide ban is unconstitutional because it "places an undue burden on the exercise of [that] constitutionally protected liberty interest." *Id.*, at 1465.[5] The District Court also decided that the Washington statute violated the Equal Protection Clause's requirement that " 'all persons similarly situated . . . be treated alike.' " *Id.*, at 1466 (quoting *Cleburne* v. *Cleburne Living Center, Inc.*, 473 U.S. 432, 439 (1985)).

A panel of the Court of Appeals for the Ninth Circuit reversed, emphasizing that "[i]n the two hundred and five years of our existence no constitutional right to aid in killing oneself has ever been asserted and upheld by a court of final jurisdiction." *Compassion in Dying* v. *Washington*, 49 F. 3d 586, 591 (1995). The Ninth Circuit reheard the case en banc, reversed the panel's decision, and affirmed the District Court. *Compassion in Dying* v. *Washington*, 79 F. 3d 790, 798 (1996). Like the District Court, the en banc Court of Appeals emphasized our *Casey* and *Cruzan* decisions. 79 F. 3d, at 813–816. The court also discussed what it described as "historical" and "current societal attitudes" toward suicide and assisted suicide, *id.*, at 806–812, and concluded that "the Constitution encompasses a due process liberty interest in controlling the time and manner of one's death—that there is, in short, a constitutionally recognized 'right to die.' " *Id.*, at 816. After "[w]eighing and then balancing" this interest against Washington's various interests, the court held that the State's assisted suicide ban was unconstitutional "as applied to terminally ill competent adults who wish to hasten their deaths with medication prescribed by their physicians." *Id.*, at 836, 837.[6] The court did not reach the District Court's equal protection holding. *Id.*, at 838.[7] We granted certiorari, 519 U. S. _____ (1996), and now reverse.

I

We begin, as we do in all due process cases, by examining our Nation's history, legal traditions, and practices. See, e.g., *Casey*, 505 U. S., at 849–850; *Cruzan*, 497 U. S., at 269–279; *Moore* v. *East Cleveland*, 431 U.S. 494, 503 (1977) (plurality opinion) (noting importance of "careful 'respect for the teachings of history' "). In almost every State—indeed, in almost every western democracy—it is a crime to assist a suicide.[8] The States' assisted suicide bans are not innovations. Rather, they are longstanding expressions of the States' commitment to the protection and preservation of all human life. *Cruzan*, 497 U. S., at 280 ("[T]he States—indeed, all civilized nations—demonstrate their commitment to life by treating homicide as a serious crime. Moreover, the majority of States in this country have laws imposing criminal penalties on one who assists another to commit suicide"); see *Stanford* v. *Kentucky*, 492 U.S. 361, 373 (1989) ("[T]he primary and most reliable indication of [a national] consensus is . . . the pattern of enacted laws"). Indeed, opposition to and condemnation of suicide—and, therefore, of assisting suicide—are consistent and enduring themes of our philosophical, legal, and cultural heritages. See generally, Marzen, O'Dowd, Crone & Balch, Suicide: A Constitutional Right?, 24 Duquesne L. Rev. 1, 17–56 (1985) (hereinafter Marzen); New York State Task Force on Life and the Law, When Death is Sought: Assisted Suicide and Euthanasia in the Medical Context 77–82 (May 1994) (hereinafter New York Task Force).

More specifically, for over 700 years, the Anglo American common law tradition has punished or otherwise disapproved of both suicide and assisting suicide.[9] *Cruzan*, 497 U. S., at 294–295 (SCALIA, J., concurring). In the 13th century, Henry de Bracton, one of the first legal treatise writers, observed that "[j]ust as a man may commit felony by slaying another so may he do so by slaying himself." 2 Bracton on Laws and Customs of England 423 (f. 150) (G. Woodbine ed., S. Thorne transl., 1968). The real and personal property of one who killed himself to avoid conviction and punishment for a crime were forfeit to the king; however, thought Bracton, "if a man slays himself in weariness of life or because he is unwilling to endure further bodily pain . . . [only] his movable goods [were] confiscated." *Id.*, at 423–424 (f. 150). Thus, "[t]he principle that suicide of a sane person, for whatever reason, was a punishable felony was . . . introduced into English common law."[10] Centuries later, Sir William Blackstone, whose Commentaries on the Laws of England not only provided a definitive summary of the common law but was also a primary legal authority for 18th and 19th century American lawyers, referred to suicide as "self murder" and "the pretended heroism, but real cowardice, of the Stoic philosophers, who destroyed themselves to avoid those ills which they had not the fortitude to endure. . . ." 4 W. Blackstone, Commentaries *189. Blackstone emphasized that "the law has . . . ranked [suicide] among the highest crimes," ibid., although, anticipating later developments, he conceded that the harsh and shameful punishments imposed for suicide "borde[r] a little upon severity." *Id.*, at *190.

For the most part, the early American colonies adopted the common law approach. For example, the legislators of the Providence Plantations, which would later become Rhode Island, declared, in 1647, that "[s]elf murder is by all agreed to be the most unnatural, and it is by this present Assembly declared, to be that, wherein he that doth it, kills himself out of a premeditated hatred against his own life or other humor: . . . his goods and chattels are the king's custom, but not his debts nor lands; but in case he be an infant, a lunatic, mad or distracted man, he forfeits nothing." The Earliest Acts and Laws of the Colony of Rhode Island and Providence Plantations 1647–1719, p. 19 (J. Cushing ed. 1977). Virginia also required ignominious burial for suicides, and their estates were forfeit to the crown. A. Scott, Criminal Law in Colonial Virginia 108, and n. 93, 198, and n. 15 (1930).

Over time, however, the American colonies abolished these harsh common law penalties. William Penn abandoned the criminal forfeiture sanction in Pennsylvania in 1701, and the other colonies (and later, the other States) eventually followed this example. *Cruzan*, 497 U. S., at 294 (SCALIA, J., concurring). Zephaniah Swift, who would later become Chief Justice of Connecticut, wrote in 1796 that

> "[t]here can be no act more contemptible, than to attempt to punish an offender for a crime, by exercising a mean act of revenge upon lifeless clay, that is insensible of the punishment. There can be no greater cruelty, than the inflicting [of] a punishment, as the forfeiture of goods, which must fall solely on the innocent offspring of the offender. . . . [Suicide] is so abhorrent to the feelings of mankind, and that strong love of life which is implanted in the human heart, that it cannot be so frequently committed, as to become dangerous to society. There can of course be no necessity of any punishment." 2 Z. Swift, A System of the Laws of the State of Connecticut 304 (1796).

This statement makes it clear, however, that the movement away from the common law's harsh sanctions did not represent an acceptance of suicide; rather, as Chief Justice Swift observed, this change reflected the growing consensus that it was unfair to punish the suicide's family for his wrongdoing. *Cruzan*, *supra*, at 294 (SCALIA, J., concurring). Nonetheless, although States moved away from Blackstone's treatment of suicide, courts continued to condemn it as a grave public wrong. See, e.g., *Bigelow* v. *Berkshire Life Ins. Co.*, 93 U.S. 284, 286 (1876) (suicide is "an act of criminal self destruction"); *Von Holden* v. *Chapman*, 87 App. Div. 2d 66, 70–71, 450 N. Y. S. 2d 623, 626–627 (1982); *Blackwood* v. *Jones*, 111 Fla. 528, 532, 149 So. 600, 601 (1933) ("No sophistry is tolerated . . . which seek[s] to justify self destruction as commendable or even a matter of personal right").

That suicide remained a grievous, though nonfelonious, wrong is confirmed by the fact that colonial and early state legislatures and courts did not retreat from prohibiting assisting suicide. Swift, in his early 19th century treatise on the laws of Connecticut, stated that "[i]f one counsels another to commit suicide, and the other by reason of the advice kills himself, the advisor is guilty of murder as principal." 2 Z. Swift, A Digest of the Laws of the State of Connecticut 270 (1823). This was the well established common law view, see In re Joseph G., 34 Cal. 3d 429, 434–435, 667 P. 2d 1176, 1179 (1983); *Commonwealth* v. *Mink*, 123 Mass. 422, 428 (1877) ("'Now if the murder of one's self is felony, the accessory is equally guilty as if he had aided and abetted in the murder'") (quoting Chief Justice Parker's charge to the jury in *Commonwealth* v. *Bowen*, 13 Mass. 356 (1816)), as was the similar principle that the consent of a homicide victim is "wholly immaterial to the guilt of the person who cause[d] [his death]," 3 J. Stephen, A History of the Criminal Law of England 16 (1883); see 1 F. Wharton, Criminal Law §§451–452 (9th ed. 1885); *Martin* v. *Commonwealth*, 184 Va. 1009, 1018–1019, 37 S. E. 2d 43, 47 (1946) ("'The right to life and to personal security is not only sacred in the estimation of the common law, but it is inalienable'"). And the prohibitions against assisting suicide never contained exceptions for those who were near death. Rather, "[t]he life of those to whom life ha[d] become a burden—of those who [were] hopelessly diseased or fatally wounded—nay, even the lives of criminals condemned to death, [were] under the protection of law, equally as the lives of those who [were] in the full tide of life's enjoyment, and anxious to continue to live." *Blackburn* v. *State*, 23 Ohio St. 146, 163 (1872); see *Bowen, supra*, at 360 (prisoner who persuaded another to commit suicide could be tried for murder, even though victim was scheduled shortly to be executed).

The earliest American statute explicitly to outlaw assisting suicide was enacted in New York in 1828, Act of Dec. 10, 1828, ch. 20, §4, 1828 N. Y. Laws 19 (codified at 2 N. Y. Rev. Stat. pt. 4, ch. 1, tit. 2, art. 1, §7, p. 661 (1829)), and many of the new States and Territories followed New York's example. Marzen 73–74. Between 1857 and 1865, a New York commission led by Dudley Field drafted a criminal code that prohibited "aiding" a suicide and, specifically, "furnish[ing] another person with any deadly weapon or poisonous drug, knowing that such person intends to use such weapon or drug in taking his own life." *Id.*, at 76–77. By the time the Fourteenth Amendment was ratified, it was a crime in most States to assist a suicide. See *Cruzan, supra*, at 294–295 (SCALIA, J., concurring). The Field Penal Code was adopted in the Dakota Territory in 1877, in New York in 1881, and its language served as a model for several other western States' statutes in the late 19th and early 20th centuries. Marzen 76–77, 205–206, 212–213. California, for example, codified its assisted suicide prohibition in 1874, using language similar to the Field Code's.[11] In this century, the Model Penal Code also prohibited "aiding" suicide, prompting many States to enact or revise their assisted suicide bans.[12] The Code's drafters observed that "the interests in the sanctity of life that are represented by the criminal homicide laws are threatened by one who expresses a willingness to participate in taking the life of another, even though the act may be accomplished with the consent, or at the request, of the suicide victim." American Law Institute, Model Penal Code §210.5, Comment 5, p. 100 (Official Draft and Revised Comments 1980).

Though deeply rooted, the States' assisted suicide bans have in recent years been reexamined and, generally, reaffirmed. Because of advances in medicine and technology, Americans today are increasingly likely to die in institutions, from chronic illnesses. President's Comm'n for the Study of Ethical Problems in Medicine and Biomedical and Behavioral Research, Deciding to Forego Life Sustaining Treatment 16–18 (1983). Public concern and democratic action are therefore sharply focused on how best to protect dignity and independence at the end of life, with the result that there have been many significant changes in state laws and in the attitudes these laws reflect. Many States, for example, now permit "living wills," surrogate health care decisionmaking, and the withdrawal or refusal of life sustaining medical treatment. See *Vacco* v. *Quill, post,* at 9–11; 79 F. 3d, at 818–820; *People* v. *Kevorkian,* 447Mich. 436, 478–480, and nn. 53–56, 527 N. W. 2d 714, 731–732, and nn. 53–56 (1994). At the same time, however, voters and legislators continue for the most part to reaffirm their States' prohibitions on assisting suicide.

TheWashington statute at issue in this case,Wash. Rev. Code §9A.36.060 (1994), was enacted in 1975 as part of a revision of that State's criminal code. Four years later, Washington passed its Natural Death Act, which specifically stated that the "withholding or withdrawal of life sustaining treatment . . . shall not, for any purpose, constitute a suicide" and that "[n]othing in this chapter shall be construed to condone, authorize, or approve mercy killing. . . ." Natural Death Act, 1979 Wash. Laws, ch. 112, §§8(1), p. 11 (codified atWash. Rev. Code §§70.122.070(1), 70.122.100 (1994)). In 1991, Washington voters rejected a ballot initiative which, had it passed, would have permitted a form of physician assisted suicide.[13] Washington then added a provision to the Natural Death Act expressly excluding physician assisted suicide. 1992 Wash. Laws, ch. 98, §10; Wash. Rev. Code §70.122.100 (1994).

California voters rejected an assisted suicide initiative similar to Washington's in 1993. On the other hand, in 1994, voters in Oregon enacted, also through ballot initiative, that State's "DeathWith Dignity Act," which legalized physician assisted suicide for competent, terminally ill adults.[14] Since the Oregon vote, many proposals to legalize assisted suicide have been and continue to be introduced in the States' legislatures, but none has been enacted.[15] And just last year, Iowa and Rhode Island joined the overwhelming majority of States explicitly prohibiting assisted suicide. See Iowa Code Ann. §§707A.2, 707A.3 (Supp. 1997); R. I. Gen. Laws §§ 11–60–1, 11–60–3 (Supp. 1996). Also, on April 30, 1997, President Clinton signed the Federal Assisted Suicide Funding Restriction Act of 1997, which prohibits the use of federal funds in support of physician assisted suicide. Pub. L. 105–12, 111 Stat. 23 (codified at 42 U.S.C. § 14401 *et seq*).[16]

Thus, the States are currently engaged in serious, thoughtful examinations of physician assisted suicide and other similar issues. For example, New York State's Task Force on Life and the Law—an ongoing, blue ribbon commission composed of doctors, ethicists, lawyers, religious leaders, and interested laymen—was convened in 1984 and commissioned with "a broad mandate to recommend public policy on issues raised by medical advances." New York Task Force vii. Over the past decade, the Task Force has recommended laws relating to end of life decisions, surrogate pregnancy, and organ donation. *Id.,* at 118–119. After studying physician assisted suicide, however, the Task Force unanimously concluded that "[l]egalizing assisted suicide and euthanasia would pose profound risks to many individuals who are ill and vulnerable. . . . [T]he potential dangers of this dramatic change in public policy would outweigh any benefit that might be achieved." *Id.,* at 120.

Attitudes toward suicide itself have changed since Bracton, but our laws have consistently condemned, and continue to prohibit, assisting suicide. Despite changes in medical technology and notwithstanding an increased emphasis on the importance of end of life decisionmaking, we have not retreated from this prohibition. Against this backdrop of history, tradition, and practice, we now turn to respondents' constitutional claim.

II

The Due Process Clause guarantees more than fair process, and the "liberty" it protects includes more than the absence of physical restraint. *Collins* v. *Harker Heights*, 503 U.S. 115, 125 (1992) (Due Process Clause "protects individual liberty against 'certain government actions regardless of the fairness of the procedures used to implement them'") (quoting *Daniels* v. *Williams*, 474 U.S. 327, 331 (1986)). The Clause also provides heightened protection against government interference with certain fundamental rights and liberty interests. *Reno* v. *Flores*, 507 U.S. 292, 301–302 (1993); *Casey*, 505 U. S., at 851. In a long line of cases, we have held that, in addition to the specific freedoms protected by the Bill of Rights, the "liberty" specially protected by the Due Process Clause includes the rights to marry, *Loving* v. *Virginia*, 388 U.S. 1 (1967); to have children, *Skinner* v. *Oklahoma ex rel. Williamson*, 316 U.S. 535 (1942); to direct the education and upbringing of one's children, *Meyer* v. *Nebraska*, 262 U.S. 390 (1923); *Pierce* v. *Society of Sisters*, 268 U.S. 510 (1925); to marital privacy, *Griswold* v. *Connecticut*, 381 U.S. 479 (1965); to use contraception, ibid; *Eisenstadt* v. *Baird*, 405 U.S. 438 (1972); to bodily integrity, *Rochin* v. *California*, 342 U.S. 165 (1952), and to abortion, *Casey*, *supra*. We have also assumed, and strongly suggested, that the Due Process Clause protects the traditional right to refuse unwanted lifesaving medical treatment. *Cruzan*, 497 U. S., at 278–279.

But we "ha[ve] always been reluctant to expand the concept of substantive due process because guide*posts* for responsible decisionmaking in this unchartered area are scarce and open ended." *Collins*, 503 U. S., at 125. By extending constitutional protection to an asserted right or liberty interest, we, to a great extent, place the matter outside the arena of public debate and legislative action. We must therefore "exercise the utmost care whenever we are asked to break new ground in this field," ibid, lest the liberty protected by the Due Process Clause be subtly transformed into the policy preferences of the members of this Court, *Moore*, 431 U. S., at 502 (plurality opinion).

Our established method of substantive due process analysis has two primary features: First, we have regularly observed that the Due Process Clause specially protects those fundamental rights and liberties which are, objectively, "deeply rooted in this Nation's history and tradition," *id.*, at 503 (plurality opinion); *Snyder* v. *Massachusetts*, 291 U.S. 97, 105 (1934) ("so rooted in the traditions and conscience of our people as to be ranked as fundamental"), and "implicit in the concept of ordered liberty," such that "neither liberty nor justice would exist if they were sacrificed," *Palko* v. *Connecticut*, 302 U.S. 319, 325, 326 (1937). Second, we have required in substantive due process cases a "careful description" of the asserted fundamental liberty interest. *Flores*, *supra*, at 302; *Collins*, *supra*, at 125; *Cruzan*, *supra*, at 277–278. Our Nation's history, legal traditions, and practices thus provide the crucial "guide*posts* for responsible decisionmaking," *Collins*, *supra*, at 125, that direct and restrain our exposition of the Due Process Clause. As we stated recently in *Flores*, the Fourteenth Amendment "forbids the government to infringe . . . 'fundamental' liberty interests *at all*, no matter what process is provided, unless the infringement is narrowly tailored to serve a compelling state interest." 507 U. S., at 302.

JUSTICE SOUTER, relying on JUSTICE HARLAN's dissenting opinion in *Poe* v. *Ullman*, would largely abandon this restrained methodology, and instead ask "whether [Washington's] statute sets up one of those 'arbitrary impositions' or 'purposeless restraints' at odds with the Due Process Clause of the Fourteenth Amendment," *post*, at 1 (quoting *Poe*, 367 U.S. 497, 543 (1961) (HARLAN, J., dissenting)).[17] In our view, however, the development of this Court's substantive due process jurisprudence, described briefly above, *supra*, at 15, has been a process whereby the outlines of the "liberty" specially protected by the Fourteenth Amendment—never fully clarified, to be sure, and perhaps not capable of being fully clarified—have at least been carefully refined by concrete examples involving fundamental rights found to be deeply rooted in our legal tradition. This approach tends to rein in the subjective elements that are necessarily present in due process judicial review. In addition, by establishing a threshold requirement—that a challenged state action implicate a fundamental right—before requiring more than a reasonable relation to a legitimate state interest to justify the action, it avoids the need for complex balancing of competing interests in every case.

Turning to the claim at issue here, the Court of Appeals stated that "[p]roperly analyzed, the first issue to be resolved is whether there is a liberty interest in determining the time and manner of one's death," 79 F. 3d, at 801, or, in other words, "[i]s there a right to die?," *id.*, at 799. Similarly, respondents assert a "liberty to choose how to die" and a right to "control of one's final days," Brief for Respondents 7, and describe the asserted liberty as "the right to choose a humane, dignified death," *id.*, at 15, and "the liberty to shape death," *id.*, at 18. As noted above, we have a tradition of carefully formulating the interest at stake in substantive due process cases. For example, although *Cruzan* is often described as a "right to die" case, see 79 F. 3d, at 799; *post*, at 9 (STEVENS, J., concurring in judgment) (*Cruzan* recognized "the more specific interest in making decisions about how to confront an imminent death"), we were, in fact, more precise: we assumed that the Constitution granted competent persons a "constitutionally protected right to refuse lifesaving hydration and nutrition." *Cruzan*, 497 U.S., at 279; *id.*, at 287 (O'CONNOR, J., concurring) ("[A] liberty interest in refusing unwanted medical treatment may be inferred from our prior decisions"). The Washington statute at issue in this case prohibits "aid[ing] another person to attempt suicide," Wash. Rev. Code §9A.36.060(1) (1994), and, thus, the question before us is whether the "liberty" specially protected by the Due Process Clause includes a right to commit suicide which itself includes a right to assistance in doing so.[18]

We now inquire whether this asserted right has any place in our Nation's traditions. Here, as discussed above, *supra*, at 4–15, we are confronted with a consistent and almost universal tradition that has long rejected the asserted right, and continues explicitly to reject it today, even for terminally ill, mentally competent adults. To hold for respondents, we would have to reverse centuries of legal doctrine and practice, and strike down the considered policy choice of almost every State. See *Jackman v. Rosenbaum Co.*, 260 U.S. 22, 31 (1922) ("If a thing has been practiced for two hundred years by common consent, it will need a strong case for the Fourteenth Amendment to affect it"); *Flores*, 507 U. S., at 303 ("The mere novelty of such a claim is reason enough to doubt that 'substantive due process' sustains it").

Respondents contend, however, that the liberty interest they assert is consistent with this Court's substantive due process line of cases, if not with this Nation's history and practice. Pointing to *Casey* and *Cruzan*, respondents read our jurisprudence in this area as reflecting a general tradition of "self sovereignty," Brief of Respondents 12, and as teaching that the "liberty" protected by the Due Process Clause includes "basic and intimate exercises of personal autonomy," *id.*, at 10; see *Casey*, 505 U. S., at 847 ("It is a promise of the Constitution that there is a realm of personal liberty which the government may not enter"). According to respondents, our liberty jurisprudence, and the broad, individualistic principles it reflects, protects the "liberty of competent, terminally ill adults to make end of life decisions free of undue government interference." Brief for Respondents 10. The question presented in this case, however, is whether the protections of the Due Process Clause include a right to commit suicide with another's assistance. With this "careful description" of respondents' claim in mind, we turn to *Casey* and *Cruzan*.

In *Cruzan*, we considered whether Nancy Beth Cruzan, who had been severely injured in an automobile accident and was in a persistive vegetative state, "ha[d] a right under the United States Constitution which would require the hospital to withdraw life sustaining treatment" at her parents' request. *Cruzan*, 497 U. S., at 269. We began with the observation that "[a]t common law, even the touching of one person by another without consent and without legal justification was a battery." *Ibid.* We then discussed the related rule that "informed consent is generally required for medical treatment." *Ibid.* After reviewing a long line of relevant state cases, we concluded that "the common law doctrine of informed consent is viewed as generally encompassing the right of a competent individual to refuse medical treatment." *Id.*, at 277. Next, we reviewed our own cases on the subject, and stated that "[t]he principle that a competent person has a constitutionally protected liberty interest in refusing unwanted medical treatment may be inferred from our prior decisions." *Id.*, at 278. Therefore, "for purposes of [that] case, we assume[d] that the United States Constitution would grant a competent person a constitutionally protected right to refuse lifesaving hydration and nutrition." *Id.*, at 279; see *id.*, at 287 (O'CONNOR, J., concurring). We concluded that, notwithstanding this right, the Constitution permitted Missouri to require clear and convincing evidence of an incompetent patient's wishes concerning the withdrawal of life sustaining treatment. *Id.*, at 280–281.

Respondents contend that in *Cruzan* we "acknowledged that competent, dying persons have the right to direct the removal of life sustaining medical treatment and thus hasten death," Brief for Respondents 23, and that "the constitutional principle behind recognizing the patient's liberty to direct the withdrawal of artificial life support applies at least as strongly to the choice to hasten impending death by consuming lethal medication," *id.*, at 26. Similarly, the Court of Appeals concluded that "*Cruzan*, by recognizing a liberty interest that includes the refusal of artificial provision of life sustaining food and water, necessarily recognize[d] a liberty interest in hastening one's own death." 79 F. 3d, at 816.

The right assumed in *Cruzan*, however, was not simply deduced from abstract concepts of personal autonomy. Given the common law rule that forced medication was a battery, and the long legal tradition protecting the decision to refuse unwanted medical treatment, our assumption was entirely consistent with this Nation's history and constitutional traditions. The decision to commit suicide with the assistance of another may be just as personal and profound as the decision to refuse unwanted medical treatment, but it has never enjoyed similar legal protection. Indeed, the two acts are widely and reasonably regarded as quite distinct. See *Quill* v. *Vacco*, *post*, at 5–13. In *Cruzan* itself, we recognized that most States outlawed assisted suicide—and even more do today— and we certainly gave no intimation that the right to refuse unwanted medical treatment could be somehow transmuted into a right to assistance in committing suicide. 497 U. S., at 280.

Respondents also rely on *Casey*. There, the Court's opinion concluded that "the essential holding of *Roe* v. *Wade* should be retained and once again reaffirmed." *Casey*, 505 U. S., at 846. We held, first, that a woman has a right, before her fetus is viable, to an abortion "without undue interference from the State"; second, that States may restrict post-viability abortions, so long as exceptions are made to protect a woman's life and health; and third, that the State has legitimate interests throughout a pregnancy in protecting the health of the woman and the life of the unborn child. *Ibid.* In reaching this conclusion, the opinion discussed in some detail this Court's substantive due process tradition of interpreting the Due Process Clause to protect certain fundamental rights and "personal decisions relating to marriage, procreation, contraception, family relationships, child rearing, and education," and noted that many of those rights and liberties "involv[e] the most intimate and personal choices a person may make in a lifetime." *Id.*, at 851.

The Court of Appeals, like the District Court, found *Casey* " 'highly instructive' " and " 'almost prescriptive' " for determining " 'what liberty interest may inhere in a terminally ill person's choice to commit suicide' ":

> "Like the decision of whether or not to have an abortion, the decision how and when to die is one of 'the most intimate and personal choices a person may make in a lifetime,' a choice 'central to personal dignity and autonomy.' " 79 F. 3d, at 813–814.

Similarly, respondents emphasize the statement in *Casey* that:

> "At the heart of liberty is the right to define one's own concept of existence, of meaning, of the universe, and of the mystery of human life. Beliefs about these matters could not define the attributes of personhood were they formed under compulsion of the State." *Casey*, 505 U. S., at 851.

Brief for Respondents 12. By choosing this language, the Court's opinion in *Casey* described, in a general way and in light of our prior cases, those personal activities and decisions that this Court has identified as so deeply rooted in our history and traditions, or so fundamental to our concept of constitutionally ordered liberty, that they are protected by the Fourteenth Amendment.[19] The opinion moved from the recognition that liberty necessarily includes freedom of conscience and belief about ultimate considerations to the observation that "though the abortion decision may originate within the zone of conscience and belief, *it is more than a philosophic exercise.*" *Casey*, 505 U. S., at 852 (emphasis added). That many of the rights and liberties protected by the Due Process Clause sound in personal autonomy does not warrant the sweeping conclusion that any and all important, intimate, and personal decisions are so protected, *San Antonio Independent School Dist.* v. *Rodriguez*, 411 U.S. 1, 33–35 (1973), and *Casey* did not suggest otherwise.

The history of the law's treatment of assisted suicide in this country has been and continues to be one of the rejection of nearly all efforts to permit it. That being the case, our decisions lead us to conclude that the asserted "right" to assistance in committing suicide is not a fundamental liberty interest protected by the Due Process Clause. The Constitution also requires, however, that Washington's assisted suicide ban be rationally related to legitimate government interests. See *Heller* v. *Doe*, 509 U.S. 312, 319–320 (1993); *Flores*, 507 U. S., at 305. This requirement is unquestionably met here. As the court below recognized, 79 F. 3d, at 816–817,[20] Washington's assisted suicide ban implicates a number of state interests.[21] See 49 F. 3d, at 592–593; Brief for State of California et al. as *Amici Curiae* 26–29; Brief for United States as *Amicus Curiae* 16–27.

First, Washington has an "unqualified interest in the preservation of human life." *Cruzan*, 497 U. S., at 282. The State's prohibition on assisted suicide, like all homicide laws, both reflects and advances its commitment to this interest. See *id.*, at 280; Model Penal Code §210.5, Comment 5, at 100 ("[T]he interests in the sanctity of life that are represented by the criminal homicide laws are threatened by one who expresses a willingness to participate in taking the life of another").[22] This interest is symbolic and aspirational as well as practical:

"While suicide is no longer prohibited or penalized, the ban against assisted suicide and euthanasia shores up the notion of limits in human relationships. It reflects the gravity with which we view the decision to take one's own life or the life of another, and our reluctance to encourage or promote these decisions." New York Task Force 131–132.

Respondents admit that "[t]he State has a real interest in preserving the lives of those who can still contribute to society and enjoy life." Brief for Respondents 35, n. 23. The Court of Appeals also recognized Washington's interest in protecting life, but held that the "weight" of this interest depends on the "medical condition and the wishes of the person whose life is at stake." 79 F. 3d, at 817. Washington, however, has rejected this sliding scale approach and, through its assisted suicide ban, insists that all persons' lives, from beginning to end, regardless of physical or mental condition, are under the full protection of the law. See *United States* v. *Rutherford*, 442 U.S. 544, 558 (1979) ("... Congress could reasonably have determined to protect the terminally ill, no less than other patients, from the vast range of self styled panaceas that inventive minds can devise"). As we have previously affirmed, the States "may properly decline to make judgments about the 'quality' of life that a particular individual may enjoy," *Cruzan*, 497 U. S., at 282. This remains true, as *Cruzan* makes clear, even for those who are near death.

Relatedly, all admit that suicide is a serious public health problem, especially among persons in otherwise vulnerable groups. See Washington State Dept. of Health, Annual Summary of Vital Statistics 1991, pp. 29–30 (Oct. 1992) (suicide is a leading cause of death in Washington of those between the ages of 14 and 54); New York Task Force 10, 23–33 (suicide rate in the general population is about one percent, and suicide is especially prevalent among the young and the elderly). The State has an interest in preventing suicide, and in studying, identifying, and treating its causes. See 79 F. 3d, at 820; *id.*, at 854 (Beezer, J., dissenting) ("The state recognizes suicide as a manifestation of medical and psychological anguish"); Marzen 107–146.

Those who attempt suicide—terminally ill or not—often suffer from depression or other mental disorders. See New York Task Force 13–22, 126–128 (more than 95% of those who commit suicide had a major psychiatric illness at the time of death; among the terminally ill, uncontrolled pain is a "risk factor" because it contributes to depression); Physician Assisted Suicide and Euthanasia in the Netherlands: A Report of Chairman Charles T. Canady to the Subcommittee on the Constitution of the House Committee on the Judiciary, 104th Cong., 2d Sess., 10–11 (Comm. Print 1996); cf. Back, Wallace, Starks, & Pearlman, Physician Assisted Suicide and Euthanasia in Washington State, 275 JAMA 919, 924 (1996) ("[I]ntolerable physical symptoms are not the reason most patients request physician assisted suicide or euthanasia"). Research indicates, however, that many people who request physician assisted suicide withdraw that request if their depression and pain are treated. H. Hendin, Seduced by Death: Doctors, Patients and the Dutch Cure 24–25 (1997) (suicidal, terminally ill patients "usually respond well to treatment for depressive illness and pain medication and are then grateful to be alive"); New York Task Force 177–178. The New York Task Force, however, expressed its concern that, because depression is difficult to diagnose, physicians and medical professionals often fail to respond adequately to seriously ill patients' needs. *Id.*, at 175. Thus, legal physician assisted suicide could make it more difficult for the State to protect depressed or mentally ill persons, or those who are suffering from untreated pain, from suicidal impulses.

The State also has an interest in protecting the integrity and ethics of the medical profession. In contrast to the Court of Appeals' conclusion that "the integrity of the medical profession would [not] be threatened in any way by [physician assisted suicide]," 79 F. 3d, at 827, the American Medical Association, like many other medical and physicians' groups, has concluded that "[p]hysician assisted suicide is fundamentally incompatible with the physician's role as healer." American Medical Association, Code of Ethics §2.211 (1994); see Council on Ethical and Judicial Affairs, Decisions Near the End of Life, 267 JAMA 2229, 2233 (1992) ("[T]he societal risks of involving physicians in medical interventions to cause patients' deaths is too great"); New York Task Force 103–109 (discussing physicians' views). And physician assisted suicide could, it is argued, undermine the trust that is essential to the doctor patient relationship by blurring the time honored line between healing and harming. Assisted Suicide in the United States, Hearing before the Subcommittee on the Constitution of the House Committee on the Judiciary, 104th Cong., 2d Sess., 355–356 (1996) (testimony of Dr. Leon R. Kass) ("The patient's trust in the doctor's whole hearted devotion to his best interests will be hard to sustain").

Next, the State has an interest in protecting vulnerable groups—including the poor, the elderly, and disabled persons—from abuse, neglect, and mistakes. The Court of Appeals dismissed the State's concern that disadvantaged persons might be pressured into physician assisted suicide as "ludicrous on its face." 79 F. 3d, at 825. We have recognized, however, the real risk of subtle coercion and undue influence in end of life situations. *Cruzan*, 497 U. S., at 281. Similarly, the New York Task Force warned that "[l]egalizing physician assisted suicide would pose profound risks to many individuals who are ill and vulnerable. . . . The risk of harm is greatest for the many individuals in our society whose autonomy and well being are already compromised by poverty, lack of access to good medical care, advanced age, or membership in a stigmatized social group." New York Task Force 120; see *Compassion in Dying*, 49 F. 3d, at 593 ("[A]n insidious bias against the handicapped—again coupled with a cost saving mentality— makes them especially in need of Washington's statutory protection"). If physician assisted suicide were permitted, many might resort to it to spare their families the substantial financial burden of end of life health care costs.

The State's interest here goes beyond protecting the vulnerable from coercion; it extends to protecting disabled and terminally ill people from prejudice, negative and inaccurate stereotypes, and "societal indifference." 49 F. 3d, at 592. The State's assisted suicide ban reflects and reinforces its policy that the lives of terminally ill, disabled, and elderly people must be no less valued than the lives of the young and healthy, and that a seriously disabled person's suicidal impulses should be interpreted and treated the same way as anyone else's. See New York Task Force 101–102; Physician Assisted Suicide and Euthanasia in the Netherlands: A Report of Chairman Charles T. Canady, at 9, 20 (discussing prejudice toward the disabled and the negative messages euthanasia and assisted suicide send to handicapped patients).

Finally, the State may fear that permitting assisted suicide will start it down the path to voluntary and perhaps even involuntary euthanasia. The Court of Appeals struck down Washington's assisted suicide ban only "as applied to competent, terminally ill adults who wish to hasten their deaths by obtaining medication prescribed by their doctors." 79 F. 3d, at 838. Washington insists, however, that the impact of the court's decision will not and cannot be so limited. Brief for Petitioners 44–47. If suicide is protected as a matter of constitutional right, it is argued, "every man and woman in the United States must enjoy it." *Compassion in Dying*, 49 F. 3d, at 591; see *Kevorkian*, 447 Mich., at 470, n. 41, 527 N. W. 2d, at 727–728, n. 41. The Court of Appeals' decision, and its expansive reasoning, provide ample support for the State's concerns. The court noted, for example, that the "decision of a duly appointed surrogate decision maker is for all legal purposes the decision of the patient himself," 79 F. 3d, at 832, n. 120; that "in some instances, the patient may be unable to self administer the drugs and . . . administration by the physician . . . may be the only way the patient may be able to receive them," *id.*, at 831; and that not only physicians, but also family members and loved ones, will inevitably participate in assisting suicide. *Id.*, at 838, n. 140. Thus, it turns out that what is couched as a limited right to "physician assisted suicide" is likely, in effect, a much broader license, which could prove extremely difficult to police and contain.[23] Washington's ban on assisting suicide prevents such erosion.

This concern is further supported by evidence about the practice of euthanasia in the Netherlands. The Dutch government's own study revealed that in 1990, there were 2,300 cases of voluntary euthanasia (defined as "the deliberate termination of another's life at his request"), 400 cases of assisted suicide, and more than 1,000 cases of euthanasia without an explicit request. In addition to these latter 1,000 cases, the study found an additional 4,941 cases where physicians administered lethal morphine overdoses without the patients' explicit consent. Physician Assisted Suicide and Euthanasia in the Netherlands: A Report of Chairman Charles T. Canady, at 12–13 (citing Dutch study). This study suggests that, despite the existence of various reporting procedures, euthanasia in the Netherlands has not been limited to competent, terminally ill adults who are enduring physical suffering, and that regulation of the practice may not have prevented abuses in cases involving vulnerable persons, including severely disabled neonates and elderly persons suffering from dementia. *Id.*, at 16–21; see generally C. Gomez, Regulating Death: Euthanasia and the Case of the Netherlands (1991); H. Hendin, Seduced By Death: Doctors, Patients, and the Dutch Cure (1997). The New York Task Force, citing the Dutch experience, observed that "assisted suicide and euthanasia are closely linked," New York Task Force 145, and concluded that the "risk of . . . abuse is neither speculative nor distant," *id.*, at 134. Washington, like most other States, reasonably ensures against this risk by banning, rather than regulating, assisting suicide. See *United States* v. *12 200-ft Reels of Super 8MM Film*, 413 U.S. 123, 127 (1973) ("Each step, when taken, appear[s] a reasonable step in relation to that which preceded it, although the aggregate or end result is one that would never have been seriously considered in the first instance").

We need not weigh exactly the relative strengths of these various interests. They are unquestionably important and legitimate, and Washington's ban on assisted suicide is at least reasonably related to their promotion and protection. We therefore hold that Wash. Rev. Code §9A.36.060(1) (1994) does not violate the Fourteenth Amendment, either on its face or "as applied to competent, terminally ill adults who wish to hasten their deaths by obtaining medication prescribed by their doctors." 79 F. 3d, at 838.[24]

*   *   *

Throughout the Nation, Americans are engaged in an earnest and profound debate about the morality, legality, and practicality of physician assisted suicide. Our holding permits this debate to continue, as it should in a democratic society. The decision of the en banc Court of Appeals is reversed, and the case is remanded for further proceedings consistent with this opinion.

It is so ordered.

JUSTICE O'CONNOR, CONCURRING.

Death will be different for each of us. For many, the last days will be spent in physical pain and perhaps the despair that accompanies physical deterioration and a loss of control of basic bodily and mental functions. Some will seek medication to alleviate that pain and other symptoms.

The Court frames the issue in this case as whether the Due Process Clause of the Constitution protects a "right to commit suicide which itself includes a right to assistance in doing so," *ante*, at 18, and concludes that our Nation's history, legal traditions, and practices do not support the existence of such a right. I join the Court's opinions because I agree that there is no generalized right to "commit suicide." But respondents urge us to address the narrower question whether a mentally competent person who is experiencing great suffering has a constitutionally cognizable interest in controlling the circumstances of his or her imminent death. I see no need to reach that question in the context of the facial challenges to the New York and Washington laws at issue here. See *ante*, at 18 ("The Washington statute at issue in this case prohibits 'aid[ing] another person to attempt suicide,' ... and, thus, the question before us is whether the 'liberty' specially protected by the Due Process Clause includes a right to commit suicide which itself includes a right to assistance in doing so"). The parties and amici agree that in these States a patient who is suffering from a terminal illness and who is experiencing great pain has no legal barriers to obtaining medication, from qualified physicians, to alleviate that suffering, even to the point of causing unconsciousness and hastening death. See Wash. Rev. Code §70.122.010 (1994); Brief for Petitioners in No. 95–1858, p. 15, n. 9; Brief for Respondents in No. 95–1858, p. 15. In this light, even assuming that we would recognize such an interest, I agree that the State's interests in protecting those who are not truly competent or facing imminent death, or those whose decisions to hasten death would not truly be voluntary, are sufficiently weighty to justify a prohibition against physician assisted suicide. *Ante*, at 27–30; *post*, at 11 (STEVENS, J., concurring in judgments); *post*, at 33–39 (SOUTER, J., concurring in judgment).

Every one of us at some point may be affected by our own or a family member's terminal illness. There is no reason to think the democratic process will not strike the proper balance between the interests of terminally ill, mentally competent individuals who would seek to end their suffering and the State's interests in protecting those who might seek to end life mistakenly or under pressure. As the Court recognizes, States are presently undertaking extensive and serious evaluation of physician assisted suicide and other related issues. *Ante*, at 11, 12–13; see *post*, at 36–39 (SOUTER, J., concurring in judgment). In such circumstances, "the ... challenging task of crafting appropriate procedures for safeguarding ... liberty interests is entrusted to the 'laboratory' of the States ... in the first instance." *Cruzan* v. *Director, Mo. Dept. of Health*, 497 U.S. 261, 292 (1990) (O'CONNOR, J., concurring) (citing *New State Ice Co. v. Liebmann*, 285 U.S. 262, 311 (1932)).

In sum, there is no need to address the question whether suffering patients have a constitutionally cognizable interest in obtaining relief from the suffering that they may experience in the last days of their lives. There is no dispute that dying patients in Washington and New York can obtain palliative care, even when doing so would hasten their deaths. The difficulty in defining terminal illness and the risk that a dying patient's request for assistance in ending his or her life might not be truly voluntary justifies the prohibitions on assisted suicide we uphold here.

JUSTICE STEVENS, CONCURRING IN THE JUDGMENTS.

The Court ends its opinion with the important observation that our holding today is fully consistent with a continuation of the vigorous debate about the "morality, legality, and practicality of physician assisted suicide" in a democratic society. *Ante*, at 32. I write separately to make it clear that there is also room for further debate about the limits that the Constitution places on the power of the States to punish the practice.

I

The morality, legality, and practicality of capital punishment have been the subject of debate for many years. In 1976, this Court upheld the constitutionality of the practice in cases coming to us from Georgia,[1] Florida,[2] and Texas.[3] In those cases we concluded that a State does have the power to place a lesser value on some lives than on others; there is no absolute requirement that a State treat all human life as having an equal right to preservation. Because the state legislatures had sufficiently narrowed the category of lives that the State could terminate, and had enacted special procedures to ensure that the defendant belonged in that limited category, we concluded that the statutes were not unconstitutional on their face. In later cases coming to us from each of those States, however, we found that some applications of the statutes were unconstitutional.[4]

Today, the Court decides that Washington's statute prohibiting assisted suicide is not invalid "on its face," that is to say, in all or most cases in which it might be applied.[5] That holding, however, does not foreclose the possibility that some applications of the statute might well be invalid.

As originally filed, this case presented a challenge to the Washington statute on its face and as it applied to three terminally ill, mentally competent patients and to four physicians who treat terminally ill patients. After the District Court issued its opinion holding that the statute placed an undue burden on the right to commit physician assisted suicide, see *Compassion in Dying* v. *Washington*, 850 F. Supp. 1454, 1462, 1465 (WD Wash. 1994), the three patients died. Although the Court of Appeals considered the constitutionality of the statute-as applied to the prescription of life ending medication for use by terminally ill, competent adult patients who wish to hasten their deaths," *Compassion in Dying* v. *Washington*, 79 F. 3d 790, 798 (CA9 1996), the court did not have before it any individual plaintiff seeking to hasten her death or any doctor who was threatened with prosecution for assisting in the suicide of a particular patient; its analysis and eventual holding that the statute was unconstitutional was not limited to a particular set of plaintiffs before it.

The appropriate standard to be applied in cases making facial challenges to state statutes has been the subject of debate within this Court. See *Janklow* v. *Planned Parenthood, Sioux Falls Clinic*, 517 U. S. (1996). Upholding the validity of the federal Bail Reform Act of 1984, the Court stated in *United States* v. *Salerno*, 481 U.S. 739 (1987), that a "facial challenge to a legislative Act is, of course, the most difficult challenge to mount successfully, since the challenger must establish that no set of circumstances exists under which the Act would be valid." *Id.*, at 745.[6] I do not believe the Court has ever actually applied such a strict standard,[7] even in *Salerno* itself, and the Court does-not appear to apply *Salerno* here. Nevertheless, the Court does conceive of respondents' claim as a facial challenge—addressing not the application of the statute to a particular set of plaintiffs before it, but the constitutionality of the statute's categorical prohibition against "aid[ing] another person to attempt suicide." *Ante*, at 18 (internal quotation marks omitted) (citing Wash. Rev. Code §9A.36.060(1) (1994)). Accordingly, the Court requires the plaintiffs to show that the interest in liberty protected by the

Fourteenth Amendment "includes a right to commit suicide which itself includes a right to assistance in doing so." *Ante*, at 18.

History and tradition provide ample support for refusing to recognize an open ended constitutional right to commit suicide. Much more than the State's paternalistic interest in protecting the individual from the irrevocable consequences of an ill advised decision motivated by temporary concerns is at stake. There is truth in John Donne's observation that "No man is an island."[8] The State has an interest in preserving and fostering the benefits that every human being may provide to the community— a community that thrives on the exchange of ideas, expressions of affection, shared memories and humorous incidents as well as on the material contributions that its members create and support. The value to others of a person's life is far too precious to allow the individual to claim a constitutional entitlement to complete autonomy in making a decision to end that life. Thus, I fully agree with the Court that the "liberty" protected by the Due Process Clause does not include a categorical "right to commit suicide which itself includes a right to assistance in doing so." *Ante*, at 18.

But just as our conclusion that capital punishment is not always unconstitutional did not preclude later decisions holding that it is sometimes impermissibly cruel, so is it equally clear that a decision upholding a general statutory prohibition of assisted suicide does not mean that every possible application of the statute would be valid. A State, like Washington, that has authorized the death penalty and thereby has concluded that the sanctity of human life does not require that it always be preserved, must acknowledge that there are situations in which an interest in hastening death is legitimate. Indeed, not only is that interest sometimes legitimate, I am also convinced that there are times when it is entitled to constitutional protection.

II

In *Cruzan v. Director, Mo. Dept. of Health*, 497 U.S. 261 (1990), the Court assumed that the interest in liberty protected by the Fourteenth Amendment encompassed the right of a terminally ill patient to direct the withdrawal of life sustaining treatment. As the Court correctly observes today, that assumption "was not simply deduced from abstract concepts of personal autonomy." *Ante*, at 21. Instead, it was supported by the common law tradition protecting the individual's general right to refuse unwanted medical treatment. *Ibid.* We have recognized, however, that this common law right to refuse treatment is neither absolute nor always sufficiently weighty to overcome valid countervailing state interests. As Justice Brennan pointed out in his *Cruzan* dissent, we have upheld legislation imposing punishment on persons refusing to be vaccinated, 497 U. S., at 312, n. 12, citing *Jacobson v. Massachusetts*, 197 U.S. 11, 26–27 (1905), and as JUSTICE SCALIA pointed out in his concurrence, the State ordinarily has the right to interfere with an attempt to commit suicide by, for example, forcibly placing a bandage on a self inflicted wound to stop the flow of blood. 497 U. S., at 298. In most cases, the individual's constitutionally protected interest in his or her own physical autonomy, including the right to refuse unwanted medical treatment, will give way to the State's interest in preserving human life.

Cruzan, however, was not the normal case. Given the irreversible nature of her illness and the progressive character of her suffering,[9] Nancy Cruzan's interest in refusing medical care was incidental to her more basic interest in controlling the manner and timing of her death. In finding that her best interests would be served by cutting off the nourishment that kept her alive, the trial court did more than simply vindicate Cruzan's interest in refusing medical treatment; the court, in essence, authorized affirmative conduct that would hasten her death. When this Court reviewed the case and upheld Missouri's requirement that there be clear and convincing evidence establishing Nancy Cruzan's intent to have life sustaining nourishment withdrawn, it made two important assumptions: (1) that there was a "liberty interest" in refusing unwanted treatment protected by the Due Process Clause; and (2) that this liberty interest did not "end the inquiry" because it might be outweighed by relevant state interests. *Id.*, at 279. I agree with both of those assumptions, but I insist that the source of Nancy Cruzan's right to refuse treatment was not just a common law rule. Rather, this right is an aspect of a far broader and more basic concept of freedom that is even older than the common law.[10] This freedom embraces, not merely a person's right to refuse a particular kind of unwanted treatment, but also her interest in dignity, and in determining the character of the memories that will survive long after her death.[11] In recognizing that the State's interests did not outweigh Nancy Cruzan's liberty interest in refusing medical treatment, *Cruzan* rested not simply on the common law right to refuse medical treatment, but—at least implicitly—on the even more fundamental right to make this "deeply personal decision," 497 U. S., at 289 (O'CONNOR, J., concurring).

Thus, the common law right to protection from battery, which included the right to refuse medical treatment in most circumstances, did not mark "the outer limits of the substantive sphere of liberty" that supported the Cruzan family's decision to hasten Nancy's death. *Planned Parenthood of Southeastern Pa.* v. *Casey*, 505 U.S. 833, 848 (1992). Those limits have never been precisely defined. They are generally identified by the importance and character of the decision confronted by the individual, *Whalen* v. *Roe*, 429 U.S. 589, 599–600, n. 26 (1977). Whatever the outer limits of the concept may be, it definitely includes protection for matters "central to personal dignity and autonomy." *Casey*, 505 U. S., at 851. It includes,

> "the individual's right to make certain unusually important decisions that will affect his own, or his family's, destiny. The Court has referred to such decisions as implicating 'basic values,' as being 'fundamental,' and as being dignified by history and tradition. The character of the Court's language in these cases brings to mind the origins of the American heritage of freedom—the abiding interest in individual liberty that makes certain state intrusions on the citizen's right to decide how he will live his own life intolerable." *Fitzgerald* v. *Porter Memorial* Hospital, 523 F. 2d 716, 719–720 (CA7 1975) (footnotes omitted), cert. denied, 425 U.S. 916 (1976).

The *Cruzan* case demonstrated that some state intrusions on the right to decide how death will be encountered are also intolerable. The now deceased plaintiffs in this action may in fact have had a liberty interest even stronger than Nancy Cruzan's because, not only were they terminally ill, they were suffering constant and severe pain. Avoiding intolerable pain and the indignity of living one's final days incapacitated and in agony is certainly "[a]t the heart of [the] liberty . . . to define one's own concept of existence, of meaning, of the universe, and of the mystery of human life." *Casey*, 505 U. S., at 851.

While I agree with the Court that *Cruzan* does not decide the issue presented by these cases, *Cruzan* did give recognition, not just to vague, unbridled notions of autonomy, but to the more specific interest in making decisions about how to confront an imminent death. Although there is no absolute right to physician assisted suicide, *Cruzan* makes it clear that some individuals who no longer have the option of deciding whether to live or to die because they are already on the threshold of death have a constitutionally protected interest that may outweigh the State's interest in preserving life at all costs. The liberty interest at stake in a case like this differs from, and is stronger than, both the common law right to refuse medical treatment and the unbridled interest in deciding whether to live or die. It is an interest in deciding how, rather than whether, a critical threshold shall be crossed.

III

The state interests supporting a general rule banning the practice of physician assisted suicide do not have the same force in all cases. First and foremost of these interests is the " 'unqualified interest in the preservation of human life,' " *ante*, at 24, (quoting *Cruzan*, 497 U. S., at 282,) which is equated with " 'the sanctity of life,' " *ante*, at 25, (quoting the American Law Institute, Model Penal Code §210.5, Comment 5, p. 100 (Official Draft and Revised Comments 1980)). That interest not only justifies—it commands—maximum protection of every individual's interest in remaining alive, which in turn commands the same protection for decisions about whether to commence or to terminate life support systems or to administer pain medication that may hasten death. Properly viewed, however, this interest is not a collective interest that should always outweigh the interests of a person who because of pain, incapacity, or sedation finds her life intolerable, but rather, an aspect of individual freedom.

Many terminally ill people find their lives meaningful even if filled with pain or dependence on others. Some find value in living through suffering; some have an abiding desire to witness particular events in their families' lives; many believe it a sin to hasten death. Individuals of different religious faiths make different judgments and choices about whether to live on under such circumstances. There are those who will want to continue aggressive treatment; those who would prefer terminal sedation; and those who will seek withdrawal from life support systems and death by gradual starvation and dehydration. Although as a general matter the State's interest in the contributions each person may make to society outweighs the person's interest in ending her life, this interest does not have the same force for a terminally ill patient faced not with the choice of whether to live, only of how to die. Allowing the individual, rather than the State, to make judgments " 'about the "quality" of life that a particular individual may enjoy.' " *ante*, at 25 (quoting *Cruzan*, 497 U. S., at 282), does not mean that the lives of terminally ill, disabled people have less value than the lives of those who are healthy, see *ante*, at 28. Rather, it gives proper recognition to the individual's interest in choosing a final chapter that accords with her life story, rather than one that demeans her values and poisons memories of her. See Brief for Bioethicists as *Amici Curiae* 11; see also R. Dworkin, Life's Dominion 213 (1993) ("Whether it is in someone's best interests that his life end in one way rather than another depends on so much else that is special about him—about the shape and character of his life and his own sense of his integrity and critical interests—that no uniform collective decision can possibly hope to serve everyone even decently").

Similarly, the State's legitimate interests in preventing suicide, protecting the vulnerable from coercion and abuse, and preventing euthanasia are less significant in this context. I agree that the State has a compelling interest in preventing persons from committing suicide because of depression, or coercion by third parties. But the State's legitimate interest in preventing abuse does not apply to an individual who is not victimized by abuse, who is not suffering from depression, and who makes a rational and voluntary decision to seek assistance in dying. Although, as the New York Task Force report discusses, diagnosing depression and other mental illness is not always easy, mental health workers and other professionals expert in working with dying patients can help patients cope with depression and pain, and help patients assess their options. See Brief for Washington State Psychological Association et al. as *Amici Curiae* 8–10.

Relatedly, the State and amici express the concern that patients whose physical pain is inadequately treated will be more likely to request assisted suicide. Encouraging the development and ensuring the availability of adequate pain treatment is of utmost importance; palliative care, however, cannot alleviate all pain and suffering. See Orentlicher, Legalization of Physician Assisted Suicide: A Very Modest Revolution, 38 Boston College L. Rev. (Galley, p. 8) (1997) ("Greater use of palliative care would reduce the demand for assisted suicide, but it will not eliminate [it]"); see also Brief for Coalition of Hospice Professionals as *Amici Curiae* 8 (citing studies showing that "[a]s death becomes more imminent, pain and suffering become progressively more difficult to treat"). An individual adequately informed of the care alternatives thus might make a rational choice for assisted suicide. For such an individual, the State's interest in preventing potential abuse and mistake is only minimally implicated.

The final major interest asserted by the State is its interest in preserving the traditional integrity of the medical profession. The fear is that a rule permitting physicians to assist in suicide is inconsistent with the perception that they serve their patients solely as healers. But for some patients, it would be a physician's refusal to dispense medication to ease their suffering and make their death tolerable and dignified that would be inconsistent with the healing role See Block & Billings, Patient Request to Hasten Death, 154 Archives Internal Med. 2039, 2045 (1994) (A doctor's refusal to hasten death "may be experienced by the [dying] patient as an abandonment, a rejection, or an expression of inappropriate paternalistic authority"). For doctors who have long standing relationships with their patients, who have given their patients advice on alternative treatments, who are attentive to their patient's individualized needs, and who are knowledgeable about pain symptom management and palliative care options, see Quill, Death and Dignity, A Case of Individualized DecisionMaking, 324 New England J. of Med. 691–694 (1991), heeding a patient's desire to assist in her suicide would not serve to harm the physician patient relationship. Furthermore, because physicians are already involved in making decisions that hasten the death of terminally ill patients—through termination of life support, withholding of medical treatment, and terminal sedation—there is in fact significant tension between the traditional view of the physician's role and the actual practice in a growing number of cases.[12]

As the New York State Task Force on Life and the Law recognized, a State's prohibition of assisted suicide is justified by the fact that the " 'ideal' " case in which "patients would be screened for depression and offered treatment, effective pain medication would be available, and all patients would have a supportive committed family and doctor" is not the usual case. New York State Task Force on Life and the Law, When Death Is Sought: Assisted Suicide and Euthanasia in the Medical Context 120 (May 1994). Although, as the Court concludes today, these *potential* harms are sufficient to support the State's general public policy against assisted suicide, they will not always outweigh the individual liberty interest of a particular patient. Unlike the Court of Appeals, I would not say as a categorical matter that these state interests are invalid as to the entire class of terminally ill, mentally competent patients. I do not, however, foreclose the possibility that an individual plaintiff seeking to hasten her death, or a doctor whose assistance was sought, could prevail in a more particularized challenge. Future cases will determine whether such a challenge may succeed.

IV

In New York, a doctor must respect a competent person's decision to refuse or to discontinue medical treatment even though death will thereby ensue, but the same doctor would be guilty of a felony if she provided her patient assistance in committing suicide.[13] Today we hold that the Equal Protection Clause is not violated by the resulting disparate treatment of two classes of terminally ill people who may have the same interest in hastening death. I agree that the distinction between permitting death to ensue from an underlying fatal disease and causing it to occur by the administration of medication or other means provides a constitutionally sufficient basis for the State's classification.[14] Unlike the Court, however, see *Vacco, ante,* at 6–7, I am not persuaded that in all cases there will in fact be a significant difference between the intent of the physicians, the patients or the families in the two situations.

There may be little distinction between the intent of a terminally ill patient who decides to remove her life support and one who seeks the assistance of a doctor in ending her life; in both situations, the patient is seeking to hasten a certain, impending death. The doctor's intent might also be the same in prescribing lethal medication as it is in terminating life support. A doctor who fails to administer medical treatment to one who is dying from a disease could be doing so with an intent to harm or kill that patient. Conversely, a doctor who prescribes lethal medication does not necessarily intend the patient's death—rather that doctor may seek simply to ease the patient's suffering and to comply with her wishes. The illusory character of any differences in intent or causation is confirmed by the fact that the American Medical Association unequivocally endorses the practice of terminal sedation—the administration of sufficient dosages of pain killing medication to terminally ill patients to protect them from excruciating pain even when it is clear that the time of death will be advanced. The purpose of terminal sedation is to ease the suffering of the patient and comply with her wishes, and the actual cause of death is the administration of heavy doses of lethal sedatives. This same intent and causation may exist when a doctor complies with a patient's request for lethal medication to hasten her death.[15]

Thus, although the differences the majority notes in causation and intent between terminating life support and assisting in suicide support the Court's rejection of the respondents' facial challenge, these distinctions may be inapplicable to particular terminally ill patients and their doctors. Our holding today in *Vacco v. Quill* that the Equal Protection Clause is not violated by New York's classification, just like our holding in *Washington v. Glucksberg* that the Washington statute is not invalid on its face, does not foreclose the possibility that some applications of the New York statute may impose an intolerable intrusion on the patient's freedom.

There remains room for vigorous debate about the outcome of particular cases that are not necessarily resolved by the opinions announced today. How such cases may be decided will depend on their specific facts. In my judgment, however, it is clear that the so called "unqualified interest in the preservation of human life," *Cruzan,* 497 U. S., at 282, *Glucksberg, ante,* at 24, is not itself sufficient to outweigh the interest in liberty that may justify the only possible means of preserving a dying patient's dignity and alleviating her intolerable suffering.

JUSTICE SOUTER, CONCURRING IN THE JUDGMENT.

Three terminally ill individuals and four physicians who sometimes treat terminally ill patients brought this challenge to the Washington statute making it a crime "knowingly ... [to] ai[d] another person to attempt suicide," Wash. Rev. Code §9A.36.060 (1994), claiming on behalf of both patients and physicians that it would violate substantive due process to enforce the statute against a doctor who acceded to a dying patient's request for a drug to be taken by the patient to commit suicide. The question is whether the statute sets up one of those "arbitrary impositions" or "purposeless restraints" at odds with the Due Process Clause of the Fourteenth Amendment. *Poe* v.

Ullman, 367 U. S. 497, 543 (1961) (Harlan, J., dissenting). I conclude that the statute's application to the doctors has not been shown to be unconstitutional, but I write separately to give my reasons for analyzing the substantive due process claims as I do, and for rejecting this one.

I

Although the terminally ill original parties have died during the pendency of this case, the four physicians who remain as respondents here[1] continue to request declaratory and injunctive relief for their own benefit in discharging their obligations to other dying patients who request their help.[2] See, *e.g., Southern Pacific Terminal Co.* v. *ICC,* 219 U. S. 498, 515 (1911) (question was capable of repetition yet evading review). The case reaches us on an order granting summary judgment, and we must take as true the undisputed allegations that each of the patients was mentally competent and terminally ill, and that each made a knowing and voluntary choice to ask a doctor to prescribe "medications . . . to be self-administered for the purpose of hastening . . . death." Complaint ¶2.3. The State does not dispute that each faced a passage to death more agonizing both mentally and physically, and more protracted over time, than death by suicide with a physician's help, or that each would have chosen such a suicide for the sake of personal dignity, apart even from relief from pain. Each doctor in this case claims to encounter patients like the original plaintiffs who have died, that is, mentally competent, terminally ill, and seeking medical help in "the voluntary self-termination of life." *Id.,* at ¶2.5–2.8. While there may be no unanimity on the physician's professional obligation in such circumstances, I accept here respondents' representation that providing such patients with prescriptions for drugs that go beyond pain relief to hasten death would, in these circumstances, be consistent with standards of medical practice. Hence, I take it to be true, as respondents say, that the Washington statute prevents the exercise of a physician's "best professional judgment to prescribe medications to [such] patients in dosages that would enable them to act to hasten their own deaths." *Id.,* at ¶2.6; see also App. 35–37, 49–51, 55–57, 73–75.

In their brief to this Court, the doctors claim not that they ought to have a right generally to hasten patients' imminent deaths, but only to help patients who have made "personal decisions regarding their own bodies, medical care, and, fundamentally, the future course of their lives," Brief for Respondents 12, and who have concluded responsibly and with substantial justification that the brief and anguished remainders of their lives have lost virtually all value to them. Respondents fully embrace the notion that the State must be free to impose reasonable regulations on such physician assistance to ensure that the patients they assist are indeed among the competent and terminally ill and that each has made a free and informed choice in seeking to obtain and use a fatal drug. Complaint ¶3.2; App. 28–41.

In response, the State argues that the interest asserted by the doctors is beyond constitutional recognition because it has no deep roots in our history and traditions. Brief for Petitioners 21–25. But even aside from that, without disputing that the patients here were competent and terminally ill, the State insists that recognizing the legitimacy of doctors' assistance of their patients as contemplated here would entail a number of adverse consequences that the Washington Legislature was entitled to forestall. The nub of this part of the State's argument is not that such patients are constitutionally undeserving of relief on their own account, but that any attempt to confine a right of physician assistance to the circumstances presented by these doctors is likely to fail. *Id.,* at 34–35, 44–47.

First, the State argues that the right could not be confined to the terminally ill. Even assuming a fixed definition of that term, the State observes that it is not always possible to say with certainty how long a person may live. *Id.*, at 34. It asserts that "[t]here is no principled basis on which [the right] can be limited to the prescription of medication for terminally ill patients to administer to themselves" when the right's justifying principle is as broad as "'merciful termination of suffering.'" *Id.*, at 45 (citing Y. Kamisar, Are Laws Against Assisted Suicide Unconstitutional?, Hastings Center Report 32, 36–37 (May–June 1993)). Second, the State argues that the right could not be confined to the mentally competent, observing that a person's competence cannot always be assessed with certainty, Brief for Petitioners 34, and suggesting further that no principled distinction is possible between a competent patient acting independently and a patient acting through a duly appointed and competent surrogate, *id.*, at 46. Next, according to the State, such a right might entail a right to or at least merge in practice into "other forms of life-ending assistance," such as euthanasia. *Id.*, at 46–47. Finally, the State believes that a right to physician assistance could not easily be distinguished from a right to assistance from others, such as friends, family, and other health-care workers. *Id.*, at 47. The State thus argues that recognition of the substantive due process right at issue here would jeopardize the lives of others outside the class defined by the doctors' claim, creating risks of irresponsible suicides and euthanasia, whose dangers are concededly within the State's authority to address.

II

When the physicians claim that the Washington law deprives them of a right falling within the scope of liberty that the Fourteenth Amendment guarantees against denial without due process of law,[3] they are not claiming some sort of procedural defect in the process through which the statute has been enacted or is administered. Their claim, rather, is that the State has no substantively adequate justification for barring the assistance sought by the patient and sought to be offered by the physician. Thus, we are dealing with a claim to one of those rights sometimes described as rights of substantive due process and sometimes as unenumerated rights, in view of the breadth and indeterminacy of the "due process" serving as the claim's textual basis. The doctors accordingly arouse the skepticism of those who find the Due Process Clause an unduly vague or oxymoronic warrant for judicial review of substantive state law, just as they also invoke two centuries of American constitutional practice in recognizing unenumerated, substantive limits on governmental action. Although this practice has neither rested on any single textual basis nor expressed a consistent theory (or, before *Poe* v. *Ullman*, a much articulated one), a brief overview of its history is instructive on two counts. The persistence of substantive due process in our cases points to the legitimacy of the modern justification for such judicial review found in Justice Harlan's dissent in *Poe*,[4] on which I will dwell further on, while the acknowledged failures of some of these cases point with caution to the difficulty raised by the present claim.

Before the ratification of the Fourteenth Amendment, substantive constitutional review resting on a theory of unenumerated rights occurred largely in the state courts applying state constitutions that commonly contained either due process clauses like that of the Fifth Amendment (and later the Fourteenth) or the textual antecedents of such clauses, repeating Magna Carta's guarantee of "the law of the land."[5] On the basis of such clauses, or of general principles untethered to specific constitutional language, state courts evaluated the constitutionality of a wide range of statutes.

Thus, a Connecticut court approved a statute legitimating a class of previous illegitimate marriages, as falling within the terms of the "social compact," while making clear its power to review constitutionality in those terms. *Goshen* v. *Stonington*, 4 Conn.

209, 225–226 (1822). In the same period, a specialized court of equity, created under a Tennessee statute solely to hear cases brought by the state bank against its debtors, found its own authorization unconstitutional as "partial" legislation violating the state constitution's "law of the land" clause. *Bank of the State* v. *Cooper,* 2 Yerg. 599, 602–608 (Tenn. 1831) (Green, J.); *id.,* at 613–615 (Peck, J.); *id.,* at 618–623 (Kennedy, J.). And the middle of the nineteenth century brought the famous *Wynehamer* case, invalidating a statute purporting to render possession of liquor immediately illegal except when kept for narrow, specified purposes, the state court finding the statute inconsistent with the state's due process clause. *Wynehamer* v. *People,* 13 N. Y. 378, 486–487 (1856). The statute was deemed an excessive threat to the "fundamental rights of the citizen" to property. *Id.,* at 398 (Comstock, J.). See generally, E. Corwin, Liberty Against Government 58–115 (1948) (discussing substantive due process in the state courts before the Civil War); T. Cooley, Constitutional Limitations *85–*129, *351–*397.

Even in this early period, however, this Court anticipated the developments that would presage both the Civil War and the ratification of the Fourteenth Amendment, by making it clear on several occasions that it too had no doubt of the judiciary's power to strike down legislation that conflicted with important but unenumerated principles of American government. In most such instances, after declaring its power to invalidate what it might find inconsistent with rights of liberty and property, the Court nevertheless went on to uphold the legislative acts under review. See, *e.g., Wilkinson* v. *Leland,* 2 Pet. 627, 656–661 (1829); *Calder* v. *Bull,* 3 Dall. 386, 386–395 (1798) (opinion of Chase, J.); see also *Corfield* v. *Coryell,* 6 F. Cas. 546, 550–552 (No. 3,230) (1823). But in *Fletcher* v. *Peck,* 6 Cranch 87 (1810), the Court went further. It struck down an act of the Georgia legislature that purported to rescind a sale of public land *ab initio* and reclaim title for the State, and so deprive subsequent, good-faith purchasers of property conveyed by the original grantees. The Court rested the invalidation on alternative sources of authority: the specific prohibitions against bills of attainder, *ex post facto* laws, laws impairing contracts in Article I, §10 of the Constitution; and "general principles which are common to our free institutions," by which Chief Justice Marshall meant that a simple deprivation of property by the State could not be an authentically "legislative" act. *Fletcher,* 6 Cranch, at 135–139.

Fletcher was not, though, the most telling early example of such review. For its most salient instance in this Court before the adoption of the Fourteenth Amendment was, of course, the case that the Amendment would in due course overturn, *Dred Scott* v. *Sandford,* 19 How. 393 (1857). Unlike *Fletcher, Dred Scott* was textually based on a due process clause (in the Fifth Amendment, applicable to the national government), and it was in reliance on that clause's protection of property that the Court invalidated the Missouri Compromise. 19 How., at 449–452. This substantive protection of an owner's property in a slave taken to the territories was traced to the absence of any enumerated power to affect that property granted to the Congress by Article I of the Constitution, *id.,* at 451–452, the implication being that the government had no legitimate interest that could support the earlier congressional compromise. The ensuing judgment of history needs no recounting here.

After the ratification of the Fourteenth Amendment, with its guarantee of due process protection against the States, interpretation of the words "liberty" and "property" as used in due process clauses became a sustained enterprise, with the Court generally describing the due process criterion in converse terms of reasonableness or arbitrariness. That standard is fairly traceable to Justice Bradley's dissent in the *Slaughter-House Cases,* 16 Wall. 36 (1873), in which he said that a person's right to choose a calling was an element of liberty (as the calling, once chosen, was an aspect of property) and declared that the liberty and property protected by due process are not truly recognized if such rights may be "arbitrarily assailed," *id.*, at 116.[6] After that, opinions comparable to those that preceded *Dred Scott* expressed willingness to review legislative action for consistency with the Due Process Clause even as they upheld the laws in question. See, *e.g., Bartemeyer* v. *Iowa*, 18 Wall. 129, 133–135 (1874); *Munn* v. *Illinois*, 94 U. S. 113, 123–135 (1877); *Railroad Comm'n Cases*, 116 U. S. 307, 331 (1886); *Mugler* v. *Kansas*, 123 U. S. 623, 659–670 (1887). See generally Corwin, Liberty Against Government, at 121–136 (surveying the Court's early Fourteenth Amendment cases and finding little dissent from the general principle that the Due Process Clause authorized judicial review of substantive statutes).

The theory became serious, however, beginning with *Allgeyer* v. *Louisiana*, 165 U. S. 578 (1897), where the Court invalidated a Louisiana statute for excessive interference with Fourteenth Amendment liberty to contract, *id.*, at 588–593, and offered a substantive interpretation of "liberty," that in the aftermath of the so-called Lochner Era has been scaled back in some respects, but expanded in others, and never repudiated in principle. The Court said that Fourteenth Amendment liberty includes "the right of the citizen to be free in the enjoyment of all his faculties; to be free to use them in all lawful ways; to live and work where he will; to earn his livelihood by any lawful calling; to pursue any livelihood or avocation; and for that purpose to enter into all contracts which may be proper, necessary and essential to his carrying out to a successful conclusion the purposes above mentioned." *Id.*, at 589. "[W]e do not intend to hold that in no such case can the State exercise its police power," the Court added, but "[w]hen and how far such power may be legitimately exercised with regard to these subjects must be left for determination to each case as it arises." *Id.*, at 590.

Although this principle was unobjectionable, what followed for a season was, in the realm of economic legislation, the echo of *Dred Scott. Allgeyer* was succeeded within a decade by *Lochner* v. *New York*, 198 U. S. 45 (1905), and the era to which that case gave its name, famous now for striking down as arbitrary various sorts of economic regulations that post-New Deal courts have uniformly thought constitutionally sound. Compare, *e.g., id.*, at 62 (finding New York's maximum-hours law for bakers "unreasonable and entirely arbitrary") and *Adkins* v. *Children's Hospital of D. C.*, 261 U. S. 525, 559 (1923) (holding a minimum wage law "so clearly the product of a naked, arbitrary exercise of power that it cannot be allowed to stand under the Constitution of the United States") with *West Coast Hotel Co.* v. *Parrish*, 300 U. S. 379, 391 (1937) (overruling *Adkins* and approving a minimum-wage law on the principle that "regulation which is reasonable in relation to its subject and is adopted in the interests of the community is due process"). As the parentheticals here suggest, while the cases in the *Lochner* line routinely invoked a correct standard of constitutional arbitrariness review, they harbored the spirit of *Dred Scott* in their absolutist implementation of the standard they espoused.

Even before the deviant economic due process cases had been repudiated, however, the more durable precursors of modern substantive due process were reaffirming this Court's obligation to conduct arbitrariness review, beginning with *Meyer* v. *Nebraska*, 262 U. S. 390 (1923). Without referring to any specific guarantee of the Bill of Rights, the Court invoked precedents from the *Slaughter-House Cases* through *Adkins* to declare that the Fourteenth Amendment protected "the right of the individual to contract, to engage in any of the common occupations of life, to acquire useful knowledge, to marry, establish a home and bring up children, to worship God according to the dictates of his own conscience, and generally to enjoy those privileges long recognized at common law as essential to the orderly pursuit of happiness by free men." *Id.*, at 399.

The Court then held that the same Fourteenth Amendment liberty included a teacher's right to teach and the rights of parents to direct their children's education without unreasonable interference by the States, *id.*, at 400, with the result that Nebraska's prohibition on the teaching of foreign languages in the lower grades was, "arbitrary and without reasonable relation to any end within the competency of the State," *id.*, at 403. See also *Pierce* v. *Society of Sisters,* 268 U. S. 510, 534–536 (1925) (finding that a statute that all but outlawed private schools lacked any "reasonable relation to some purpose within the competency of the State"); *Palko* v. *Connecticut,* 302 U. S. 319, 327–238 (1937) ("even in the field of substantive rights and duties the legislative judgment, if oppressive and arbitrary, may be overridden by the courts"; "Is that [injury] to which the statute has subjected [the appellant] a hardship so acute and shocking that our polity will not endure it? Does it violate those fundamental principles of liberty and justice which lie at the base of all our civil and political institutions?") (citation and internal quotation marks omitted).

After *Meyer* and *Pierce,* two further opinions took the major steps that lead to the modern law. The first was not even in a due process case but one about equal protection, *Skinner* v. *Oklahoma ex rel. Williamson,* 316 U. S. 535 (1942), where the Court emphasized the "fundamental" nature of individual choice about procreation and so foreshadowed not only the later prominence of procreation as a subject of liberty protection, but the corresponding standard of "strict scrutiny," in this Court's Fourteenth Amendment law. See *id.*, at 541. *Skinner,* that is, added decisions regarding procreation to the list of liberties recognized in *Meyer* and *Pierce* and loosely suggested, as a gloss on their standard of arbitrariness, a judicial obligation to scrutinize any impingement on such an important interest with heightened care. In so doing, it suggested a point that Justice Harlan would develop, that the kind and degree of justification that a sensitive judge would demand of a State would depend on the importance of the interest being asserted by the individual. *Poe,* 367 U. S., at 543.

The second major opinion leading to the modern doctrine was Justice Harlan's *Poe* dissent just cited, the conclusion of which was adopted in *Griswold* v. *Connecticut,* 381 U. S. 478 (1965), and the authority of which was acknowledged in *Planned Parenthood of Southeastern Pa.* v. *Casey,* 505 U. S. 833 (1992). See also n. 4, *supra.* The dissent is important for three things that point to our responsibilities today. The first is Justice Harlan's respect for the tradition of substantive due process review itself, and his acknowledgement of the Judiciary's obligation to carry it on. For two centuries American courts, and for much of that time this Court, have thought it necessary to provide some degree of review over the substantive content of legislation under constitutional standards of textual breadth. The obligation was understood before *Dred Scott* and has continued after the repudiation of *Lochner's* progeny, most notably on the subjects of segregation in public education, *Bolling* v. *Sharpe,* 347 U. S. 497, 500 (1954), interracial marriage, *Loving* v. *Virginia,* 388 U. S. 1, 12 (1967), marital privacy and contraception, *Carey* v. *Population Services Int'l,* 431 U. S. 678, 684–691 (1977), *Griswold* v. *Connecticut, supra,* at 481–486, abortion, *Planned Parenthood of Southeastern Pa.* v. *Casey,* 505 U. S. 833, 849, 869–879 (1992) (joint opinion of O'CONNOR, KENNEDY, and SOUTER, JJ.), *Roe* v. *Wade,* 410 U. S. 113, 152–166 (1973), personal control of medical treatment, *Cruzan* v. *Director, Mo. Dept. of Health,* 497 U. S. 261, 287–289 (1990) (O'CONNOR, J., concurring); *id.*, at 302 (Brennan, J., dissenting); *id.*, at 331 (STEVENS, J., dissenting); see also *id.*, at 278 (majority opinion), and physical confinement, *Foucha* v. *Louisiana,* 504 U. S. 71, 80–83 (1992). This enduring tradition of American constitutional practice is, in Justice Harlan's view, nothing more than what is required by the judicial authority and obligation to construe constitutional text and review legislation for conformity to that text. See *Marbury* v. *Madison,* 1 Cranch 137 (1803). Like many judges who preceded him and many who followed, he found it impossible to construe the text of due process without recognizing substantive, and not merely procedural, limitations. "Were due process merely a procedural safeguard it would fail to reach those situations where the deprivation of life, liberty or property was accomplished by legislation which by operating in the future could, given even the fairest possible procedure in application to individuals, nevertheless destroy the enjoyment of all three." *Poe,* 367 U. S., at 541.[7] The text of the Due Process Clause thus imposes nothing less than an obligation to give substantive content to the words "liberty" and "due process of law."

Following the first point of the *Poe* dissent, on the necessity to engage in the sort of examination we conduct today, the dissent's second and third implicitly address those cases, already noted, that are now condemned with virtual unanimity as disastrous mistakes of substantive due process review. The second of the dissent's lessons is a reminder that the business of such review is not the identification of extratextual absolutes but scrutiny of a legislative resolution (perhaps unconscious) of clashing principles, each quite possibly worthy in and of itself, but each to be weighed within the history of our values as a people. It is a comparison of the relative strengths of opposing claims that informs the judicial task, not a deduction from some first premise. Thus informed, judicial review still has no warrant to substitute one reasonable resolution of the contending positions for another, but authority to supplant the balance already struck between the contenders only when it falls outside the realm of the reasonable. Part III, below, deals with this second point, and also with the dissent's third, which takes the form of an object lesson in the explicit attention to detail that is no less essential to the intellectual discipline of substantive due process review than an understanding of the basic need to account for the two sides in the controversy and to respect legislation within the zone of reasonableness.

III

My understanding of unenumerated rights in the wake of the *Poe* dissent and subsequent cases avoids the absolutist failing of many older cases without embracing the opposite pole of equating reasonableness with past practice described at a very specific level. See *Planned Parenthood of Southeastern Pa.* v. *Casey,* 505 U. S. 833, 847–849 (1992). That understanding begins with a concept of "ordered liberty," *Poe,* 367 U. S., at 549 (Harlan, J.); see also *Griswold,* 381 U. S., at 500, comprising a continuum of rights to be free from "arbitrary impositions and purposeless restraints," *Poe,* 367 U. S., at 543 (Harlan, J., dissenting).

> "Due Process has not been reduced to any formula; its content cannot be determined by reference to any code. The best that can be said is that through the course of this Court's decisions it has represented the balance which our Nation, built upon postulates of respect for the liberty of the individual, has struck between that liberty and the demands of organized society. If the supplying of content to this Constitutional concept has of necessity been a rational process, it certainly has not been one where judges have felt free to roam where unguided speculation might take them. The balance of which I speak is the balance struck by this country, having regard to what history teaches are the traditions from which it developed as well as the traditions from which it broke. That tradition is a living thing. A decision of this Court which radically departs from it could not long survive, while a decision which builds on what has survived is likely to be sound. No formula could serve as a substitute, in this area, for judgment and restraint." *Id.,* at 542.

See also *Moore* v. *East Cleveland,* 431 U. S. 494, 503 (1977) (plurality opinion of Powell, J.) ("Appropriate limits on substantive due process come not from drawing arbitrary lines but rather from careful 'respect for the teachings of history [and] solid recognition of the basic values that underlie our society'") (quoting *Griswold,* 481 U. S., at 501 (Harlan, J., concurring)).

After the *Poe* dissent, as before it, this enforceable concept of liberty would bar statutory impositions even at relatively trivial levels when governmental restraints are undeniably irrational as unsupported by any imaginable rationale. See, *e.g., United States* v. *Carolene Products Co.,* 304 U. S. 144, 152 (1938) (economic legislation "not ... unconstitutional unless ... facts ... preclude the assumption that it rests upon some rational basis"); see also *Poe,* 367 U. S., at 545, 548 (Harlan, J., dissenting) (referring to usual "presumption of constitutionality" and ordinary test "going merely to the plausibility of [a statute's] underlying rationale"). Such instances are suitably rare. The claims of arbitrariness that mark almost all instances of unenumerated substantive rights are those resting on "certain interests requir[ing] particularly careful scrutiny of the state needs asserted to justify their abridgment. Cf. *Skinner* v. *Oklahoma* [*ex rel. Williamson,* 316 U. S. 535 (1942)]; *Bolling* v. *Sharpe,* [347 U. S. 497 (1954)]," *id.,* at 543; that is, interests in liberty sufficiently important to be judged "fundamental," *id.,* at 548; see also *id.,* at 541 (citing *Corfield* v. *Coryell,* 4 Wash. C. C. 371, 380 (CC ED Pa. 1825)). In the face of an interest this powerful a State may not rest on threshold rationality or a presumption of constitutionality, but may prevail only on the ground of an interest sufficiently compelling to place within the realm of the reasonable a refusal to recognize the individual right asserted. *Poe, supra,* at 548 (Harlan, J., dissenting) (an "enactment involv[ing] ... a most fundamental aspect of 'liberty' ... [is] subjec[t] to 'strict scrutiny'") (quoting *Skinner* v. *Oklahoma ex rel. Williamson,* 316 U. S., at 541);[8] *Reno* v. *Flores,* 507 U. S. 292, 301–302 (1993) (reaffirming that due process "forbids the government to infringe certain 'fundamental' liberty interests ... unless the infringement is narrowly tailored to serve a compelling state interest").[9]

This approach calls for a court to assess the relative "weights" or dignities of the contending interests, and to this extent the judicial method is familiar to the common law. Common law method is subject, however, to two important constraints in the hands of a court engaged in substantive due process review. First, such a court is bound to confine the values that it recognizes to those truly deserving constitutional stature, either to those expressed in constitutional text, or those exemplified by "the traditions from which [the Nation] developed," or revealed by contrast with "the traditions from which it broke." *Poe,* 367 U. S., at 542 (Harlan, J., dissenting). "'We may not draw on our merely personal and private notions and disregard the limits ... derived from considerations that are fused in the whole nature of our judicial process ...[,] considerations deeply rooted in reason and in the compelling traditions of the legal profession.'" *Id.,* at 544–545 (quoting *Rochin* v. *California,* 342 U. S. 165, 170–171 (1952)); see also *Palko* v. *Connecticut,* 302 U. S., at 325 (looking to "'principle[s] of justice so rooted in the traditions and conscience of our people as to be ranked as fundamental'") (quoting *Snyder* v. *Massachusetts,* 291 U. S. 97, 105 (1934)).

The second constraint, again, simply reflects the fact that constitutional review, not judicial lawmaking, is a court's business here. The weighing or valuing of contending interests in this sphere is only the first step, forming the basis for determining whether the statute in question falls inside or outside the zone of what is reasonable in the way it resolves the conflict between the interests of state and individual. See, *e.g., Poe, supra,* at 553 (Harlan, J., dissenting); *Youngberg* v. *Romeo,* 457 U. S. 307, 320–321 (1982). It is no justification for judicial intervention merely to identify a reasonable resolution of contending values that differs from the terms of the legislation under review. It is only when the legislation's justifying principle, critically valued, is so far from being commensurate with the individual interest as to be arbitrarily or pointlessly applied that the statute must give way. Only if this standard points against the statute can the individual claimant be said to have a constitutional right. See *Cruzan* v. *Director, Mo. Dept. of Health,* 497 U. S., at 279 ("[D]etermining that a person has a 'liberty interest' under the Due Process Clause does not end the inquiry; 'whether [the individual's] constitutional rights have been violated must be determined by balancing his liberty interests against the relevant state interests'") (quoting *Youngberg* v. *Romeo, supra,* at 321).[10]

The *Poe* dissent thus reminds us of the nature of review for reasonableness or arbitrariness and the limitations entailed by it. But the opinion cautions against the repetition of past error in another way as well, more by its example than by any particular statement of constitutional method: it reminds us that the process of substantive review by reasoned judgment, *Poe,* 367 U. S., at 542–544, is one of close criticism going to the details of the opposing interests and to their relationships with the historically recognized principles that lend them weight or value.

Although the *Poe* dissent disclaims the possibility of any general formula for due process analysis (beyond the basic analytic structure just described), see *id.,* at 542, 544, Justice Harlan of course assumed that adjudication under the Due Process Clauses is like any other instance of judgment dependent on common-law method, being more or less persuasive according to the usual canons of critical discourse. See also *Casey,* 505 U. S., at 849 ("The inescapable fact is that adjudication of substantive due process claims may call upon the Court in interpreting the Constitution to exercise that same capacity which by tradition courts always have exercised: reasoned judgment"). When identifying and assessing the competing interests of liberty and authority, for example, the breadth of expression that a litigant or a judge selects in stating the competing principles will have much to do with the outcome and may be dispositive. As in any process of rational argumentation, we recognize that when a generally accepted principle is challenged, the broader the attack the less likely it is to succeed. The principle's defenders will, indeed, often try to characterize any challenge as just such a broadside, perhaps by couching the defense as if a broadside attack had occurred. So the Court in *Dred Scott* treated prohibition of slavery in the Territories as nothing less than a general assault on the concept of property. See *Dred Scott* v. *Sandford,* 19 How., at 449–452.

Just as results in substantive due process cases are tied to the selections of statements of the competing interests, the acceptability of the results is a function of the good reasons for the selections made. It is here that the value of common-law method becomes apparent, for the usual thinking of the common law is suspicious of the all-or-nothing analysis that tends to produce legal petrification instead of an evolving boundary between the domains of old principles. Common-law method tends to pay respect instead to detail, seeking to understand old principles afresh by new examples and new counterexamples. The "tradition is a living thing," *Poe,* 367 U. S., at 542 (Harlan, J., dissenting), albeit one that moves by moderate steps carefully taken. "The decision of an apparently novel claim must depend on grounds which follow closely on well-accepted principles and criteria. The new decision must take its place in relation to what went before and further [cut] a channel for what is to come." *Id.,* at 544 (Harlan, J., dissenting) (internal quotation marks omitted). Exact analysis and characterization of any due process claim is critical to the method and to the result.

So, in *Poe*, Justice Harlan viewed it as essential to the plaintiffs' claimed right to use contraceptives that they sought to do so within the privacy of the marital bedroom. This detail in fact served two crucial and complementary functions, and provides a lesson for today. It rescued the individuals' claim from a breadth that would have threatened all state regulation of contraception or intimate relations; extramarital intimacy, no matter how privately practiced, was outside the scope of the right Justice Harlan would have recognized in that case. See *id.,* at 552–553. It was, moreover, this same restriction that allowed the interest to be valued as an aspect of a broader liberty to be free from all unreasonable intrusions into the privacy of the home and the family life within it, a liberty exemplified in constitutional provisions such as the Third and Fourth Amendments, in prior decisions of the Court involving unreasonable intrusions into the home and family life, and in the then-prevailing status of marriage as the sole lawful locus of intimate relations. *Id.,* at 548, 551.[11] The individuals' interest was therefore at its peak in *Poe,* because it was supported by a principle that distinguished of its own force between areas in which government traditionally had regulated (sexual relations outside of marriage) and those in which it had not (private marital intimacies), and thus was broad enough to cover the claim at hand without being so broad as to be shot-through by exceptions.

On the other side of the balance, the State's interest in *Poe* was not fairly characterized simply as preserving sexual morality, or doing so by regulating contraceptive devices. Just as some of the earlier cases went astray by speaking without nuance of individual interests in property or autonomy to contract for labor, so the State's asserted interest in *Poe* was not immune to distinctions turning (at least potentially) on the precise purpose being pursued and the collateral consequences of the means chosen, see *id.,* at 547–548. It was assumed that the State might legitimately enforce limits on the use of contraceptives through laws regulating divorce and annulment, or even through its tax policy, *ibid.,* but not necessarily be justified in criminalizing the same practice in the marital bedroom, which would entail the consequence of authorizing state enquiry into the intimate relations of a married couple who chose to close their door, *id.,* at 548–549. See also *Casey,* 505 U. S., at 869 (strength of State's interest in potential life varies depending on precise context and character of regulation pursuing that interest).

The same insistence on exactitude lies behind questions, in current terminology, about the proper level of generality at which to analyze claims and counter-claims, and the demand for fitness and proper tailoring of a restrictive statute is just another way of testing the legitimacy of the generality at which the government sets up its justification.[12] We may therefore classify Justice Harlan's example of proper analysis in any of these ways: as applying concepts of normal critical reasoning, as pointing to the need to attend to the levels of generality at which countervailing interests are stated, or as examining the concrete application of principles for fitness with their own ostensible justifications. But whatever the categories in which we place the dissent's example, it stands in marked contrast to earlier cases whose reasoning was marked by comparatively less discrimination, and it points to the importance of evaluating the claims of the parties now before us with comparable detail. For here we are faced with an individual claim not to a right on the part of just anyone to help anyone else commit suicide under any circumstances, but to the right of a narrow class to help others also in a narrow class under a set of limited circumstances. And the claimants are met with the State's assertion, among others, that rights of such narrow scope cannot be recognized without jeopardy to individuals whom the State may concededly protect through its regulations.

IV

A

Respondents claim that a patient facing imminent death, who anticipates physical suffering and indignity, and is capable of responsible and voluntary choice, should have a right to a physician's assistance in providing counsel and drugs to be administered by the patient to end life promptly. Complaint ¶3.1. They accordingly claim that a physician must have the corresponding right to provide such aid, contrary to the provisions of Wash. Rev. Code §9A.36.060 (1994). I do not understand the argument to rest on any assumption that rights either to suicide or to assistance in committing it are historically based as such. Respondents, rather, acknowledge the prohibition of each historically, but rely on the fact that to a substantial extent the State has repudiated that history. The result of this, respondents say, is to open the door to claims of such a patient to be accorded one of the options open to those with different, traditionally cognizable claims to autonomy in deciding how their bodies and minds should be treated. They seek the option to obtain the services of a physician to give them the benefit of advice and medical help, which is said to enjoy a tradition so strong and so devoid of specifically countervailing state concern that denial of a physician's help in these circumstances is arbitrary when physicians are generally free to advise and aid those who exercise other rights to bodily autonomy.

1

The dominant western legal codes long condemned suicide and treated either its attempt or successful accomplishment as a crime, the one subjecting the individual to penalties, the other penalizing his survivors by designating the suicide's property as forfeited to the government. See 4 W. Blackstone, Commentaries *188–*189 (commenting that English law considered suicide to be "ranked ... among the highest crimes" and deemed persuading another to commit suicide to be murder); see generally Marzen, O'Dowd, Crone, & Balch, Suicide: A Constitutional Right?, 24 Duquense L. Rev. 1, 56–63 (1985). While suicide itself has generally not been considered a punishable crime in the United States, largely because the common-law punishment of forfeiture was rejected as improperly penalizing an innocent family, see *id.*, at 98–99, most States have consistently punished the act of assisting a suicide as either a common-law or statutory crime and some continue to view suicide as an unpunishable crime. See generally *id.*, at 67–100, 148–242.[13] Criminal prohibitions on such assistance remain widespread, as exemplified in the Washington statute in question here.[14]

The principal significance of this history in the State of Washington, according to respondents, lies in its repudiation of the old tradition to the extent of eliminating the criminal suicide prohibitions. Respondents do not argue that the State's decision goes further, to imply that the State has repudiated any legitimate claim to discourage suicide or to limit its encouragement. The reasons for the decriminalization, after all, may have had more to do with difficulties of law enforcement than with a shift in the value ascribed to life in various circumstances or in the perceived legitimacy of taking one's own. See, *e.g.*, Kamisar, Physician-Assisted Suicide: The Last Bridge to Active Voluntary Euthanasia, in Euthanasia Examined 225, 229 (J. Keown ed. 1995); CeloCruz, Aid-in-Dying: Should We Decriminalize Physician-Assisted Suicide and Physician-Committed Euthanasia?, 18 Am. J. L. & Med. 369, 375 (1992); Marzen, O'Dowd, Crone, & Balch 24 Duquesne L. Rev. *supra*, at 98–99. Thus it may indeed make sense for the State to take its hands off suicide as such, while continuing to prohibit the sort of assistance that would make its commission easier. See, *e.g.*, American Law Institute, Model Penal Code §210.5, Comment 5 (1980). Decriminalization does not, then, imply the existence of a constitutional liberty interest in suicide as such; it simply opens the door to the assertion of a cognizable liberty interest in bodily integrity and associated medical care that would otherwise have been inapposite so long as suicide, as well as assisting a suicide, was a criminal offense.

This liberty interest in bodily integrity was phrased in a general way by then-Judge Cardozo when he said, "[e]very human being of adult years and sound mind has a right to determine what shall be done with his own body" in relation to his medical needs. *Schloendorff* v. *Society of New York Hospital*, 211 N. Y. 125, 129, 105 N.E. 92, 93 (1914). The familiar examples of this right derive from the common law of battery and include the right to be free from medical invasions into the body, *Cruzan* v. *Director, Mo. Dept. of Health*, 497 U. S., at 269–279, as well as a right generally to resist enforced medication, see *Washington* v. *Harper*, 494 U. S. 210, 221–222, 229 (1990). Thus "[i]t is settled now . . . that the Constitution places limits on a State's right to interfere with a person's most basic decisions about . . . bodily integrity." *Casey*, 505 U. S., at 849 (citations omitted); see also *Cruzan*, 497 U. S., at 278; *id.*, at 288 (O'CONNOR, J., concurring); *Washington* v. *Harper, supra*, at 221–222; *Winston* v. *Lee*, 470 U. S. 753, 761–762 (1985); *Rochin* v. *California*, 342 U. S., at 172. Constitutional recognition of the right to bodily integrity underlies the assumed right, good against the State, to require physicians to terminate artificial life support, *Cruzan, supra*, at 279 ("we assume that the United States Constitution would grant a competent person a constitutionally protected right to refuse lifesaving hydration and nutrition"), and the affirmative right to obtain medical intervention to cause abortion, see *Casey, supra*, at 857, 896; cf. *Roe* v. *Wade*, 410 U. S., at 153.

It is, indeed, in the abortion cases that the most telling recognitions of the importance of bodily integrity and the concomitant tradition of medical assistance have occurred. In *Roe* v. *Wade*, the plaintiff contended that the Texas statute making it criminal for any person to "procure an abortion," *id.*, at 117, for a pregnant woman was unconstitutional insofar as it prevented her from "terminat[ing] her pregnancy by an abortion 'performed by a competent, licensed physician, under safe, clinical conditions,'" *id.*, at 120, and in striking down the statute we stressed the importance of the relationship between patient and physician, see *id.*, at 153, 156.

The analogies between the abortion cases and this one are several. Even though the State has a legitimate interest in discouraging abortion, see *Casey*, 505 U. S., at 871 (joint opinion of O'CONNOR, KENNEDY, and SOUTER, JJ.) *Roe*, 410 U. S., at 162, the Court recognized a woman's right to a physician's counsel and care. Like the decision to commit suicide, the decision to abort potential life can be made irresponsibly and under the influence of others, and yet the Court has held in the abortion cases that physicians are fit assistants. Without physician assistance in abortion, the woman's right would have too often amounted to nothing more than a right to self-mutilation, and without a physician to assist in the suicide of the dying, the patient's right will often be confined to crude methods of causing death, most shocking and painful to the decedent's survivors.

There is, finally, one more reason for claiming that a physician's assistance here would fall within the accepted tradition of medical care in our society, and the abortion cases are only the most obvious illustration of the further point. While the Court has held that the performance of abortion procedures can be restricted to physicians, the Court's opinion in *Roe* recognized the doctors' role in yet another way. For, in the course of holding that the decision to perform an abortion called for a physician's assistance, the Court recognized that the good physician is not just a mechanic of the human body whose services have no bearing on a person's moral choices, but one who does more than treat symptoms, one who ministers to the patient. See *id.*, at 153; see also *Griswold* v. *Connecticut*, 381 U. S., at 482 ("This law . . . operates directly on an intimate relation of husband and wife and their physician's role in one aspect of that relation"); see generally R. Cabot, Ether Day Address, Boston Medical and Surgical J. 287, 288 (1920). This idea of the physician as serving the whole person is a source of the high value traditionally placed on the medical relationship. Its value is surely as apparent here as in the abortion cases, for just as the decision about abortion is not directed to correcting some pathology, so the decision in which a dying patient seeks help is not so limited. The patients here sought not only an end to pain (which they might have had, although perhaps at the price of stupor) but an end to their short remaining lives with a dignity that they believed would be denied them by powerful pain medication, as well as by their consciousness of dependency and helplessness as they approached death. In that period when the end is imminent, they said, the decision to end life is closest to decisions that are generally accepted as proper instances of exercising autonomy over one's own body, instances recognized under the Constitution and the State's own law, instances in which the help of physicians is accepted as falling within the traditional norm.

Respondents argue that the State has in fact already recognized enough evolving examples of this tradition of patient care to demonstrate the strength of their claim. Washington, like other States, authorizes physicians to withdraw life-sustaining medical treatment and artificially delivered food and water from patients who request it, even though such actions will hasten death. See Wash. Rev. Code §§70.122.110, 70.122.051 (1994); see generally Notes to Uniform Rights of the Terminally Ill Act, 9B U. L. A. 168–169 (Supp. 1997) (listing state statutes). The State permits physicians to alleviate anxiety and discomfort when withdrawing artificial life-supporting devices by administering medication that will hasten death even further. And it generally permits physicians to administer medication to patients in terminal conditions when the primary intent is to alleviate pain, even when the medication is so powerful as to hasten death and the patient chooses to receive it with that understanding. See Wash. Rev. Code §70.122.010 (1994); see generally P. Rousseau, Terminal Sedation in the Care of Dying Patients, 156 Archives of Internal Medicine 1785 (1996); Truog, Berde, Mitchell, & Grier, Barbiturates in the Care of the Terminally Ill, 327 New Eng. J. Med. 1678 (1992).[15]

2

The argument supporting respondents' position thus progresses through three steps of increasing forcefulness. First, it emphasizes the decriminalization of suicide. Reliance on this fact is sanctioned under the standard that looks not only to the tradition retained, but to society's occasional choices to reject traditions of the legal past. See *Poe* v. *Ullman*, 367 U. S., at 542 (Harlan, J., dissenting). While the common law prohibited both suicide and aiding a suicide, with the prohibition on aiding largely justified by the primary prohibition on self-inflicted death itself, see, *e.g.*, American Law Institute, Model Penal Code §210.5, Comment 1, pp. 92–93, and n. 7 (1980), the State's rejection of the traditional treatment of the one leaves the criminality of the other open to questioning that previously would not have been appropriate. The second step in the argument is to emphasize that the State's own act of decriminalization gives a freedom of choice much like the individual's option in recognized instances of bodily autonomy. One of these, abortion, is a legal right to choose in spite of the interest a State may legitimately invoke in discouraging the practice, just as suicide is now subject to choice, despite a state interest in discouraging it. The third step is to emphasize that respondents claim a right to assistance not on the basis of some broad principle that would be subject to exceptions if that continuing interest of the State's in discouraging suicide were to be recognized at all. Respondents base their claim on the traditional right to medical care and counsel, subject to the limiting conditions of informed, responsible choice when death is imminent, conditions that support a strong analogy to rights of care in other situations in which medical counsel and assistance have been available as a matter of course. There can be no stronger claim to a physician's assistance than at the time when death is imminent, a moral judgment implied by the State's own recognition of the legitimacy of medical procedures necessarily hastening the moment of impending death.

In my judgment, the importance of the individual interest here, as within that class of "certain interests" demanding careful scrutiny of the State's contrary claim, see *Poe, supra,* at 543, cannot be gainsaid. Whether that interest might in some circumstances, or at some time, be seen as "fundamental" to the degree entitled to prevail is not, however, a conclusion that I need draw here, for I am satisfied that the State's interests described in the following section are sufficiently serious to defeat the present claim that its law is arbitrary or purposeless.

B

The State has put forward several interests to justify the Washington law as applied to physicians treating terminally ill patients, even those competent to make responsible choices: protecting life generally, Brief for Petitioners 33, discouraging suicide even if knowing and voluntary, *id.,* at 37–38, and protecting terminally ill patients from involuntary suicide and euthanasia, both voluntary and nonvoluntary, *id.,* at 34–35.

It is not necessary to discuss the exact strengths of the first two claims of justification in the present circumstances, for the third is dispositive for me. That third justification is different from the first two, for it addresses specific features of respondents' claim, and it opposes that claim not with a moral judgment contrary to respondents', but with a recognized state interest in the protection of nonresponsible individuals and those who do not stand in relation either to death or to their physicians as do the patients whom respondents describe. The State claims interests in protecting patients from mistakenly and involuntarily deciding to end their lives, and in guarding against both voluntary and involuntary euthanasia. Leaving aside any difficulties in coming to a clear concept of imminent death, mistaken decisions may result from inadequate palliative care or a terminal prognosis that turns out to be error; coercion and abuse may stem from the large medical bills that family members cannot bear or unreimbursed hospitals decline to shoulder. Voluntary and involuntary euthanasia may result once doctors are authorized to prescribe lethal medication in the first instance, for they might find it pointless to distinguish between patients who administer their own fatal drugs and those who wish not to, and their compassion for those who suffer may obscure the distinction between those who ask for death and those who may be unable to request it. The argument is that a progression would occur, obscuring the line between the ill and the dying, and between the responsible and the unduly influenced, until ultimately doctors and perhaps others would abuse a limited freedom to aid suicides by yielding to the impulse to end another's suffering under conditions going beyond the narrow limits the respondents propose. The State thus argues, essentially, that respondents' claim is not as narrow as it sounds, simply because no recognition of the interest they assert could be limited to vindicating those interests and affecting no others. The State says that the claim, in practical effect, would entail consequences that the State could, without doubt, legitimately act to prevent.

The mere assertion that the terminally sick might be pressured into suicide decisions by close friends and family members would not alone be very telling. Of course that is possible, not only because the costs of care might be more than family members could bear but simply because they might naturally wish to see an end of suffering for someone they love. But one of the points of restricting any right of assistance to physicians, would be to condition the right on an exercise of judgment by someone qualified to assess the patient's responsible capacity and detect the influence of those outside the medical relationship.

The State, however, goes further, to argue that dependence on the vigilance of physicians will not be enough. First, the lines proposed here (particularly the requirement of a knowing and voluntary decision by the patient) would be more difficult to draw than the lines that have limited other recently recognized due process rights. Limiting a state from prosecuting use of artificial contraceptives by married couples posed no practical threat to the State's capacity to regulate contraceptives in other ways that were assumed at the time of *Poe* to be legitimate; the trimester measurements of *Roe* and the viability determination of *Casey* were easy to make with a real degree of certainty. But the knowing and responsible mind is harder to assess.[16] Second, this difficulty could become the greater by combining with another fact within the realm of plausibility, that physicians simply would not be assiduous to preserve the line. They have compassion, and those who would be willing to assist in suicide at all might be the most susceptible to the wishes of a patient, whether the patient were technically quite responsible or not. Physicians, and their hospitals, have their own financial incentives, too, in this new age of managed care. Whether acting from compassion or under some other influence, a physician who would provide a drug for a patient to administer might well go the further step of administering the drug himself; so, the barrier between assisted suicide and euthanasia could become porous, and the line between voluntary and involuntary euthanasia as well.[17] The case for the slippery slope is fairly made out here, not because recognizing one due process right would leave a court with no principled basis to avoid recognizing another, but because there is a plausible case that the right claimed would not be readily containable by reference to facts about the mind that are matters of difficult judgment, or by gatekeepers who are subject to temptation, noble or not.

Respondents propose an answer to all this, the answer of state regulation with teeth. Legislation proposed in several States, for example, would authorize physician-assisted suicide but require two qualified physicians to confirm the patient's diagnosis, prognosis, and competence; and would mandate that the patient make repeated requests witnessed by at least two others over a specified time span; and would impose reporting requirements and criminal penalties for various acts of coercion. See App. to Brief for State Legislators as *Amici Curiae* 1a–2a.

But at least at this moment there are reasons for caution in predicting the effectiveness of the teeth proposed. Respondents' proposals, as it turns out, sound much like the guidelines now in place in the Netherlands, the only place where experience with physician-assisted suicide and euthanasia has yielded empirical evidence about how such regulations might affect actual practice. Dutch physicians must engage in consultation before proceeding, and must decide whether the patient's decision is voluntary, well considered, and stable, whether the request to die is enduring and made more than once, and whether the patient's future will involve unacceptable suffering. See C. Gomez, Regulating Death 40–43 (1991). There is, however, a substantial dispute today about what the Dutch experience shows. Some commentators marshall evidence that the Dutch guidelines have in practice failed to protect patients from involuntary euthanasia and have been violated with impunity. See, *e.g.*, H. Hendin, Seduced By

Death 75–84 (1997) (noting many cases in which decisions intended to end the life of a fully competent patient were made without a request from the patient and without consulting the patient); Keown, Euthanasia in the Netherlands: Sliding Down the Slippery Slope?, in Euthanasia Examined 261, 289 (J. Keown ed. 1995) (guidelines have "proved signally ineffectual; non-voluntary euthanasia is now widely practised and increasingly condoned in the Netherlands"); Gomez, *supra*, at 104–113. This evidence is contested. See, *e.g.*, R. Epstein, Mortal Peril 322 (1997) ("Dutch physicians are not euthanasia enthusiasts and they are slow to practice it in individual cases"); R. Posner, Aging and Old Age 242, and n. 23 (1995) (noting fear of "doctors' rushing patients to their death" in the Netherlands "has not been substantiated and does not appear realistic"); Van der Wal, Van Eijk, Leenen, & Spreeuwenberg, Euthanasia and Assisted Suicide, 2, Do Dutch Family Doctors Act Prudently?, 9 Family Practice 135 (1992) (finding no serious abuse in Dutch practice). The day may come when we can say with some assurance which side is right, but for now it is the substantiality of the factual disagreement, and the alternatives for resolving it, that matter. They are, for me, dispositive of the due process claim at this time.

I take it that the basic concept of judicial review with its possible displacement of legislative judgment bars any finding that a legislature has acted arbitrarily when the following conditions are met: there is a serious factual controversy over the feasibility of recognizing the claimed right without at the same time making it impossible for the State to engage in an undoubtedly legitimate exercise of power; facts necessary to resolve the controversy are not readily ascertainable through the judicial process; but they are more readily subject to discovery through legislative factfinding and experimentation. It is assumed in this case, and must be, that a State's interest in protecting those unable to make responsible decisions and those who make no decisions at all entitles the State to bar aid to any but a knowing and responsible person intending suicide, and to prohibit euthanasia. How, and how far, a State should act in that interest are judgments for the State, but the legitimacy of its action to deny a physician the option to aid any but the knowing and responsible is beyond question.

The capacity of the State to protect the others if respondents were to prevail is, however, subject to some genuine question, underscored by the responsible disagreement over the basic facts of the Dutch experience. This factual controversy is not open to a judicial resolution with any substantial degree of assurance at this time. It is not, of course, that any controversy about the factual predicate of a due process claim disqualifies a court from resolving it. Courts can recognize captiousness, and most factual issues can be settled in a trial court. At this point, however, the factual issue at the heart of this case does not appear to be one of those. The principal enquiry at the moment is into the Dutch experience, and I question whether an independent front-line investigation into the facts of a foreign country's legal administration can be soundly undertaken through American courtroom litigation. While an extensive literature on any subject can raise the hopes for judicial understanding, the literature on this subject is only nascent. Since there is little experience directly bearing on the issue, the most that can be said is that whichever way the Court might rule today, events could overtake its assumptions, as experimentation in some jurisdictions confirmed or discredited the concerns about progression from assisted suicide to euthanasia.

Legislatures, on the other hand, have superior opportunities to obtain the facts necessary for a judgment about the present controversy. Not only do they have more flexible mechanisms for factfinding than the Judiciary, but their mechanisms include the power to experiment, moving forward and pulling back as facts emerge within their own jurisdictions. There is, indeed, good reason to suppose that in the absence of a judgment for respondents here, just such experimentation will be attempted in some of the States. See, *e.g.*, Ore. Rev. Stat. Ann. §§127.800 *et seq.* (Supp. 1996); App. to Brief for State Legislators as *Amici Curiae* 1a (listing proposed statutes).

I do not decide here what the significance might be of legislative foot-dragging in ascertaining the facts going to the State's argument that the right in question could not be confined as claimed. Sometimes a court may be bound to act regardless of the institutional preferability of the political branches as forums for addressing constitutional claims. See, e.g., *Bolling v. Sharpe*, 347 U. S. 497 (1954). Now, it is enough to say that our examination of legislative reasonableness should consider the fact that the Legislature of the State of Washington is no more obviously at fault than this Court is in being uncertain about what would happen if respondents prevailed today. We therefore have a clear question about which institution, a legislature or a court, is relatively more competent to deal with an emerging issue as to which facts currently unknown could be dispositive. The answer has to be, for the reasons already stated, that the legislative process is to be preferred. There is a closely related further reason as well.

One must bear in mind that the nature of the right claimed, if recognized as one constitutionally required, would differ in no essential way from other constitutional rights guaranteed by enumeration or derived from some more definite textual source than "due process." An unenumerated right should not therefore be recognized, with the effect of displacing the legislative ordering of things, without the assurance that its recognition would prove as durable as the recognition of those other rights differently derived. To recognize a right of lesser promise would simply create a constitutional regime too uncertain to bring with it the expectation of finality that is one of this Court's central obligations in making constitutional decisions. See *Casey*, 505 U. S., at 864–869.

Legislatures, however, are not so constrained. The experimentation that should be out of the question in constitutional adjudication displacing legislative judgments is entirely proper, as well as highly desirable, when the legislative power addresses an emerging issue like assisted suicide. The Court should accordingly stay its hand to allow reasonable legislative consideration. While I do not decide for all time that respondents' claim should not be recognized, I acknowledge the legislative institutional competence as the better one to deal with that claim at this time.

JUSTICE GINSBURG, CONCURRING IN THE JUDGMENTS.

I concur in the Court's judgments in these cases substantially for the reasons stated by Justice O'Connor in her concurring opinion.

JUSTICE BREYER, CONCURRING IN THE JUDGMENTS.

I believe that JUSTICE O'CONNOR's views, which I share, have greater legal significance than the Court's opinion suggests. I join her separate opinion, except insofar as it joins the majority. And I concur in the judgments. I shall briefly explain how I differ from the Court.

I agree with the Court in *Vacco v. Quill, ante,* that the articulated state interests justify the distinction drawn between physician assisted suicide and withdrawal of life support. I also agree with the Court that the critical question in both of the cases before us is whether "the 'liberty' specially protected by the Due Process Clause includes a right" of the sort that the respondents assert. *Washington v. Glucksberg, ante,* at 19. I do not agree, however, with the Court's formulation of that claimed "liberty" interest.

The Court describes it as a "right to commit suicide with another's assistance." *Ante*, at 20. But I would not reject the respondents' claim without considering a different formulation, for which our legal tradition may provide greater support. That formulation would use words roughly like a "right to die with dignity." But irrespective of the exact words used, at its core would lie personal control over the manner of death, professional medical assistance, and the avoidance of unnecessary and severe physical suffering—combined.

As JUSTICE SOUTER points out, *ante* at 13–16 (Souter, J., concurring in the judgment), Justice Harlan's dissenting opinion in *Poe* v. *Ullman*, 367 U.S. 497 (1961), offers some support for such a claim. In that opinion, Justice Harlan referred to the "liberty" that the Fourteenth Amendment protects as including "a freedom from all substantial arbitrary impositions and purposeless restraints" and also as recognizing that "*certain interests* require particularly careful scrutiny of the state needs asserted to justify their abridgment." *Id.*, at 543. The "certain interests" to which Justice Harlan referred may well be similar (perhaps identical) to the rights, liberties, or interests that the Court today, as in the past, regards as "fundamental." *Ante*, at 15; see also *Planned Parenthood of Southeastern Pa.* v. *Casey*, 505 U.S. 833 (1992); *Eisenstadt* v. *Baird*, 405 U.S. 438 (1972); *Griswold* v. *Connecticut*, 381 U.S. 479 (1965); *Rochin* v. *California*, 342 U.S. 165 (1952); *Skinner* v. *Oklahoma ex rel. Williamson*, 316 U.S. 535 (1942).

JUSTICE HARLAN concluded that marital privacy was such a "special interest." He found in the Constitution a right of "privacy of the home"—with the home, the bedroom, and "intimate details of the marital relation" at its heart—by examining the protection that the law had earlier provided for related, but not identical, interests described by such words as "privacy," "home,"and "family." 367 U. S., at 548, 552; cf. *Casey*, *supra*, at 851. The respondents here essentially ask us to do the same. They argue that one can find a "right to die with dignity" by examining the protection the law has provided for related, but not identical, interests relating to personal dignity, medical treatment, and freedom from state inflicted pain. See *Ingraham* v. *Wright*, 430 U.S. 651 (1977); *Cruzan* v. *Director, Mo. Dept. of Health*, 497 U.S. 261 (1990); *Casey*, *supra*.

I do not believe, however, that this Court need or now should decide whether or not such a right is "fundamental." That is because, in my view, the avoidance of severe physical pain (connected with death) would have to comprise an essential part of any successful claim and because, as JUSTICE O'CONNOR points out, the laws before us do not force a dying person to undergo that kind of pain. *Ante*, at 2 (O'CONNOR, J., concurring). Rather, the laws of New York and of Washington do not prohibit doctors from providing patients with drugs sufficient to control pain despite the risk that those drugs themselves will kill. Cf. New York State Task Force on Life and the Law, When Death Is Sought: Assisted Suicide and Euthanasia in the Medical Context 163, n. 29 (May 1994). And under these circumstances the laws of New York and Washington would overcome any remaining significant interests and would be justified, regardless.

Medical technology, we are repeatedly told, makes the administration of pain relieving drugs sufficient, except for a very few individuals for whom the ineffectiveness of pain control medicines can mean, not pain, but the need for sedation which can end in a coma. Brief for National Hospice Organization 8; Brief for the American Medical Association (AMA) et al. as *Amici Curiae* 6; see also Byock, Consciously Walking the Fine Line: Thoughts on a Hospice Response to Assisted Suicide and Euthanasia, 9 J. Palliative Care 25, 26 (1993); New York State Task Force, at 44, and n. 37. We are also told that there are many instances in which patients do not receive the palliative care that, in principle, is available, *Id.*, at 43–47; Brief for AMA as *Amici Curiae* 6; Brief for Choice in Dying, Inc., as *Amici Curiae* 20, but that is so for institutional reasons or inadequacies or obstacles, which would seem possible to overcome, and which do *not* include *a prohibitive set of laws. Ante*, at 2 (O'Connor, J., concurring); see also 2 House of Lords, Session 1993–1994 Report of Select Committee on Medical Ethics 113 (1994) (indicating that the number of palliative care centers in the United Kingdom, where physician assisted suicide is illegal, significantly exceeds that in the Netherlands, where such practices are legal).

This legal circumstance means that the state laws before us do not infringe directly upon the (assumed) central interest (what I have called the core of the interest in dying with dignity) as, by way of contrast, the state anticontraceptive laws at issue in *Poe* did interfere with the central interest there at stake—by bringing the State's police powers to bear upon the marital bedroom.

Were the legal circumstances different—for example, were state law to prevent the provision of palliative care, including the administration of drugs as needed to avoid pain at the end of life—then the law's impact upon serious and otherwise unavoidable physical pain (accompanying death) would be more directly at issue. And as Justice O'Connor suggests, the Court might have to revisit its conclusions in these cases.

NOTES

Notes to Justice Rehnquist's Opinion

1. Act of Apr. 28, 1854, §17, 1854 Wash. Laws 78 ("Every person deliberately assisting another in the commission of self murder, shall be deemed guilty of manslaughter"); see also Act of Dec. 2, 1869, §17, 1869 Wash. Laws 201; Act of Nov. 10, 1873, §19, 1873 Wash. Laws 184; Criminal Code, ch. 249, §§135–136, 1909 Wash. Laws, 11th sess., 929.

2. Under Washington's Natural Death Act, "adult persons have the fundamental right to control the decisions relating to the rendering of their own health care, including the decision to have life sustaining treatment withheld or withdrawn in instances of a terminal condition or permanent unconscious condition." Wash. Rev. Code §70.122.010 (1994). In Washington, "[a]ny adult person may execute a directive directing the withholding or withdrawal of life sustaining treatment in a terminal condition or permanent unconscious condition," §70.122.030, and a physician who, in accordance with such a directive, participates in the withholding or withdrawal of life sustaining treatment is immune from civil, criminal, or professional liability. §70.122.051.

3. Glucksberg Declaration, App. 35; Halperin Declaration, *id.*, at 49–50; Preston Declaration, *id.*, at 55–56; Shalit Declaration, *id.*, at 73–74.

4. John Doe, Jane Roe, and James *Poe*, plaintiffs in the District Court, were then in the terminal phases of serious and painful illnesses. They declared that they were mentally competent and desired assistance in ending their lives. Declaration of Jane Roe, *id.*, at 23–25; Declaration of John Doe, *id.*, at 27–28; Declaration of James *Poe, id.*, at 30–31; *Compassion in Dying*, 850 F. Supp., at 1456–1457.

5. The District Court determined that *Casey's* "undue burden" standard, 505 U. S., at 874 (joint opinion), not the standard from *United States* v. *Salerno*, 481 U.S. 739, 745 (1987) (requiring a showing that "no set of circumstances exists under which the [law] would be valid"), governed the plaintiffs' facial challenge to the assisted suicide ban. 850 F. Supp., at 1462–1464.

6. Although, as JUSTICE STEVENS observes, *post*, at 2–3 (opinion concurring in judgment), "[the court's] analysis and eventual holding that the statute was unconstitutional was not limited to a particular set of plaintiffs before it," the court did note that "[d]eclaring a statute unconstitutional as applied to members of a group is atypical but not uncommon." 79 F. 3d, at 798, n. 9, and emphasized that it was "not deciding the facial validity of [the Washington statute]," *id.*, at 797–798, and nn. 8–9. It is therefore the court's holding that

Washington's physician assisted suicide statute is unconstitutional as applied to the "class of terminally ill, mentally competent patients," *post*, at 14 (STEVENS, J., concurring in judgment), that is before us today.

7. The Court of Appeals did note, however, that "the equal protection argument relied on by [the District Court] is not insubstantial," 79 F. 3d., at 838, n. 139, and sharply criticized the opinion in a separate case then pending before the Ninth Circuit, *Lee* v. *Oregon*, 891 F. Supp. 1429 (Ore. 1995) (Oregon's Death With Dignity Act, which permits physician assisted suicide, violates the Equal Protection Clause because it does not provide adequate safeguards against abuse), vacated, *Lee* v. *Oregon*, 107 F. 3d 1382 (CA9 1997) (concluding that plaintiffs lacked Article III standing). *Lee*, of course, is not before us, any more than it was before the Court of Appeals below, and we offer no opinion as to the validity of the Lee courts' reasoning. In *Vacco* v. *Quill*, *post*, however, decided today, we hold that New York's assisted suicide ban does not violate the Equal Protection Clause.

8. See *Compassion in Dying* v. *Washington*, 79 F. 3d 790, 847, and nn. 10–13 (CA9 1996) (Beezer, J., dissenting) ("In total, forty four states, the District of Columbia and two territories prohibit or condemn assisted suicide") (citing statutes and cases); *Rodriguez* v. *British Columbia* (Attorney General), 107 D. L. R. (4th) 342, 404 (Can. 1993) ("[A] blanket prohibition on assisted suicide ... is the norm among western democracies") (discussing assisted suicide provisions in Austria, Spain, Italy, the United Kingdom, the Netherlands, Denmark, Switzerland, and France). Since the Ninth Circuit's decision, Louisiana, Rhode Island, and Iowa have enacted statutory assisted suicide bans. La. Rev. Stat. Ann. §14:32.12 (Supp. 1997); R. I. Gen. Laws §§11–60–1, 11–60–3 (Supp. 1996); Iowa Code Ann. §§707A.2, 707A.3 (Supp. 1997). For a detailed history of the States' statutes, see Marzen, O'Dowd, Crone & Balch, Suicide: A Constitutional Right?, 24 Duquesne L. Rev. 1, 148–242 (1985) (Appendix) (hereinafter Marzen).

9. The common law is thought to have emerged through the expansion of pre-Norman institutions sometime in the 12th century. J. Baker, An Introduction to English Legal History 11 (2d ed. 1979). England adopted the ecclesiastical prohibition on suicide five centuries earlier, in the year 673 at the Council of Hereford, and this prohibition was reaffirmed by King Edgar in 967. See G. Williams, The Sanctity of Life and the Criminal Law 257 (1957).

10. Marzen 59. Other late medieval treatise writers followed and restated Bracton; one observed that "man slaughter" may be "[o]f [one]self; as in case, when people hang themselves or hurt themselves, or otherwise kill themselves of their own felony" or "[o]f others; as by beating, famine, or other punishment; in like cases, all are man slayers." A. Horne, The Mirrour of Justices, ch. 1, §9, pp. 41–42 (W. Robinson ed. 1903). By the mid 16th century, the Court at Common Bench could observe that "[suicide] is an Offence against Nature, against God, and against the King.... [T]o destroy one's self is contrary to Nature, and a Thing most horrible." *Hales* v. *Petit*, 1 Plowd. Com. 253, 261, 75 Eng. Rep. 387, 400 (1561–1562).

    In 1644, Sir Edward Coke published his Third Institute, a lodestar for later common lawyers. See T. Plucknett, A Concise History of the Common Law 281–284 (5th ed. 1956). Coke regarded suicide as a category of murder, and agreed with Bracton that the goods and chattels—but not, for Coke, the lands—of a sane suicide were forfeit. 3 E. Coke, Institutes *54. William Hawkins, in his 1716 Treatise of the Pleas of the Crown, followed Coke, observing that "our laws have always had ... an abhorrence of this crime." 1 W. Hawkins, Pleas of the Crown, ch. 27, §4, p. 164 (T. Leach ed. 1795).

11. In 1850, the California legislature adopted the English common law, under which assisting suicide was, of course, a crime. Act of Apr. 13, 1850, ch. 95, 1850 Cal. Stats. 219. The provision adopted in 1874 provided that "[e]very person who deliberately aids or advises, or encourages another to commit suicide, is guilty of a felony." Act of Mar. 30, 1874, ch. 614, §13, 400, 255 (codified at Cal. Penal Code §400 (T. Hittel ed. 1876)).

12. "A person who purposely aids or solicits another to commit suicide is guilty of a felony in the second degree if his conduct causes such suicide or an attempted suicide, and otherwise

of a misdemeanor." American Law Institute, Model Penal Code §210.5(2) (Official Draft and Revised Comments 1980).

13. Initiative 119 would have amended Washington's Natural Death Act, Wash. Rev. Code §70.122.010 *et seq.* (1994), to permit "aid in dying," defined as "aid in the form of a medical service provided in person by a physician that will end the life of a conscious and mentally competent qualified patient in a dignified, painless and humane manner, when requested voluntarily by the patient through a written directive in accordance with this chapter at the time the medical service is to be provided." App. H to Pet. for Cert. 3–4.

14. Ore. Rev. Stat. §§127.800 *et seq.* (1996); *Lee* v. *Oregon,* 891 F. Supp.1429 (Ore. 1995) (Oregon Act does not provide sufficient safeguards for terminally ill persons and therefore violates the Equal Protection Clause), vacated, *Lee* v. *Oregon,* 107 F. 3d 1382 (CA9 1997).

15. See, *e.g.,* Alaska H. B. 371 (1996); Ariz. S. B. 1007 (1996); Cal. A. B. 1080, A. B. 1310 (1995); Colo. H. B. 1185 (1996); Colo. H. B. 1308 (1995); Conn. H. B. 6298 (1995); Ill. H. B. 691, S. B. 948 (1997); Me. H. P. 663 (1997); Me. H. P. 552 (1995); Md. H. B. 474 (1996); Md. H. B. 933 (1995); Mass. H. B. 3173 (1995); Mich. H. B. 6205 (1996); Mich. S. B. 556 (1996); Mich. H. B. 4134 (1995); Miss. H. B. 1023 (1996); N. H. H. B. 339 (1995); N. M. S. B. 446 (1995); N. Y. S. B. 5024 (1995); N. Y. A. B. 6333 (1995); Neb. L. B. 406 (1997); Neb. L. B. 1259 (1996); R. I. S. 2985 (1996);Vt. H. B. 109 (1997);Vt. H. B. 335 (1995);Wash. S. B. 5596 (1995); Wis. A. B. 174, S. B. 90 (1995); Senate of Canada, Of Life and Death, Report of the Special Senate Committee on Euthanasia and Assisted Suicide A—156 (June 1995) (describing unsuccessful proposals, between 1991–1994, to legalize assisted suicide).

16. Other countries are embroiled in similar debates: The Supreme Court of Canada recently rejected a claim that the Canadian Charter of Rights and Freedoms establishes a fundamental right to assisted suicide, *Rodriguez* v. *British Columbia (Attorney General),* 107 D. L. R. (4th) 342 (1993); the British House of Lords Select Committee on Medical Ethics refused to recommend any change in Great Britain's assisted suicide prohibition, House of Lords, Session 1993–94 Report of the Select Committee on Medical Ethics, 12 Issues in Law & Med. 193, 202 (1996) ("We identify no circumstances in which assisted suicide should be permitted"); New Zealand's Parliament rejected a proposed "Death With Dignity Bill" that would have legalized physician assisted suicide in August 1995, Graeme, MPs Throw out Euthanasia Bill, The Dominion (Wellington), Aug. 17, 1995, p. 1; and the Northern Territory of Australia legalized assisted suicide and voluntary euthanasia in 1995. See Shenon, Australian Doctors Get Right to Assist Suicide, N.Y. Times, July 28, 1995, p. A8. As of February 1997, three persons had ended their lives with physician assistance in the Northern Territory. Mydans, Assisted Suicide: Australia Faces a Grim Reality, N.Y. Times, Febr. 2, 1997, p. A3. On March 24, 1997, however, the Australian Senate voted to overturn the Northern Territory's law. Thornhill, Australia Repeals Euthanasia Law, Washington Post, March 25, 1997, p. A14; see Euthanasia Laws Act 1997, No. 17, 1997 (Austl.). On the other hand, on May 20, 1997, Colombia's Constitutional Court legalized voluntary euthanasia for terminally ill people. Sentencia No. C 239/97 (Corte Constitucional, Mayo 20, 1997); see Colombia's Top Court Legalizes Euthanasia, Orlando Sentinel, May 22, 1997, p. A18.

17. In JUSTICE SOUTER's opinion, Justice Harlan's *Poe* dissent supplies the "modern justification" for substantive due process review. Post, at 5, and n. 2 (Souter, J., concurring in judgment). But although Justice Harlan's opinion has often been cited in due process cases, we have never abandoned our fundamental rights based analytical method. Just four Terms ago, six of the Justices now sitting joined the Court's opinion in *Reno* v. *Flores,* 507 U.S. 292, 301–305 (1993); *Poe* was not even cited. And in *Cruzan,* neither the Court's nor the concurring opinions relied on *Poe*; rather, we concluded that the right to refuse unwanted medical treatment was so rooted in our history, tradition, and practice as to require special protection under the Fourteenth Amendment. *Cruzan* v. Director, Mo. Dept. of Health, 497 U.S. 261, 278–279 (1990); *id.,* at 287–288 (O'CONNOR, J., concurring). True, the Court relied on Justice HARLAN's dissent in *Casey,* 505 U. S., at 848–850, but, as *Flores* demon-

strates, we did not in so doing jettison our established approach. Indeed, to read such a radical move into the Court's opinion in *Casey* would seem to fly in the face of that opinion's emphasis on *stare decisis.* 505 U. S., at 854–869.

18. See, e.g., *Quill* v. *Vacco,* 80 F. 3d 716, 724 (CA2 1996) ("right to assisted suicide finds no cognizable basis in the Constitution's language or design"); *Compassion in Dying* v. *Washington,* 49 F. 3d 586, 591 (CA9 1995) (referring to alleged "right to suicide," "right to assistance in suicide," and "right to aid in killing oneself"); *People* v. *Kevorkian,* 447 Mich. 436, 476, n. 47, 527 N. W. 2d 714, 730, n. 47 (1994) ("[T]he question that we must decide is whether the [C]onstitution encompasses a right to commit suicide and, if so, whether it includes a right to assistance").

19. See *Moore* v. *East Cleveland,* 431 U.S. 494, 503 (1977) ("[T]he Constitution protects the sanctity of the family precisely because the institution of the family is deeply rooted in this Nation's history and tradition") (emphasis added); *Griswold* v. *Connecticut,* 381 U.S. 479, 485–486 (1965) (intrusions into the "sacred precincts of marital bedrooms" offend rights "older than the Bill of Rights"); *id.,* at 495–496 (Goldberg, J., concurring) (the law in question "disrupt[ed] the traditional relation of the family—a relation as old and as fundamental as our entire civilization"); *Loving* v. *Virginia,* 388 U.S. 1, 12 (1967) ("The freedom to marry has long been recognized as one of the vital personal rights essential to the orderly pursuit of happiness"); *Turner* v. *Safley,* 482 U.S. 78, 95 (1987) ("[T]he decision to marry is a fundamental right"); *Roe* v. *Wade,* 410 U.S. 113, 140 (1973) (stating that at the Founding and throughout the nineteenth century, "a woman enjoyed a substantially broader right to terminate a pregnancy"); *Skinner* v. *Oklahoma ex rel. Williamson,* 316 U.S. 535, 541 (1942) ("Marriage and procreation are fundamental"); *Pierce* v. *Society of Sisters,* 268 U.S. 510, 535 (1925); *Meyer* v. *Nebraska,* 262 U.S. 390, 399 (1923) (liberty includes "those privileges long recognized at common law as essential to the orderly pursuit of happiness by free men").

20. The court identified and discussed six state interests: (1) preserving life; (2) preventing suicide; (3) avoiding the involvement of third parties and use of arbitrary, unfair, or undue influence; (4) protecting family members and loved ones; (5) protecting the integrity of the medical profession; and (6) avoiding future movement toward euthanasia and other abuses. 79 F. 3d, at 816–832.

21. Respondents also admit the existence of these interests, Brief for Respondents 28–39, but contend that Washington could better promote and protect them through regulation, rather than prohibition, of physician assisted suicide. Our inquiry, however, is limited to the question whether the State's prohibition is rationally related to legitimate state interests.

22. The States express this commitment by other means as well:

"[N]early all states expressly disapprove of suicide and assisted suicide either in statutes dealing with durable powers of attorney in health care situations, or in 'living will' statutes. In addition, all states provide for the involuntary commitment of persons who may harm themselves as the result of mental illness, and a number of states allow the use of nondeadly force to thwart suicide attempts." *People* v. *Kevorkian,* 447 Mich., at 478–479, and nn. 53–56, 527 N. W. 2d, at 731–732, and nn. 53–56.

23. JUSTICE SOUTER concludes that "[t]he case for the slippery slope is fairly made out here, not because recognizing one due process right would leave a court with no principled basis to avoid recognizing another, but because there is a plausible case that the right claimed would not be readily containable by reference to facts about the mind that are matters of difficult judgment, or by gatekeepers who are subject to temptation, noble or not." Post, at 36–37 (opinion concurring in judgment). We agree that the case for a slippery slope has been made out, but—bearing in mind Justice Cardozo's observation of "[t]he tendency of a principle to expand itself to the limit of its logic," The Nature of the Judicial Process 51 (1932)—we also recognize the reasonableness of the widely expressed skepticism about the lack of a principled basis for confining the right. See Brief for United States as *Amicus Curiae* 26 ("Once a legislature abandons a categorical prohibition against physician assisted suicide,

there is no obvious stopping point"); Brief for Not Dead Yet et al. as *Amici Curiae* 21–29; Brief for Bioethics Professors as *Amici Curiae* 23–26; Report of the Council on Ethical and Judicial Affairs, App. 133, 140 ("[I]f assisted suicide is permitted, then there is a strong argument for allowing euthanasia"); New York Task Force 132; Kamisar, The "Right to Die": On Drawing (and Erasing) Lines, 35 Duquesne L. Rev. 481 (1996); Kamisar, Against Assisted Suicide—Even in a Very Limited Form, 72 U. Det. Mercy L. Rev. 735 (1995).

24. JUSTICE STEVENS states that "the Court does conceive of respondents' claim as a facial challenge—addressing not the application of the statute to a particular set of plaintiffs before it, but the constitutionality of the statute's categorical prohibition. . . ." *Post*, at 4 (opinion concurring in judgment). We emphasize that we today reject the Court of Appeals' specific holding that the statute is unconstitutional "as applied" to a particular class. See n. 6, *supra*. JUSTICE STEVENS agrees with this holding, see *post*, at 14, but would not "foreclose the possibility that an individual plaintiff seeking to hasten her death, or a doctor whose assistance was sought, could prevail in a more particularized challenge," ib*id*. Our opinion does not absolutely foreclose such a claim. However, given our holding that the Due Process Clause of the Fourteenth Amendment does not provide heightened protection to the asserted liberty interest in ending one's life with a physician's assistance, such a claim would have to be quite different from the ones advanced by respondents here.

Notes to Justice O'Connor's Concurring Opinion

Justice Ginsburg concurs in the Court's judgments substantially for the reasons stated in this opinion. Justice Breyer joins this opinion except insofar as it joins the opinions of the Court.

Notes to Justice Stevens's Concurring Opinion

1. *Gregg* v. *Georgia*, 428 U.S. 153 (1976)
2. *Proffitt* v. *Florida*, 428 U.S. 242 (1976).
3. *Jurek* v. *Texas*, 428 U.S. 262 (1976).
4. See, e.g., *Godfrey* v. *Georgia*, 446 U.S. 420 (1980); *Enmund* v. *Florida*, 458 U.S. 782 (1982); *Penry* v. *Lynaugh*, 492 U.S. 302 (1989).
5. See *ante*, at 3, n. 5.
6. If the Court had actually applied the *Salerno* standard in this action, it would have taken only a few paragraphs to identify situations in which the Washington statute could be validly enforced. In *Salerno* itself, the Court would have needed only to look at whether the statute could be constitutionally applied to the arrestees before it; any further analysis would have been superfluous. See Dorf, Facial Challenges to State and Federal Statutes, 46 Stan. L. Rev. 235, 239–240 (1994) (arguing that if the *Salerno* standard were taken literally, a litigant could not succeed in her facial challenge unless she also succeeded in her as applied challenge).
7. In other cases and in other contexts, we have imposed a significantly lesser burden on the challenger. The most lenient standard that we have applied requires the challenger to establish that the invalid applications of a statute "must not only be real, but substantial as well, judged in relation to the statute's plainly legitimate sweep." *Broadrick* v. *Oklahoma*, 413 U.S. 601, 615 (1973). As the Court's opinion demonstrates, Washington's statute prohibiting assisted suicide has a "plainly legitimate sweep." While that demonstration provides a sufficient justification for rejecting respondents' facial challenge, it does not mean that every application of the statute should or will be upheld.
8. "Who casts not up his eye to the sun when it rises? but who takes off his eye from a comet when that breaks out? Who bends not his ear to any bell which upon any occasion rings? but who can remove it from that bell which is passing a piece of himself out of this world? No man is an island, entire of itself; every man is a piece of the continent, a part of the main. If a clod be washed away by the sea, Europe is the less, as well as if a promontory were, as well as if a manor of thy friend's or of thine own were; any man's death diminishes me, because I am involved in mankind; and therefore never send to know for whom the bell tolls;

it tolls for thee." J. Donne, Meditation No. 17, Devotions Upon Emergent Occasions 86, 87 (A. Raspa ed. 1987).

9. See 497 U. S., at 332, n. 2.

10. "[N]either the Bill of Rights nor the laws of sovereign States create the liberty which the Due Process Clause protects. The relevant constitutional provisions are limitations on the power of the sovereign to infringe on the liberty of the citizen. The relevant state laws either create property rights, or they curtail the freedom of the citizen who must live in an ordered society. Of course, law is essential to the exercise and enjoyment of individual liberty in a complex society. But it is not the source of liberty, and surely not the exclusive source.

"I had thought it self evident that all men were endowed by their Creator with liberty as one of the cardinal unalienable rights. It is that basic freedom which the Due Process Clause protects, rather than the particular rights or privileges conferred by specific laws or regulations." *Meachum* v. *Fano*, 427 U.S. 215, 230 (1976) (STEVENS, J., dissenting).

11. "Nancy *Cruzan*'s interest in life, no less than that of any other person, includes an interest in how she will be thought of after her death by those whose opinions mattered to her. There can be no doubt that her life made her dear to her family and to others. How she dies will affect how that life is remembered." *Cruzan* v. *Director, Mo. Dept. of Health*, 497 U.S. 261, 344 (1990) (STEVENS, J., dissenting).

"Each of us has an interest in the kind of memories that will survive after death. To that end, individual decisions are often motivated by their impact on others. A member of the kind of family identified in the trial court's findings in this case would likely have not only a normal interest in minimizing the burden that her own illness imposes on others, but also an interest in having their memories of her filled predominantly with thoughts about her past vitality rather than her current condition." *Id.*, at 356.

12. I note that there is evidence that a significant number of physicians support the practice of hastening death in particular situations. A survey published in the New England Journal of Medicine, found that 56% of responding doctors in Michigan preferred legalizing assisted suicide to an explicit ban. Bachman et al., Attitudes of Michigan Physicians and the Public Toward Legalizing Physician Assisted Suicide and Voluntary Euthanasia, 334 New England J. Med. 303–309 (1996). In a survey of Oregon doctors, 60% of the responding doctors supported legalizing assisted suicide for terminally ill patients. See Lee et al., Legalizing Assisted Suicide—Views of Physicians in Oregon, 335 New England J. Med. 310–315 (1996). Another study showed that 12% of physicians polled in Washington State reported that they had been asked by their terminally ill patients for prescriptions to hasten death, and that, in the year prior to the study, 24% of those physicians had complied with such requests. See Back, Wallace, Starks, & Perlman, Physician Assisted Suicide and Euthanasia in Washington State, 275 JAMA 919–925 (1996); see also Doukas, Waterhouse, Gorenflo, & Seld, Attitudes and Behaviors on Physician Assisted Death: A Study of Michigan Oncologists, 13 J. Clinical Oncology 1055 (1995) (reporting that 18% of responding Michigan oncologists reported active participation in assisted suicide); Slome, Moulton, Huffine, Gorter, & Abrams, Physicians' Attitudes Toward Assisted Suicide in AIDS, 5 J. Acquired Immune Deficiency Syndromes 712 (1992) (reporting that 24% of responding physicians who treat AIDS patients would likely grant a patient's request for assistance in hastening death).

13. See *Vacco* v. *Quill, ante,* at 1, nn. 1 and 2.

14. The American Medical Association recognized this distinction when it supported Nancy *Cruzan* and continues to recognize this distinction in its support of the States in these cases.

15. If a doctor prescribes lethal drugs to be self administered by the patient, it not at all clear that the physician's intent is that the patient "be made dead," *ante,* at 7 (internal quotation marks omitted). Many patients prescribed lethal medications never actually take them; they merely acquire some sense of control in the process of dying that the availability of those medications provides. See Back, *supra* n. 12, at 922; see also Quill, 324 New England J. Med., at 693 (describing how some patients fear death less when they feel they have the option of physician assisted suicide).

Notes to Justice Souter's Concurring Opinion

1. A nonprofit corporation known as Compassion in Dying was also a plaintiff and appellee below but is not a party in this Court.

2. As I will indicate in some detail below, I see the challenge to the statute not as facial but as applied, and I understand it to be in narrower terms than those accepted by the Court.

3. The doctors also rely on the Equal Protection Clause, but that source of law does essentially nothing in a case like this that the Due Process Clause cannot do on its own.

4. The status of the Harlan dissent in *Poe* v. *Ullman*, 367 U. S. 497 (1961), is shown by the Court's adoption of its result in *Griswold* v. *Connecticut*, 381 U. S. 479 (1965), and by the Court's acknowledgment of its status and adoption of its reasoning in *Planned Parenthood of Southeastern Pa.* v. *Casey*, 505 U. S. 833, 848–849 (1992). See also *Youngberg* v. *Romeo*, 457 U. S. 307, 320 (1982) (citing Justice Harlan's *Poe* dissent as authority for the requirement that this Court balance "the liberty of the individual" and "the demands of an organized society"); *Roberts* v. *United States Jaycees*, 468 U. S. 609, 619 (1984); *Moore* v. *East Cleveland*, 431 U. S. 494, 500–506, and n. 12 (1977) (plurality opinion) (opinion for four Justices treating Justice Harlan's *Poe* dissent as a central explication of the methodology of judicial review under the Due Process Clause).

5. Coke indicates that prohibitions against deprivations without "due process of law" originated in an English statute that "rendred" Magna Carta's "law of the land" in such terms. See 2 E. Coke, Institutes 50 (1797); see also E. Corwin, Liberty Against Government 90–91 (1948).

6. The *Slaughter-House Cases* are important, of course, for their holding that the Privileges or Immunities Clause was no source of any but a specific handful of substantive rights. *Slaughter-House Cases*, 16 Wall., at 74–80. To a degree, then, that decision may have led the Court to look to the Due Process Clause as a source of substantive rights. In *Twining* v. *New Jersey*, 211 U. S. 78, 95–97 (1908), for example, the Court of the Lochner Era acknowledged the strength of the case against *Slaughter-House's* interpretation of the Privileges or Immunities Clause but reaffirmed that interpretation without questioning its own frequent reliance on the Due Process Clause as authorization for substantive judicial review. See also J. Ely, Democracy and Distrust 14–30 (1980) (arguing that the Privileges or Immunities Clause and not the Due Process Clause is the proper warrant for courts' substantive oversight of state legislation). But the courts' use of due process clauses for that purpose antedated the 1873 decision, as we have seen, and would in time be supported in the *Poe* dissent, as we shall see.

7. Judge Johnson of the New York Court of Appeals had made the point more obliquely a century earlier when he wrote that, "the form of this declaration of right, 'no person shall be deprived of life, liberty or property, without due process of law,' necessarily imports that the legislature cannot make the mere existence of the rights secured the occasion of depriving a person of any of them, even by the forms which belong to 'due process of law.' For if it does not necessarily import this, then the legislative power is absolute." And, "To provide for a trial to ascertain whether a man is in the enjoyment of [any] of these rights, and then, as a consequence of finding that he is in the enjoyment of it, to deprive him of it, is doing indirectly just what is forbidden to be done directly, and reduces the constitutional provision to a nullity." *Wynehamer* v. *People*, 13 N. Y. 378, 420 (1856).

8. We have made it plain, of course, that not every law that incidentally makes it somewhat harder to exercise a fundamental liberty must be justified by a compelling counterinterest. See *Casey*, 505 U. S., at 872–876 (joint opinion of O'CONNOR, KENNEDY, and SOUTER, JJ.); *Carey* v. *Population Services Int'l*, 431 U. S. 678, 685–686 (1977) ("[A]n individual's [constitutionally protected] liberty to make choices regarding contraception does not . . . automatically invalidate every state regulation in this area. The business of manufacturing and selling contraceptives may be regulated in ways that do not [even] infringe protected individual choices"). But a state law that creates a "substantial obstacle," *Casey*, *supra*, at 877, for the exercise of a fundamental liberty interest requires a commensurably substantial justification in order to place the legislation within the realm of the reasonable.

9. Justice Harlan thus recognized just what the Court today assumes, that by insisting on a

threshold requirement that the interest (or, as the Court puts it, the right) be fundamental before anything more than rational basis justification is required, the Court ensures that not every case will require the "complex balancing" that heightened scrutiny entails. See *ante,* at 17–18.

10. Our cases have used various terms to refer to fundamental liberty interests, see, *e.g., Poe,* 367 U. S., at 545 (Harlan, J., dissenting) ("'basic liberty'") (quoting *Skinner* v. *Oklahoma ex rel. Williamson,* 316 U. S. 535, 541 (1942)); *Poe, supra,* at 543 (Harlan, J., dissenting) ("certain interests" must bring "particularly careful scrutiny"); *Casey,* 505 U. S., at 851 ("protected liberty"); *Cruzan* v. *Director, Mo. Dept. of Health,* 497 U. S. 261, 278 (1990) ("constitution-ally protected liberty interest"); *Youngberg* v. *Romeo,* 457 U. S., at 315 ("liberty interests"), and at times we have also called such an interest a "right" even before balancing it against the government's interest, see, *e.g., Roe* v. *Wade,* 410 U. S. 113, 153–154 (1973); *Carey* v. *Population Services Int'l, supra,* at 686, 688, and n. 5; *Poe,* 367 U. S., at 541 ("rights 'which are ... fundamental'") (quoting *Corfield* v. *Coryell,* 4 Wash. C.C. 371, 380 (CC ED Pa. 1825)). Precision in terminology, however, favors reserving the label "right" for instances in which the individual's liberty interest actually trumps the government's countervailing interests; only then does the individual have anything legally enforceable as against the state's attempt at regulation.

11. Thus, as the *Poe* dissent illustrates, the task of determining whether the concrete right claimed by an individual in a particular case falls within the ambit of a more generalized protected liberty requires explicit analysis when what the individual wants to do could arguably be characterized as belonging to different strands of our legal tradition requiring different degrees of constitutional scrutiny. See also Tribe & Dorf, Levels of Generality in the Definition of Rights, 57 U. Chi. L. Rev. 1057, 1091 (1990) (abortion might conceivably be assimilated either to the tradition regarding women's reproductive freedom in general, which places a substantial burden of justification on the State, or to the tradition regarding protection of fetuses, as embodied in laws criminalizing feticide by someone other than the mother, which generally requires only rationality on the part of the State). Selecting among such competing characterizations demands reasoned judgment about which broader prin-ciple, as exemplified in the concrete privileges and prohibitions embodied in our legal tra-dition, best fits the particular claim asserted in a particular case.

12. The dual dimensions of the strength and the fitness of the government's interest are suc-cinctly captured in the so-called "compelling interest test," under which regulations that substantially burden a constitutionally protected (or "fundamental") liberty may be sus-tained only if "narrowly tailored to serve a compelling state interest," *Reno* v. *Flores,* 507 U. S. 292, 302 (1993); see also, *e.g., Roe* v. *Wade,* 410 U. S., at 155; *Carey* v. *Population Services Int'l,* 431 U. S., at 686. How compelling the interest and how narrow the tailoring must be will depend, of course, not only on the substantiality of the individual's own liberty inter-est, but also on the extent of the burden placed upon it, see *Casey,* 505 U. S., at 871–874 (opinion of O'CONNOR, KENNEDY, and SOUTER, JJ.); *Carey, supra,* at 686.

13. Washington and New York are among the minority of States to have criminalized attempted suicide, though neither State still does so. See Brief for Members of the New York and Wash-ington State Legislatures as *Amicus Curiae* 15, n. 8 (listing state statutes). The common law governed New York as a colony and the New York Constitution of 1777 recognized the com-mon law, N. Y. Const. of 1777, Art. XXXV, and the state legislature recognized common-law crimes by statute in 1788. See Act of Feb. 21, 1788, ch. 37, §2, 1788 N.Y. Laws 664 (codified at 2 N. Y. Laws 242) (Jones & Varick 1789). In 1828, New York changed the com-mon law offense of assisting suicide from murder to manslaughter in the first degree. See 2 N. Y. Rev. Stat. pt. 4, ch. 1, tit. 2, art. 1, §7, p. 661 (1829). In 1881, New York adopted a new penal code making attempted suicide a crime punishable by two years in prison, a fine, or both, and retaining the criminal prohibition against assisting suicide as manslaughter in the first degree. Act of July 26, 1881, ch. 676, §§ 172–178, 1881 N. Y. Laws (3 Penal Code), pp. 42–43 (codified at 4 N. Y. Consolidated Laws, Penal Law §§2300 to 2306, pp. 2809–2810 (1909)). In 1919, New York repealed the statutory provision making attempted suicide a crime. See Act of May 5, 1919, ch. 414, §1, 1919 N.Y. Laws 1193. The 1937 New York Report

of the Law Revision Commission found that the history of the ban on assisting suicide was "traceable into the ancient common law when a suicide or *felo de se* was guilty of crime punishable by forfeiture of his goods and chattels." State of New York, Report of the Law Revision Commission for 1937, p. 830. The Report stated that since New York had removed "all stigma [of suicide] as a crime" and that "[s]ince liability as an accessory could no longer hinge upon the crime of a principal, it was necessary to define it as a substantive offense." *Id.*, at 831. In 1965, New York revised its penal law, providing that a "person is guilty of manslaughter in the second degree when . . . he intentionally causes or aids another person to commit suicide." Penal Law, ch. 1030, 1965 N.Y. Laws at 2387 (codified at N. Y. Penal Law §125.15(3) (McKinney 1975)).

Washington's first territorial legislature designated assisting another "in the commission of self-murder" to be manslaughter, see Act of Apr. 28, 1854, §17, 1854 Wash. Laws 78, and re-enacted the provision in 1869 and 1873, see Act of Dec. 2, 1869, §17, 1869 Wash. Laws 201; Act of Nov. 10, 1873, §19, 1873 Wash. Laws 184 (codified at Wash. Code §794 (1881)). In 1909, the state legislature enacted a law based on the 1881 New York law and a similar one enacted in Minnesota, see Marzen, O'Dowd, Crone, & Balch, 24 Duquesne L. Rev., at 206, making attempted suicide a crime punishable by two years in prison or a fine, and retaining the criminal prohibition against assisting suicide, designating it manslaughter. See Criminal Code, ch. 249, §§133–137, 1909 Wash. Laws, 11th Sess. 890, 929 (codified at Remington & Ballinger's Wash. Code §§2385–2389 (1910)). In 1975, the Washington Legislature repealed these provisions, see Wash. Crim. code, 1975, ch. 260, §9A.92.010 (213–217) 1975 Wash. Laws 817, 858, 866, and enacted the ban on assisting suicide at issue in this case, see Wash. Crim. code, 1975, ch. 260, §9A.36.060 1975 Wash. Laws 817, 836, codified at Rev. Wash. Code §§9A.36.060 (1977). The decriminalization of attempted suicide reflected the view that a person compelled to attempt it should not be punished if the attempt proved unsuccessful. See *Compassion in Dying* v. *Washington*, 850 F. Supp. 1454, 1464, n. 9 (WD Wash. 1994) (citing Legislative Council Judiciary Committee, Report on the Revised Washington Criminal Code 153 (Dec. 3, 1970).

14. Numerous States have enacted statutes prohibiting assisting a suicide. See, *e.g.*, Alaska Stat. Ann. §11.41.120(a)(2) (1996); Ariz. Rev. Stat. Ann. §13–1103(A)(3) (West Supp. 1996–1997); Ark. Code Ann. §5–10–104(a)(2) (1993); Cal. Penal Code Ann. §401 (West 1988); Colo. Rev. Stat. §18–3–104(1)(b) (Supp. 1996); Conn. Gen. Stat. §53a-56(a)(2) (1997); Del. Code Ann. Tit. 11, §645 (1995); Fla. Stat. §782.08 (1991); Ga. Code Ann. §16–5–5(b) (1996); Haw. Rev. Stat. §707–702(1)(b) (1993); Ill. Comp. Stat., ch. 720, §5/12–31 (1993); Ind. Stat. Ann. §§35–42–1–2 to 35–42–1–2.5 (1994 and Supp. 1996); Iowa Code Ann. §707A.2 (West Supp. 1997); Kan. Stat. Ann. §21–3406 (1995); Ky. Rev. Stat. Ann. §216.302 (Michie 1994); La. Rev. Stat. Ann. §14:32.12 (West Supp. 1997); Me. Rev. Stat. Ann., Tit. 17–A, §204 (1983); Mich. Comp. Laws Ann. §752.1027 (West Supp. 1997–1998); Minn. Stat. §609.215 (1996); Miss. Code Ann. §97–3–49 (1994); Mo. Stat. §565.023.1(2) (1994); Mont. Code Ann. §45–5–105 (1995); Neb. Rev. Stat. §28–307 (1995); N. H. Rev. Stat. Ann. §630:4 (1996); N. J. Stat. Ann. §2C:11–6 (West 1995); N. M. Stat. Ann. §30–2–4 (1996); N. Y. Penal Law §120.30 (McKinney 1987); N. D. Cent. Code §12.1–16–04 (Supp. 1995); Okla. Stat. Tit. 21, §§813–815 (1983); Ore. Rev. Stat. §163.125(1)(b) (1991); Pa. Cons. Stat. Ann., Tit. 18 Purdon §2505 (1983); R. I. Gen. Laws §§11–60–1 through 11–60–5 (Supp. 1996); S. D. Codified Laws §22–16–37 (1988); Tenn. Code Ann. §39–13–216 (Supp. 1996); Tex. Penal Code Ann. §22.08 (1994); Wash. Rev. Code §9A.36.060 (1994); Wis. Stat. §940.12 (1993–1994). See also P. R. Law Ann., Tit. 33, § 4009 (1984).

15. Other States have enacted similar provisions, some categorically authorizing such pain treatment, see, *e.g.*, Ind. Code Ann. §35–42–1–2.5(a)(1) (Supp. 1996) (ban on assisted suicide does not apply to licensed health care provider who administers or dispenses medications or procedures to relieve pain or discomfort, even if such medications or procedures hasten death, unless provider intends to cause death); Iowa Code Ann. §707A.3.1 (West Supp. 1997) (same); Ky. Rev. Stat. Ann. §216.304 (Michie 1997) (same); Minn. Stat. Ann. §609.215(3) (West Supp. 1997) (same); Ohio Rev. Code Ann. §§2133.11(A)(6), 2133.12(E)(1) (1994); R. I. Gen. Laws §11–60–4 (Supp. 1996) (same); S. D. Codified Laws §22–16–37.1 (Supp. 1997);

see Mich. Comp. Laws Ann. §752.1027(3) (West Supp. 1997); Tenn. Code Ann. §39–13–216(b)(2) (1996); others permit patients to sign health-care directives in which they authorize pain treatment even if it hastens death. See, *e.g.*, Me. Rev. Stat. Ann., Tit. 18–A, §§5–804, 5–809 (1996); N. M. Stat. Ann. §§24–7A–4, 24–7A–9 (Supp. 1995); S. C. Code Ann. §62–5–504 (Supp. 1996); Va. Code Ann. §§54.1–2984, 4.1–2988 (1994).

16. While it is also more difficult to assess in cases involving limitations on life incidental to pain medication and the disconnection of artificial life support, there are reasons to justify a lesser concern with the punctilio of responsibility in these instances. The purpose of requesting and giving the medication is presumably not to cause death but to relieve the pain so that the State's interest in preserving life is not unequivocally implicated by the practice; and the importance of pain relief is so clear that there is less likelihood that relieving pain would run counter to what a responsible patient would choose, even with the consequences for life expectancy. As for ending artificial life support, the State again may see its interest in preserving life as weaker here than in the general case just because artificial life support preserves life when nature would not; and, because such life support is a frequently offensive bodily intrusion, there is a lesser reason to fear that a decision to remove it would not be the choice of one fully responsible. Where, however, a physician writes a prescription to equip a patient to end life, the prescription is written to serve an affirmative intent to die (even though the physician need not and probably does not characteristically have an intent that the patient die but only that the patient be equipped to make the decision). The patient's responsibility and competence are therefore crucial when the physician is presented with the request.

17. Again, the same can be said about life support and shortening life to kill pain, but the calculus may be viewed as different in these instances, as noted just above.

Appendix B

Vacco et al. v. Quill et al.

Text of the Supreme Court Decision Delivered by Chief Justice Rehnquist, in which O'Connor, Scalia, Kennedy, and Thomas, JJ., joined. O'Connor, J., filed a concurring opinion, in which Ginsburg and Breyer, JJ., joined in part. Stevens, J., Souter, J., Ginsburg, J., and Breyer, J., filed opinions concurring in the judgment.

Vacco, Attorney General of New York, et al. No. 95–1858 v. *Quill et al.*, 117 S.Ct.2293 (1997)

ON WRIT OF CERTIORARI TO THE UNITED STATES COURT OF APPEALS FOR THE SECOND CIRCUIT

Argued January 8, 1997—Decided June 26, 1977

CHIEF JUSTICE REHNQUIST DELIVERED THE OPINION OF THE COURT.

In New York, as in most States, it is a crime to aid another to commit or attempt suicide,[1] but patients may refuse even lifesaving medical treatment.[2] The question presented by this case is whether New York's prohibition on assisting suicide therefore violates the Equal Protection Clause of the Fourteenth Amendment. We hold that it does not.

Petitioners are various New York public officials. Respondents Timothy E. Quill, Samuel C. Klagsbrun, and Howard A. Grossman are physicians who practice in New York. They assert that although it would be "consistent with the standards of [their] medical practice[s]" to prescribe lethal medication for "mentally competent, terminally ill patients" who are suffering great pain and desire a doctor's help in taking their own lives, they are deterred from doing so by New York's ban on assisting suicide. App. 25–26.[3] Respondents, and three gravely ill patients who have since died,[4] sued the State's Attorney General in the United States District Court. They urged that because New York permits a competent person to refuse life sustaining medical treatment, and because the refusal of such treatment is "essentially the same thing" as physician assisted suicide, New York's assisted suicide ban violates the Equal Protection Clause. *Quill* v. *Koppell*, 870 F. Supp. 78, 84–85 (SDNY 1994).

The District Court disagreed: "[I]t is hardly unreasonable or irrational for the State to recognize a difference between allowing nature to take its course, even in the most severe situations, and intentionally using an artificial death producing device." *Id.*, at 84. The court noted New York's "obvious legitimate interests in preserving life, and in protecting vulnerable persons,"and concluded that "[u]nder the United States Constitution and the federal system it establishes, the resolution of this issue is left to the normal democratic processes within the State." *Id.*, at 84–85.

The Court of Appeals for the Second Circuit reversed. 80 F. 3d 716 (1996). The court determined that, despite the assisted suicide ban's apparent general applicability, "New York law does not treat equally all competent persons who are in the final stages of fatal illness and wish to hasten their deaths," because "those in the final stages of terminal illness who are on life support systems are allowed to hasten their deaths by directing the removal of such systems; but those who are similarly situated, except for the previous attachment of life sustaining equipment, are not allowed to hasten death by self administering prescribed drugs." *Id.*, at 727, 729. In the court's view, "[t]he ending of life by [the withdrawal of life support systems] is *nothing more nor less than assisted suicide.*" *Id.*, at 729 (emphasis added) (citation omitted). The Court of Appeals then examined whether this supposed unequal treatment was rationally related to any legitimate state interests,[5] and concluded that "to the extent that [New York's statutes] prohibit a physician from prescribing medications to be self administered by a mentally competent, terminally ill person in the final stages of his terminal illness, they are not rationally related to any legitimate state interest." *Id.*, at 731. We granted certiorari, 518 U. S. –_____ (1996), and now reverse.

The Equal Protection Clause commands that no State shall "deny to any person within its jurisdiction the equal protection of the laws." This provision creates no substantive rights. *San Antonio Independent School Dist.* v. *Rodriguez*, 411 U.S. 1, 33 (1973); *Id.*, at 59 (Stewart, J., concurring). Instead, it embodies a general rule that States must treat like cases alike but may treat unlike cases accordingly. *Plyler* v. *Doe*, 457 U.S. 202, 216 (1982) ("'[T]he Constitution does not require things which are different in fact or opinion to be treated in law as though they were the same'") (quoting *Tigner* v. *Texas*, 310 U.S. 141, 147 (1940)). If a legislative classification or distinction "neither burdens a fundamental right nor targets a suspect class, we will uphold [it] so long as it bears a rational relation to some legitimate end." *Romer* v. *Evans*, 517 U. S. _____, _____ (slip op., at 10) (1996).

New York's statutes outlawing assisting suicide affect and address matters of profound significance to all New Yorkers alike. They neither infringe fundamental rights nor involve suspect classifications. *Washington* v. *Glucksberg, ante*, at 15–24; see 80 F. 3d, at 726; San Antonio School Dist., 411 U. S., at 28 ("The system of alleged discrimination and the class it defines have none of the traditional indicia of suspectness"); *Id.*, at 33–35 (courts must look to the Constitution, not the "importance" of the asserted right, when deciding whether an asserted right is "fundamental"). These laws are therefore entitled to a "strong presumption of validity." *Heller* v. *Doe*, 509 U.S. 312, 319 (1993).

On their faces, neither New York's ban on assisting suicide nor its statutes permitting patients to refuse medical treatment treat anyone differently than anyone else or draw any distinctions between persons. Everyone, regardless of physical condition, is entitled, if competent, to refuse unwanted lifesaving medical treatment; no one is permitted to assist a suicide. Generally speaking, laws that apply evenhandedly to all "unquestionably comply" with the Equal Protection Clause. *New York City Transit Authority* v. *Beazer*, 440 U.S. 568, 587 (1979); see *Personnel Administrator of Mass.* v. *Feeney*, 442 U.S. 256, 271–273 (1979) ("[M]any [laws] affect certain groups unevenly, even though the law itself treats them no differently from all other members of the class described by the law").

The Court of Appeals, however, concluded that some terminally ill people—those who are on life support systems—are treated differently than those who are not, in that the former may "hasten death" by ending treatment, but the latter may not "hasten death" through physician assisted suicide. 80 F. 3d, at 729. This conclusion depends on the submission that ending or refusing lifesaving medical treatment "is nothing more nor less than assisted suicide." *Ibid.* Unlike the Court of Appeals, we think the distinction between assisting suicide and withdrawing life sustaining treatment, a distinction widely recognized and endorsed in the medical profession[6] and in our legal traditions, is both important and logical; it is certainly rational. See *Feeney, supra*, at 272 ("When the basic classification is rationally based, uneven effects upon particular groups within a class are ordinarily of no constitutional concern").

The distinction comports with fundamental legal principles of causation and intent. First, when a patient refuses life sustaining medical treatment, he dies from an underlying fatal disease or pathology; but if a patient ingests lethal medication prescribed by a physician, he is killed by that medication. See, e.g., *People* v. *Kevorkian*, 447 Mich. 436, 470–472, 527 N. W. 2d 714, 728 (1994), cert. denied, 514 U.S. 1083 (1995); *Matter of Conroy*, 98 N. J. 321, 355, 486 A. 2d 1209, 1226 (1985) (when feeding tube is removed, death "result[s] . . . from [the patient's] underlying medical condition"); *In re Colyer*, 99 Wash. 2d 114, 123, 660 P. 2d 738, 743 (1983) ("[D]eath which occurs after the removal of life sustaining systems is from natural causes"); American Medical Association, Council on Ethical and Judicial Affairs, Physician Assisted Suicide, 10 Issues in Law & Medicine 91, 92 (1994) ("When a life sustaining treatment is declined, the patient dies primarily because of an underlying disease").

Furthermore, a physician who withdraws, or honors a patient's refusal to begin, life sustaining medical treatment purposefully intends, or may so intend, only to respect his patient's wishes and "to cease doing useless and futile or degrading things to the patient when [the patient] no longer stands to benefit from them." Assisted Suicide in the United States, Hearing before the Subcommittee on the Constitution of the House Committee on the Judiciary, 104th Cong., 2d Sess., 368 (1996) (testimony of Dr. Leon R. Kass). The same is true when a doctor provides aggressive palliative care; in some cases, painkilling drugs may hasten a patient's death, but the physician's purpose and intent is, or maybe, only to ease his patient's pain. A doctor who assists a suicide, however, "must, necessarily and indubitably, intend primarily that the patient be made dead." *Id.*, at 367. Similarly, a patient who commits suicide with a doctor's aid necessarily has the specific intent to end his or her own life, while a patient who refuses or discontinues treatment might not. See, *e.g.*, *Matter of Conroy*, *supra*, at 351, 486 A. 2d, at 1224 (patients who refuse life sustaining treatment "may not harbor a specific intent to die" and may instead "fervently wish to live, but to do so free of unwanted medical technology, surgery, or drugs"); *Superintendent of Belchertown State School* v. *Saikewicz*, 373 Mass. 728, 743, n. 11, 370 N. E. 2d 417, 426, n. 11 (1977) ("[I]n refusing treatment the patient may not have the specific intent to die").

The law has long used actors' intent or purpose to distinguish between two acts that may have the same result. See, e.g., *United States* v. *Bailey*, 444 U.S. 394, 403–406 (1980) ("[T]he . . . common law of homicide often distinguishes . . . between a person who knows that another person will be killed as the result of his conduct and a person who acts with the specific purpose of taking another's life"); *Morissette* v. *United States*, 342 U.S. 246, 250 (1952) (distinctions based on intent are "universal and persistent in mature systems of law"); M. Hale, 1 Pleas of the Crown 412 (1847) ("If A., with an intent to prevent gangrene beginning in his hand doth without any advice cut off his hand, by which he dies, he is not thereby *felo de se* for tho it was a voluntary act, yet it was not with an intent to kill himself"). Put differently, the law distinguishes actions taken "because of" a given end from actions taken "in spite of" their unintended but foreseen consequences. *Feeney*, 442 U. S., at 279; *Compassion in Dying* v. *Washington*, 79 F. 3d 790, 858 (CA9 1996) (Kleinfeld, J., dissenting) ("When General Eisenhower ordered American soldiers onto the beaches of Normandy, he knew that he was sending many American soldiers to certain death. . . . His purpose, though, was to . . . liberate Europe from the Nazis").

Given these general principles, it is not surprising that many courts, including New York courts, have carefully distinguished refusing life sustaining treatment from suicide. See, *e.g.*, *Fosmire* v. *Nicoleau*, 75 N. Y. 2d 218, 227, and n. 2, 551 N. E. 2d 77, 82, and n. 2 (1990) ("[M]erely declining medical . . . care is not considered a suicidal act").[7]

In fact, the first state court decision explicitly to authorize withdrawing lifesaving treatment noted the "real distinction between the self infliction of deadly harm and a self determination against artificial life support." In re Quinlan, 70 N. J. 10, 43, 52, and n. 9, 355 A. 2d 647, 665, 670, and n. 9, cert. denied sub nom. Garger v. New Jersey, 429 U.S. 922 (1976). And recently, the Michigan Supreme Court also rejected the argument that the distinction "between acts that artificially sustain life and acts that artificially curtail life" is merely a "distinction without constitutional significance—a meaningless exercise in semantic gymnastics," insisting that "the Cruzan majority disagreed and so do we." Kevorkian, 447 Mich., at 471, 527 N. W. 2d, at 728.[8]

Similarly, the overwhelming majority of state legislatures have drawn a clear line between assisting suicide and withdrawing or permitting the refusal of unwanted lifesaving medical treatment by prohibiting the former and permitting the latter. Glucksberg, ante, at 4–6, 11–15. And "nearly all states expressly disapprove of suicide and assisted suicide either in statutes dealing with durable powers of attorney in health care situations, or in 'living will' statutes." Kevorkian, 447 Mich., at 478–479, and nn. 53–54, 527 N. W. 2d, at 731–732, and nn. 53–54.[9] Thus, even as the States move to protect and promote patients' dignity at the end of life, they remain opposed to physician assisted suicide.

New York is a case in point. The State enacted its current assisted suicide statutes in 1965.[10] Since then, New York has acted several times to protect patients' common law right to refuse treatment. Act of Aug. 7, 1987, ch. 818, §1, 1987 N. Y. Laws 3140 ("Do Not Resuscitate Orders") (codified as amended at N. Y. Pub. Health Law §§2960–2979 (McKinney 1994 and Supp. 1997)); Act of July 22, 1990, ch. 752, §2, 1990 N. Y. Laws 3547 ("Health Care Agents and Proxies") (codified as amended at N. Y. Pub. Health Law §§2980–2994 (McKinney 1994 and Supp. 1997)). In so doing, however, the State has neither endorsed a general right to "hasten death" nor approved physician assisted suicide. Quite the opposite: The State has reaffirmed the line between "killing" and "letting die." See N. Y. Pub. Health Law §2989(3) (McKinney 1994) ("This article is not intended to permit or promote suicide, assisted suicide, or euthanasia"); New York State Task Force on Life and the Law, Life Sustaining Treatment: Making Decisions and Appointing a Health Care Agent 36–42 (July 1987); Do Not Resuscitate Orders: The Proposed Legislation and Report of the New York State Task Force on Life and the Law 15 (Apr. 1986). More recently, the New York State Task Force on Life and the Law studied assisted suicide and euthanasia and, in 1994, unanimously recommended against legalization. When Death is Sought: Assisted Suicide and Euthanasia in the Medical Context vii (1994). In the Task Force's view, "allowing decisions to forego life sustaining treatment and allowing assisted suicide or euthanasia have radically different consequences and meanings for public policy." Id., at 146.

This Court has also recognized, at least implicitly, the distinction between letting a patient die and making that patient die. In Cruzan v. Director, Mo. Dept. of Health, 497 U.S. 261, 278 (1990), we concluded that "[t]he principle that a competent person has a constitutionally protected liberty interest in refusing unwanted medical treatment may be inferred from our prior decisions," and we assumed the existence of such a right for purposes of that case, Id., at 279. But our assumption of a right to refuse treatment was grounded not, as the Court of Appeals supposed, on the proposition that patients have a general and abstract "right to hasten death," 80 F. 3d, at 727–728, but on well established, traditional rights to bodily integrity and freedom from unwanted touching, Cruzan, 497 U. S., at 278–279; Id., at 287–288 (O'CONNOR, J., concurring). In fact, we observed that "the majority of States in this country have laws imposing criminal penalties on one who assists another to commit suicide." Id., at 280. Cruzan therefore provides no support for the notion that refusing life sustaining medical treatment is "nothing more nor less than suicide."

For all these reasons, we disagree with respondents' claim that the distinction between refusing lifesaving medical treatment and assisted suicide is "arbitrary" and "irrational." Brief for Respondents 44.[11] Granted, in some cases, the line between the two may not be clear, but certainty is not required, even were it possible.[12] Logic and contemporary practice support New York's judgment that the two acts are different, and New York may therefore, consistent with the Constitution, treat them differently. By permitting everyone to refuse unwanted medical treatment while prohibiting anyone from assisting a suicide, New York law follows a longstanding and rational distinction.

New York's reasons for recognizing and acting on this distinction—including prohibiting intentional killing and preserving life; preventing suicide; maintaining physicians' role as their patients' healers; protecting vulnerable people from indifference, prejudice, and psychological and financial pressure to end their lives; and avoiding a possible slide towards euthanasia—are discussed in greater detail in our opinion in *Glucksberg, ante*. These valid and important public interests easily satisfy the constitutional requirement that a legislative classification bear a rational relation to some legitimate end.[13]

The judgment of the Court of Appeals is reversed.

It is so ordered.

JUSTICE O'CONNOR CONCURRING IN THE JUDGMENTS.

See Justice O'Connor's opinion in *Washington v. Glucksberg* (pp. 388–89).

JUSTICE STEVENS CONCURRING IN THE JUDGMENTS.

Even though I do not conclude that assisted suicide is a fundamental right entitled to recognition at this time, I accord the claims raised by the patients and physicians in this case and *Washington v. Glucksberg* a high degree of importance, requiring a commensurate justification. See *Washington v. Glucksberg, ante*, at 24–41 (SOUTER, J., concurring in judgment). The reasons that lead me to conclude in Glucksberg that the prohibition on assisted suicide is not arbitrary under the due process standard also support the distinction between assistance to suicide, which is banned, and practices such as termination of artificial life support and death hastening pain medication, which are permitted. I accordingly concur in the judgment of the Court.

JUSTICE SOUTER CONCURRING IN THE JUDGMENTS.

See Justice Souter's opinion in *Washington v. Glucksberg* (pp. 395–411).

JUSTICE GINSBURG CONCURRING IN THE JUDGMENTS.

See Justice Ginsburg's opinion in *Washington v. Glucksberg* (p. 411).

JUSTICE BREYER CONCURRING IN THE JUDGMENTS.

See Justice Breyer's opinion in *Washington v. Glucksberg* (pp. 411–13).

Notes to Justice Rehnquist's Opinion

1. N. Y. Penal Law §125.15 (McKinney 1987) ("Manslaughter in the second degree") provides: "A person is guilty of manslaughter in the second degree when ... (3) He intentionally causes or aids another person to commit suicide. Manslaughter in the second degree is a class C felony." Section 120.30 ("Promoting a suicide attempt") states: "A person is guilty of promoting a suicide attempt when he intentionally causes or aids another person to attempt suicide. Promoting a suicide attempt is a class E felony." See generally, *Washington* v. *Glucksberg*, ___ U. S. ___ (1997), *ante*, at 4–15.

2. "It is established under New York law that a competent person may refuse medical treatment, even if the withdrawal of such treatment will result in death." *Quill* v. *Koppell*, 870 F. Supp. 78, 84 (SDNY 1994); see N. Y. Pub. Health Law, Art. 29-B, §§2960–2979 (McKinney 1993 & Supp. 1997) ("Orders Not to Resuscitate") (regulating right of "adult with capacity" to direct issuance of orders not to resuscitate); *id.*, §§2980–2994 ("Health Care Agents and Proxies") (allowing appointment of agents "to make ... Health care decisions on the principal's behalf," including decisions to refuse lifesaving treatment).

3. Declaration of Timothy E. Quill, M. D., App. 42–49; Declaration of Samuel C. Klagsbrun, M. D., *id.*, at 68–74; Declaration of Howard A. Grossman, M. D., *id.*, at 84–89; 80 F. 3d 716, 719 (CA2 1996).

4. These three patients stated that they had no chance of recovery, faced the "prospect of progressive loss of bodily function and integrity and increasing pain and suffering," and desired medical assistance in ending their lives. App. 25–26; Declaration of William A. Barth, *id.*, at 96–98; Declaration of George A. Kingsley, *id.*, at 99–102; Declaration of Jane Doe, *id.*, at 105–109.

5. The court acknowledged that because New York's assisted suicide statutes "do not impinge on any fundamental rights [or] involve suspect classifications," they were subject only to rational basis judicial scrutiny. 80 F. 3d, at 726–727.

6. The American Medical Association emphasizes the "fundamental difference between refusing life sustaining treatment and demanding a life ending treatment." American Medical Association, Council on Ethical and Judicial Affairs, Physician Assisted Suicide, 10 Issues in Law & Medicine 91, 93 (1994); see also American Medical Association, Council on Ethical and Judicial Affairs, Decisions Near the End of Life, 267 JAMA 2229, 2230–2231, 2233 (1992) ("The withdrawing or withholding of life sustaining treatment is not inherently contrary to the principles of beneficence and nonmaleficence," but assisted suicide "is contrary to the prohibition against using the tools of medicine to cause a patient's death"); New York State Task Force on Life and the Law, When Death is Sought: Assisted Suicide and Euthanasia in the Medical Context 108 (1994) ("[Professional organizations] consistently distinguish assisted suicide and euthanasia from the withdrawing or withholding of treatment, and from the provision of palliative treatments or other medical care that risk fatal side effects"); Brief for the American Medical Association et al. as *Amici Curiae* 18–25. Of course, as respondents' lawsuit demonstrates, there are differences of opinion within the medical profession on this question. See New York Task Force, When Death is Sought, *supra*, at 104–109.

7. Thus, the Second Circuit erred in reading New York law as creating a "right to hasten death"; instead, the authorities cited by the court recognize a right to refuse treatment, and nowhere equate the exercise of this right with suicide. *Schloendorff* v. *Society of New York Hospital*, 211 N. Y. 125, 129–130, 105 N. E. 92, 93 (1914), which contains Justice Cardozo's famous statement that "[e]very human being of adult years and sound mind has a right to determine what shall be done with his own body," was simply an informed consent case. See also *Rivers* v. *Katz*, 67 N. Y. 2d 485, 495, 495 N. E. 2d 337, 343 (1986) (right to refuse antipsychotic medication is not absolute, and may be limited when "the patient presents a danger to himself"); *Matter of Storar*, 52 N. Y. 2d 363, 377, n. 6, 420 N. E. 2d 64, 71, n. 6, cert. denied, 454 U.S. 858 (1981).

8. Many courts have recognized this distinction. See, e.g., *Kevorkian* v. *Thompson*, 947 F. Supp. 1152, 1178, and nn. 20–21 (ED Mich. 1997); *In re Fiori*, 543 Pa. 592, 602, 673 A. 2d 905, 910 (1996); *Singletary* v. *Costello*, 665 So. 2d 1099, 1106 (Fla. App. 1996); *Laurie* v. *Senecal*, 666 A. 2d 806, 808–809 (R. I. 1995); *State ex rel. Schuetzle* v. *Vogel*, 537 N. W. 2d 358, 360

(N. D. 1995); *Thor* v. *Superior Court*, 5 Cal. 4th 725, 741–742, 855 P. 2d 375, 385–386 (1993); *DeGrella* v. *Elston*, 858 S. W. 2d 698, 707 (Ky. 1993); *People* v. *Adams*, 216 Cal. App. 3d 1431, 1440, 265 Cal. Rptr. 568, 573–574 (1990); *Guardianship of Jane Doe*, 411 Mass. 512, 522–523, 583 N. E. 2d 1263, 1270, cert. denied sub nom. *Doe* v. *Gross*, 503 U.S. 950 (1992); *In re L. W.*, 167 Wis. 2d 53, 83, 482 N. W. 2d 60, 71 (1992); *In re Rosebush*, 195 Mich. App. 675, 681, n. 2, 491 N. W. 2d 633, 636, n. 2 (1992); *Donaldson* v. *Van de Kamp*, 2 Cal. App. 4th 1614, 1619–1625, 4 Cal. Rptr. 2D 59, 61–64 (1992); *In re Lawrance*, 579 N. E. 2d 32, 40, n. 4 (Ind. 1991); *McKay* v. *Bergstedt*, 106 Nev. 808, 822–823, 801 P. 2d 617, 626–627 (1990); *In re Browning*, 568 So. 2d 4, 14 (Fla. 1990); *McConnell* v. *Beverly Enterprises Connecticut, Inc.*, 209 Conn. 692, 710, 553 A. 2d 596, 605 (1989); *State* v. *McAfee*, 259 Ga. 579, 581, 385 S. E. 2d 651, 652 (1989); *In re Grant*, 109 Wash. 2d 545, 563, 747 P. 2d 445, 454–455 (1987); *In re Gardner*, 534 A. 2d 947, 955–956 (Me. 1987); *Matter of Farrell*, 108 N. J. 335, 349–350, 529 A. 2d 404, 411 (1987); *Rasmussen* v. *Fleming*, 154 Ariz. 207, 218, 741 P. 2d 674, 685 (1987); *Bouvia* v. *Superior Court*, 179 Cal. App. 3d 1127, 1144–1145, 225 Cal. Rptr. 297, 306 (1986); *Von Holden* v. *Chapman*, 87 App. Div. 2d 66, 70, 450 N. Y. S. 2d 623, 627 (1982); *Bartling* v. *Superior Court*, 163 Cal. App. 3d 186, 196–197, 209 Cal. Rptr. 220, 225–226 (1984); *Foody* v. *Manchester Memorial Hospital*, 40 Conn. Sup. 127, 137, 482 A. 2d 713, 720 (1984); *In re P. v. W.*, 424 So. 2d 1015, 1022 (La. 1982); *Leach* v. *Akron General Medical Center*, 68 Ohio Misc. 1, 10, 426 N. E. 2d 809, 815 (Ohio Comm. Pleas 1980); *In re Severns*, 425 A. 2d 156, 161 (Del. Ch. 1980); *Satz* v. *Perlmutter*, 362 So. 2d 160, 162–163 (Fla. App. 1978); *Application of the President and Directors of Georgetown College*, 331 F. 2d 1000, 1009 (CADC), cert. denied, 377 U.S. 978 (1964); *Brophy* v. *New England Sinai Hospital*, 398 Mass. 417, 439, 497 N. E. 2d 626, 638 (1986). The British House of Lords has also recognized the distinction. *Airedale N. H. S. Trust* v. *Bland*, 2 W. L. R. 316, 368 (1993).

9. See Ala. Code §22–8A—10 (1990); Alaska Stat. Ann. §§18.12.080(a), (f) (1996); Ariz. Rev. Stat. Ann. §36–3210 (Supp. 1996); Ark. Code Ann. §§20–13–905(a), (f), 20–17–210(a),(g) (1991 and Supp. 1995); Cal. Health & Safety Code Ann. §§7191.5(a), (g) (West Supp. 1997); Cal. Prob. Code Ann. §4723 (West. Supp. 1997); Colo. Rev. Stat. §§15–14–504(4), 15–18–112(1), 15–18.5–101(3), 15–18.6–108 (1987 and Supp. 1996); Conn. Gen. Stat. §19a—575 (Supp. 1996); Del. Code Ann., Tit. 16, §2512 (Supp. 1996); D. C. Code Ann. §§6–2430, 21–2212 (1995 and Supp. 1996); Fla. Stat. §§765.309(1), (2) (Supp. 1997); Ga. Code Ann. §§31–32–11(b), 31–36–2(b) (1996); Haw. Rev. Stat. §327D—13 (1996); Idaho Code §39–152 (Supp. 1996); Ill. Comp. Stat., ch. 755, §§35/9(f), 40/5, 40/50, 45/2–1 (1992); Ind. Code §§16–36–1-13, 16–36–4-19, 30–5-5-17 (1994 and Supp. 1996); Iowa Code §§144A.11.1–144A.11.6, 144B.12.2 (1989 and West Supp. 1997); Kan. Stat. Ann. §65–28,109 (1985); Ky. Rev. Stat. Ann. §311.638 (Baldwin Supp. 1992); La. Rev. Stat. Ann. 40: §§1299.58.10(A), (B) (West 1992); Me. Rev. Stat. Ann., Tit. 18-A, §§5–813(b), (c) (West Supp. 1996); Mass. Gen. Laws 201D, §12 (Supp. 1997); MD. Health Code Ann. §5–611(c) (1994); Mich. Comp. Laws Ann. §700.496(20) (West 1995); Minn. Stat. §§145B.14, 145C.14 (Supp. 1997); Miss. Code Ann. §§41–41–117(2),41–41–119(1) (Supp. 1992); Mo. Rev. Stat. §§459.015.3, 459.055(5) (1992); Mont. Code Ann. §§50–9-205(1), (7), 50–10–104(1), (6) (1995); Neb. Rev. Stat. §§20–412(1), (7), 30–3401(3) (1995); N. H. Rev. Stat. Ann. §§137-H:10, 137-H:13, 137 J:1 (1996); N. J. Stat. Ann. §§26:2H—54(d), (e), 26:2H—77 (West 1996); N. M. Stat. Ann. §§24–7A—13(B)(1), (C) (Supp. 1995); N. Y. Pub. Health Law §2989(3) (1993); Nev. Rev. Stat. §449.670(2) (1996); N. C. Gen. Stat. §§90–320(b), 90–321(f) (1993); N. D. Cent. Code §§23–06.4–01, 23–06.5–01 (1991); Ohio Rev. Code Ann. §2133.12(A), (D) (Supp. 1996); Okla. Stat. Ann., Tit. 63, §§3101.2(C),3101.12(A),(G) (1996); 20 Pa. Cons. Stat. §5402(b) (Supp. 1996); R. I. Gen. Laws §§23–4.10–9(a), (f), 23–4.11–10(a), (f) 1996); S. C. Code Ann. §§44–77–130, 44–78–50(A), (C), 62–5-504(O) (Supp. 1996); S. D. Codified Laws §§34–12D—14, 34–12D—20 (1994); Tenn. Code Ann. §§32–11–110(a), 39–13–216 (Supp. 1996); Tex. Health & Safety Code Ann. §§672.017, 672.020, 672.021 (1992); Utah Code Ann. §§75–2-1116,75–2-1118 (1993); Va. Code Ann. §54.1–2990 (1994); Vt. Stat. Ann., Tit. 18, §5260 (1987); V. I. Code Ann.,Tit. 19, §§198(a), (g) (1995); Wash. Rev. Code §§70.122.070(1), 70.122.100 (Supp. 1997); W. Va. Code §§16–30–10, 16–30A—16(a), 16–30B—2(b), 16–30B—13, 16–30C—14 (1995); Wis. Stat.

§§154.11(1), (6), 154.25(7), 155.70(7) (Supp. 1996); Wyo. Stat. §§3–5-211, 35–22–109, 35–22–208 (1994 & Supp. 1996). See also, 42 U.S.C. § 14402(b)(1), (2), (4) ("Assisted Suicide Funding Restriction Act of 1997").

10. It has always been a crime, either by statute or under the common law, to assist a suicide in New York. See Marzen, O'Dowd, Crone, & Balch, Suicide: A Constitutional Right?, 24 Duquesne L. Rev. 1, 205–210 (1985) (Appendix).

11. Respondents also argue that the State irrationally distinguishes between physician assisted suicide and "terminal sedation," a process respondents characterize as "induc[ing] barbiturate coma and then starv[ing] the person to death." Brief for Respondents 48–50; see 80 F. 3d, at 729. Petitioners insist, however, that " '[a]lthough proponents of physician assisted suicide and euthanasia contend that terminal sedation is covert physician assisted suicide or euthanasia, the concept of sedating pharmacotherapy is based on informed consent and the principle of double effect.' " Reply Brief for Petitioners 12 (quoting P. Rousseau, Terminal Sedation in the Care of Dying Patients, 156 Archives Internal Med. 1785, 1785–1786 (1996)). Just as a State may prohibit assisting suicide while permitting patients to refuse unwanted lifesaving treatment, it may permit palliative care related to that refusal, which may have the foreseen but unintended "double effect" of hastening the patient's death. See New York Task Force, When Death is Sought, *supra*, n. 6, at 163 ("It is widely recognized that the provision of pain medication is ethically and professionally acceptable even when the treatment may hasten the patient's death, if the medication is intended to alleviate pain and severe discomfort, not to cause death").

12. We do not insist, as JUSTICE STEVENS suggests, *ante*, at 14–15 (concurring opinion), that "in all cases there will in fact be a significant difference between the intent of the physicians, the patients or the families [in withdrawal of treatment and physician assisted suicide cases]." See 6–7, *supra* ("[A] physician who withdraws, or honors a patient's refusal to begin, life sustaining medical treatment purposefully intends, or may so intend, only to respect his patient's wishes.... The same is true when a doctor provides aggressive palliative care; ... The physician's purpose and intent is, *or may be,* only to ease his patient's pain") (emphasis added). In the absence of omniscience, however, the State is entitled to act on the reasonableness of the distinction.

13. JUSTICE STEVENS observes that our holding today "does not foreclose the possibility that some applications of the New York statute may impose an intolerable intrusion on the patient's freedom." *Ante*, at 16 (concurring opinion). This is true, but, as we observe in *Glucksberg, ante,* at 31–32, n. 24, a particular plaintiff hoping to show that New York's assisted suicide ban was unconstitutional in his particular case would need to present different and considerably stronger arguments than those advanced by respondents here.

Appendix C

The Philosophers' Brief

RONALD DWORKIN, THOMAS NAGEL, ROBERT NOZICK, JOHN RAWLS, THOMAS SCANLON, AND JUDITH JARVIS THOMSON

State of *Washington* v. *Glucksberg*; *Vacco* v. *Quill*, nos. 95–1858, 96–110, October term, 1996, December 10, 1996, Brief for Ronald Dworkin, Thomas Nagel, Robert Nozick, John Rawls, Thomas Scanlon, and Judith Jarvis Thompson as amici curiae in support of respondents

The Brief of the Amici Curiae

Interest of the Amici Curiae

Amici are six moral and political philosophers who differ on many issues of public morality and policy. They are united, however, in their conviction that respect for fundamental principles of liberty and justice, as well as for the American constitutional tradition, requires that the decisions of the Courts of Appeals be affirmed.

Introduction and Summary of Argument

These cases do not invite or require the Court to make moral, ethical, or religious judgments about how people should approach or confront their death or about when it is ethically appropriate to hasten one's own death or to ask others for help in doing so. On the contrary, they ask the Court to recognize that individuals have a constitutionally protected interest in making those grave judgments for themselves, free from the imposition of any religious or philosophical orthodoxy by court or legislature. States have a constitutionally legitimate interest in protecting individuals from irrational, ill-informed, pressured, or unstable decisions to hasten their own death. To that end, states may regulate and limit the assistance that doctors may give individuals who express a wish to die. But states may not deny people in the position of the patient-plaintiffs in these cases the opportunity to demonstrate, through whatever reasonable procedures the state might institute—even procedures that err on the side of caution—that their decision to die is indeed informed, stable, and fully free. Denying that opportunity to terminally ill patients who are in agonizing pain or otherwise doomed to an existence they regard as intolerable could only be justified on the basis of a religious or ethical conviction about the value or meaning of life itself. Our Constitution forbids government to impose such convictions on its citizens.

Petitioners [i.e., the state authorities of Washington and New York] and the amici who support them offer two contradictory arguments. Some deny that the patient-plaintiffs have any constitutionally protected liberty interest in hastening their own deaths. But that liberty interest flows directly from this Court's previous decisions. It flows from the right of people to make their own decisions about matters "involving the most intimate and personal choices a person may make in a lifetime, choices central to personal dignity and autonomy." *Planned Parenthood* v. *Casey*, 505 U.S. 833, 851 (1992).

The Solicitor General, urging reversal in support of Petitioners, recognizes that the patient-plaintiffs do have a constitutional liberty interest at stake in these cases. See Brief for the United States as *Amicus Curiae* Supporting Petitioners at 12, *Washington v. Vacco* [hereinafter Brief for the United States] ("The term 'liberty' in the Due Process Clause . . . is broad enough to encompass an interest on the part of terminally ill, mentally competent adults in obtaining relief from the kind of suffering experienced by the plaintiffs in this case, which includes not only severe physical pain, but also the despair and distress that comes from physical deterioration and the inability to control basic bodily functions."); see also id. at 13 ("*Cruzan* . . . supports the conclusion that a liberty interest is at stake in this case.).

The Solicitor General nevertheless argues that Washington and New York properly ignored this profound interest when they required the patient-plaintiffs to live on in circumstances they found intolerable. He argues that a state may simply declare that it is unable to devise a regulatory scheme that would adequately protect patients whose desire to die might be ill-informed or unstable or foolish or not fully free, and that a state may therefore fall back on a blanket prohibition. This Court has never accepted that patently dangerous rationale for denying protection altogether to a conceded fundamental constitutional interest. It would be a serious mistake to do so now. If that rationale were accepted, an interest acknowledged to be constitutionally protected would be rendered empty.

I. The Liberty Interest Asserted Here Is Protected by the Due Process Clause

The Due Process Clause of the Fourteenth Amendment protects the liberty interest asserted by the patient-plaintiffs here.

Certain decisions are momentous in their impact on the character of a person's life—decisions about religious faith, political and moral allegiance, marriage, procreation, and death, for example. Such deeply personal decisions pose controversial questions about how and why human life has value. In a free society, individuals must be allowed to make those decisions for themselves, out of their own faith, conscience, and convictions. This Court has insisted, in a variety of contexts and circumstances, that this great freedom is among those protected by the Due Process Clause as essential to a community of "ordered liberty"; *Palko* v. *Connecticut*, 302 U.S. 319, 325 (1937). In its recent decision in *Planned Parenthood v.Casey*, 505 U.S. 833, 851 (1992), the Court offered a paradigmatic statement of that principle:

> matters [] involving the most intimate and personal choices a person may make in a lifetime, choices central to a person's dignity and autonomy, are central to the liberty protected by the Fourteenth Amendment.

That declaration reflects an idea underlying many of our basic constitutional protections.[1] As the Court explained in *West Virginia State Board of Education* v. *Barnette*, 319 U.S. 624, 642 (1943):

> If there is any fixed star in our constitutional constellation, it is that no official . . . can prescribe what shall be orthodox in politics, nationalism, religion, or other matters of opinion or force citizens to confess by word or act their faith therein.

A person's interest in following his own convictions at the end of life is so central a part of the more general right to make; "intimate and personal choices"; for himself that a failure to protect that particular interest would undermine the general right altogether. Death is, for each of us, among the most significant events of life. As the Chief

Justice said in *Cruzan v. Missouri*, 497 U.S. 261, 281(1990), "[t]he choice between life and death is a deeply personal decision of obvious and overwhelming finality." Most of us see death—whatever we think wills follow it—as the final act of life's drama, and we want that last act to reflect our own convictions, those we have tried to live by, not the convictions of others forced on us in our most vulnerable moment.

Different people, of different religious and ethical beliefs, embrace very different convictions about which way of dying confirms and which contradicts the value of their lives. Some fight against death with every weapon their doctors can devise. Others will do nothing to hasten death even if they pray it will come soon. Still others, including the patient-plaintiffs in these cases, want to end their lives when they think that living on, in the only way they can, would disfigure rather than enhance the lives they had created. Some people make the latter choice not just to escape pain. Even if it were possible to eliminate all pain for a dying patient—and frequently that is not possible—that would not end or even much alleviate the anguish some would feel at remaining alive, but intubated, helpless, and often sedated near oblivion.

None of these dramatically different attitudes about the meaning of death can be dismissed as irrational. None should be imposed, either by the pressure of doctors or relatives or by the fiat of government, on people who reject it. Just as it would be intolerable for government to dictate that doctors never be permitted to try to keep someone alive as long as possible. When that is what the patient wishes, so it is intolerable for government to dictate that doctors may never, under any circumstances, help someone to die who believes that further life means only degradation. The Constitution insists that people must be free to make these deeply personal decisions for themselves and must not be forced to end their lives in a way that appalls them, just because that is what some majority thinks proper.

II. This Court's Decisions in *Casey* and *Cruzan* Compel Recognition of a Liberty Interest Here

A. Casey Supports the Liberty Interest Asserted Here

In *Casey*, this Court, in holding that a state cannot constitutionally proscribe abortion in all cases, reiterated that the Constitution protects a sphere of autonomy in which individuals must be permitted to make certain decisions for themselves. The Court began its analysis by pointing out that "[a]t the heart of liberty is the right to define one's own concept of existence, of meaning, of the universe, and of the mystery of human life." 505 U.S. at 851. Choices flowing out of these conceptions, on matters "involving the most intimate and personal choices a person may make in a lifetime, choices central to personal dignity and autonomy, are central to the liberty protected by the Fourteenth Amendment. *Id.* "Beliefs about these matters," the Court continued, "could not define the attributes of personhood were they formed under compulsion of the State." *Id.*

In language pertinent to the liberty interest asserted here, the Court explained why decisions about abortion fall within this category of "personal and intimate" decisions. A decision whether or not to have an abortion, "originat[ing] within the zone of conscience and belief," involves conduct in which "the liberty of the woman is at stake in a sense unique to the human condition and so unique to the law." *Id.* at 852. As such, the decision necessarily involves the very "destiny of the woman" and is inevitably "shaped to a large extent on her own conception of her spiritual imperatives and her place in society." *Id.* Precisely because of these characteristics of the decision, "the State is [not] entitled to proscribe [abortion] in all instances." *Id.* Rather, to allow a total prohibition on abortion would be to permit a state to impose one conception of the meaning and value of human existence on all individuals. This the Constitution forbids.

The Solicitor General nevertheless argues that the right to abortion could be supported on grounds other than this autonomy principle, grounds that would not apply here. He argues, for example, that the abortion right might flow from the great burden an unwanted child imposes on its mother's life. Brief for the United States at 14–15. But whether or not abortion rights could be defended on such grounds, they were not the grounds on which this Court in fact relied. To the contrary, the Court explained at length that the right flows from the constitutional protection accorded all individuals to "define one's own concept of existence, of meaning, of the universe, and of the mystery of human life." *Casey*, 505 U.S. at 851.

The analysis in *Casey* compels the conclusion that the patient-plaintiffs have a liberty interest in this case that a state cannot burden with a blanket prohibition. Like a woman's decision whether to have an abortion, a decision to die involves one's very "destiny" and inevitably will be "shaped to a large extent on [one's] own conception of [one's] spiritual imperatives and [one's] place in society." *Id.* at 852. Just as a blanket prohibition on abortion would involve the improper imposition of one conception of the meaning and value of human existence on all individuals, so too would a blanket prohibition on assisted suicide. The liberty interest asserted here cannot be rejected without undermining the rationale of *Casey*. Indeed, the lower court opinions in the Washington case expressly recognized the parallel between the liberty interest in Casey and the interest asserted here. See *Compassion in Dying* v. *Washington*, 79 F.3d 790, 801 (9th Cir. 1996) (en banc) ("In deciding right-to-die cases, we are guided by the Court's approach to the abortion cases. *Casey* in particular provides a powerful precedent, for in that case the Court had the opportunity to evaluate its past decisions and to determine whether to adhere to its original judgment."), *aff'g*, 850 F. Supp. 1454, 1459 (W.D. Wash. 1994) ("[T]he reasoning in *Casey* [is] highly instructive and almost prescriptive . . ."). This Court should do the same.

B. Cruzan Supports the Liberty Interest Asserted Here

We agree with the Solicitor General that this Court's decision in "*Cruzan* ... supports the conclusion that a liberty interest is at stake in this case." Brief for the United States at 8. Petitioners, however, insist that the present cases can be distinguished because the right at issue in *Cruzan* was limited to a right to reject an unwanted invasion of one's body.[2] But this Court repeatedly has held that in appropriate circumstances a state may require individuals to accept unwanted invasions of the body. *See, e.g., Schmerber* v. *California* , 384 U.S. 757 (1966) (extraction of blood sample from individual suspected of driving while intoxicated, notwithstanding defendant's objection, does not violate privilege against self-incrimination or other constitutional rights); *Jacobson v. Massachusetts*, 197 U.S. 11 (1905) (upholding compulsory vaccination for smallpox as reasonable regulation for protection of public health).

The liberty interest at stake in *Cruzan* was a more profound one. If a competent patient has a constitutional right to refuse life-sustaining treatment, then, the Court implied, the state could not override that right. The regulations upheld in *Cruzan* were designed only to ensure that the individual's wishes were ascertained correctly. Thus, if *Cruzan* implies a right of competent patients to refuse life-sustaining treatment, that implication must be understood as resting not simply on a right to refuse bodily invasions but on the more profound right to refuse medical intervention when what is at stake is a momentous personal decision, such as the timing and manner of one's death. In her concurrence, Justice O'Connor expressly recognized that the right at issue involved a "deeply personal decision"; that is "inextricably intertwined" with our notion of "self-determination." 497 U.S. at 287—89.

Cruzan also supports the proposition that a state may not burden a terminally ill patient's liberty interest in determining the time and manner of his death by prohibiting doctors from terminating life support. Seeking to distinguish *Cruzan*, Petitioners insist that a state may nevertheless burden that right in a different way by forbidding doctors to assist in the suicide of patients who are not on life-support machinery. They argue that doctors who remove life support are only allowing a natural process to end in death whereas doctors who prescribe lethal drugs are intervening to cause death. So, according to this argument, a state has an independent justification for forbidding doctors to assist in suicide that it does not have for forbidding them to remove life support. In the former case though not the latter, it is said, the state forbids an act of killing that is morally much more problematic than merely letting a patient die.

This argument is based on a misunderstanding of the pertinent moral principles. It is certainly true that when a patient does not wish to die, different acts, each of which foreseeably results in his death, nevertheless have very different moral status. When several patients need organ transplants and organs are scarce, for example, it is morally permissible for a doctor to deny an organ to one patient, even though he will die without it, in order to give it to another. But it is certainly not permissible for a doctor to kill one patient in order to use his organs to save another. The morally significant difference between those two acts is not, however, that killing is a positive act and not providing an organ is a mere omission, or that killing someone is worse than merely allowing a "natural" process to result in death. It would be equally impermissible for a doctor to let an injured patient bleed to death, or to refuse antibiotics to a patient with pneumonia—in each case the doctor would have allowed death to result from a 'natural" process—in order to make his organs available for transplant to others. A doctor violates his patient's rights whether the doctor acts or refrains from acting, against the patient's wishes, in a way that is designed to cause death.

When a competent patient does want to die, the moral situation is obviously different, because then it makes no sense to appeal to the patient's right not to be killed as a reason why an act designed to cause his death is impermissible. From the patient's point of view, there is no morally pertinent difference between a doctor's terminating treatment that keeps him alive, if that is what he wishes, and a doctor's helping him to end his own life by providing lethal pills he may take himself, when ready, if that is what he wishes—except that the latter may be quicker and more humane. Nor is that a pertinent difference from the doctor's point of view. If and when it is permissible for him to act with death in view, it does not matter which of those two means he and his patient choose. If it is permissible for a doctor deliberately to withdraw medical treatment in order to allow death to result from a natural process, then it is equally permissible for him to help his patient hasten his own death more actively, if that is the patient's express wish.

It is true that some doctors asked to terminate life support are reluctant and do so only in deference to a patient's right to compel them to remove unwanted invasions of his body. But other doctors, who believe that their most fundamental professional duty is to act in the patient's interests and that, in certain circumstances, it is in their patient's best interests to die, participate willingly in such decisions: they terminate life support to cause death because they know that is what their patient wants. *Cruzan* implied that a state may not absolutely prohibit a doctor from deliberately causing death, at the patient's request, in that way and for that reason. If so, then a state may not prohibit doctors from deliberately using more direct and often more humane means to the same end when that is what a patient prefers. The fact that failing to provide life-sustaining treatment may be regarded as "only letting nature take its course" is no more morally significant in this context, when the patient wishes to die, than in the other, when he wishes to live. Whether a doctor turns off a respirator in accordance with the patient's request or prescribes pills that a patient may take when he is ready to kill himself, the doctor acts with the same intention: to help the patient die.

The two situations do differ in one important respect. Since patients have a right not to have life-support machinery attached to their bodies, they have, in principle, a right to compel its removal. But that is not true in the case of assisted suicide: patients in certain circumstances have a right that the state not forbid doctors to assist in their deaths, but they have no right to compel a doctor to assist them. The right in question, that is, is only a right to the help of a willing doctor.

III. State Interests Do Not Justify a Categorical Prohibition on All Assisted Suicide

The Solicitor General concedes that "a competent, terminally ill adult has a constitutionally cognizable liberty interest in avoiding the kind of suffering experienced by the plaintiffs in this case." Brief for the United States at 8. He agrees that this interest extends not only to avoiding pain, but to avoiding an existence the patient believes to be one of intolerable indignity or incapacity as well. *Id* . at 12. The Solicitor General argues, however, that states nevertheless have the right to "override" this liberty interest altogether, because a state could reasonably conclude that allowing doctors to assist in suicide, even under the most stringent regulations and procedures that could be devised, would unreasonably endanger the lives of a number of patients who might ask for death in circumstances when it is plainly not in their interests to die or when their consent has been improperly obtained.

This argument is unpersuasive, however, for at least three reasons. *First* , in *Cruzan*, this Court noted that its various decisions supported the recognition of a general liberty interest in refusing medical treatment, even when such refusal could result in death. 497 U.S. At 278—79. The various risks described by the Solicitor General apply equally to those situations. For instance, a patient kept alive only by an elaborate and disabling life-support system might well become depressed, and doctors might be equally uncertain whether the depression is curable: such a patient might decide for death only because he has been advised that he will die soon anyway or that he will never live free of the burdensome apparatus, and either diagnosis might conceivably be mistaken. Relatives or doctors might subtly or crudely influence that decision, and state provision for the decision may (to the same degree in this case as if it allowed assisted suicide) be thought to encourage it.

Yet there has been no suggestion that states are incapable of addressing such dangers through regulation. In fact, quite the opposite is true. In *McKay* v. *Bergstedt*, 106 Nev. 808, 801 P.2d 617 (1990), for example, the Nevada Supreme Court held that "competent adult patients desiring to refuse or discontinue medical treatment" must be examined by two non-attending physicians to determine whether the patient is mentally competent, understands his prognosis and treatment options, and appears free of coercion or pressure in making his decision. See also: *Id*. At 827—28, 801 P.2d at 630. *Id.* See also: (in the case of terminally-ill patients with natural life expectancy of less than six months, [a] patient's right of self-determination shall be deemed to prevail over state interests, whereas [a] non-terminal patient's decision to terminate life-support systems must first be weighed against relevant state interests by trial judge); [and] *In re Farrell*, 108 N.J. 335, 354, 529 A.2d 404, 413 (1987) ([which held that a] terminally-ill patient requesting termination of life-support must be determined to be competent and properly informed about [his] prognosis, available treatment options and

risks, and to have made the decision voluntarily and without coercion). Those protocols served to guard against precisely the dangers that the Solicitor General raises. The
case law contains no suggestion that such protocols are inevitably insufficient to prevent deaths that should have been prevented.

Indeed, the risks of mistake are overall greater in the case of terminating life support. *Cruzan* implied that a state must allow individuals to make such decisions
through an advance directive stipulating either that life support be terminated (or not
initiated) in described circumstances when the individual was no longer competent to
make such a decision himself, or that a designated proxy be allowed to make that decision. All the risks just described are present when the decision is made through or pursuant to such an advance directive, and a grave further risk is added: that the directive,
though still in force, no longer represents the wishes of the patient. The patient might
have changed his mind before he became incompetent, though he did not change the
directive, or his proxy may make a decision that the patient would not have made himself if still competent. In *Cruzan*, this Court held that a state may limit these risks
through reasonable regulation. It did not hold—or even suggest—that a state may avoid
them through a blanket prohibition that, in effect, denies the liberty interest altogether.

Second, nothing in the record supports the [Solicitor General's] conclusion that no
system of rules and regulations could adequately reduce the risk of mistake. As discussed above, the experience of states in adjudicating requests to have life-sustaining
treatment removed indicates the opposite.[3] The Solicitor General has provided no persuasive reason why the same sort of procedures could not be applied effectively in the
case of a competent individual's request for physician-assisted suicide.

Indeed, several very detailed schemes for regulating physician-assisted suicide have
been submitted to the voters of some states[4] and one has been enacted.[5] In addition,
concerned groups, including a group of distinguished professors of law and other professionals, have drafted and defended such schemes. *See, e.g., Charles H. Baron, et. al.,
A Model State Act to Authorize and Regulate Physician-Assisted Suicide,* 33 Harv. J. Legis.
1 (1996). Such draft statutes propose a variety of protections and review procedures
designed to insure against mistakes, and neither Washington nor New York attempted
to show that such schemes would be porous or ineffective. Nor does the Solicitor General's brief: it relies instead mainly on flat and conclusory statements. It cites a New
York Task Force report, written before the proposals just described were drafted, whose
findings have been widely disputed and were implicitly rejected in the opinion of the
Second Circuit below. *See generally Quill v. Vacco,* 80 F.3d 716 (2d Cir. 1996). The weakness of the Solicitor General's argument is signaled by his strong reliance on the experience in the Netherlands which, in effect, allows assisted suicide pursuant to published
guidelines. Brief for the United States at 23—24. The Dutch guidelines are more permissive than the proposed and model American statutes, however. The Solicitor General deems the Dutch practice of ending the lives of people like neo-nates who cannot
consent particularly noteworthy, for example, but that practice could easily and effectively be made illegal by any state regulatory scheme without violating the Constitution.

The Solicitor General's argument would perhaps have more force if the question
before the Court were simply whether a state has any rational basis for an absolute prohibition; if that were the question, then it might be enough to call attention to risks a
state might well deem not worth running. But as the Solicitor General concedes, the
question here is a very different one: whether a state has interests sufficiently compelling to allow it to take the extraordinary step of altogether refusing the exercise of a
liberty interest of constitutional dimension. In those circumstances, the burden is
plainly on the state to demonstrate that the risk of mistakes is very high, and that no

alternative to complete prohibition would adequately and effectively reduce those risks. Neither of the Petitioners has made such a showing.

Nor could they. The burden of proof on any state attempting to show this would be very high. Consider, for example, the burden a state would have to meet to show that it was entitled altogether to ban public speeches in favor of unpopular causes because it could not guarantee, either by regulations short of an outright ban or by increased police protection, that such speeches would not provoke a riot that would result in serious injury or death to an innocent party. Or that it was entitled to deny those accused of crime the procedural rights that the Constitution guarantees, such as the right to a jury trial, because the security risk those rights would impose on the community would be too great. One can posit extreme circumstances in which some such argument would succeed. *See, e.g., Korematsu* v. *United States*, 323 U.S. 214 (1944) (permitting United States to detain individuals of Japanese ancestry during wartime). But these circumstances would be extreme indeed, and the *Korematsu* ruling has been widely and severely criticized.

Third, it is doubtful whether the risks the Solicitor General cites are even of the right character to serve as justification for an absolute prohibition on the exercise of an important liberty interest. The risks fall into two groups. The first is the risk of medical mistake, including a misdiagnosis of competence or terminal illness. To be sure, no scheme of regulation, no matter how rigorous, can altogether guarantee that medical mistakes will not be made. But the Constitution does not allow a state to deny patients a great variety of important choices, for which informed consent is properly deemed necessary, just because the information on which the consent is given may, in spite of the most strenuous efforts to avoid mistake, be wrong. Again, these identical risks are present in decisions to terminate life support, yet they do not justify an absolute prohibition on the exercise of the right.

The second group consists of risks that a patient will be unduly influenced by considerations that the state might deem it not in his best interests to be swayed by, for example, the feelings and views of close family members. Brief for the United States at 20. But what a patient regards as proper grounds for such a decision normally reflects exactly the judgments of personal ethics—of why his life is important and what affects its value—that patients have a crucial liberty interest in deciding for themselves. Even people who are dying have a right to hear and, if they wish, act on what others might wish to tell or suggest or even hint to them, and it would be dangerous to suppose that a state may prevent this on the ground that it knows better than its citizens when they should be moved by or yield to particular advice or suggestion in the exercise of their right to make fateful personal decisions for themselves. It is not a good reply that some people may not decide as they really wish—as they would decide, for example, if free from the "pressure" of others. That possibility could hardly justify the most serious pressure of all—the criminal law which tells them that they may not decide for death if they need the help of a doctor in dying, no matter how firmly they wish it.

There is a fundamental infirmity in the Solicitor General's argument. He asserts that a state may reasonably judge that the risk of "mistake" to some persons justifies a prohibition that not only risks but insures and even aims at what would undoubtedly be a vastly greater number of "mistakes" of the opposite kind—preventing many thousands of competent people who think that it disfigures their lives to continue living, in the only way left to them, from escaping that—to them—terrible injury. A state grievously and irreversibly harms such people when it prohibits that escape. The Solicitor General's argument may seem plausible to those who do not agree that individuals are harmed by being forced to live on in pain and what they regard as indignity. But many other people plainly do think that such individuals are harmed, and a state may not take one side in that essentially ethical or religious controversy as its justification for denying a crucial liberty.

Of course, a state has important interests that justify regulating physician-assisted suicide. It may be legitimate for a state to deny an opportunity for assisted suicide when it acts in what it reasonably judges to be the best interests of the potential suicide, and when its judgment on that issue does not rest on contested judgments about "matters involving the most intimate and personal choices a person may make in a lifetime, choices central to personal dignity and autonomy." *Casey*, 505 U.S. At 851. A state might assert, for example, that people who are not terminally ill, but who have formed a desire to die, are, as a group, very likely later to be grateful if they are prevented from taking their own lives. It might then claim that it is legitimate, out of concern for such people, to deny any of them a doctor's assistance [in taking their own lives].

This Court need not decide now the extent to which such paternalistic interests might override an individual's liberty interest. No one can plausibly claim, however— and it is noteworthy that neither Petitioners nor the Solicitor General does claim—that any such prohibition could serve the interests of any significant number of terminally ill patients. On the contrary, any paternalistic justification for an absolute prohibition of assistance to such patients would of necessity appeal to a widely contested religious or ethical conviction many of them, including the patient-plaintiffs, reject. Allowing *that* justification to prevail would vitiate the liberty interest.

Even in the case of terminally ill patients, a state has a right to take all reasonable measures to insure that a patient requesting such assistance has made an informed, competent, stable and uncoerced decision. It is plainly legitimate for a state to establish procedures through which professional and administrative judgments can be made about these matters, and to forbid doctors to assist in suicide when its reasonable procedures have not been satisfied. States may be permitted considerable leeway in designing such procedures. They may be permitted, within reason, to err on what they take to be the side of caution. But they may not use the bare possibility of error as justification for refusing to establish any procedures at all and relying instead on a flat prohibition.

Conclusion

Each individual has a right to make the "most intimate and personal choices central to personal dignity and autonomy." That right encompasses the right to exercise some control over the time and manner of one's death.

The patient-plaintiffs in these cases were all mentally competent individuals in the final phase of terminal illness and died within months of filing their claims.

Jane Doe described how her advanced cancer made even the most basic bodily functions such as swallowing, coughing, and yawning extremely painful and that it was "not possible for [her] to reduce [her] pain to an acceptable level of comfort and to retain an alert state." Faced with such circumstances, she sought to be able to "discuss freely with [her] treating physician [her] intention of hastening [her] death through the consumption of drugs prescribed for that purpose." *Quill* v. *Vacco*, 80 F.2d 716, 720 (2d Cir. 1996) (quoting declaration of Jane Doe).

George A. Kingsley, in advanced stages of AIDS which included, among other hardships, the attachment of a tube to an artery in his chest which made even routine functions burdensome and the development of lesions on his brain, sought advice from his doctors regarding prescriptions which could hasten his impending death. *Id.*

Jane Roe, suffering from cancer since 1988, had been almost completely bedridden since 1993 and experienced constant pain which could not be alleviated by medication. After undergoing counseling for herself and her family, she desired to hasten her death by taking prescription drugs. *Compassion in Dying* v. *Washington*, 850 F. Supp. 1454, 1456 (1994).

John Doe, who had experienced numerous AIDS-related ailments since 1991, was "especially cognizant of the suffering imposed by a lingering terminal illness because he was the primary caregiver for his long-term companion who died of AIDS" and sought prescription drugs from his physician to hasten his own death after entering the terminal phase of AIDS. *Id.* at 1456—57.

James Poe suffered from emphysema which caused him "a constant sensation of suffocating" as well as a cardiac condition which caused severe leg pain. Connected to an oxygen tank at all times but unable to calm the panic reaction associated with his feeling of suffocation even with regular doses of morphine, Mr. Poe sought physician-assisted suicide. *Id.* at 1457.

A state may not deny the liberty claimed by the patient-plaintiffs in these cases without providing them an opportunity to demonstrate, in whatever way the state might reasonably think wise and necessary, that the conviction they expressed for an early death is competent, rational, informed, stable, and uncoerced.

Affirming the decisions by the Courts of Appeals would establish nothing more than that there is such a constitutionally protected right in principle. It would establish only that some individuals, whose decisions for suicide plainly cannot be dismissed as irrational or foolish or premature, must be accorded a reasonable opportunity to show that their decision for death is informed and free. It is not necessary to decide precisely which patients are entitled to that opportunity. If, on the other hand, this Court reverses the decisions below, its decision could only be justified by the momentous proposition—a proposition flatly in conflict with the spirit and letter of the Court's past decisions—that an American citizen does not, after all, have the right, even in principle, to live and die in the light of his own religious and ethical beliefs, his own convictions about why his life is valuable and where its value lies.

> has been determined by the attending physician and consulting physician to be suffering from a terminal disease, and who has voluntarily expressed his or her wish to die, may make a written request for medication for the purpose of ending his life in a human and dignified manner in accordance with [the provisions of the Act].

Notes

1. In *Cohen v. California*, 403 U.S. 15, 24 (1971), for example, this Court held that the First Amendment guarantee of free speech and expression derives from "the belief that no other approach would comport with the premise of individual dignity and choice upon which our political system rests." Interpreting the religion clauses of the First Amendment, this Court has explained that "[t]he victory for freedom of thought recorded in our Bill of Rights recognizes that in the domain of conscience there is a moral power higher than the State." *Girouard v. United States*, 328 U.S. 61, 68 (1946). And, in a number of Due Process cases, this Court has protected this conception of autonomy by carving out a sphere of personal family life that is immune from government intrusion. See, e.g., *Cleveland Bd. of Educ. v. LeFleur*, 414 U.S. 632, 639 (1974) "This Court has long recognized that freedom of personal choice in matters of marriage and family life is one of the liberties protected by the Due Process Clause of the Fourteenth Amendment." *Eisenstadt v. Baird*, 405 U.S. 438, 453 (1973) (recognizing right "to be free from unwarranted governmental intrusion into matters so fundamentally affecting a person as the decision to bear and beget a child"); *Skinner v. Oklahoma*, 316 U.S. 535, 541(1942) (holding unconstitutional a state statute requiring the ster-

ilization of individuals convicted of three offenses, in large part because the state's actions unwarrantedly intruded on marriage and procreation, "one of the basic civil rights of man"); *Loving v. Virginia*, 388 U.S. 1, 12 (1967) (striking down the criminal prohibition of interracial marriages as an infringement of the right to marry and holding that "[t]he freedom to marry has long been recognized as one of the vital personal rights essential to the orderly pursuit of happiness by free men").

These decisions recognize as constitutionally immune from state intrusion that realm in which individuals make "intimate and personal" decisions that define the very character of their lives. See Charles Fried, *Right and Wrong* 146—47 (1978) ("What a person is, what he wants, the determination of his life plan, of his concept of the good, are the most intimate expressions of self-determination, and by asserting a person's responsibility for the results of this self-determination, we give substance to the concept of liberty."

2. In that case, the parents of Nancy Cruzan, a woman who was in a persistent vegetative state following an automobile accident, asked the Missouri courts to authorize doctors to end life support and therefore her life. The Supreme Court held that Missouri was entitled to demand explicit evidence that Ms. Cruzan had made a decision that she would not wish to be kept alive in those circumstances, and to reject the evidence the family had offered as inadequate. But a majority of justices assumed, for the sake of the argument, that a competent patient has a right to reject life-preserving treatment, and it is now widely assumed that the Court would so rule in an appropriate case.

3. When state protocols are observed, sometimes the patient is permitted to die and sometimes not. *See, e.g., In re Tavel*, 661 A.2d 1061 (Del. 1995) (affirming finding that petitioner-daughter had proven by clear and convincing evidence that incompetent patient would want life-support systems removed); *In re Martin*, 450 Mich. 204, 538 N.W.2d 399 (1995) (holding that wife's testimony and affidavit did not constitute clear and convincing evidence of incompetent patient's pre-injury decision to decline life-sustaining medical treatment in patient's present circumstances); *DiGrella v. Elston*, 858 S.W.2d 698, 710 (Ky. 1993) ("If the attending physician, the hospital or nursing home ethics committee where the patient resides, and the legal guardian or next of kin all agree and document the patient's wishes and condition, and if no one disputes their decision, no court order is required to proceed to carry out [an incompetent] patient's wishes"); *Mack v. Mack*, 329 Md. 188, 618 A.2d 744 (1993) (holding that wife failed to provide clear and convincing evidence that incompetent husband would want life support removed); *In re Doe*, 411 Mass. 512, 583 N.E.2d 1263 (applying doctrine of substituted judgment and holding that evidence supported finding that, if incompetent patient were capable of making a choice, she would remove life support).

4. For example, 46 percent of California voters supported Proposition 161, which would have legalized physician-assisted suicide, in November 1992. The measure was a proposed amendment to Cal. Penal Code ° 401 (1992) which currently makes assisted suicide a felony. Those who did not vote for the measure cited mainly religious reasons or concerns that the proposed law was flawed because it lacked safeguards against abuse and needed more restrictions that might be easily added, such as a waiting period and a psychological examination. Alison C. Hall, *To Die With Dignity: Comparing Physician-Assisted Suicide in the United States, Japan, and the Netherlands*, 74 Wash. U.L.Q. 803, 817 n.84 (1996).

5. In November 1994, Oregon voters approved the Oregon Death With Dignity Act through voter initiative, legalizing physician-assisted suicide under limited circumstances. Oregon Death With Dignity Act, Or. Rev. Stat. °° 127.800-.827 (1995). The Act provides specific definitions of essential terms such as "incapable" and "terminal disease." The Act also provides numerous other regulations designed to safeguard the integrity of the process.

Appendix D

The Oregon Death With Dignity Act

Ballot Measure No. 16

Oregon Revised Statutes, 1996 Supplement §127.800–127.897

Section I: General Provisions

1.01 Definitions

The following words and phrases, whenever used in this Act, shall have the following meanings:

(1) "Adult" means an individual who is 18 years of age or older.

(2) "Attending physician" means the physician who has primary responsibility for the care of the patient and treatment of the patient's disease.

(3) "Consulting physician" means the physician who is qualified by specialty or experience to make a professional diagnosis and prognosis regarding the patient's disease.

(4) "Counseling" means a consultation between a state licensed psychiatrist or psychologist and a patient for the purpose of determining whether the patient is suffering from a psychiatric or psychological disorder, or depression causing impaired judgment.

(5) "Health care provider" means a person licensed, certified, or otherwise authorized or permitted by the law of this State to administer health care in the ordinary course of business or practice of a profession, and includes a health care facility.

(6) "Incapable" means that in the opinion of a court or in the opinion of the patient's attending physician or consulting physician, a patient lacks the ability to make and communicate health care decisions to health care providers, including communication through persons familiar with the patient's manner of communicating if those persons are available. Capable means not incapable.

(7) "Informed decision" means a decision by a qualified patient, to request and obtain a prescription to end his or her life in a humane and dignified manner, that is based on an appreciation of the relevant facts and after being fully informed by the attending physician of:

(a) his or her medical diagnosis;

(b) his or her prognosis:

(c) the potential risks associated with taking the medication to be prescribed;

(d) the probable result of taking the medication to be prescribed;

(e) the feasible alternatives, including, but not limited to, comfort care, hospice care and pain control.

(8) "Medically confirmed" means the medical opinion of the attending physician has been confirmed by a consulting physician who has examined the patient and the patient's relevant medical records.

(9) "Patient" means a person who is under the care of a physician.

(10) "Physician" means a doctor of medicine or osteopathy licensed to practice medicine by the Board of Medical Examiners for the State of Oregon.

(11) "Qualified patient" means a capable adult who is a resident of Oregon and has satisfied the requirements of this Act in order to obtain a prescription for medication to end his or her life in a humane and dignified manner.

(12) "Terminal disease" means an incurable and irreversible disease that has been medically confirmed and will, within reasonable medical judgment, produce death within six (6) months.

Section 2: Written Request for Medication to End One's Life in a Humane and Dignified Manner

2.01 Who may initiate a written request for medication

An adult who is capable, is a resident of Oregon, and has been determined by the attending physician and consulting physician to be suffering from a terminal disease, and who has voluntarily expressed his or her wish to die, may make a written request for medication for the purpose of ending his or her life in a humane and dignified manner in accordance with this Act.

2.02 Form of the written request

(1) A valid request for medication under this Act shall be in substantially the form described in Section 6 of this Act, signed and dated by the patient and witnessed by at least two individuals who, in the presence of the patient, attest that to the best of their knowledge and belief the patient is capable, acting voluntarily, and is not being coerced to sign the request.

(2) One of the witnesses shall be a person who is not:

(a) A relative of the patient by blood, marriage or adoption;
(b) A person who at the time the request is signed would be entitled to any portion of the estate of the qualified patient upon death under any will or by operation of law; or
(c) An owner, operator or employee of a health care facility where the qualified patient is receiving medical treatment or is a resident.

(3) The patient's attending physician at the time the request is signed shall not be a witness.

(4) If the patient is a patient in a long term care facility at the time the written request is made, one of the witnesses shall be an individual designated by the facility and having the qualifications specified by the Department of Human Resources by rule.

Section 3: Safeguards

3.01 Attending physician responsibilities

The attending physician shall:

(1) Make the initial determination of whether a patient has a terminal disease, is capable, and has made the request voluntarily;

(2) Inform the patient of;

(a) his or her medical diagnosis;
(b) his or her prognosis;
(c) the potential risks associated with taking the medication to be prescribed;
(d) the probable result of taking the medication to be prescribed;
(e) the feasible alternatives, including, but not limited to, comfort care, hospice care and pain control.

(3) Refer the patient to a consulting physician for medical confirmation of the diagnosis, and for determination that the patient is capable and acting voluntarily;

(4) Refer the patient for counseling if appropriate pursuant to Section 3.03;

(5) Request that the patient notify next of kin;

(6) Inform the patient that he or she has an opportunity to rescind the request at any time and in any manner, and offer the patient an opportunity to rescind at the end of the 15 day waiting period pursuant to Section 3.06;

(7) Verify, immediately prior to writing the prescription for medication under this Act, that the patient is making an informed decision;

(8) Fulfill the medical record documentation requirements of Section 3.09;

(9) Ensure that all appropriate steps are carried out in accordance with this Act prior to writing a prescription for medication to enable a qualified patient to end his or her life in a humane and dignified manner.

3.02 Consulting Physician Confirmation

Before a patient is qualified under this Act, a consulting physician shall examine the patient and his or her relevant medical records and confirm, in writing, the attending physician's diagnosis that the patient is suffering from a terminal disease, and verify that the patient is capable, is acting voluntarily and has made an informed decision.

3.03 Counseling Referral

If in the opinion of the attending physician or the consulting physician a patient may be suffering from a psychiatric or psychological disorder, or depression causing impaired judgment, either physician shall refer the patient for counseling. No medication to end a patient's life in a humane and dignified manner shall be prescribed until the person performing the counseling determines that the person is not suffering from a psychiatric or psychological disorder, or depression causing impaired judgment.

3.04 Informed decision

No person shall receive a prescription for medication to end his or her life in a humane and dignified manner unless he or she has made an informed decision as defined in Section 1.01(7). Immediately prior to writing a prescription for medication under this Act, the attending physician shall verify that the patient is making an informed decision.

3.05 Family notification

The attending physician shall ask the patient to notify next of kin of his or her request for medication pursuant to this Act. A patient who declines or is unable to notify next of kin shall not have his or her request denied for that reason.

3.06 Written and oral requests

In order to receive a prescription for medication to end his or her life in a humane and dignified manner, a qualified patient shall have made an oral request and a written request, and reiterate the oral request to his or her attending physician no less than fifteen (15) days after making the initial oral request. At the time the qualified patient makes his or her second oral request, the attending physician shall offer the patient an opportunity to rescind the request.

3.07 Right to rescind request

A patient may rescind his or her request at any time and in any manner without regard to his or her mental state. No prescription for medication under this Act may be written without the attending physician offering the qualified patient an opportunity to rescind the request.

3.08 Waiting periods

No less than fifteen (15) days shall elapse between the patient's initial and oral request and the writing of a prescription under this Act. No less than 48 hours shall elapse between the patient's written request and the writing of a prescription under this Act.

3.09 Medical record documentation requirements

The following shall be documented or filed in the patient's medical record:

(1) All oral requests by a patient for medication to end his or her life in a humane and dignified manner;

(2) All written requests by a patient for medication to end his or her life in a humane and dignified manner;

(3) The attending physician's diagnosis and prognosis, determination that the patient is capable, acting voluntarily and has made an informed decision.

(4) The consulting physician's diagnosis and prognosis, and verification that the patient is capable, acting voluntarily and has made an informed decision;

(5) A report of the outcome and determinations made during counseling, of performed;

(6) The attending physician's offer to the patient to rescind his or her request at the time of the patient's second oral request pursuant to Section 3.06; and

(7) A note by the attending physician indicating that all requirements under this Act have been met and indicating the steps taken to carry out the request, including a notation of the medication prescribed.

3.10 Residency requirements

Only requests made by Oregon residents, under this Act, shall be granted.

3.11 Reporting requirements

(1) The Health Division shall annually review a sample of records maintained pursuant to this Act.

(2) The Health Division shall make rules to facilitate the collection of information regarding compliance with this Act. The information collected shall not be a public record and may not be made available for inspection by the public.

(3) The Health Division shall generate and make available to the public an annual statistical report of information collected under Section 3.11(2) of this Act.

3.12 Effect on construction of wills, contracts and statutes

(1) No provision in a contract, will or other agreement, whether written or oral, to the extent the provision would affect whether a person may make or rescind a request for medication to end his or her life in a humane and dignified manner, shall be valid.

(2) No obligation owing under any currently existing contract shall be conditioned or affected by the making or rescinding of a request, by a person, for medication to end his or her life in a humane and dignified manner.

3.13 Insurance or annuity policies

The sale, procurement, or issuance of any life, health, or accident insurance or annuity policy or the rate charged for any policy shall not be conditioned upon or affected by the making or rescinding of a request, by a person, for medication to end his or her life in a humane and dignified manner. Neither shall a qualified patient's act of ingesting medication to end his or her life in a humane and dignified manner have an effect upon a life, health, or accident insurance or annuity policy.

3.14 Construction of act

Nothing in this Act shall be construed to authorize a physician or any other person to end a patient's life by lethal injection, mercy killing or active euthanasia. Actions taken in accordance with this Act shall not, for any purpose, constitute suicide, assisted suicide, mercy killing or homicide, under the law.

Section 4: Immunities and Liabilities

4.01 Immunities

Except as provided in Section 4.02:

(1) No person shall be subject to civil or criminal liability or professional disciplinary action for participating in good faith compliance with this Act. This includes being present when a qualified patient takes the prescribed medication to end his or her life in a humane and dignified manner.

(2) No professional organization or association, or health care provider, may subject a person to censure, discipline, suspension, loss of license, loss of privileges, loss of membership or other penalty for participating or refusing to participate in good faith compliance with this Act.

(3) No request by a patient for or provision by an attending physician of medication in good faith compliance with the provisions of this Act shall constitute neglect for any purpose of law or provide the sole basis for the appointment of a guardian or conservator.

(4) No health care provider shall be under any duty, whether by contract, by statute or by any other legal requirement to participate in the provision to a qualified patient of medication to end his or her life in a humane and dignified manner. If a health care provider is unable or unwilling to carry out a patient's health care provider shall transfer, upon request, a copy of the patient's relevant medical records to the new health care provider.

4.02 Liabilities

(1) A person who without authorization of the patient willfully alters or forges a request for medication or conceals or destroys a rescission of that request with the intent or effect of causing the patient's death shall be guilty of a Class A felony.

(2) A person who coerces or exerts undue influence on a patient to request medication for the purpose of ending the patient's life, or to destroy a rescission of such a request, shall be guilty of a Class A felony.

(3) Nothing in this Act limits further liability for civil damages resulting from other negligent conduct or intentional misconduct by any persons.

(4) The penalties in this Act do not preclude criminal penalties applicable under other law for conduct which is inconsistent with the provisions of this Act.

Section 5: Severability

5.01 Severability

Any section of this Act being held invalid as to any person or circumstance shall not affect the application of any other section of this Act which can be given full effect without the invalid section or application.

Section 6: Form of the Request

6.01 Form of the request

A request for a medication as authorized by this Act shall be in substantially the following form:

REQUEST FOR MEDICATION
TO END MY LIFE IN A HUMANE AND DIGNIFIED MANNER

I, _____, am an adult of sound mind.

I am suffering from _____, which by my attending physician has determined is a terminal disease and which has been medically formed by a consulting physician.

I have been fully informed of my diagnosis, prognosis, the nature of medication to be prescribed and potential associated risks, the expected result, and the feasible alternatives, including comfort

care, hospice care and pain control.

I request that my attending physician prescribe medication that will end my life in a humane and dignified manner.

INITIAL ONE:

_____ I have informed my family of my decision and taken their opinions into consideration.

_____ I have decided not to inform my family of my decision.

_____ I have no family to inform of my decision.

I understand that I have the right to rescind this request at any time.

I understand the full import of this request and I expect to die when I take the medication to be prescribed.

I make this request voluntarily and without reservation, and I accept full moral responsibility for my actions.

Signed: _____

Dated: _____

DECLARATION OF WITNESSES

We declare that the person signing this request:

(a) Is personally known to us or has provided proof of identity;

(b) Signed this request in our presence;

(c) Appears to be of sound mind and not under duress, fraud or undue influence;

(d) Is not a patient for whom either of us is attending physician.

_____ Witness
1/ Date

_____ Witness
2/ Date

NOTE: One witness shall not be a relative (by blood, marriage or adoption) of the person signing this request, shall not be entitled to any portion of the person's estate upon death and shall not own, operate or be employed at a health care facility where the person is a patient or resident. If the patient is an inpatient at a health care facility, one of the witnesses shall be an individual designated by the facility.

Contributors

Felicia Ackerman is Professor of Philosophy at Brown University. Her philosophy publications range over various areas, including medical ethics, philosophy in literature, methodology of analytic philosophy, philosophy of language, epistemology, and metaphysics. She is also a writer whose short stories, many of which deal with illness and medical treatment, have appeared in ten magazines and one O. Henry Awards collection.

John D. Arras is Porterfield Professor of Bioethics and Professor of Philosophy at the University of Virginia, where he directs the undergraduate bioethics program. A Fellow of the Hastings Center and former member of the New York State Task Force on Life and the Law, Professor Arras's current work focuses on problems of method in practical ethics. In addition to authoring numerous articles on a broad range of issues in bioethics, he is the editor of *Bringing the Hospital Home: Ethical and Social Implications of High-Tech Home Care* (Johns Hopkins) and coeditor with Bonnie Steinbock of *Ethical Issues in Modern Medicine*, 4th ed. (Mayfield). He has previously taught philosophy and bioethics at the Albert Einstein College of Medicine–Montefiore Medical Center, Barnard College, SUNY-Purchase, and the University of Redlands.

Margaret Pabst Battin is Professor of Philosophy and Adjunct Professor of Internal Medicine, Division of Medical Ethics, at the University of Utah. She is a graduate of Bryn Mawr College, and holds an M.F.A. in fiction-writing and a Ph.D. in philosophy from the University of California at Irvine. The author of prize-winning short stories, she has authored, edited, or coedited eleven books, among them a study of philosophical issues in suicide; a scholarly edition of John Donne's *Biathanatos*; a collection on age-rationing of medical care; *Puzzles About Art*, a volume of case-puzzles in aesthetics; a text on professional ethics; and *Ethics in the Sanctuary*, a study of ethical issues in organized religion. She has also been engaged in research on active euthanasia and assisted suicide in the Netherlands. A collection of her essays on end-of-life issues written over the last fifteen years is entitled, *The Least Worst Death*, and she has recently published *Ethical Issues in Suicide*, trade-titled *The Death Debate*, as well as an edited collection *Drug Use in Euthanasia and Assited Suicide*. She is currently at work on a book on world population growth and reproductive rights.

Bernard (Stefan) Baumrin is Professor of Philosophy at the City University of New York. He teaches at the Graduate School, Lehman College, and Mount Sinai School of Medicine. He took his Ph.D. at the Johns Hopkins University, and his J.D. at

Columbia School of Law, and is a partner in the law firm of Baumrin, Galub, and Volkomer in New York. His primary work has been in philosophy of science and in ethical theory and its history.

Jerome E. Bickenbach teaches in the Department of Philosophy, the Faculties of Law and Medicine, and the School of Physical Rehabilitation at Queen's University, Kingston, Canada. He is the author of *Physical Disability and Social Policy* (Toronto, 1993) and focus his research interests entirely on social policy aspects of physical and mental disablement.

K. Danner Clouser is University Professor of Humanities Emeritus at Penn State University College of Medicine. He is a Senior Member of the Institute of Medicine and a recipient of The Hastings Center Henry Beecher Award. A charter member of the Editorial Board of *The Journal of Medicine and Philosophy*, Professor Clouser was also an editor of the *Encyclopedia of Bioethics* (1978) and the *Encyclopedia of Philosophy Supplement* (1996). He is the author of *Teaching Bioethics: Strategies, Problems, and Resources* (1980), and the coauthor of *Morality and the New Genetics: A Guide for Students and Health Care Providers* (1996), and *Bioethics: A Return to Fundamentals* (1997).

Cynthia B. Cohen, Ph.D., J.D. is a Senior Research Fellow at the Kennedy Institute of Ethics at Georgetown University and a member of the Standing Commission on National Concerns of the Protestant Episcopal Church. She has served as Associate for Ethical Studies at The Hastings Center, Executive Director of the National Advisory Board on Ethics in Reproduction, and Chair of the Philosophy Department at the University of Denver. Dr. Cohen has published numerous articles and books on ethical and legal questions that arise at the beginning and end of life.

Charles M. Culver is Professor of Medical Education in the School of Graduate Medical Science at Barry University in Miami Shores, Florida. He is also Adjunct Professor of Psychiatry and Behavioral Science at the University of Miami School of Medicine, and Adjunct Professor of Public Health in the School of Public Health at Florida International University. He is the editor of *Ethics at the Bedside* (1990); and the coauthor of *Philosophy in Medicine: Conceptual and Medical Issues in Medicine and Psychiatry* (1982), *Morality and the New Genetics: A Guide for Students and Health Care Providers* (1996), and *Bioethics: A Return to Fundamentals* (1997).

Dena S. Davis, J.D., Ph.D., is an Associate Professor at Cleveland-Marshall College of Law, Cleveland State University. She has been a Fulbright Scholar in India and an Ethics Fellow at the Cleveland Clinic. She is the author of numerous articles on death and dying, as well as on genetic ethics, and writes the "Legal Trends in Bioethics" column for *The Journal of Clinical Ethics*.

Leslie Pickering Francis is a Professor of Law, Professor of Philosophy, and a member of the Division of Medical Ethics in the Department of Internal Medicine at the University of Utah. She received her Ph.D. in philosophy from the University of Michigan in 1974 and her J.D from the University of Utah in 1981. She was a law clerk to Judge Abner Mikva of the United States Court of Appeals for the District of Columbia Circuit in 1981–82. Professor Francis specializes in health law, bioethics, and legal ethics. She is the author of a number of articles on issues in philosophy of law, healthcare, and professional ethics. She is currently a member of the American Law Institute, of the American Bar Association's Commission on the Legal Problems of the Elderly, of the Executive Committee of the Pacific Division of the American Philosophical Association, and of the Utah State Bar's Ethics Advisory Opinion Committee. She also chairs the American Philosophical Association's Committee for the Defense of the Professional Rights of Philosophers.

Bernard Gert is Eunice and Julian Cohen Professor for the Study of Ethics and Human Values at Dartmouth College and Adjunct Professor of Psychiatry at Dartmouth Medical School. He is author of *The Moral Rules: A New Rational Foundation for Morality* (1970, 1973, and 1975, German edition, 1983), *Morality: A New Justification of the Moral Rules* (1988), and *Morality: Its Nature and Justification* (1998); editor of *Man and Citizen* by Thomas Hobbes, (1972, 1978, 1991); co-author of *Philosophy in Medicine: Conceptual and Ethical Issues In Medicine and Psychiatry* (1982, Japanese edition, 1984), *Morality and the New Genetics: A Guide for Students and Health Care Providers* (1996), and *Bioethics: A Return to Fundamentals*, (1997).

F. M. Kamm is Professor of Philosophy and Adjunct Professor of Law at New York University and Visiting Professor of Philosophy at UCLA. She has published many articles on normative ethical theory and practical ethics and is the author of three books, *Creation and Abortion* (Oxford University Press, 1992); *Morality, Mortality, vol. 1: Death and Whom to Save From It*; and *Morality, Mortality, vol. 2: Rights, Duties, and Status* (Oxford University Press, 1993 and 1996 respectively).

Patricia A. King is the Carmack Waterhouse Professor of Law, Medicine, Ethics, and Public Policy at Georgetown University Law Center in Washington, DC. She received a J.D. from Harvard Law School in1969 and a B.A. from Wheaton College in 1963.

Helga Kuhse is Associate Professor at Monash University in Melbourne, Australia and Director of the Monash University Centre for Human Bioethics. She has published widely in the field of bioethics, and her books include: *The Sanctity-of-Life Doctrine in Medicine: A Critique* (Oxford University Press, 1987); *Should the Baby Live?: The Problem of Handicapped Infants*, with Peter Singer (Oxford University Press, 1984); *Caring: Nurses, Women and Ethics* (Blackwell, 1997); and the collection *Willing to Listen—Wanting to Die* (Penguin Books, 1994). Helga Kuhse is editor of *Monash Bioethics Review* and, with Peter Singer, coeditor of *Bioethics*. Professor Kuhse is a member of a number of ethics committees and has acted as an Expert Witness for the Northern Territory of Australia on the Rights of the Terminally Ill Act, and for the Australian Senate, in its Inquiry into the Euthanasia Laws Bill.

Patricia S. Mann is in the Philosophy Department at Hofstra University. Her book, *Micro-Politics: Agency in a Postfeminist Era* (Minnesota, 1994), analyzes the dynamics of women's empowerment over the last twenty-five years. In *Unmoored in the*

Twenty-First Century, Mann will show how changing gender relations provide a key for rethinking modern theories of selfhood and agency, thereby enabling a better grasp of contemporary issues such as assisted suicide.

Don Marquis is Professor of Philosophy at the University of Kansas. He was chair of the American Philosophical Association Committee on Philosophy and Medicine from 1995 to 1998. He has published a widely reprinted essay on abortion.

Merrill Matthews, Jr., Ph.D., is Vice President of Domestic Policy and director of the Center for Health Policy Studies at the National Center for Policy Analysis. He regularly travels to Washington, D.C., to brief members of Congress on healthcare issues and testifies frequently before congressional committees. He is a frequent guest on numerous radio and television talk venues, including C-SPAN, CNN, and Fox News. Articles and reviews written by Dr. Matthews have been published in the *Wall Street Journal, Investor's Business Daily, The Washington Times*, and several other magazines and newspapers. Dr. Matthews received a B.B.A. in economics from the University of Texas at Arlington, a master's degree in divinity from Southwest Baptist Theological Seminary, and a Ph.D. in philosophy and humanities from the University of Texas at Dallas.

Michael P. Moreland, a graduate of the University of Notre Dame, is a doctoral candidate in theological ethics at Boston College.

David Orentlicher is an Associate Professor and codirector of the Center for Law and Health at the Indiana University School of Law, Indianapolis, where he teaches courses in bioethics, constitutional law, and professional responsibility. He is also an Adjunct Associate Professor of Medicine at Indiana University School of Medicine. Previously, he served as the Director of the Division of Medical Ethics at the American Medical Association, drafting guidelines for the medical profession on a wide range of issues, including end-of-life decision-making, healthcare access and rationing, organ transplantation, genetic testing, and physicians' conflicts of interests. During the 1997–98 academic year, he was the Visiting DeCamp Professor of Bioethics at Princeton University. He is a member of the American Law Institute, was a George E. Allen Professor of Law at the University of Richmond's T.C. Williams School of Law, and served on the founding board of the American Association of Bioethics. He is a coauthor of *Health Care Law and Ethics* and authored or coauthored numerous articles in leading medical and legal journals. He has most recently written about physician-assisted suicide, healthcare rationing, and the impact of managed care on the patient-physician relationship. He has an A.B. From Brandeis University and an M.D. and J.D. from Harvard University.

Rev. John J. Paris, S.J., is the Michael P. Walsh Professor of Bioethics at Boston College. He is also Clinical Professor of Family Medicine and Community Health at Tufts Medical School and Adjunct Professor of Medicine at the University of Massachusetts Medical School. He has served as consultant to the President's Commission for the Study of Ethics in Medicine, the United States Senate Committee on Aging, and the Congressional Office of Technology Assessment. Fr. Paris has published over 100 articles on law, medicine, and ethics. He has served as a consultant and expert witness in many of the landmark biomedical cases including *Quinlan*, *Brophy*, *Jobes*, *Baby K*, and *Gilgunn*.

Rosamond Rhodes, Ph.D., is Associate Professor of Medical Education and Director of Bioethics Education at the Mount Sinai School of Medicine, CUNY. Outside of Mount Sinai, she teaches in the CUNY Graduate School MALS Program in Bioethics, Science, and Society. Dr. Rhodes also serves as editor of the American Philosophical Association's *Newsletter on Philosophy and Medicine*. In her own writing she has focused on the work of Hobbes and Aristotle and a variety of bioethical issues relating to the doctor-patient relationship, transplantation, genetics, reproduction, and psychiatry.

Anita Silvers, Professor of Philosophy at San Francisco State University, is the author of more than fifty academic publications in ethics and bioethics, disability studies, aesthetics, and public policy. She is a long-time disability advocate who also writes for the popular press. She is a member of the Board of Officers of the American Philosophical Association, a former member of the National Endowment for the Humanities' National Council, and a former Trustee of the American Society for Aesthetics. In 1978 she was California's Distinguished Humanist and in 1989 the first recipient of the California Faculty Association's Equal Rights Award.

Lance Stell is the Charles A. Dana Professor of Philosophy and Department Chair at Davidson College. He is also the Medical Ethicist at the Carolinas Medical Center. He has published in the fields of ethics, philosophy of law, and political philosophy.

Michael Teitelman, Ph.D., M.D., is an Assistant Professor in the Department of Psychiatry of Mount Sinai Medical School. For the last seven years, he has served as a clinical psychiatrist in the AIDS Center of Mount Sinai Hospital in New York City.

Allen Verhey, Ph.D. is the Evert J. And Hattie E. Blekkink Professor of Religion at Hope College in Holland, Michigan. His most recent book is *Religion and Medical Ethics*, which he edited.

Leslie E. Wolf is a Greenwall Fellow in Bioethics and Health Policy, Georgetown University and Johns Hopkins University. She has a J.D. from Harvard Law School, 1991; M.P.H. Johns Hopkins School of Hygiene and Public Health, 1997 and an A.B. from Stanford University, 1988.

Noam Zohar, Ph.D., is Senior Lecturer in the Department of Philosophy, Bar Ilan University, teaching rabbinic thought, moral and political philosophy, and courses in ethics and *Halakha*. He is Director of the Graduate Program in Bioethics. He is the author of several journal articles in the above fields, and of *Alternatives in Jewish Bioethics* (SUNY Press, 1997); and coeditor (with Michael Walzer and others) of a multivolume work, *The Jewish Political Tradition*, forthcoming in Yale University Press.

Index

AARP, 76

abortion, 4, 15, 26n.12, 64, 94, 115–16, 207–8, 218, 280, 288, 294, 323, 382, 384–5, 407, 433–4

abuse: of African-Americans, 96–7; of assisted suicide, 3, 25, 92, 339, 388; of persons with disabilities, 124–5, 144, 154; of vulnerable groups, 75, 94, 135, 341, 387, 393; risk of, 63, 340

Ackerman, F., 10

acts: moral significance of, 51; causing death, 233, 235, 254–5, 259–61, 263–4

acts/omissions distinction, 29, 51, 183, 231, 256

African-American(s), 90–122, 151; access to healthcare, 99–105; and medical experimentation, 97–8; and medical research, 97; and PAS, 91–122; and the healthcare system, 91; attitudes regarding death, health and illness, 95; autonomy, 95, 98, 104; community, 74, 99, 218; distrust of the healthcare system, 95–9, 103, 218; experience with the healthcare system, 93–100, 103–4; genocide, 99; health status of, 99, 103; medical schools, 100; mortality rate, 101; patients, 94, 102–3; physicians, 99

age, 97, 100

agency, 14, 18–22; human, 12–13, 244, 289; individual, 18–19; of medical doctors, 22; of women, 18

agency relations, 11, 19–25

AIDS, 68, 99, 101, 110n.61, 150, 221, 282, 315, 317, 318, 439–40

Airedale N.H.S. Trust v. *Bland,* 131

allowing to die, 4, 196, 254, 280, 289, 327, 341, 353

Alzheimer's disease, 68, 114–15, 118, 231, 273, 291

American Bar Association: Commission on the Legal Problems of the Elderly, 75–6, 80, 83, 86

American Medical Association, 183, 386, 395, 418n.14, 425, 428n.6; Council on Ethical and Judicial Affairs, 331; Principles of Ethics, 170

Americans with Disabilities Act of 1990 (ADA), 129, 137–40, 144

amicus curiae briefs, 6, 14, 50, 125, 132n.7, 133, 137, 139–40, 225, 247, 374, 385, 389, 393, 412, 431–41

Amundson, R., 147

Angell, M., 154

Annas, G., 328

Aristotle, 18

Arras, J., 95, 134, 224

artificial nutrition and hydration, 4, 64, 66, 69, 226, 236, 244, 280, 303

assisted suicide, 4, 7, 10, 11, 14–17, 19–25, 29, 51–2, 66, 75–90, 92, 113, 115, 118, 121n.24, 125–6, 129–30, 134, 136, 139, 149–62, 165–6, 173–5, 177, 182, 188, 191, 194–6, 198, 200, 205–8, 210, 213–14, 216, 219, 221, 227–9, 234–6, 238, 245, 252–3, 258, 264, 267, 288–90, 301–6, 306–8, 325, 330–1, 375, 378, 384–5, 387–8, 390, 393–5, 405, 409–10, 423–7, 433, 436–9; and the elderly, 75–90; and the Supreme Court's deci-

sions, 302–3; arguments against, 339–42; arguments for, 337–42; Christian views on, 323–61; constitutional right to, 14–15, 50; Jewish views on, 362–72; legalization of, 16, 253, 328; locus of, 205–6; prohibitions against, 381, 385, 389, 421n.14, 423, 427

Australia and PAS, 5, 224, 252–3, 262–3

autonomy, 3, 14, 17–19, 25, 26n.19, 55, 63, 75, 77–80, 92–3, 96, 105, 114, 123–6, 128–32, 150–1, 158, 165, 169–71, 174, 205, 208–11, 219, 281, 283, 284, 326, 331, 337, 348, 350, 387, 391–2, 404–5, 407, 432–4; and moral issues, 26n.18, 340, 353, 359; individual, 11, 15–16, 24, 324, 329, 360, 364, 384, 391, 431, 439; inequality of, 126–31; patient's. *See* patient, autonomy; values of, 3, 24

Back et al., 319, 320n.7

Bacon, F., 355–6

Barber v. *Superior Court,* 238

barbituates, 211–12, 236, 243, 289, 303

Barrington, M. R., 117

Battin, M., 10, 25, 26n.7, 27n.25, 176n.16

Baumrin, B., 163

beneficence, 165, 169–71, 181

Bergstedt, K., 141

Bernadin, J. C., 327–8, 332

Bible, the, 335. *See* Scripture, Torah

Bickenbach, J., 10, 74

bioethics, 68, 82d, 371, 374, 393

Blackstone, W., 230–2, 378–9, 405

Blanchot, M., 24
Bland, Mr., 131
body, 46, 113, 115; integrity of, 406, 426; invasion of, 405, 434–5; loss of control over one's, 81, 338, 308; right to control one's, 116, 123, 239–40, 382, 396, 405, 407, 426, 435–6
Book of Common Prayer, 337, 340
Bouvier v. *Superior Court*, 249n.15
Bouvier, E., 141, 191, 194
Bradley, Justice, 398
Brandt, K., 136–7
Brandt, R., 249n.20
Brennan, Justice, 227, 391
Breyer, Justice, 302–3, 325, 374, 377, 411, 423, 427
Brock, D., 55–6, 56n.1, 250n.23, 268, 271, 341
Brody, B., 242–3
burden: desire to not be a, 154–8, 268, 276; of end of life healthcare costs, 387; of living, 43, 45, 275
Burt, S., 232
Bush administration, 317

California: and PAS, 2, 203, 229, 381; Natural Death Act of 1976, 66
Callahan, D., 61n.40, 64, 72n.2, 158, 241, 269, 328, 330
Callahan, S., 115, 118
Campbell, 343
Canada, 5, 131; criminal code regarding assisted suicide, 123
Canadian Charter of Rights and Freedom, 123
cancer, 65, 67–8, 101, 114–15, 209, 282–3, 286, 303, 315, 439
Cantor, N., 248n.3
capitation systems, 143, 213, 285
Cardozo, Judge, 405
care, 4, 16, 23, 68, 187, 347, 354–7; comfort, 5, 85; costs of, 6, 206, 312–22; home, 206, 219; long-term, 81, 314; medical, 118, 157, 171, 206–7, 221, 239, 272–4, 282, 302, 355, 391, 396, 406–7; of the dying, 4, 6, 91, 104,

312–13, 327, 328, 339, 350; palliative. *See* palliative care; quality of, 213, 317
caregivers, 69, 142, 331, 440
Catholic(s): church, 2, 7, 207; hospitals, 7, 208; patients, 7; views on death, 326–7; views on PAS, 208, 324–33
Christian(s), 115, 334–6, 338–9, 350, 353–4; communities, 348, 352–4; moral principles, 335, 343; perspectives on PAS, 334–46; traditions, 335–9, 342, 359
Civil Rights Act of 1964, 100
Clinton, President Bill, 64, 317, 381
Clouser, K.D., 10, 164
Coalition of Provincial Organizations of the Handicap (COPOH), 124–6, 129–30
coercion, 127–8, 393; and assisted suicide, 75, 91, 126, 437; of vulnerable groups, 135, 387; risks of, 76, 92
cognitive capacities, 77–80, 83, 139
Cohen, C., 323
coma, 49–50, 64, 152, 180, 211, 303–4
Committee on Medical Ethics of the Episcopal Diocese of Washington, 334
common law, 378–80, 384, 391–2, 402–3, 405, 414n.9, 425–6
Commonweatlh Euthanasia Laws Bill 1996, 252–3
communitarian: ethics, 134, 147; perspectives, 73, 156
community, 133–5, 144, 147, 156–7, 274, 336, 347, 390; welfare, 73, 338, 340, 343
compassion, 349, 350, 409
Compassion in Dying v. *Washington*, 6–7, 62n.49, 93–4, 115–16, 238, 255, 287, 373, 377–8, 390, 414n.8, 415n.18, 418n.1, 434, 440
competence, 75, 77–81, 84, 87–8, 91, 130–1, 134, 138–9, 141, 144–6, 149–50, 155, 226, 229, 263, 271, 273, 396, 424
competent adults, 378, 381, 383–4, 389–90, 396, 423, 426, 432, 437–8
consent, 37, 46, 97–8, 252–66,

307, 318, 384, 438; informed, 184, 237–8, 247, 384
constitutional law, 1, 287–8
contraception, 15, 66, 113–22, 382, 384, 403–4, 409
Coronary Artery Surgery Study, 102–3
Critchley, Simon, 11, 24
Cruzan v. *Missouri*, 4, 50, 53, 141, 225–8, 377–80, 383–5, 387, 389, 391–2, 395, 400, 402, 405–6, 412, 418n.11, 419n.10, 426, 433–6, 437
Cruzan, N., 62n.45, 226, 383, 391–2, 418, 441n.2
cultural: changes, 65, 69, 86; contexts, 9, 11, 65, 94, 96; differences, 102, 104, 262; expectations, 23–4; practices, 69–71, 97
culture, 13, 20, 25, 66, 69, 96, 338
Culver, C., 10, 164
Curran, C., 117

Daniels, N., 85, 89n.29
Davis, D., 10, 74
death, 4, 12, 14, 17, 20, 23, 28–9, 31, 32–3, 35, 37–9, 42–9, 56, 63, 66–8, 70–1, 84, 86–7, 95, 114, 128–9, 132, 134, 142, 150, 165, 172, 179, 190, 192, 195, 197, 200, 227, 229, 235, 239, 244, 254, 260, 267, 270, 281, 282, 287–8, 290, 306, 323, 330, 338, 343, 351, 353, 356, 360, 374, 378, 388, 396, 408, 431, 433, 435, 438; as a lesser evil, 48, 50, 53–4, 196; as a side effect of drugs, 47–8, 50, 60n.32; as suicide, 230–6; attitudes about, 9, 11, 66, 70; cause of, 30, 40, 51, 195, 226, 230, 241–3, 255–6, 289, 301, 435; choices regarding, 70, 357, 360, 365; comprehending, 11–14; foreseeing, 42–3, 46, 51, 327; good, 205, 329, 343; hastening of, 166, 168, 171–3, 194–5, 198–200, 217, 228, 258, 260–2, 280, 288, 307, 337, 378, 384, 387, 391, 393–4, 396, 407, 418n.12, 423–7, 431, 435, 439; imminence of, 35, 180, 219, 342,

366, 389, 396, 404, 407–8; intended, 28–62, 226, 234, 236, 327, 425; meaning of, 11–27, 281, 323, 325, 327, 334; means of, 28, 301; mystery of, 13, 20, 24; natural, 73, 225–6, 240–4, 366; unnatural, 225–6, 244; with dignity, 92, 149; wrongful, 125, 168, 320

Death With Dignity Act, 1, 2, 83–4, 145, 229, 375, 381, 441n.5, 443–8

Declaration of Independence, 353

dementia, 49, 79, 113–15, 119, 139, 208, 220, 388

dependency, 24–5, 81, 118, 151, 359, 393, 407

depression, 3, 65, 75, 77, 139–40, 145, 185, 208–11, 269, 271, 282, 285, 288, 291, 307, 318, 324, 386, 393–4, 436; and the elderly, 79–83; clinical, 113, 150, 172, 209–10, 220, 247, 270, 274, 282, 285, 293, 295; major, 82, 84, 87, 209; suicidal, 210; treatment of. *See* psychotherapeutic intervention

Derrida, J., 12–13, 20

Descartes, R., 18

DeVries, P., 347–8

diabetes, 101, 146

dignity, 43, 48, 91, 94, 104, 114, 123, 125, 171, 281, 290, 331, 354, 391, 396, 432; human, 151–2, 159n.9, 170, 337, 426, 431, 439; loss of, 151–2, 269

disability(ies), 137–41, 146–7, 327; advocacy groups, 123–5, 127, 147, 154, 158; and despair, 139–41; and life-ending decisions, 123–32, 133–48; people with, 5, 74, 80, 92–3, 119, 124–32, 133–48, 149–62, 193, 274, 341, 387, 393; rights, 138; severe, 74, 130, 149–62, 195, 388

Disability-Adjusted Life Year, 127

discrimination: against people with disabilities, 74, 124–5, 128, 133–48, 154, 292; against terminally ill people,

257–8; against the poor, 285; lethal, 125; regarding assisted suicide, 74, 293

disease, 65, 67, 70, 79, 98, 117, 127, 168, 179, 193, 209, 215–17, 221, 225–6, 230, 242, 268, 307, 319, 355, 395; chronic, 146, 208; terminal, 209, 325, 331, 440, 444; underlying, 255, 258, 301–6, 325, 425

DNR (Do Not Resuscitate) orders, 66, 76–77, 229, 237, 239

do no harm, 37, 179, 242, 353

Doctors Without Borders, 179

doctrine of creation, 337, 339

Doctrine of the Faith, 326

Doe v. *Bolton,* 288

Doerflinger, R., 16

Donne, J., 336, 390

Double Effect, 33–4, 256–9, 261, 305

drug(s), 44–5, 48–9, 63–4, 181, 196, 255, 303, 413; pain-relieving, 69, 194, 280, 425; suicide, 178, 228, 260–1, 264, 306, 387, 396, 424, 440

Due Process Clause, 15, 92, 292, 381–5, 388–91, 397–403, 409, 411, 417n.10, 418n.3, 432–6, 440n.1

Dutch Royal Society of Medicine, the, 318

duty: of beneficence, 170–1; to die, 156; to live, 36, 45, 275; to prolong life, 184–5, 281, 324, 326; to protect, 73, 133–48, 326; to relieve pain, 35, 281–2; to relieve suffering, 36, 281–2; to respect patients, 170; to treat, 186

Dworkin et al., 51–3, 133, 271, 297n.33, 431–41

Dworkin, R., 19–20, 26n.14, 28, 50, 53, 130, 133, 153, 160n.23, 271, 281, 330, 393. *See also* Philosophers' Brief; *Life's Dominion,* 15, 17, 271

dying, 23–4, 64, 66–8, 213, 268, 270, 272, 295, 323, 328, 331, 336–7, 341, 343, 347, 349–55, 408; aid in, 75, 178; assisted, 69, 71; cost of, 22–4, 312, 313–15, 387, 409; manner of, 66, 69; patients. *See* patients, dying; person,

16, 17, 22, 206, 337, 384, 412, 438; process of, 15, 21, 23, 25, 86, 332, 338; self-directed, 63, 66, 70; with dignity, 94, 105

elderly, the, 5, 23–4, 73–7, 92, 135, 139, 146–7, 151, 193, 230, 274, 285, 324, 341, 386–8; advocates for, 75–6; and assisted suicide, 75–90; autonomy of, 80–3

Emanuel, E., 236–7, 269, 314–15

Emanuel, L.L., 314–15

end of life, 43, 77, 91–3, 219, 340, 387, 413; agency at the, 17–19; care, 4, 91, 104–5, 219–20; decisions, 91, 94–5, 104–5, 117, 123–32, 204, 211, 252, 254–7, 259, 261–2, 263–4, 273–4, 381, 383, 389, 391, 407; decisions and physician responsibility, 171–3; medical request form, 448; treatment, 95, 260

Epicurus, 12

Episcopal Diocese of Newark: *Newark Report,* 337–40

Epstein, R., 228, 249n.15

Equal Protection Clause, 92, 228, 280, 288–9, 292, 373, 377, 394–5, 400, 418n.3, 423–4

equality, 125–6, 131, 137

euthanasia, 2, 3, 4, 28–62, 67, 95, 143, 165–6, 169, 171–2, 174–5, 199, 202n.22, 211–13, 217, 252–66, 279–80, 281–2, 287, 290–1, 301–9, 310n.13, 318–19, 324, 330, 334–46, 366, 373, 385–6, 393, 397, 408–10, 426–7; active, 28, 30, 55–6, 76, 183–5, 293–4, 327–31, 366, 372n.7; active voluntary, 91, 94; arguments against, 282–6, 339–42; arguments for, 32–6, 47–50, 281–2, 337–42; Christian view on, 334–46; duty to perform, 35–6; involuntary, 124, 178, 193, 211–12, 217–18, 262, 318, 324, 338, 387–8, 408–9; Jewish views on, 362–72; legalization of, 253, 258–9, 328; moral responsibility for, 54–6;

euthanasia *(cont.)*
  passive, 28, 30, 183–4, 327, 329, 366; terminal sedation as a form of, 304–6; voluntary, 30, 76, 124, 178, 193, 211–13, 217, 252–3, 256, 258–9, 262–4, 324, 341, 349, 358, 366, 387–8, 408–9; voluntary active, 182–4, 187–8, 192, 196, 198–9; voluntary passive, 182–4, 187, 192, 196, 198–9
Euthanasia Laws Act, 258, 262
exploitation: of African-Americans, 96–7, 218; of vulnerable groups, 93–4

family members, 4, 55, 69, 81, 205–6, 214, 216–17, 273, 275, 285–6, 289, 291, 317, 320, 330, 353, 387, 389, 393, 397
Farley, W., 338
Farrakhan, L., 98–9
Federal Assisted Suicide Funding Restriction Act of 1997, 381
federal social spending, 81, 100
feminist(s), 18, 115–6, 118–19, 120n.7; views on PAS, 113–22
Fifth Amendment, 281, 397–8
Final Exit, 2
First Amendment, 440n.1
Fletcher, J., 336
food and fluids: refusal of, 182, 192–3, 195, 197–200, 201n.16, 230, 273, 384; witholding of, 187, 190, 194, 196, 301, 304–5, 308–9, 391, 407
Foot, P., 174
Foucault, 138
Fourteenth Amendment, 15, 92, 271, 281, 377, 382–3, 385, 390–1, 395, 397–400, 412, 423, 432–6, 440n.1
Fourth Amendment, 403
Francis, L., 74
freedom, 347, 357–60, 392, 412, 426; individual, 145, 274, 343, 393, 395; of choice, 214, 340, 343, 407
Freud, S., 18

Gamble, V.N., 97, 99, 103
gender, 18, 97

Genesis Rabbah, 364
Gert, B., 10, 164
Gill, C., 128, 159n.22
Ginsberg, Justice, 303, 374, 377, 411, 417, 423, 427
Glucksberg, H., 377, 395
greater: evil, 33, 42, 44, 49; good, 32–3, 36, 42, 46–8, 53–4, 339
Griswold v. *Connecticut,* 116
Grossman, H.A., 423

Halakha, the, 362. *See* Hebrew tradition, Jewish tradition, Mishna, Torah
Hall, C.E., 150
Hall, T., 62n.48
Halperin, A., 377
Hanina, Rabbi, 365–8
Hardwig, J., 156
Harlan, Justice, 100, 382, 397, 400, 403–4, 411–12, 415n.17, 419n.9
harm, 37–8, 94, 189, 197, 220, 387, 395; greater, 196; lesser, 38, 196; risk of, 6, 92, 387; social, 143, 279
Harrison, B., 119
Harvey, D., 157
Hawking, S., 153
healing, 347, 354–7, 387, 394, 426
health: insurance, 101, 138, 217, 295, 312, 313, 316, 341, 446; professionals, 5, 94, 96, 105, 117; status, 94, 130
Health Care Financing Administration (HCFA), 314
healthcare, 2, 92, 94, 101–2, 137, 154, 164, 204, 272, 318, 426; access to, 6, 81, 83–4, 92, 100–2, 125, 285–6, 293–4, 341, 387; costs, 6, 94, 312–22, 338–9, 387; delivery of, 94, 105; home, 172; insurers, 6, 143; national, 316; organizations, 16, 21–2, 25, 102; preventive, 84; providers, 5, 23, 25, 84, 100, 102, 104–5, 170, 213, 224, 306, 312, 315–17, 343, 443; rationing of, 84–5, 139, 316; system, 5, 91, 93, 95–6, 100–1, 104–5, 141, 217, 286, 293–4, 317–18, 320, 328; workers, 103, 178, 200, 397; zero-sum system of, 316–17
Hebrew tradition, 335. *See* Ha-

lakha, Jewish tradition Mishna, Torah
Hegel, 138
Hehir, J. B., 326–7
Heidegger, M., 13, 14
Hemlock Society, 2, 181, 357
Hendin, H., 269
Hill, T., 61n.33
Hippocratic tradition, 20, 21, 178–9, 213, 328, 331, 354
HIV, 291
HMOs (health maintenance organizations), 22–3, 95, 117, 181, 213, 217, 285, 293, 317, 341, 409
Hobbes, T., 18, 166
Hochschild, A., 23–4
homicide, 166, 168, 212, 227, 229, 230–1, 244–6, 330, 378–9, 385, 425
hospice, 22, 26n.14, 64, 172, 219; care, 16, 23, 84, 294, 313, 315, 351; philosophy, 152
Hospital Survey and Construction Act (Hill-Burton Act), 99–100
hospitalization, 206, 208–11, 214, 219
hospitals, 6, 163, 173, 203, 217–21, 225, 341, 384, 409; and PAS, 203–20; black-controlled, 97
House of Lords Select Committee on Medical Ethics, 253, 257
Humphrey, D., 2
Huntington Disease, 118

illness, 94, 128, 131, 146–7, 206, 208–9, 217, 221, 230, 241, 291, 306, 309, 338, 340–1, 380, 408, 423
immorality, 115, 116
immortality, 12, 13
independent living, 81, 140–1
individualism, 18, 73, 156, 348
Inge, W.R., 336, 337
intended death. *See* death, intended
intention, 40–1, 234, 237–8, 242, 245, 252–66, 289, 302, 304, 325, 394, 425, 436

Jehovah's Witness, 233
Jewish: traditions 208, 362–72. *See* Hebrew tradition, Jewish tradition, Mishna, Torah

Johnson, J.W., 91
Judaeo-Christian tradition, 13, 256
justice, 141, 143, 223, 237, 279, 343, 347, 348–52;
justification, 41, 128, 189, 191, 197, 230, 238, 342, 359, 396; legal, 384, 438; moral, 51, 291

Kamisar, Y., 95, 150, 158, 161n.39, 241
Kamm, F., 10, 86–7
Kant, I., 39, 61n.33, 275
Kass, Dr. L., 325, 331
Kastenbaum, R., 66
Kaveny, M. C., 326
Kemp, E., Jr., 137
Kennedy, Justice, 423
Keown, J., 262
Kevorkian, J., 2, 68, 95, 118, 136, 206, 222n.8, 246, 293, 309, 313, 320, 321, 328, 357
killing, 4, 28, 38, 40–7, 51–2, 54, 166, 168–9, 180, 182–3, 187, 191–2, 201n.9, 242–3, 254, 267, 283, 290, 330, 336, 339–40, 341, 349, 435; analysis of, 187–90; assisted, 47, 50–4; consensual, 351; intentional, 40, 42, 44, 46, 49, 53, 218, 252–3, 324, 330–1, 426; mercy, 143, 229, 256, 330, 349, 381; passive, 29; sanctions against, 323
killing/letting die distinction, 4, 28–9, 168–9, 173, 183–4, 186–7, 240–4, 289–92, 325, 327, 329–30, 341, 347–8, 354, 426
King Saul, 365–9
King, P., 74
Kirk, Bishop, 343
Klagsbrun, S.C., 423
Kleinfeld, Judge A., 238
Kuhse, H., 223, 264n.1

Lamm, Governor, 84
Law Professors' Brief, 247
Lawrence, C., 96
legal restraint, 293–4
Legislative Assembly of the Northern Territory of Australia, 252
lesser evil, 32–6, 41–2, 49, 58n.15, 59n.22; death as a, 48, 50, 53–4

lethal: doses, 178, 188, 226, 229, 235, 246, 273–4, 289–90, 302, 330, 368, 388; drugs, 1, 2, 30–1, 40, 47, 55, 150, 172, 178, 194, 199, 211, 239, 245, 247, 257, 259, 280, 282, 302, 325, 369, 394–5, 408, 418n.15, 423, 435; injection, 28–9, 36, 40, 48, 217, 255, 329–30
letting die, 28, 30, 40–1, 51–3, 168–9, 228, 231–2, 239, 242, 267, 299n.70, 435
letting die/killing distinction. See killing/letting die distinction
Levinas, E., 11, 12–14, 20
Lewin-VHI, 315
liberal tradition, 15, 18, 274, 283
liberty, 166–7, 195, 245, 291, 381–3, 385, 390, 397–403, 411–12, 417n.10, 420n.11, 432, 439–40; interests, 120, 227, 249n.13, 271, 279, 288, 292, 324, 377–8, 382, 384–5, 391–2, 405, 419n.10, 426, 432–6, 437–8
life, 39, 70, 173, 288, 339, 343, 364, 390, 432; destruction of, 337, 355; meaning of, 134, 281, 325, 334; mystery of, 385, 392; preservation of, 124, 143, 227, 324, 355, 378, 385, 392, 395, 426; prolongation of, 15, 63–6, 71, 86, 262, 335–9; quality of, 49, 123, 127–9, 131, 143–4, 151–2, 153, 316, 393; sanctity of, 336, 391–2; span, 65, 68, 85–6, 88, 131, 150; termination of, 69, 124, 252–3, 256, 257–8, 261–3, 267, 365, 396; value of, 144, 256, 271, 362
life-support, 30, 40, 141, 194, 228, 235–6, 257, 280, 373, 384, 393–5, 423–4, 426; termination of, 30, 406, 421n.16, 427, 435–8
lifesaving treatment. See treatment, lifesaving
living wills, 2, 95, 380, 426. See powers of attorney
Lou Gehrig's disease (ALS), 123, 153
Luker, K., 115
Lynn, J., 117, 276

Magna Carta, 397
Maimonides, 336, 364
Malory, Sir T., 149, 153
managed care organizations. See HMOs
mandatory retirement, 79, 81
Mann, P., 9; Micro-Politics, 17
marginalized groups, 135, 142
Marquis, D., 224
Marshall, Chief Justice, 398
martyrdom, 365–7
Marx, K., 138
Matthews, M., 224
May, W.F., 114
McAfee, L., 140–1, 144
McCormick, R., 326
Measure 16, 1, 2, 6, 120, 246, 375, 443–8
Medicaid, 81, 316–17
medical: assistance, 45–6, 94, 117, 228, 267, 406; institutions, 94–5, 97, 104; interventions, 95, 125, 168, 172, 293–4, 302, 304, 308, 329, 387, 406, 434; practice, 4, 68, 92, 168, 204, 206, 208, 213, 217, 220, 263, 291, 356, 396; practitioner, 123, 125; procedures, 117, 407; system, 114, 216; technology, 14–15, 23, 330, 338, 381, 412
medical ethics, 154, 196, 207, 213–17, 242, 312, 318; ethics of the profession, 3, 124, 213, 281, 289, 324, 386, 394
medical profession, 21, 97, 117–18, 136–7, 168, 193, 319, 325, 354, 374, 424
Medicare, 81, 100–1, 110n.53, 314–15; spending, 81, 314
medication, 44, 47, 79, 171, 195, 216, 287, 302–3; fatal effects of, 53, 212, 220, 390. See also lethal drugs; prescription, 50, 387
medicine, 5, 64, 65, 163, 223, 328, 348; distrust of, 97, 104; emergency, 76, 358
mental: health, 77; illness, 65, 139. See also depression
mercy, 54, 267, 281, 283, 284, 291, 347–52; argument for, 268–71
mercy killing. See killing, mercy
Micah, 348

Mill, J.S., 130

Miner, Judge, 280, 289–90, 292

minorities, 5–6, 94–6, 100, 134, 218, 285, 293; disabled, 133; ethnic, 95–6; racial, 95–6

Mishna, the, 363. *See* Talmud

moral: principles, 77, 119, 123, 131, 165, 169, 207, 257

moral difference, 186; between killing and letting die, 51–3

moral responsibility, 54–6, 166, 169, 203, 253–4, 307

morality, 38, 42, 54, 167, 172, 197, 199, 207, 215, 275, 279, 287, 343, 347, 369, 389; and law, 174–5, 279

More, T., 336

morphine, 4, 7, 32–3, 35, 41, 47, 64, 69, 188, 211, 216, 260–1, 268, 440; for death (MD), 33–4, 38–9, 46, 51, 388; for pain relief (MPR), 32–3, 35–7, 41–8, 51

Morris, J., 136

mortality, 76, 100, 128, 350

MPR. *See* morphine for pain relief

Muir, Judge R., 330

murder. *See* homicide

Mwaria, C., 23

Nagel, T., 50, 57n.13, 58n.16, 133, 271, 431

Nahmanides, 367–8

narcotics, 63, 66, 303, 340

Nation of Islam, 98

National: Center for Health Statistics, 314; Hospice Organization, 152; Legislative Council (NLC), 76

Natural Death Act, 377, 381

natural law theory, 34, 114

Nazis, the, 137, 143, 177, 179, 181, 279

neglect, 92, 283, 288; of African-Americans, 96; of persons with disabilities, 125; of vulnerable groups, 135, 387

Netherlands, 5, 47, 67, 71, 72n.5, 224, 248n.8, 251n.48, 252, 262–3, 294, 318–19, 331, 388, 409, 437

New York, 193, 228, 245, 374, 389, 412, 420n.13, 423–30, 431–2

New York State Task Force on

Life and the Law, 6, 92, 119, 253, 282, 285, 290, 292, 296n.13, 378, 381, 385–8, 393–4, 412, 426

Nickens, H., 96, 103

Nietzsche F., 324

Ninth Circuit Court of Appeals, 115–16, 193, 229, 238, 255, 279, 292, 326, 373, 378

Nitschke, P., 259

North Carolina and PAS, 246, 248n.5

Northern Territory Rights of the Terminally Ill Bill, 252, 258–9, 264

Not Dead Yet, 2, 125–6, 129–31, 132n.7

Novak, D., 114

Nozick, R., 50, 133, 271, 431

nursing homes, 114, 140–1, 143–4, 172, 273, 314–15, 341

O'Brien, M., 136

O'Connor, Justice, 195, 302–3, 325, 374, 377, 388, 411–13, 417, 423, 427, 434

Oath of Maimonides, 170

omissions, 28–30, 38, 51, 186, 189–92, 227, 233, 235; causing death, 51, 188, 254, 259–61, 263–4, 327

Oregon, 2, 6, 8, 15–16, 120, 328, 375, 381; and rationed healthcare, 139, 317; *See* Death With Dignity Act; Health Sciences University, 6, 84; law, 2, 203, 375; *See* Measure 16

Orentlicher, D., 224, 241, 244, 258, 393

organ donation, 51, 84, 152, 218, 312, 316, 381, 435; and African-Americans, 98, 103

pain, 4, 12, 15, 31, 39–41, 43–5, 48, 53, 64, 66, 77, 114, 119, 130–1, 143, 146, 153, 165, 167, 172, 175, 185, 189, 192, 197, 204, 216, 285, 290, 302–3, 324, 328, 393, 407, 423, 431, 433, 438, 440; control, 64–6, 70–1, 120, 207, 254–5, 282, 288, 295, 412; management, 4, 172, 204, 268–9, 293, 386, 421n.15; medication, 16, 36, 182, 195, 200, 286, 393, 395,

406, 427; physical, 47, 270, 306, 338, 388, 393, 413, 432; relief, 4, 33, 35–6, 40–1, 45, 48, 75, 191, 259–60, 293, 295, 412; severe, 32, 34, 46–7, 134, 150–1, 193, 200, 204, 258, 268, 283, 386, 392

pain and suffering, 47, 63–4, 68–9, 184, 187, 190–1, 197, 200, 259, 267, 284–5, 288, 303, 306, 334, 335, 337, 339, 341–3, 393

pain control, 3, 4, 6, 7, 16, 44, 47, 63; techniques, 63, 204, 268, 282

palliative care, 75–6, 83–5, 88, 92, 94, 105, 128, 173, 185, 188, 190–3, 198–200, 214, 219, 252–4, 258–60, 263–4, 265n.10, 268, 282, 286, 294–5, 303, 306–7, 341, 389, 393, 408, 412–13, 425

Paris, J., 323

paternalism, 93, 124, 125, 135–6, 145, 147, 157, 185, 329, 390, 394, 439

Patient Self-Determination Act, 174, 329

patient(s), 4, 5, 29, 30, 34–6, 47–9, 64–5, 70, 73, 91–5, 118, 139, 155–7, 166, 171, 179–80, 214, 217, 219, 223, 254, 257, 259, 279–80, 284, 295, 312, 327, 356, 369, 387, 396, 412, 436, 443–4; African-American, 94, 104; agency, 17, 29; agent for, 54–6; AIDS, 209. *See also* AIDS; autonomy, 16, 54, 62n.48, 76, 77, 93, 181, 264, 281, 283, 293, 329; competent, 52, 92–3, 183, 185, 186, 188–91, 194, 200, 231, 264, 272, 279, 390, 394, 396, 408–9, 423, 434; consent, 29, 35–6, 39, 50, 52–5, 196, 252–4, 262, 264, 388; death of, 28, 41, 50, 54–5, 144, 183, 187, 190–1, 194, 216, 229, 234, 236, 238–40, 241–2, 254–7, 263, 301–2, 304–6, 309, 317, 325, 338, 387, 395; decisions of, 47, 55, 173, 184; desire to die, 47, 52, 55, 185, 194; dying, 7, 11, 22, 24–5, 65, 114, 208, 212, 215, 219, 221, 257, 259, 261, 268, 272, 276, 291,

301–3, 306, 308, 320, 389, 393–5, 433; family. See family; killing of, 44, 50, 55, 183, 196–9, 224, 252, 280, 305, 331; letting die, 53, 228; requests for treatment, 184, 190, 196, 285; right to die. See rights; right to life, 36, 435; right to pain control. See rights; right to refuse treatment. See rights; right to self-determination, 70, 181, 246, 436; rights of, 52, 62n.48, 253, 329, 435. See also rights; suicides of, 10, 173, 214, 224, 234–5, 239, 304; terminally ill. See also terminally ill, the, 1, 5, 6, 32, 47, 63, 66, 70, 75, 84, 92, 104, 128, 134, 182, 198–200, 206, 227–8, 245–6, 253, 257, 268, 279, 281, 284, 288, 291, 312, 318, 320, 366, 373, 389, 391, 393–6, 408, 423, 431, 439; welfare, 16, 52–3, 307; wishes, 52, 182

People v. Kevorkian, 381, 415n.18, 425

Philosphers' Brief, 14–17, 50–4, 151, 153–7, 160n.23, 296n.23, 329, 330, 331, 374, 431–41. See also Dworkin, R.

Physician-Assisted Suicide, 2, 4, 7–8, 9, 16, 28–62, 62–72, 73, 75, 77, 92, 94–5, 113, 117–20, 123, 125–6, 129–32, 136, 142, 147–8, 149, 151, 163, 165–76, 177–81, 182–202, 219, 223, 235–6, 239, 271, 272–8, 279–300, 373–5, 377, 381, 386–7, 389, 392, 394, 397, 409, 423–6, 430n.11, 437, 439–40, 441n.4; African-Americans and, 91–122; arguments against, 213, 339–42; arguments for, 32–6, 47–50, 281–2, 337–42; as a tragic choice, 279–300; Catholic perspective on, 324–33; Christian views on, 334–46; debate, 2, 4–5, 92, 93–7, 180, 203, 205–6; decriminalization of, 245–8; duty to perform, 35–6; equality and, 123–6; healthcare costs and, 312–22, 409; hospitals and, 203–20; Jewish views on,

362–72; legalization of, 2, 3, 5, 8, 9, 11, 14, 63–4, 76, 84, 86, 91, 95, 104, 117, 119, 149–51, 154–7, 163, 165, 175, 181, 182, 197–9, 203–9, 211–13, 217–18, 220, 223–4, 225–51, 267–78, 279, 282, 284, 287–8, 290, 292–5; legalized but strictly regulated225–6, 280; locus of, 205–8; medical ethics and, 213–17; moral responsibility for, 54–6, 182; persons with disabilties and, 133–48; philosophical debate about, 3–4, 5; policy of exclusion from hospitals and, 208–19; prohibition of, 3, 124, 152, 206, 281; protecting vulnerable groups from, 133–48; Protestant views on, 347–61; regulation of, 203, 208, 280, 288–9, 388, 446; religious issues and, 7–8; risk of abuse of, 3, 192, 200, 203, 268–9, 280, 283, 284–6, 288, 290, 292, 294, 306–7, 388

Physician's Desk Reference, 178

physician(s), 3, 4, 5, 6, 23, 28, 35–7, 51, 66, 70, 104, 118, 130, 134, 151, 154, 165–76, 184, 187, 211, 214–15, 223, 226, 228, 236, 239, 241, 279, 281, 285, 288, 290, 294, 312, 318, 354, 362, 370, 374, 387, 395, 397, 405, 408–9, 425; -facilitated suicide, 235–6, 238, 245; -patient relationship, 102, 105, 235, 261, 283, 286, 294, 307, 371, 394, 406; American, 223, 320; and assisted suicide, 177–81, 267; attending, 443–5; Australian, 261, 263; distrust of, 95, 218; Dutch, 143, 262, 263, 264n.2, 320, 409; duty of, 165, 184–6, 227, 239, 281; intention of, 252–3; responsibility of, 165, 170–3, 243; role of, 163, 253, 324, 426

Planned Parenthood v. Casey, 53, 116, 377–8, 383, 384–5, 392, 400–1, 412, 431–2, 433–6

Plato, 18

Plessey v. Ferguson, 100

policy: public. See public policy

poor, the, 92, 94, 193, 293, 387

Pope Pius XI: Casti Connubii, 116

Pope Pius XII, 7

poverty, 6, 81, 96, 104, 117, 153, 387

powers of attorney, 2, 272. See living wills

Preston, T. A., 377

privacy, 150–1, 215, 403, 412

Protestant(s), 208, 347–61

psychotherapeutic intervention, 82, 140, 209, 270–1, 282, 293–4, 307, 309

public: debate about PAS, 3, 8, 274, 279, 293–4, 313, 323, 327, 334, 343, 388; health, 135, 139, 218, 324; policy on PAS, 2, 5, 8, 73, 75–6, 80, 84, 87–8, 92, 95, 118, 135, 138–9, 142–3, 207–8, 223–4, 252–3, 256–7, 263–4, 279, 290, 338, 347–8, 357, 360, 381, 426

quadriplegic(s), 140–1, 231

Quality of Life Adjusted Year (QALY), 127

Quill v. New York, 257

Quill, T., 2, 30, 64, 151, 245, 318, 423, 428n.3

Quinlan case, 4, 330

Quinn, W., 37, 59n.24

Rachels, J., 2, 168, 240, 329–30

racial: biases, 103, 286; differences in healthcare, 96–7, 100–2; ideology, 97; stereotypes, 103

Rashdall, H., 336

rationality, 43–4, 117, 158

Rawls, J., 50, 133, 271, 275

Regina v. Dudley and Stephens, 243

Rehnquist, Justice, 16, 124, 135–6, 139, 143, 145, 193–5, 226, 228–9, 325, 373–4, 377, 413, 423, 428

Reinhardt, Judge, 256, 279–80, 287–9

religious: beliefs, 70, 207, 323, 332, 343; issues, 2; morality, 208, 218; perspectives on PAS, 323–33, 334–46, 347–61, 362–72, 393; practices, 70

respirator: removal of, 52, 66, 69, 183, 186–8, 190, 192, 219, 230, 234, 236–7, 245,

247, 289, 302, 304, 330, 436
Reynolds, P.P., 99
Rhodes, R., 10, 163
Richman, 82
Right To Life Committee, 145
right(s), 166, 168, 175n.3,
    176n.17, 193, 281, 288, 353,
    382, 384, 398–9, 402, 405,
    412, 424, 438; analysis, 169;
    Bill of, 382, 399; civil, 65,
    137–8; constitutional, 50,
    72, 130, 193, 227, 271, 279,
    308, 318, 378, 387, 434; dis-
    ability, 138; Divine, 166; in-
    dividual, 348; legal, 166;
    natural, 166, 177; negative,
    169, 286; positive, 169; to
    abortion, 116; to assisted
    suicide, 50, 53, 115, 130,
    178, 239, 271–2, 274–6,
    279–80, 288, 303, 308, 318,
    324, 350, 373–4, 378, 383,
    385, 387–8, 391–2, 404, 411;
    to avoid suffering, 3; to bod-
    ily integrity. *See* body, right
    to integrity; to choose time,
    method of death, 383, 434;
    to commit suicide, 383,
    388–91; to contraception,
    117; to die, 82, 137, 165–76,
    193, 207, 225, 306–7, 339,
    353, 373, 378, 383, 412; to
    life, 37, 165–6, 353, 378; to
    live, 82, 165–76; to pain
    control, 47; to privacy, 150,
    280; to refuse treatment, 50,
    53, 66, 168, 226, 263, 272–3,
    308, 329, 374, 382, 384,
    391–2, 405–6, 426, 434; to
    self-determination, 53,
    65–6, 124, 271–4, 276, 281
Rivlin, D., 141
Rodriquez v. *British Columbia*,
    123
Rodriquez, S., 123–7, 129,
    130–1
Roe v. *Wade*, 4, 26n.12, 218,
    288, 384, 400, 406, 409,
    416n.19
Rothstein, Judge, 115

safeguards, 93, 129–30, 139,
    197, 200, 288–9, 292, 400,
    444–5
Sanderson, R., 343
Savitt, T., 97
Scalia, Justice, 227–8, 423
Scanlon, T., 50, 133, 271, 431

Scitovsky, A., 314–15
scripture, 335, 352–3, 357, 362
Second Circuit Court of Ap-
    peals, 193, 228, 280, 288–9,
    325, 330, 373, 419n.7
sedation, 29–30, 303, 309, 393,
    412; terminal, 64, 66, 69,
    183, 216–17, 258–9, 301–2,
    303–8, 393–5, 428n.11
segregation, 96, 100; in health-
    care, 100
self: -destruction, 230–1, 233,
    364, 378; -determination,
    15, 17, 74, 93, 98, 123, 128,
    130–2, 134–5, 138–9, 141–6,
    171, 239, 247, 267, 271–6,
    332, 337, 340, 373, 426, 434;
    -sacrifice, 118; harm, 364,
    366; respect, 43, 104, 125
Shalit, P., 377
sickle cell anemia, 99
Silvers, A., 10, 74
Sims, Dr. M., 107n.29
Siegler, M 330
Singer, P., 47–8, 330
Sixth Commandment, 335,
    337
slavery, 96–8, 107n.29, 276,
    398
slippery slope, 25, 63, 262,
    279, 283–4, 289–90, 294,
    307, 341, 409, 416n.23
social: agency relations, 22, 24;
    change, 66, 147; factors, 25,
    270; policy, 5, 24, 281, 285,
    286–94, 296n.22, 343, 360;
    practices, 11, 69–70, 92–3,
    127–9, 284, 290–1; reform,
    138, 295; relations, 9, 23–5,
    341, 370–1; services, 81,
    141; structures, 94, 102; val-
    ues, 23–5, 138
Social Security, 81
societal: attitudes about suicide
    and PAS, 378; indifference,
    91–2, 104, 387
society, 91–2, 97, 105, 120,
    134, 151, 312; American, 25,
    279, 374; democratic, 1,
    325, 388–9; pluralistic, 158,
    343, 348
Socrates, 178; *Apology,* 12
Souter, Justice, 374, 377, 382,
    395, 411, 415n.17, 416n.23,
    418, 423, 427
sovereignty: divine, 339, 343,
    367–8
Soylent Green, 70

St. Augustine, 327, 335, 357
St. Paul, 335, 338, 340
Steinbock, B., 134
Stell, L., 10, 223
stereotypes, 92, 96, 104, 133;
    of African-Americans,
    98–99, 103; of persons with
    disabilities, 125, 135
sterilization, 113–14, 117;
    forced, 117
Stevens, Justice, 143–5, 194–5,
    325, 374, 377, 389, 413,
    416n.24, 423, 427, 430n.12
stewardship, 326, 331, 340
suffering, 66–8, 73, 95, 141,
    147, 165, 171, 175, 185,
    197–9, 206, 208, 216–17,
    220, 270–1, 281, 283–4,
    287–8, 302–3, 305, 307–8,
    328, 330, 336–8, 340, 343,
    347, 349–54, 356, 358,
    362–3, 365, 366, 368, 370,
    389, 391–3, 395–6, 423, 432,
    436; duty to relieve, 36; in-
    tolerable, 141–5, 303, 308,
    338, 409; meaning of, 339;
    non-redemptive, 338, 340;
    physical, 36, 47, 268–9, 272,
    303, 367, 404; psychological,
    48, 61n.39, 270–2, 282, 386;
    relief of, 54, 144, 191, 356,
    389, 394
suicidal ideation, 208–10, 282,
    387
suicide, 2, 6, 21, 23–4, 28, 30,
    43, 47, 55, 65, 67, 69, 73–4,
    77, 78, 113–22, 123–4,
    129–30, 135–6, 139, 142,
    151, 155–7, 163, 167, 171,
    173, 177–8, 180, 191–2,
    194–5, 199–200, 203, 206,
    209–10, 214–15, 217,
    219–21, 223–4, 225–30,
    230–7, 241, 244–7, 271, 273,
    279–80, 282, 309, 324, 327,
    329, 347, 349, 351, 373, 375,
    377, 378–9, 381, 385–6,
    394–7, 405, 407–8, 423,
    426–7, 439–40; active, 30,
    45, 123, 168; among the el-
    derly, 77, 80–1, 87. *See also*
    elderly attempts, 118, 172;
    ban on, 377–8, 386; com-
    mitting, 130, 199, 227, 275,
    289, 307, 330, 334, 342,
    378–9, 384–5, 393–4, 404,
    406, 414n.12, 426; defini-
    tion of, 230–6; facilitated,

234–6; feminist view regarding, 113–22; in-hospital, 214–16; Jewish views on, 362–72; means of, 211–12; moral status of, 335; passive, 31, 168, 174; prevention, 82, 125, 141, 225, 228, 280, 289, 393, 426; prohibition against, 143, 362, 364–5, 368, 373, 380, 405; rational, 113, 117, 119–20; religious conceptions of, 70, 323–61; risks, 81, 140; social regulation of, 205, 358

SUPPORT study, 4, 63, 68, 72n.1, 120n.6, 328

Supreme Court, 1, 2, 3, 6, 7–8, 9, 14, 15, 25, 50, 61n.40, 71–2, 76, 92, 115, 118–19, 124, 133, 141, 143–5, 153, 165, 182, 195, 200, 203, 258, 271, 279–80, 288–90, 292, 295, 304, 318, 325, 373–4; and legislation on PAS, 193–5, 301–11, 318, 324, 327, 329–30, 373–5; Canadian, 129; Justices, 53, 92, 281, 295, 308, 374; of British Columbia, 123–4

symptom(s), 64, 67, 209, 219, 258, 303, 386, 388; control, 5, 6, 63, 254–5; relief, 207, 260

syphilis, 98–9

Talmud, the, 362, 364, 366. See Mishna, Jewish tradition

Taylor, J., 336

Teitelman, M., 163

terminal: disease, 66, 185, 203, 207, 219–20; illness, 67, 70, 87, 113–14, 139, 149–62, 187, 205, 228, 267, 274, 280, 287, 289, 291, 303, 340, 389

terminally ill, the, 2, 65, 73–4, 87–8, 92, 95, 115, 135, 140, 144, 149–62, 180, 229, 246, 282–3, 287, 302, 306, 308, 331, 368, 377–8, 381, 383, 385, 386, 387, 390, 392–6, 424, 435, 436, 438–9

Third Amendment, 403

Thomas, Justice, 423

Thomson, J.J., 50, 133, 271,

431

Three-Step Argument, 28, 35, 36–40, 48–50, 53–4, 58n.18

Tong, R., 120n.7

Torah, the, 362–3, 366. See Bible, Scripture

treatment, 50, 64, 68, 95, 124, 209, 226; forced, 52, 54, 193, 405; invasive, 102, 291; life-prolonging, 92, 94–5, 172, 188, 190–1, 199, 260, 330; life-sustaining, 102, 124, 126, 131, 154, 184–5, 188, 191–2, 194, 199, 219, 225–30, 236, 238, 241–2, 246–7, 252, 254, 256, 257, 264, 280, 288, 290, 301, 304, 330, 338, 377, 381, 425, 435; lifesaving, 15, 29, 172–3, 185–6, 193, 235, 244; medical, 53, 94, 139, 187, 194, 227, 291, 316, 325, 329–30, 341, 384, 394, 426; psychological. See psychotherapeutic intervention; refusal of, 4, 52–3, 66, 168, 184–95, 197–9, 201n.16, 225–30, 233, 236–7, 239, 241, 306, 308–9, 325, 394, 423–4, 426–7, 428n.2, 436. See also right, to refuse treatment; termination of, 41–2, 45–6, 50, 54, 66, 183, 225, 247; withdrawing, 4, 38, 40, 69, 174, 186, 241, 258, 260, 263, 301–2, 305, 308, 325, 377, 381, 384, 426–7; witholding, 4, 29, 51, 69, 125, 165–6, 168, 174, 245, 253, 256, 260, 263, 288, 291, 377, 394

Tuskegee Syphilis Study, 98–9, 218. See also African–American

U.S. Equal Opportunities Commission, 137

United States, 5, 68, 125, 152, 254, 431; Constitution, 150, 226, 271, 280, 292, 301, 377, 384–5, 388–9, 403, 406–7, 424, 437–8; healthcare system, 83, 100; Public Health Service (PHS), 98. See Supreme Court

utilitarianism, 275, 281, 339, 352

Vacco v. Quill, 1, 9, 71, 92, 123–4, 133, 141, 144, 165, 228, 287–8, 324, 330, 373–5, 381, 384, 394, 411, 415n.18, 423–430, 432

van der Maas et al., 319

Vatican's Declaration on Euthanasia, 256, 324, 329, 330–1

Velleman, D., 154–6, 158

Verhey, A., 323

vulnerable groups, 5–6, 65, 73, 75, 77, 92–3, 129, 134–6, 139, 145–8, 223, 247, 262, 280, 293–4, 324, 341, 359, 373, 381, 386–8, 393, 426; duty to protect, 124, 133–48; exploitation of, 93–4

waiting period, 211, 289, 445–6

Waldenberg, Rabbi E., 364–7

Washington state: and Natural Death Act, 377, 381, 413, 414n.13; and PAS, 2, 193, 229, 248n.8, 251n.49, 319, 328, 331, 377–422, 431–2

Washington v. Glucksberg, 1, 9, 25, 71, 92, 123–4, 133, 145, 165, 229, 324, 373–5, 377–422, 424, 427

Wendell, S., 146–7

Wennberg, R., 342

Wild, E., 258–9

Williams, B., 86

Wolf, S.M., 118–19, 239–40

women, 5, 117; of color, 103; oppression of, 116; poor, 117

World Bank, 127

World Health Organization, 127

Zohar, N., 323